a LANGE medical book

CURRENT
Practice Guidelines
in Primary Care
2018

Joseph S. Esherick, MD, FAAFP
Director of Medicine
Ventura County Medical Center
Associate Clinical Professor of Family Medicine
David Geffen School of Medicine
Los Angeles, California

Evan D. Slater, MD
Ventura County Medical Center
Assistant Clinical Professor of Medicine
David Geffen School of Medicine
Los Angeles, California

Jacob A. David, MD, FAAFP
Associate Program Director
Family Medicine Residency Program
Ventura County Medical Center
Clinical Instructor
UCLA School of Medicine
Los Angeles, California

New York   Chicago   San Francisco   Athens   London   Madrid
Mexico City   Milan   New Delhi   Singapore   Sydney   Toronto

CURRENT Practice Guidelines in Primary Care, 2018

ISBN 978-1-260-03106-5
MHID 1-260-03106-3
ISSN 1528-1612

Notice

This book was set in Minion Pro by MPS Limited.
The editors were Amanda Fielding and Kim J. Davis.
The production supervisor was Richard Ruzycka.
Project management was provided by Nikhil, MPS Limited.

This book is printed on acid-free paper.

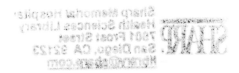

McGraw-Hill Education books are available at special quantity discounts to use as premiums and sales promotions, or for use in corporate training programs. To contact a representative please visit the Contact Us pages at www.mhprofessional.com.

This book is dedicated to all of our current and former residents at the Ventura County Medical Center.

Contents

√ denotes major 2018 updates.
+ denotes new topic for 2018.

2. DISEASE PREVENTION 103

√ denotes major 2018 updates.
+ denotes new topic for 2018.

CONTENTS

√ denotes major 2018 updates.
+ denotes new topic for 2018.

√ denotes major 2018 updates.
+ denotes new topic for 2018.

√ denotes major 2018 updates.
+ denotes new topic for 2018.

√ denotes major 2018 updates.
+ denotes new topic for 2018.

√ denotes major 2018 updates.
+ denotes new topic for 2018.

4. APPENDICES

√ denotes major 2018 updates.
+ denotes new topic for 2018.

Preface

Current Practice Guidelines in Primary Care, 2018 is intended for all clinicians interested in updated, evidence-based guidelines for primary care topics in both the ambulatory and hospital settings. This pocket-sized reference consolidates information from nationally recognized medical associations and government agencies into concise recommendations and guidelines of virtually all ambulatory care topics. This book is organized into topics related to disease screening, disease prevention, and disease management for quick reference to the evaluation and treatment of the most common primary care disorders.

The 2018 edition of *Current Practice Guidelines in Primary Care* contains updates or new chapters in over 80 primary care topics. It is a great resource for residents, medical students, midlevel providers, and practicing physicians in family medicine, internal medicine, pediatrics, and obstetrics and gynecology.

Although painstaking efforts have been made to find all errors and omissions, some errors may remain. If you find an error or wish to make a suggestion, please e-mail us at EditorialServices@mheducation.com.

Joseph S. Esherick, MD, FAAFP
Evan D. Slater, MD
Jacob A. David, MD, FAAFP

Disease Screening

ABDOMINAL AORTIC ANEURYSM

Population
–Men age 65–75 y who have ever smoked.

Recommendations
▶ USPSTF 2014, ACC/AHA 2006, Canadian Society for Vascular Surgery 2006
–Screen once, with ultrasounography.
–In men in this age group who have never smoked, no recommendation for or against screening.

Sources
–*Ann Intern Med.* 2014;161(4):281-90
–*J Vasc Surg.* 2007;45:1268-1276

Population
–Men/women at high risk.

Recommendations
▶ Canadian Society for Vascular Surgery 2008
–All men age 65–75 y be screened for AAA.
–Individual selective screening for those at high risk for AAA:
  a. Women older than 65 y at high risk secondary to smoking, cerebro-vascular disease, and family history.
  b. Men younger than 65 y with positive family history.

Source
–*Can J Surg.* 2008;51(1):23-34

Population

–Women who have never smoked.

Recommendation

▶ USPSTF 2014

–Routine screening is not recommended.

Source

–*Ann Intern Med.* 2014;161(4):281-90

Population

–Women age 65–75 y who have ever smoked.

Recommendation

▶ UPSTF 2014

–Current evidence is insufficient to assess the balance of benefits and harms.

Source

–*Ann Intern Med.* 2014;161(4):281-90

Population

–Men age 65–75 y who have smoked at least 100 cigarettes in their lifetime or people at risk who have a family history of AAA.

Recommendation

▶ ESVS 2011

–Men should be screened with a single scan at age 65 y. Screening should be considered at an earlier age in those at higher risk for AAA.

Source

–Moll FL, Powell JT, Fraedrich G, et al. Management of abdominal aortic aneurysms clinical practice guidelines of the European Society for Vascular Surgery. *Eur J Vasc Endovasc Surg.* 2011;(41):S1-S58

Comments

1. Cochrane review (2007): Significant decrease in AAA-specific mortality in men (OR, 0.60, 95% CI 0.47–0.99) but not for women. (*Cochrane Database Syst Rev.* 2007;2:CD002945; http://www. thecochranelibrary.com)
2. Early mortality benefit of screening (men age 65–74 y) maintained at 7-y follow-up. Cost-effectiveness of screening improves over time. (*Ann Intern Med.* 2007;146:699)
3. Surgical repair of AAA should be considered if diameter ≥5.5 cm or if AAA expands ≥0.5 cm over 6 mo to reduce higher risk of rupture. Meta-analysis: endovascular repair associated with fewer postoperative adverse events and lower 30-d and aneurysm-related

mortality but not all-cause mortality compared with open repair. (*Br J Surg.* 2008;95(6):677)

4. Asymptomatic AAA between 4.4 and 5.5 cm should have regular ultrasound surveillance with surgical intervention when AAA expands >1 cm in a year or diameter reaches 5.5 cm. (*Cochrane Database Syst Rev.* 2008, CD001835; http://www.thecochranelibrary.com)

5. Medicare covers one-time limited screening. (http://www.medicare. gov/coverage/ab-aortic-aneurysm-screening.html)

Populations

–Male >65 y.

–Female >65 y.

Recommendations

▶ ESC 2014

–Ultrasound screening is recommended in all men > 65 y of age.

–Ultrasound screening may be considered if history of current/past smoking is present.

–Screening is not recommended in female nonsmokers without family history of AAA.

–Targeted screening for AAA with ultrasound should be considered in first-degree siblings of a patient with AAA.

Sources

–Erbel R, Aboyans V, Boileau C, et al. 2014 ESC guidelines on the diagnosis and treatment of aortic diseases. *Eur Heart J. doi:10.1093/ eurheartj/ehu281 Eur Heart J.* doi:10.1093/eurheartj/ehu281

Comment

–Abdominal echocardiography used for mass screening in subgroups at risk was associated with a significant 45% decreased risk of AAA-related mortality at 10 y.

Populations

–Male ≥65 y.

–Female ≥ 65 y with cardiovascular risk factors.

Recommendations

▶ ACR[a]/AIUM/SRU 2014

–Ultrasound screening is recommended in all men ≥ 65 y and women ≥ 65 y with cardiovascular risk factors.

–Patients ≥ 50 y with a family history of aortic and/or peripheral vascular aneurysmal disease.

[a]ACR, American College of Radiology

–Patients with a personal history of peripheral vascular aneurysmal disease.

–Groups with additional risk include patients with a history of smoking, hypertension, or certain connective tissue diseases (eg, Marfan syndrome).

Source
–ACR-AIUM-SRU Practice Parameter for the Performance of Diagnostic and Screening Ultrasound of the Abdominal Aorta in Adults. 2014.

ADENOCARCINOMA OF GASTROESOPHAGEAL JUNCTION

Population
–Diagnosis—Barrett esophagus with or without gastroesophageal reflux disease. (*N Engl J Med*. 2014;371:836)

Recommendation
▶ ASGE 2011

–**Barrett's Follow-up**
  • No dysplasia—scope every 3 y.
  • Mild dysplasia—scope in 6 mo, then yearly.
  • High-grade dysplasia—surgery or endoscopic therapy. (*Gastrointest Cancer Res*. 2012;5:49)

Source
–*Gastrointest Endosc*. 2006;63:570

Comments
–In 2016, 16,910 Americans diagnosed with esophageal cancer and 15,690 died from this malignancy. Fourfold increase in males compared to females.

–Adenocarcinoma most common (4:1 versus squamous cell CA). Squamous cell cancer most common in African Americans (6:1).

–Risk of adeno CA increases with gastroesophageal reflux disease (GERD) and high BMI (>30kg/m2) Squamous cell related to tobacco use, alcohol, malnutrition and HPV infection.

–*Benefits:* There is fair evidence that screening would result in no decrease in gastric CA mortality in the United States. *Harms:* There is good evidence that esophagogastroduodenoscopy screening would result in rare but serious side effects, such as perforation, cardiopulmonary events, aspiration pneumonia, and bleeding. (*NCI*, 2008)

ALCOHOL ABUSE AND DEPENDENCE

Population
–Adults older than 18 y of age.

Recommendation
▶ AAFP 2010, USPSTF 2013, VA/DOD 2009, ICSI 2010
- –Screen all adults in primary care settings, including pregnant women, for alcohol misuse.
- –Provide persons engaged in risky or hazardous drinking with brief behavioral counseling interventions to reduce alcohol misuse.
- –Provide brief intervention to those who have a positive alcohol misuse screen. Brief interventions during future visits.

Sources
- –ISCI Preventive Services for Adults, 20th ed. 2014.
- –Management of Substance Use Disorders Work Group. VA/DoD clinical practice guideline for the management of substance use disorders. Version 3.0. Washington (DC): Department of Veterans Affairs, Department of Defense; 2015.
- –USPSTF: Alcohol Misuse: Screening and Behavioral Counseling in Primary Care. 2013.

Comments
1. Screen annually using validated tool.
2. AUDIT[a] score ≥4 for men and ≥3 for women and SASQ reporting of ≥5 drinks in a day (men) or ≥4 drinks in a day (women) in the past year are valid and reliable screening instruments for identifying unhealthy alcohol use.
3. The TWEAK and the T-ACE are designed to screen pregnant women for alcohol misuse.

Population
–Children and adolescents.

Recommendation
▶ AAFP 2010, USPSTF 2013, ICSI 2010
- –Insufficient evidence to recommend for or against screening or counseling interventions to prevent or reduce alcohol misuse by adolescents.

Sources
- –USPSTF: Alcohol Misuse: Screening and Behavioral Counseling Interventions in Primary Care. 2013.

[a]AUDIT, alcohol use disorders identification test; SASQ, single alcohol screening question.

–https://www.icsi.org/guidelines__more/catalog_guidelines_and_more/catalog_guidelines/
–Alcohol Misuse: Screening and Behavioral Counseling Interventions in Primary Care

Comments

1. AUDIT and CAGE questionnaires have not been validated in children or adolescents.
2. Reinforce not drinking and driving or riding with any driver under the influence.
3. Reinforce to women the harmful effects of alcohol on fetuses.

ANEMIA

Population

–Infants age 6–24 mo.

Recommendation

▶ USPSTF 2015, AAFP 2015

–Current evidence is insufficient to recommend for or against screening.
–Consider selective screening in high-risk children[a] with malnourishment, low birth weight, or symptoms of anemia.

Sources

–AAFP Clinical Recommendations: Iron Deficiency Anemia
–USPSTF: Iron Deficiency in Young Children: Screening. 2015.

Comment

–Reticulocyte hemoglobin content is a more sensitive and specific marker than is serum hemoglobin level for iron deficiency.
–One-third of patients with iron deficiency will have a hemoglobin level >11 g/dL.

Population

–Infants and young children 0–3 y.

Recommendation

▶ AAP 2010

–Universal screening of Hgb at 12 mo. If anemic, measure ferritin, C-reactive protein, and reticulocyte hemoglobin content.

---

[a]Includes infants living in poverty, Blacks, Native Americans, Alaska natives, immigrants from developing countries, preterm and low-birth-weight infants, and infants whose principal dietary intake is unfortified cow's milk or soy milk. Less than two servings per day of iron-rich foods (iron-fortified breakfast cereals or meats).

Source
    –*Pediatrics*. 2010;126(5):1040-1050

Comment
    –Use of transferring receptor 1 (TfR$_1$) assay as screening for iron deficiency is under investigation.

Population
    –Pregnant women.

Recommendation

▶ **USPSTF 2015, AAFP 2015**
    –Screen all women with hemoglobin or hematocrit at first prenatal visit.

Sources
    –http://www.ahrq.gov/clinic/cpgsix.htm
    –*Ann Intern Med*. 2015;162:566

Comments
    –Insufficient evidence to recommend for or against routine use of iron supplements for non-anemic pregnant women (USPSTF).
    –When acute stress or inflammatory disorders are not present, a serum ferritin level is the most accurate test for evaluating iron deficiency anemia. Among women of childbearing age, a cutoff of 30 ng/mL has sensitivity of 92%, specificity of 98%. (*Blood*. 1997;89:1052-1057).
    –Severe anemia (hemoglobin <6) associated with abnormal fetal oxygenation and transfusion should be considered. In iron-deficient women intolerant of oral iron or non compliant, intravenous iron sucrose or iron dextran should be given.
    –IV iron preferred in 3rd trimester with hemoglobin less than 10 g/dL. Cobalamin and folate deficiency should be excluded. (*Blood*. 2017; 129:940)

ATTENTION-DEFICIT/HYPERACTIVITY DISORDER

Population
–Children age 4–18 y with academic or behavioral problems and inattention, hyperactivity, or impulsivity.

Recommendation

▶ **AAFP 2016, AAP 2011**

–Initiate an evaluation for ADHD. Diagnosis requires the child meet DSM-IV criteria[a] and direct supporting evidence from parents or caregivers and classroom teacher.

–Evaluation of a child with ADHD should include assessment for coexisting disorders and alternative causes of the behavior.

Source
–AAFP Clinical Recommendation: ADHD in Children and Adolescents. AAFP. 2016

–*Pediatrics*. 2011;128(5):1007

–*Pediatrics*. 2000;105(5):1158

[a]DSM-IV Criteria for ADHD:

I: Either A or B.

A: *Six or more of the following symptoms of inattention have been present for at least 6 mo to a point that is disruptive and inappropriate for developmental level.* Inattention: (1) Often does not give close attention to details or makes careless mistakes in schoolwork, work, or other activities. (2) Often has trouble keeping attention on tasks or play activities. (3) Often does not seem to listen when spoken to directly. (4) Often does not follow instructions and fails to finish schoolwork, chores, or duties in the workplace (not due to oppositional behavior or failure to understand instructions). (5) Often has trouble organizing activities. (6) Often avoids, dislikes, or does not want to do things that take a lot of mental effort for a long period of time (such as schoolwork or homework). (7) Often loses things needed for tasks and activities (eg, toys, school assignments, pencils, books, or tools). (8) Is often easily distracted. (9) Is often forgetful in daily activities.

B: *Six or more of the following symptoms of hyperactivity-impulsivity have been present for at least 6 mo to an extent that is disruptive and inappropriate for developmental level.* Hyperactivity: (1) Often fidgets with hands or feet or squirms in seat. (2) Often gets up from seat when remaining in seat is expected. (3) Often runs about or climbs when and where it is not appropriate (adolescents or adults may feel very restless). (4) Often has trouble playing or enjoying leisure activities quietly. (5) Is often "on the go" or often acts as if "driven by a motor." (6) Often talks excessively.

Impulsivity: (1) Often blurts out answers before questions have been finished. (2) Often has trouble waiting one's turn. (3) Often interrupts or intrudes on others (eg, butts into conversations or games).

II: Some symptoms that cause impairment were present before age 7 y.

III: Some impairment from the symptoms is present in two or more settings (eg, at school/work and at home).

IV: There must be clear evidence of significant impairment in social, school, or work functioning.

V: The symptoms do not happen only during the course of a pervasive developmental disorder, schizophrenia, or other psychotic disorder. The symptoms are not better accounted for by another mental disorder (eg, mood disorder, anxiety disorder, dissociative disorder, or a personality disorder).

Comments
1. Stimulant prescription rates continue to rise. (*Lancet.* 2016.387(10024); 1240-1250)
2. Current estimates are that 7.2% of children/adolescents meet criteria for ADHD. (*Pediatrics.* 2015;135(4):e994.)
3. The U.S. Food and Drug Administration (FDA) approved a "black box" warning regarding the potential for cardiovascular side effects of ADHD stimulant drugs. (*N Engl J Med.* 2006;354:1445)

AUTISM SPECTRUM DISORDER

Population
–Children, age 12–36 mo.

Recommendation
▶ USPST 2016
–Insufficient evidence to screen routinely.

Source
–*JAMA.* 2016;315(7):691-6

Recommendation
▶ AAP 2014
–General developmental screening at routine 9-, 18-, and 24-mo visits, with autism-specific tool at 18 mo (M-CHAT is most commonly use— see Appendix).

Source
–*Pediatrics.* 2006;118(1):405. *Pediatrics.* 2014;135(5);e1520.

Comment
–Listen & respond to concerns raised by caregivers; signs may be identifiable by 9 mo of age.
–Prevalence is 1 in 68; 4.5:1 male:female ratio. (*MMWR Surveill Summ.* 2016;65(3):1–23.)

BACTERIURIA, ASYMPTOMATIC

Population
–Pregnant women.

Recommendation
▶ USPSTF 2008
–Recommend screening for bacteriuria at first prenatal visit or at 12 16 wk' gestation.

Population
–Men and nonpregnant women.

Recommendation
▶ USPSTF 2008
–Recommend against routine screening for bacteriuria.

Sources
–USPSTF. Asymptomatic Bacteriuria in Adults: Screening. 2008.

BACTERIAL VAGINOSIS

Population
–Pregnant women at high risk[a] for preterm delivery

Recommendation
▶ USPSTF 2008
–Insufficient evidence to recommend for or against routine screening.

Population
–Low-risk pregnant women.

Recommendation
▶ USPSTF 2008
–Do not screen routinely.

Sources
–USPSTF. Bacterial Vaginosis in Pregnancy to Prevent Preterm Delivery: Screening. 2008.

BARRETT ESOPHAGUS (BE)

Populations
–General population with GERD.
–High-risk population with GERD (multiple risk factors including age >50, male gender, white, chronic GERD, hiatal hernia, BMI >30, intra-abdominal body fat distribution or tobacco use.)

Recommendations
▶ AGA 2011
–Against screening general population with GERD for BE (strong recommendation).

---

[a]Risk factors: African-American race or ethnicity, body mass index less than 20 kg/m², previous preterm delivery, vaginal bleeding, shortened cervix <2.5 cm, pelvic infection, bacterial vaginosis.

–**High Risk Factors**
- Screening should be strongly considered in this population, especially patients with multiple risk factors (weak recommendation).
- If Barrett's found without dysplasia follow-up endoscopy in 1 y then every 3–5 y. (*JAMA. 2013;310(6):627-636*) (*Gastroenterology. 2016;151:822*)
- If low grade dysplasia confirmed by endoscopy eradication therapy is indicated.
- high grade dysplasia should be treated with endoscopic eradication rather than esophagectomy. (*N Engl J Med. 2014;371:836*)

Source
–*Gastroenterology*. 2011;140:1084-1091.

Comment
–**Clinical Aspects**
- Despite lack of evidence for benefit of screening general population with GERD for BE, endoscopic screening is common and widespread.
- 40% of patients with BE and esophageal cancer have not had chronic GERD symptoms.
- The diagnosis of dysplasia in BE should be confirmed by at least one additional pathologist, preferably one who is an expert in esophageal pathology. (*Gastroenterology*. 2011;140:1084) (*N Engl J Med*. 2014;371:836)
- All patients with BE should be treated with a protein pump inhibitor even if not symptomatic. (*Gut*. 2014;63:1229)

CANCER, BLADDER

Population
–Asymptomatic persons.

Recommendation
▶ AAFP 2011, USPSTF 2016
–Recommends against routine screening for bladder cancer (CA) in adults. Evidence is insufficient to assess balance of benefits and harms of screening for bladder CA in asymptomatic adults. (No major organization recommends screening for bladder cancer in asymptomatic adults).

Sources
–http://www.aafp.org/online/en/home/clinical/exam.html
–http://www.ahrq.gov/clinic/uspstf/uspsblad.htm
–http://www.cancer.gov

Comments
–Benefits and Harms
- There is inadequate evidence to determine whether screening for bladder CA would have any impact on mortality. Based on fair evidence, screening for bladder CA would result in unnecessary diagnostic procedures and over diagnosis (70% of bladder CA is in situ) with attendant morbidity. (NCI, 2017)

–Clinical Awareness
- Urinary biomarkers (nuclear matrix protein 22, tumor associated antigen p300, presence of DNA ploidy) do not have significant sensitivity or specificity to be utilized in clinical practice. Microscopic hematuria leads to a diagnosis of bladder cancer in only 5% of patients.
- There are 79,000 of bladder expected in 2017 in the United States with the majority being non-invasive (70%) but still 16,900 americans are expected to die of bladder cancer in 2017. (*Ann Inter Med.* 2010;153:461) (*Eur Urol.* 2013;63:4)
- A high index of suspicion should be maintained in anyone with a history of smoking (4- to 7-fold increased risk[a]), an exposure to industrial toxins (aromatic amines, benzene), therapeutic pelvic radiation, cyclophosphamide chemotherapy, a history of *Schistosoma haematobium* cystitis, hereditary nonpolyposis colon CA (Lynch syndrome), and history of transitional cell carcinoma of ureter (50% risk of subsequent bladder CA). Large screening studies in these high-risk populations have not been performed.
- Voided urine cytology with sensitivity of 40% but only 10% positive predictive value, urinary biomarkers (nuclear matrix protein 22, telomerase) with suboptimal sensitivity and specificity. Screening for microscopic hematuria has <10% positive predictive value.

[a]Individuals who smoke are 4–7 times more likely to develop bladder CA than are individuals who have never smoked. Additional environmental risk factors: exposure to aminobiphenyls; aromatic amines; azo dyes; combustion gases and soot from coal; chlorination by-products in heated water; aldehydes used in chemical dyes and in the rubber and textile industries; organic chemicals used in dry cleaning, paper manufacturing, rope and twine making, and apparel manufacturing; contaminated Chinese herbs; arsenic in well water. Additional risk factors: prolonged exposure to urinary S. *haematobium* bladder infections, cyclophosphamide, or pelvic radiation therapy for other malignancies.

CANCER, BREAST

Population
–Women age 20–44 y.

Recommendations
▶ ACS 2016

–Inform women of benefits and limitations of breast self-examination (BSE). Educate concerning reporting a lump or breast symptoms.

–Breast imaging not indicated for average-risk women. Women 40–44 y old should have the opportunity to begin annual screening if they desire.

Source

–http://www.cancer.org

Population
–Women age 40–49 y.

Recommendation
▶ USPSTF 2012

–Perform individualized assessment of breast CA risk; base screening decision on benefits and harms of screening as well as on a woman's preferences and CA risk profile. (*Ann Intern Med.* 2012;156:635) (*Ann Intern Med.* 2012;156:662)

Sources

–*Ann Intern Med.* 2012;156:609

–*Ann Intern Med.* 2014;160:864

Comment
–**Harm and Benefit of Mammography Screening**

• *Benefits:* Based on fair evidence, screening mammography in women age 40–70 y decreases breast CA mortality. The benefit is higher in older women (reduction in risk of death in women age 40–49 y = 15%–20%, 25%–30% in women age ≥50 y) but still remains controversial. *BMJ.* 2014; 348:366. *Ann Intern Med.* 2009; 151:727.

• *Harms:* Based on solid evidence, screening mammography may lead to potential harm by overdiagnosis (indolent tumors that are not life-threatening) and unnecessary biopsies for benign disease. It is estimated that 20%–25% of diagnosed breast cancers are indolent and unlikely to be clinically significant. (*CA Cancer J Clin.* 2012;62:5) (*Ann Intern Med.* 2012;156:491)

- BSE does not improve breast CA mortality (*Br J Cancer.* 2003;88:1047) and increases the rate of false-positive biopsies. (*J Natl Cancer Inst.* 2002;94:1445)
- Twenty-five percent of breast CAs diagnosed before age 40 y are attributable to *BRCA1* or *2* mutations.
- The sensitivity of annual screening of young (age 30–49 y) high-risk women with magnetic resonance imaging (MRI) and mammography is superior to either alone, but MRI is associated with a significant increase in false positives. (*Lancet.* 2005;365:1769) (*Lancet Oncol.* 2011;378:1804)
- Computer-aided detection in screening mammography appears to reduce overall accuracy (by increasing false-positive rate), although it is more sensitive in women age <50 y with dense breasts. (*N Engl J Med.* 2007;356:1399)
- Digital mammography vs. film screen mammography equal in women 50–79 y old but digital more accurate in women 40–49 y old. (*Ann Intern Med.* 2011;155:493).
- Estimated 252,710 new cases of invasive breast cancer (63,400 with DCIS) expected in 2017 with 40,600 expected deaths (NCI: 2017)
- Future cancer screening—circulating tumor DNA (ctDNA)— mutations identified consistent with specific underlying malignancy. Promising preliminary data. (*Nat Med.* 2014;20:548) (*J Clin Onc.* 2014;82:5)

Population

–Women age ≥40 y.

Recommendation

▶ AAFP 2013

–Mammography, with or without Clinical Breast Exam, every 1–2 y after counseling about potential risks and benefits.

Source

–http://www.aafp.org/online/en/home/clinical/exam.html

Comments

1. Evidence is insufficient to recommend for or against routine CBE alone, or teaching or performing a routine BSE; recommend against screening women >75 y old.
2. Breast MRI annually for *BRCA 1* and *2* mutation carriers or women with therapeutic chest radiation between ages 15–35.

Population

–Women age 45–54 y.

Recommendation

▶ ACS 2016

–Women with an average risk of breast cancer should undergo regular screening mammography annually at age 45 to 54 (*CA Cancer J Clin.* 2016; 66:95) (*JAMA.* 2015; 314:1599)

Source

–http://www.cancer.org

Comment

–In 2016, 246,000 new invasive breast cancer cases per year with 40,500 deaths. Mortality rates have declined by 1.9%/year from 1998-2012. Will these guidelines increase the risk of breast cancer deaths?

–It is estimated that 1.6 million breast biopsies are performed each year in the U.S. with the overwhelming majority having benign disease. *JAMA.* 2015; 313:1122.

Population

–Average risk women ≥55 y.

Recommendations

▶ ACS 2016

–Women age ≥55 y should transition to biannual screening or have the opportunity to continue screening annually.

–Women should continue screening mammography as long as their overall health is good and they have a life expectancy ≥10 y.

–The ACS does not recommend clinical breast examination for breast cancer screening among average risk women at any age.

Comment

–How do we classify average vs. high risk? *BRCA1 and 2*, mediastinal chest radiation for Hodgkin treatment in young females is easy but what about high BMI, lack of exercise, never pregnant, early menses, breast biopsy with atypical hyperplasia, dense breasts, breast cancer in the family, and much more—how many of these variables do you need to call a patient high risk? (*JAMA.* 2015; 314:1615) (*J Natl Cancer Inst.* 2010; 102:665) (*J Natl Compr Netw.* 2016; 14:651)

Population

–High-risk patients.
–Women with family history associated with increased risk for deleterious mutations in BRCA 1 or 2.

Recommendations

▶ ACS 2016

–If >20% risk of breast CA, annual mammogram alternating in 6 mo intervals with MRI is recommended. *BRCA1* and *2* mutation-positive women should begin MRI and mammogram screening at age 30 y or younger, depending on family history. Lymphoma survivors with a history of mediastinal radiation should begin mammography and MRI yearly 10 y after radiation.
–Dense breasts (>50%) by itself is not yet an indication for MRI screening. Adding full breast ultrasound to routine mammogram willin these patients increase early detection of breast cancer. Ultrasound has been shown to be superior to Tomosynthesis in this population. Tomosynthesis doubles the radiation exposure compared to routine mammogram.

Sources

–*CA Cancer J Clin.* 2015;65:30
–*N Engl J Med.* 2015;372:2353
–*J Clin Oncol.* 2016; 34:1882
–*JAMA.* 2012; 307:1394
–*J Clin Oncol.* 2016; 34:1840

Comment

–**High Risk Clinical Issues**
  • In high-risk women, probability of breast CA when mammogram is negative = 1.4% (1.2%–1.6%) vs. when mammogram plus MRI are negative = 0.3% (0.1%–0.8%). (*Ann Intern Med.* 2008;148:671) MRI is 2–3 times as sensitive as mammogram, but 2-fold increase in false positives—use in selected high-risk population only. (*J Clin Oncol.* 2005;23:8469) (*J Clin Oncol.* 2009;27:6124) (*J Clin Oncol.* 2011; 29:1664).
  • Tomosynthesis (three-dimensional mammography) under study with increase in sensitivity and specificity and reduction in false positives vs. film or digital mammography. There is double the dose of radiation compared to mammogram which may limit its use. (*JAMA.* 2014;311:2499) (*JAMA.* 2014;311:2488) (Effectiveness of Tomosynthesis: *JAMA.* 2016;2:737)

- If lifetime risk of breast CA is between 15% and 20%, women should discuss risks/benefits of adding annual MRI to mammography screening. Sensitivity of MRI is superior to mammography, especially in higher-risk women age <50 y with dense breasts (increasing breast density increases risk of breast CA and lowers sensitivity of mammogram). A >75% breast density increases risk of breast CA 5-fold. (*J Clin Oncol.* 2010;28:3830) (*N Engl J Med.* 2015;372:2243) (*Ann Inter Med.* 2015;162:157)
- Genetic evaluation increasing with more women tested for *BRCA 1* or *2* mutations as well as mutations in PALB2, CHEK 2, TP53, PTEN, DNA mismatch repair and others through use of next generation gene sequencing panels. (*Curr Opin Genet Dev.* 2010;20:268) (*Genet Med.* 2013;15:733) (*N Engl J Med.* 2015;372:2243)

Population

–Women age 50–74 y.
–Women age 40–50 y.

Recommendations

▶ USPSTF 2016

–Biennial screening mammography for women aged 50–74 y.
–Breast Self Exam teaching not recommended.
–Inconclusive data for screening women age >75 y.
–Decision to begin screening mammography before age 50 y should be individualized according to benefit vs. harm for each unique patient. (*Ann Intern Med.* 2012;156:609) (*Ann Intern Med.* 2009;151:727) (*Ann Intern Med.* 2016; 164:279)
–At present insufficient evidence to assess benefits and harms of tomosynthesis, ultrasound and MRI imaging for women with dense breasts.

Source

–http://www.ahrq.gov/clinic/uspstfix.htm

Comment

–These recommendations for women age 40–50 y have been widely criticized and largely ignored by other advisory organizations as inconsistent with available data. Subsequent trial from Norway showed significant benefit in mortality reduction (28%) in the age 40–49 y subset. Analysis of data sets continues, but there has been no major change in practice patterns. (*AJR Am J Roentgenol.* 2011;196:112) (*J Am Coll Radiol.* 2010;7:18) (*Cancer.* 2011;117:7) (*Eur J Cancer.* 2010;46:3137) (*CA Cancer J Clin.* 2012;62:129)

Populations

–Age 25–40 y (average risk).

–Age >40 y (average risk).

–Acquired increased risk—prior thoracic radiation therapy.

Recommendations

▶ NCCN 2016

–CBE every 1–3 y—breast awareness education in patients <40 with average risk.

–Annual CBE, mammogram yearly but MRI not recommended in average-risk patients. Women older than 80 or with limited life expectancy should not be screened.

–CBE q 6–12 mo, annual mammogram and annual MRI beginning 8–10 y after radiation therapy or age 40 y, whichever comes first.

–Breast MRI should be performed days 7–15 of menstrual cycle to maximize accuracy.

–BRCA 1 or 2 patients hould be followed with CBE q 3–6 mo with alternating mammogram and MRI every 6 mo.

–BRCA 1 and 2 patients should be referred for genetic counseling.

Source

–www.nccn.org

Comment

–**Continued Controversy Over Screening**

• The Canadian National Breast Screening study began in 1980 found no survival benefit for mammography in 40–59 y old women but the study is thought to be flawed by most experts in the United States because of study design. (*BMJ.* 2014;348:g366) (*N Engl J Med.* 2014;370:1965)

• A recent meta-analysis (*JAMA.* 2014; 311:1327) from Harvard found an overall reduction of breast cancer mortality of 19% (15% for women in their 40s and 32% for women in their 60s). They were concerned about over diagnosis and other potential harms of screening including false positive findings and unnecessary biopsies. (*N Engl J Med.* 2016; 375: 1438).

• Recent trials have led to an increase in further screening studies based on the predicted individual risk of breast cancer occurrence. These also include a history of lobular carcinoma in situ, atypical hyperplasia or history of breast CA (invasive and DCIS). *Ann Intern Med.* 2016; 165:700. *Ann Intern Med.* 2016; 165:737.

- A woman with mediastinal radiation at age 10–30 y will have a 75-fold increased risk of breast CA at age 35 y vs. age-matched controls.
- Salpingo-oophorectomy will decrease risk of breast CA in *BRCA1* and *2* carriers by 50% and decrease risk of ovarian CA by 90%–95%.

Populations

–Lifetime risk of breast CA >20% based on personal and family history (utilize Gail model, BRCAPRO model, or Tyrer-Cuzick model) and genetic predisposition (BRCA 1 or 2), PALB 2, CHEK 2 (http://www.cancer.gov/bcrisktool/).

Recommendations

▶ NCCN 2015

–Age <25 y, annual CBE, breast awareness education, and referral to genetic counselor.

–Age >25 y, annual mammogram, and MRI, CBE q 6–12 mo, consider risk-reducing strategies (surgery, chemoprevention).

Source

–www.nccn.org

Comments

1. Tamoxifen or raloxifene have not been studied as de novo chemo prevention in *BRCA1* or *2* patients, but tamoxifen will decrease risk of contralateral breast CA by 50% in *BRCA*-mutated breast CA patients. (*Int J Cancer.* 2006;118:2281)

2. Risk-reducing bilateral mastectomy in *BRCA1* and *2* mutation carriers results in a 90% risk reduction in incidence of breast CA and a 90% rate of satisfaction among patients who underwent risk-reducing surgery at 10 y follow-up. (*N Engl J Med.* 2001;345:159) (*JAMA.* 2010;304:967)

CANCER, BREAST <TESTING FOR BRCA 1 AND 2 MUTATIONS>

Population

–Women <60 y old.

Recommendations

▶ NCCN 2016

–**Who to screen – patients without cancer**

- Individual from a family with known deleterious *BRCA1* and *2* gene mutation
- Test only for the known mutation, not full genetic evaluation.
- If strong family history (FH) but unable to test family member with cancer (not alive or unavailable to be tested) then do full genetic evaluation—strong FH includes 2 primary breast cancers in a single close relative (1st, 2nd, and 3rd degree relatives) Breast cancer (BC), primaries on same side of family with at least one diagnosis occurring in a patient <50 y old, and ovarian cancer or male breast cancer at any age.

–**Who to screen – patients with breast, ovarian, pancreas and prostate cancer.**

- A known mutation in a cancer susceptibility gene within a family.
- Early age onset of breast CA (<50 y old).
- Triple negative (ER-PR-, Her2-) breast cancer diagnosed <60 y old.
- An individual of Ashkenazi Jewish descent with breast, ovarian or pancreatic cancer at any age.
- All women with ovarian cancer (epithelial and non-mucinous) at any age should be tested for *BRCA 1* and *2* mutations.

Comments

1. BRCA 2 related breast cancer is more like sporadic BC with 75% of patients with hormonal receptor positivity and significant decrease in aggressive growth. Only 15% of BRCA2 patients will develop ovarian cancer with the average time of onset being in the mid 50's.
2. One in forty Ashkenazi Jewish men and women carry a deleterious BRCA1 or 2 gene (BRCA1-185del AG, 5382inse mutations, and BRCA2 - 6174 delT mutation).
3. Some experts believe all men and women of Ashkenazi descent should be tested for these 3 genes even with no personal or family history of malignancy. (*N Engl J Med.* 2016; 374:454)

CANCER, BREAST
TABLE A: HARMS OF SCREENING MAMMOGRAPHY

Harm (*Ann Intern Med. 2016; 164:256*)	Internal Validity	Consistency	Magnitude of Effects	External Validity
Treatment of insignificant CAs (overdiagnosis of indolent cancer) can result in breast deformity, lymphedema, thromboembolic events, and chemotherapy-induced toxicities. (*Ann Intern Med. 2016; 164:215*)	Good	Good	Approximately 20%–30% of breast CAs detected by screening mammograms represent overdiagnosis. (*BMJ. 2009;339:2587*) Oncotype DX (a predictive panel of 15 breast CA genes) can reduce the use of chemotherapy by 50% in node-negative hormone receptor-positive patients. (*N Engl J Med. 2015;375:2005*)	Good
Additional testing (false positives)	Good	Good	Estimated to occur in 30% of women screened annually for 10 y, 7%–10% of whom will have biopsies. This creates anxiety and negative quality of life impact. (*Ann Intern Med. 2011;155:481*) (*Br J Cancer. 2013; 108:2205*)	Good
False sense of security, delay in CA diagnosis (false negatives) (*Ann Intern Med. 2016; 164:268*)	Good	Good	Approximately 10%–30% of women with invasive CA will have negative mammogram results, especially if young with dense breasts or with lobular or high-grade CAs. (*Radiology. 2005;235:775*) All suspicious lumps should be biopsied even with negative mammogram. (*Ann Intern Med. 2016; 164:226*)	Good
Radiation-induced mutation can cause breast CA, especially if exposed before age 30 y. Latency is more than 10 y, and the increased risk persists lifelong. (*Ann Intern Med. 2016; 164:205*)	Good	Good	In women beginning screening at age 40 y, benefits far outweigh risks of radiation-inducing breast CA. Women should avoid unnecessary CT scanning. (*Br J Cancer. 2005;93:590*) (*Ann Intern Med. 2012;156:662*)	Good

CANCER, CERVICAL

Populations
–Women <21 y old: no screening.[a]
–Women between 21 and 29 y old.
–Average-risk women 30–65 y old.

Recommendation
▶ ACS 2017
–**Guidelines ACS**
- Cytology alone (PAP smear) every 3 y until age 30 y.
- Human papillomavirus (HPV) DNA testing not recommended if age <30 y (majority of young patients will clear the infection).
- HPV and cytology "cotesting" every 5 y (preferred) or cytology alone every 3 y (acceptable). If HPV positive/cytology negative— either 12-mo follow-up with cotesting or test for HPV 16 or 18 genotypes with referral to colposcopy if positive. Continue to screen more frequently if high-risk factors present.[b,c,d]
- 10% of women age 30–34 y will have normal cytology but a positive HPV test and will need more frequent testing. In women 60–65 y old only 2.5% will have negative cytology but positive HPV testing.

Population
–Age >65 y after hysterectomy.

Recommendations
▶ ACS 2015
–No screening following adequate prior screening with negative results.
–No screening in women without a cervix and no history of CIN2 or worse in last 20 y or cervical CA ever.

Sources
–http://www.cancer.org
–http://www.survivorshipguidelines.org
–*CA Cancer J Clin.* 2012;62:147-172
–*N Engl Med.* 2013;369:2324.

[a]Sexual history in patients <21 y old not considered in beginning cytologic screening, which should start at age 21.
[b]New tests to improve CA detection include liquid-based/thin-layer preparations, computer-assisted screening methods, and HPV testing (*Am Fam Physician.* 2001;64:729. *N Engl J Med.* 2007;357:1579. *JAMA.* 2009;302:1757).
[c]High-risk factors include DES exposure before birth, HIV infection, or other forms of immunosuppression, including chronic steroid use.
[d]Women with a history of cervical CA, DES exposure, HIV infection, or a weakened immune system should continue to have screenings as long as they are in >5-y life expectancy.

Populations
–Women 21–29 y.
–Women 30–65 y.
–Women younger than 21 y.
–Women younger than 30 y.

Recommendation
▶ USPSTF 2015
–**Screening by Age**
  • Screen with cytology (Pap smear) every 3 y (age 21-29 y).
  • Screen with cytology every 3 y or co-testing (cytology/HPV testing) every 5 y (age 30-65 y).
  • Do not screen (age less than 21 y).
  • Do not screen with HPV testing alone or with cytology in 21–29 y old women.

Sources
–http://www.uspreventiveservicestaskforce.org/
–*Ann Intern Med.* 2012;156:880

Comments
–**Clinical Concerns**
–In the U.S. in 2017 it is estimated that 12,820 cases of invasive cervical cancer will be diagnosed and 4210 women die of disease (American Cancer Society: facts and figures 2017).
  • Cervical CA is causally related to infection with HPV (>70% associated with either HPV-18 or HPV-16 genotype).
  • Immunocompromised women (organ transplantation, chemotherapy, chronic steroid therapy, or human immunodeficiency virus [HIV]) should be tested twice during the first year after initiating screening and annually thereafter. (*CA Cancer J Clin.* 2011;61:8) (*Ann Intern Med.* 2011;155:698)
  • Women with a history of cervical CA or in utero exposure to diethylstilbestrol (DES) should continue average-risk protocol for women age <30 y indefinitely.
  • HPV vaccination of young women is now recommended by ACIP, UK-NHS, and others. Cervical CA screening recommendations have not changed for women receiving the vaccine because the vaccine covers only 70% of HPV serotypes that cause cervical CA. (*MMWR.* 2007;56(RR-2):1-24) (*CA cancer J Clin.* 2014;64:30) (*N Engl J Med.* 2015;372:711)
  • Long-term use of oral contraceptives may increase risk of cervical CA in women who test positive for cervical HPV DNA (*Lancet.* 2002;359:1085). Smoking increases risk of cervical CA 4-fold. (*Am J Epidemiol.* 1990;131:945)

- A vaccine against HPV-16 and HPV-18 significantly reduces the risk of acquiring transient and persistent infection. (*N Engl J Med.* 2002;347:1645) (*Obstet Gynecol.* 2006;107(1):4). New dosing schedule for HPV vaccinations - 2 dose schedules for girls and boys who initiate vaccination series at age 9–14. 3 doses are recommended for ages 15–26 y old and for immunosuppressed persons. (*CA Cancer J Clin.* 2017; 67:100).
- *Benefits:* Based on solid evidence, regular screening of appropriate women with the Pap test reduces mortality from cervical CA. Screening is effective when starting at age 21 y. *Harms:* Based on solid evidence, regular screening with the Pap test leads to additional diagnostic procedures and treatment for low-grade squamous intraepithelial lesions (LSILs), with uncertain long-term consequences on fertility and pregnancy. Harms are greatest for younger women, who have a higher prevalence of LSILs. LSILs often regress without treatment. False positives in postmenopausal women are a result of mucosal atrophy. (*NCI,* 2008)
- A study with 43,000 women ages 29–61 with both HPV DNA and cervical cytology cotesting every 5 y found the cumulative incidence of cervical cancer in women negative for both tests at baseline was 0.01% at 9 y and 0.07% after 14 y. (*BMJ.* 2016; 355:4924).
- There is basically now no significant difference in guidelines for screening for cervical cancer in average-risk women among ACOG, ACS, USPSTF.
- The risk of developing invasive cervical cancer is 3–10 times greater in women who have not been screened. (*CA Cancer J Clin.* 2017; 67:106).

Population
–Begin at age 21 y independent of sexual history.

Recommendation
▶ ACOG 2009
–Every 2 y from age 21 to 29.

Source
–ACOG Practice bulletin: *Obstet Gynecol.* 2009;114:1409-1420

Comment
–**ACOG SUMMARY**
- Women age ≥30 y can extend interval to every 2–3 y if three consecutive negative screens, no history of cervical intraepithelial neoplasia 2 or 3, not immunocompromised, no HIV, and not exposed to DES.
- No more often than 3 y if cervical cytology and HPV testing combined.

Population

–Women age >65 y.

Recommendation

▶ USPSTF 2015

–Recommends against routine screening if woman has had adequate recent screening and normal Pap smear results and is not otherwise at high risk for cervical CA.[c]

Source

–http://www.ahrq.gov/clinic/uspstf/uspscerv.htm

Population

–Women age ≥70 y.

Recommendation

▶ ACS 2016

–Discontinue screening if ≥3 normal Pap smear results in a row and no abnormal Pap smear results in the last 10 y.[d]

Source

–http://www.cancer.org

Comment

–Beyond age 70 y, there is little evidence for or against screening women who have been regularly screened in previous y. Individual circumstances, such as the patient's life expectancy, ability to undergo treatment if CA is detected, and ability to cooperate with and tolerate the Pap smear procedure, may obviate the need for cervical CA screening.

Population

–Women without a cervix and no history of high-grade pre-cancer or cervical cancer.

Recommendation

▶ ACS 2016, ACOG 2009, USPSTF 2015

–Recommends against routine Pap smear screening in women who have had a total hysterectomy or removal of the cervix for benign disease and no history of abnormal cell growth.

Sources

–http://www.cancer.org
–http://www.ahrq.gov/clinic/uspstf/uspscerv.htm
–ACOG practice bulletin-109 12/09

CANCER, COLORECTAL (CRC)

Recommendation
▶ ACS 2013, USMTFCC[a] 2012

–See table on page 29. Tests that find polyps and CA are preferred.

Sources
–*CA Cancer J Clin.* 2013;63:87-105
–*CA Cancer J Clin.* 2012;62:124-142

Comment
–**Screening Works**
  • Although colonoscopy is the de facto gold standard for colon CA screening, choice of screening technique depends on risk, comorbidities, insurance coverage, patient preference, and availability. Above all, do something to screen for colon CA. (*CA Cancer J Clin.* 2016; 66:95)
  • There is a rising incidence of CRC in younger patients (<50 y old) - beware of symptoms and strong family history. (*JAMA Surgery.* 2015; 150:17).

Population
–Age ≥50 y at average risk.[b]

Recommendations
▶ AAFP 2015, USPSTF 2016
  –**Screen with one of the following strategies**[c,d,e]
    • Fecal occult blood test (gFOBT-guaiac based or iFOBT-immunochemical based—iFOBT is preferred) annually.[f]

[a]U.S. Multisociety Task Force on Colorectal Cancer (ACG, ACP, AGA, ASGE).
[b]Risk factors indicating need for earlier/more frequent screening: personal history of CRC or adenomatous polyps or hepatoblastoma, CRC or polyps in a first-degree relative age <60 y or in 2 first-degree relatives of any age, personal history of chronic inflammatory bowel disease, and family with hereditary CRC syndromes (*Ann Intern Med.* 1998;128(1):900. *Am J Gastroenterol.* 2009;104:739. *N Engl J Med.* 1994;331(25):1669. *N Engl J Med.* 1995;332(13):861). Additional high-risk group: history of ≥30 Gy radiation to whole abdomen; all upper abdominal fields; pelvic, thoracic, lumbar, or sacral spine. Begin monitoring 10 y after radiation or at age 35 y, whichever occurs last (http://www.survivorshipguidelines.org). Screening colonoscopy in those age ≥80 y results in only 15% of the expected gain in life expectancy seen in younger patients (*JAMA.* 2006;295:2357). ACG treats African Americans as high-risk group. See separate recommendation above.
[c]A positive result on an FOBT should be followed by colonoscopy. An alternative is flexible sigmoidoscopy and air-contrast barium enema.
[d]FOBT should be performed on 2 samples from 3 consecutive specimens obtained at home. A single stool guaiac during annual physical examination is not adequate.
[e]USPSTF did not find direct evidence that a screening colonoscopy is effective in reducing CRC mortality rates.
[f]Use the guaiac-based test with dietary restriction, or an immunochemical test without dietary restriction. Two samples from each of three consecutive stools should be examined without rehydration. Rehydration increases the false-positive rate.

- Flexible sigmoidoscopy every 5 y with reflex colonoscopy if abnormal.
- FOBT^d annually plus flexible sigmoidoscopy every 5 y.
- Colonoscopy every 10 y.^{g}
- CT colonoscopy.
- (*N Engl J Med.* 2017; 376:2)
- Multi-targeted stool DNA testing (cologuard)—now approved—92% colon cancers detected in asymptomatic average risk persons but <50% of polyps detected, 10% false positives and cost $600/test. Circulating methylated 5EPT9 DNA test also available for screening tested on peripheral blood but low sensitivity (48%). (*GYT.* 2014; 63:317) (*JAMA.* 2014;312:2566)

–**Follow-up colonoscopy according to findings**
- Normal or small hyperplastic polyps—10 y.
- 1 or 2 <10 mm tubular adenomas—5–10 y.
- Small serrated polyps without dysplasia—5 y.
- 3–10 tubular adenomas, a tubular adenoma, or serrated polyp >10 mm, adenoma with high-grade dysplasia—3 y. (*N Engl J Med.* 2014;370:1298)

Sources
–http://www.aafp.org/online/en/home/clinical/exam.html
–*JAMA.* 2016;315:2564.
–http://www.cancer.org
–*Gastrointest Endosc.* 2006;63:546

Population
–Women at average risk age ≥50 y.

Recommendations
▶ ACOG 2007
–**Preferred Method Guidelines**
- Colonoscopy every 10 y.

–Other appropriate methods:
- FOBT annually.
- Flexible sigmoidoscopy every 5 y.
- FOBT annually plus flexible sigmoidoscopy every 5 y.
- Double-contrast barium enema every 5 y.

Sources
–*Ann Intern Med.* 2012;156:378
–*Gastroenterology.* 2003;124:544
–http://www.ahrq.gov/clinic/uspstf/uspscolo.htm
–ACOG Committee Opinion, No. 357, Nov 2007

^{g}Population-based retrospective analysis: risk of developing CRC remains decreased for >10 y following negative colonoscopy findings (*JAMA.* 2006;295:2366).

–N Engl J Med. 2013;369:1095

–JAMA Intern Med. 2016; 176:894.

Population

–Persons at increased risk based on family history but without a definable genetic syndrome.

Recommendations

▶ ACS 2016, USMTFCC[a] 2012

–*Group I:* Screening colonoscopy at age 40 y, or 10 y younger than the earliest diagnosis in the immediate family, and repeat every 5 y.[h]

–*Group II:* Follow average-risk recommendations, but begin at age 40 y.[h]

Source

–CA Cancer J Clin. 2008;58:130

Comment

–**Practical Points of CRC Screening**

- The USPSTF "strongly recommends" colorectal cancer (CRC) screening in this group up to age 75 y.
- Screening patients >75 should be individualized based on overall health and risk.
- Flexible sigmoidoscopy and one-time FOBT mandating a colonoscopy if either yields positive results will miss 25% of significant proximal neoplasia. This strategy should include yearly FOBT. (*N Engl J Med.* 2001;345:555) (*N Engl J Med.* 2012;366:2345)
- FOBT alone decreased CRC mortality by 33% compared with those who were not screened. (*Gastroenterology.* 2004;126:1674)
- Accuracy of colonoscopy is operator dependent—rapid withdrawal time, poor prep, and lack of experience will increase false negatives. (*N Engl J Med.* 2006;355:2533) (*Ann Intern Med.* 2012;156:692) (*Gastroenterol.* 2015; 110:72)
- Multi-targeted DNA stool testing vs. iFOBT with more cancers detected (92.3% vs. 73.8%) but more false positives with DNA test. (*N Engl J Med.* 2014;370:1287-1297) (*N Engl J Med.* 2014;370: 1298-1306)
- Percentage of U.S. adults receiving some form of CRC screening increased from 44% in 1999 to 63% in 2008. The goal is 80%

[h]Group I: First-degree relative with colon CA or adenomatous polyps at age <60 y or 2 first-degree relatives with CRC or adenomatous polyps at any time. *Group II*: First-degree relative with CRC or adenomatous polyps at age ≥60 y or 2 second-degree relatives with CRC. Revised Bethesda criteria for testing for HNPCC (Lynch syndrome)—screen for tumor microsatellite instability if CRC diagnosed in a patient age <50 y, presence of synchronous, metachronous CRC or other HNPCC defining tumor at any age. CRC with microsatellite unstable-type histology (mucinous, signet ring, infiltrating lymphocytes) in patients age <60 y. CRC diagnosed in 1 or more first-degree relatives with HNPCC-related tumor with one of the cancers diagnosed at age <50 y. CRC diagnosed younger than age 50 y. CRC diagnosed in 2 or more first-degree or second-degree relatives with HNPCC-related tumors regardless of age. Confirmation of HNPCC is made by genetic evaluation of the involved genes (*J Natl Cancer Inst.* 2004;96:261).

by 2018. (*CA Cancer J Clin.* 2015;65:30) (*Arch Intern Med.* 2011;171:647) (*Arch Intern Med.* 2012;172:575) In 2016, it is estimated that 134,000 new cases of CRC will be diagnosed and 49,000 Americans will die from CRC. Median age of diagnosis is 68. (*CA Cancer J Clin.* 2016;66:7)

- Colonoscopy vs. iFOBT testing in CRC with similar detection of cancer but more adenomas identified in colonoscopy group. (*N Engl J Med.* 2012;366:697) (*N Engl J Med.* 2012;366:687)

Populations

–*Very-high-risk** hereditary nonpolyposis colorectal cancer (HNPCC or Lynch syndrome); 5% of patients with CRC will have HNPCC.

–Evaluate if the patient <50 y old or Bethesda or Amsterdam criteria met.[h]

–Test for microstellite instability (MSI - high) or immunohistochemistry to identify missing genes.

Recommendation

▶ ACS 2016, USMTFCC[a] 2012

–Colonoscopy every 2 y beginning at age 20–25 y then yearly at age 40 y.[h] If a colorectal cancer occurs total colectomy is favored. (*A J Gastroenterol.* 2014; 109:1159)

Comments

1. In follow-up with curable CRC, CEA every 3 mo for 2 y followed by every 6 mo for 3 y was equivalent to CT scans every 6 mo for 2 y and then every 12 mo for 3 y in discovering recurrence of CRC and length of overall survival. (*JAMA.* 2014;311:263)
2. Increased risk of non-CRC (endometrial, ovary, upper gastrointestinal, pancreas, renal pelvis, ureter, breast) requires systematic screening. (*J Clin Oncol.* 2000;18:11) (*J Clin Oncol.* 2012;30:1058)
3. NCCN recommends screening for Lynch syndrome in all patients with CRC <70 y old. Do DNA mismatch repair analysis or immunohistochemistry followed by PCR study to confirm.
4. Lynch syndrome with right-sided lesions, poorly differentiated with lymphocyte infiltration—better outcome compared to sporadic CRC. (*JAMA.* 2012; 308:1555)

Population

–Classic familial adenomatous polyposis (FAP).

Recommendation

▶ ACS 2016, USMTFCC[a] 2012

–**Preferred Approach**
- At-risk children should be offered genetic testing at age 10–12 y.

- Flexible sigmoidoscopy or colonoscopy every 12 mo starting at age 10–12 y.
- Elective colectomy based on number and histology of polyps—usually done by early 20s.
- upper endoscopy every 5 y if no gastric or duodenal polyps starting in early 20s.

Sources
–*Am J Gastroenterol.* 2009;104:739
–*J Clin Oncol.* 2003;21:2397
–*Gut.* 2008;57:704
–*JAMA.* 2006;296:1507

Comment
–Broad Spectrum of Cancers
- Extraintestinal tumors in FAP include hepatoblastoma (AFP screening recommended in families with this tumor), adrenal tumors, osteomas, brain tumors, skin CA, and thyroid CA.

CANCER, COLORECTAL

The following options are acceptable choices for CRC screening in average-risk adults beginning at age 50 y. As each of the following tests has inherent characteristics related to prevention potential, accuracy, costs, and potential harms, individuals should have an opportunity to make an informed decision when choosing one of the following options.

In the opinion of the guidelines development committee, *colon CA prevention* should be the primary goal of CRC screening. Tests that are designed to detect both early CA and adenomatous polyps should be encouraged if resources are available and patients are willing to undergo an invasive test.

Chart of Tests that Detect Adenomatous Polyps and Cancer

Test	Interval	Key Issues for Informed Decisions
FSIG with insertion to 40 cm or to the splenic flexure	Every 5 y	Complete or partial bowel prep is required. Because sedation usually is not used, there may be some discomfort during the procedure. The protective effect of sigmoidoscopy is primarily limited to the portion of the colon examined. NCI study of 77,000 patients showed a significant decrease in CRC incidence (both distal and proximal) and a 50% reduction in mortality (distal only) (*J Natl Cancer Inst.* 2012;104:1). Twenty-five percent of colon cancers are missed by this strategy. Patients should understand that positive findings on sigmoidoscopy usually result in a referral for colonoscopy.

Colonoscopy	Every 10 y	Complete bowel prep is required. Procedural sedation is used in most centers; patients will miss a day of work and will need a chaperone for transportation from the facility. Risks include perforation and bleeding, which are rare but potentially serious; most of the risk is associated with polypectomy (*Ann Intern Med.* 2009;150;1).
Double Contrast Barium Enema (DCBE)	Every 5 y	Complete bowel prep is required. If patients have one or more polyps ≥6 mm, colonoscopy will still be needed for biopsy or polyp removal; follow-up colonoscopy will require complete bowel prep. Risks of DCBE are low; rare cases of perforation have been reported—radiation exposure is a concern. USPSTF does not recommend DCBE because of lower sensitivity than other methods. (*N Engl J Med.* 2007;357:1403)
CT Colonoscopy (CTC)	Every 5 y	Complete bowel prep usually required. (*Ann Intern Med.* 2012;156:692) If patients have one or more polyps ≥6 mm, colonoscopy will be recommended; if same-day colonoscopy is not available, a second complete bowel prep will be required before colonoscopy. Risks of CTC are low; rare cases of perforation have been reported. Extracolonic abnormalities may be identified on CTC that could require further evaluation (7%–15% of CT examinations). Not as sensitive as colonoscopy for polyps <1 cm, especially for polyps ≤6 mm that are flat or serrated polyps.

TESTS THAT PRIMARILY DETECT CANCER

Test	Interval	Key Issues for Informed Decisions
gFOBT with high sensitivity for CA	Annual	Depending on manufacturer's recommendations, 2–3 stool samples collected at home are needed to complete testing; a single stool gathered during a digital examination in the clinical setting is not an acceptable stool test and should not be done. Any positive result from stool samples collected at home should lead to early colonoscope evaluation
FIT (iFOBT) with high sensitivity for CA	Annual	Specificity of iFOBT superior to gFOBT but more expensive. Positive test results are associated with an increased risk of colon CA and advanced neoplasia; colonoscopy should be recommended if the test results are positive. If the test result is negative, it should be repeated annually. Patients should understand that one-time testing is likely to be ineffective.

TESTS THAT PRIMARILY DETECT CANCER *(Continued)*		
sDNA with high sensitivity for CA	Interval uncertain	An adequate stool sample must be obtained and packaged with appropriate preservative agents for shipping to the laboratory. New data (*N Engl J Med.* 2014;370:1287) is impressive and is being more widely used. The unit cost of the currently available test is significantly higher than that of other forms of stool testing ($600 vs. $23). If the test result is positive, colonoscopy will be recommended. If the test result is negative, the appropriate interval for a repeat test is uncertain. sDNA testing is becoming more widely used at this time. (*Ann Intern Med.* 2008;149:441) (*N Engl J Med.* 2014;370:1350).

CA, cancer; CRC, colorectal cancer; CT, computed tomography; CTC, computed tomography colonography; DCBE, double-contrast barium enema; FIT, fecal immunochemical test; FSIG, flexible sigmoidoscopy; gFOBT, guaiac-based fecal occult blood test; sDNA, stool DNA.

CANCER, ENDOMETRIAL

Population
  –All postmenopausal women.

Recommendation
▶ ACS 2008
  –**No Routine Screening**
  • Inform women about risks and symptoms of endometrial CA and strongly encourage them to report any unexpected bleeding or spotting. This is especially important for women with an increased risk of endometrial CA (history of unopposed estrogen therapy, tamoxifen therapy, late menopause, nulliparity, infertility or failure to ovulate, obesity, diabetes, or hypertension).

Source
  –http://www.cancer.org

Comment
  –**Clinical Facts**
  • *Benefits:* There is inadequate evidence that screening with endometrial sampling or transvaginal ultrasound (TVU) decreases mortality. *Harms:* Based on solid evidence, screening with TVU will result in unnecessary additional exams because of low specificity. Based on solid evidence, endometrial biopsy may result in discomfort, bleeding, infection, and, rarely, uterine perforation. (NCI, 2008)
  • Presence of atypical glandular cells on Pap test from postmenopausal (age >40 y) women not taking exogenous hormones is abnormal and

requires further evaluation (TVU and endometrial biopsy). Pap test is not sensitive for endometrial screening.

- Endometrial thickness of <4 mm on TVU is associated with low risk of endometrial CA. (*Am J Obstet Gynecol.* 2001;184:70)
- Most cases of endometrial CA are diagnosed as a result of symptoms reported by patients (uterine bleeding), and a high proportion of these cases are diagnosed at an early stage and have high rates of cure. Type II endometrial CA accounts for 15% of patients. Histology is serous or clear cell with 5 y survival 55% vs. 85% at 5 y compared to endometrial Type I cancer (NCI, 2008) (*Lancet.* 2016; 387:1094)
- Tamoxifen use for 5 y raises the risk of endometrial CA 2- to 3-fold, but CAs are low stage, low grade, with high cure rates. (*J Natl Cancer Inst.* 1998; 90:1371)
- In 2016, there were 60,050 new cases of endometrial cancer with 10,170 deaths. The mean age at diagnosis is 60 y old.

Population

–All women at high risk for endometrial CA[a] (patients with known or high suspicion for HNPCC mutation carrier).

Recommendations

▶ ACS 2016

–Annual screening beginning at age 35 y with endometrial biopsy.
–International guidelines advise transvaginal ultrasound and annual endometrial biopsy beginning at 25 y old.

Source

–*CA Cancer J Clin.* 2005; 55:31
–*JAMA.* 1997; 277:915
– http://www.cancer.org

Comment

–**High Risk Women – Lynch Syndrome - lifetime risk 60%**
- Variable screening with ultrasound among women (age 25–65 y; $n = 292$) at high risk for HNPCC mutation detected no CAs from ultrasound. Two endometrial cancers occurred in the cohort that presented with symptoms. (*Cancer.* 2002;94:1708) (*Gynecol Oncol.* 2007; 107:159).
- The death rate from sporadic endometrial cancer and Lynch syndrome related uterine cancer is the same.
- The Women's Health Initiative (WHI) demonstrated that combined estrogen and progestin did not increase the risk of endometrial CA but did increase the rate of endometrial biopsies and ultrasound exams prompted by abnormal uterine bleeding. (*JAMA.* 2003:290)

[a]High-risk women are those known to carry HNPCC-associated genetic mutations, or at high risk to carry a mutation, or who are from families with a suspected autosomal dominant predisposition to colon CA (15%–50% lifetime risk of endometrial CA).

CANCER, GASTRIC

Population
- Average-risk population.
- In the United States there were 22,370 patients diagnosed with gastric cancer with 10,990 deaths. 95% of these cancers were adenocarcinoma.
- Lynch syndrome patients should consider upper endoscopy baseline repeated every 5–10 y.
- Heliobacter pylori infections, atrophic gastritis, pernicious anemia, and partial gastrectomy patients have a higher risk of gastric CA.

Recommendation
▶ NCI 2015
- There are currently no recommendations regarding screening for gastric CA.

Comment
- **Clinical Considerations in Gastric Cancer**
  - Endoscopic screening for gastric CA in moderate- to high-risk population subgroups is cost-effective but not shown to be beneficial in the United States. (*Clin Gastroenterol Hepatol.* 2006;4:709)
  - Beware of hereditary gastric cancer *CDH1* gene which regulates mutation of E-cadherin, an adhesion protein which increases risk of gastric cancer to >70%. Risk reduction gastrectomy recommended at 20-30 y old. (*J Med Genet.* 2015; 52:361)
  - No randomized trials evaluating impact of screening on mortality from gastric cancer have been reported. (*NEJM.* 2014; 371:2499) (https://www.cancer.gove/types/esophageal/hp/esophageal-screening-pdq

CANCER, LIVER (HEPATOCELLULAR CARCINOMA [HCC])

Population
- Adults at high risk for HCC,[b] especially those awaiting liver transplantation, should be entered into surveillance programs.

Recommendation
▶ AASLD[a] 2010 Update
- **Screening Tests**
  - Surveillance with ultrasound at 6-mo intervals.

Sources
- *Hematology.* 2005;42:1208
- *J Hepatol.* 2015; 63:1156

Population

–Adults

Recommendations

▶ British Society of Gastroenterology[a] 2003

–Surveillance with abdominal ultrasound and alfa-fetoprotein (AFP) every 6 mo should be considered for high-risk groups.[b]

–This is low strength recommendation for screening. It identifies early-stage HCC but whether overall survival is improved is not known. (*Ann Intern Med.* 2014;161:261)

Sources

–*Gut.* 2003;52 (suppl III):iii

–http://www.bsg.org.uk/

Comment

1. HCC is the 5th most common cancer in the world. There will be 39,230 new cases of hepatocellular cancer (HCC) and 27,170 deaths due to this disease in the U.S. (NCI. February update 2017).

2. AFP alone should not be used for screening unless ultrasound is not available (low sensitivity —60% positive).

3. *Benefits:* Based on fair evidence, screening would result in a decrease in HCC-related mortality. *Harms:* Based on fair evidence, screening would result in rare, but serious, side effects associated with needle biopsy, such as needle-track seeding, hemorrhage, bile peritonitis, and pneumothorax. (NCI, 2008. *Ann Intern Med.* 2012;156:387) (*Ann Int Med.* 2014; 161:261).

▼ CANCER, LUNG

Population

–Asymptomatic persons with >30 pack-year smoking history.

Recommendation

▶ ACCP and ASCO 2013

–**Survival Benefit with CT Screening**

• Based on good evidence, routine screening for lung CA with chest x-ray (CXR) and sputum cytology is not recommended.

• Screening with low-dose CT (LDCT) is now recommended following the strict eligibility criteria of the National Lung Screening Trial (NLST). This includes age 50–74 y with a 30 pack-year smoking

---

[a]Only two organizations recommending screening for HCC in high-risk populations (low-level evidence).
[b]HBsAg+ *persons* (*carriers*): Asian males age ≥40 y, Asian females age ≥40 y; all cirrhotics; family history of HCC; Africans age >20 y. *Nonhepatitis B carriers:* hepatitis C; alcoholic cirrhosis; genetic hemochromatosis; primary biliary cirrhosis, alpha-1-antitrypsin deficiency with cirrhosis, hepatitis C with cirrhosis; hemochromatosis with cirrhosis, NASH (steatosis) with cirrhosis. (*Hepatol* 2014;60:1767) (*Clin Gastroenterol Hepatol.* 2011;9:428)

history. People who have not smoked in the last 15 y or who have
significant comorbidities are excluded.

Sources
–http://www.ahrq.gov/clinic/uspstf/uspslung.htm
–http://www.guideline.gov/summaries/summary/43894
–*CA Cancer J Clin.* 2004;54:41

Population
–Asymptomatic persons with >30-pack-year smoking history.

Recommendations

▶ ACS 2013, NCCN 2013

–Guidance in shared decision making regarding screening of high-risk
persons.
–Screening with LDCT for 3 consecutive y is recommended for patients
meeting the eligibility criteria for the NLST (>30 pack-year smoking
history, age 50–74 y, no major medical comorbidities) and the presence
of a minimum of a highly skilled support team to evaluate LDCT scans,
schedule appropriate follow-ups, and perform lung biopsies safely
when indicated. (Most patients receiving low-dose CT screening repeat
the study yearly as long as they meet criteria.)

Sources
–http://www.cancer.org
–http://www.cancer.gov/nlst

Comment
–**Clinical Insight**
  • Counsel all patients against tobacco use, even when age >50 y.
    Smokers who quit gain ~10 y of increased life expectancy and have
    maximum reduction in risk of lung CA after 15 y of no tobacco use.
    (*Br Med J.* 2004:328)
  • Spiral CT screening can detect greater number of lung CAs
    in smokers with a >10-pack-year exposure. (*N Engl J Med.*
    2006;355:1763-1771)
  • The NCI has reported data from the NLST, a randomized controlled
    trial comparing LDCT and CXR yearly × 3 with 8-y follow-up. A
    total of 53,500 men and women age 50–74 y, 30-pack/year smokers
    were randomized. A 20.3% reduction in deaths from lung CA was
    reported for the LDCT group (estimated that 10,000–15,000 lives
    could be saved per year). Problems with false-positives (25% have
    lung nodules <1 cm that are not cancer) and cost of workup were
    noted, but benefits have led to a change in guidelines. ACS 2013
    guidelines on lung cancer screening recommends adults between the
    ages of 55 and 74 y (80 y/o for USPSTF) who meet eligibility criteria

of NLST may consider LDCT screening for lung cancer. This should take place in the setting where appropriate resources and expertise are available to minimize morbidity. Less than 1 in 1000 patients with a false positive result experience a major complication resulting from diagnostic work-up. Patients with a 30-pack-year smoking history but nonsmoking for >15 y are excluded. The ACCP, ACS, NCCN, and ASCO formally recommend LDCT screening for patients who meet the criteria of the NLST study. (It is estimated that 8.6 million Americans meet NLST criteria for screening, which would save 12,000 lives annually). There is an increasing concern regarding the cost of lung cancer screening. Twenty-five percent of patients screened willhave indeterminate abnormal findings requiring repeat imaging at intervals and in a significant number of patients biopsied are done showing benign disease. Also many patients are being screened yearly instead of just 3 consecutive y of screening that was done in the randomized trials. (*Ann Intern Med.* 2011;155:540) (*N Engl J Med.* 2011;365:395) (*CA Cancer J Clin.* 2013;63:87) (*N Engl J Med.* 2013;368:1980-1991) (*N Engl J Med.* 2014;369:910) (*N Engl J Med.* 2015;372:2083) (*N Engl J Med.* 2015;372:387) (*Ann Intern Med.* 2014; 160:330) (*Lancet Onc.* 2016;17:543) (*Lancet Onc.* 2016;17:590)

- Problem with overdiagnosis and potential harm in surgical resertion of small slow growing cancers. (*JAMA Intern Med*) published online 1/30/2017) (*JAMA Intern Med.* 2014; 174:269).
- There is an increasing concern regarding the cost of lung cancer screening. Twenty-five percent of patients screened will have indeterminate abnormal findings requiring repeat imaging at intervals and in a significant number of patients biopsies are done showing benign disease. Also many patients are screened yearly instead of just 3 consecutive years of screening that was done in the randomized trials. (*JAMA.* 2012; 307:2418) (*JAMA Intern Med.* 2014; 174:269).
- Lung cancer prediction models will help designate who needs to be screened and how often. (*J Clin Oncol.* 2017; 35:861).

CANCER, ORAL

Population
–Asymptomatic persons.

Recommendation
▶ AAFP 2008, USPSTF 2014

–**No Screening**
- Evidence is insufficient to recommend for or against routinely screening adults for oral asymptomatic CA.

Sources
- http://www.aafp.org/online/en/home/clinical/exam.html
- http://www.ahrq.gov/clinic/uspstf/uspsoral.htm

Comment
- Risk factors: regular alcohol or tobacco use.
- A randomized controlled trial of visual screening for oral CA (at 3-y intervals) showed decreased oral CA mortality among screened males (but not females) who were tobacco and/or alcohol users over an 8-y period. (*Lancet.* 2005;365:1927)
- 48,370 new cases of oral cancer in 2016 with 9570 deaths

Comments
- Significant increase in HPV (subtypes 16 and 18)-related squamous cell cancer of the oropharynx (base of tongue and tonsil) in nonsmokers.
- There is a 30%–40% improvement in cure rate in HPV positive non-smokers vs. cure for smoking-related cancers. (*N Engl J Med.* 2010;363:24)
- >70% of oropharyngeal squamous cell cancers are HPV positive. (*J Clin Onc.* 2013;31:2708) (*J Clin Onc.* 2010;28:4142)
- Prevalence of oral HPV infection in the United States is 6.9%. (*JAMA.* 2012;307:693)
- Studies ongoing to determine if less therapy in HPV-positive patients will result in the same curability with less long-term and short-term toxicity. (*J Natl Cancer Inst.* 2008;180:261) (*Compr Canc Netw.* 2011;9:665)

CANCER, OVARIAN

Population
- Asymptomatic women at average risk.[a]

Recommendation
▶ USPSTF 2012
- No Benefit from Screening
  - Recommends against routine screening. Beware of symptoms of ovarian CA that can be present in early-stage disease (abdominal, pelvic, and back pain; bloating and change in bowel habits; urinary symptoms). (*Ann Intern Med.* 2012;157:900-904) (*J Clin Oncol.* 2005;23:7919) (*Ann Intern Med.* 2012;156:182)

[a]Lifetime risk of ovarian CA in a woman with no affected relatives is 1 in 70. If 1 first-degree relative has ovarian CA, lifetime risk is 5%. If 2 or more first-degree relatives have ovarian CA, lifetime risk is 7%. Women with 2 or more family members affected by ovarian cancer have a 3% chance of having a hereditary ovarian cancer syndrome. If *BRCA1* mutation, lifetime risk of ovarian CA is 45%–50%; if *BRCA2* mutation, lifetime risk is 15%–20%. Lynch syndrome = 8%–10% lifetime risk of ovarian CA.
[b]USPSTF recommends against routine referral for genetic counseling or routine BRCA testing of women whose family history is not associated with increased risk for deleterious mutation in *BRCA1* or *2* genes.

Sources

  –http://www.aafp.org/online/en/home/clinical/exam.html

  –http://www.ahrq.gov/clinic/uspstf/uspsovar.htm

Population

  –Women whose family history is associated with an increased risk for deleterious mutations in *BRCA1* or *2* genes.[b]

Recommendations

▶ USPSTF 2013

  –Recommends referral for genetic counseling and evaluation for *BRCA* testing. Does not recommend routine screening in this group.

  –Screening with CA-125, TVU, and pelvic exam can be considered, but there is no evidence in this population that screening reduces risk of death from ovarian CA.

  –*A woman with ovarian cancer at any age should be tested for BRCA1 and 2 mutations. (USPSTF-publication#12 Dec. 2013) (NCCN guideline version 2; 2017)*

Source

  –http://www.ahrq.gov/clinic/uspstf/uspsbrgen.htm

Population

  –High-risk patients with *BRCA1* or *2* mutations or strong family history of ovarian CA.

Recommendations

▶ ACOG 2009, NCCN 2011

  –Recommends screening with CA-125 and TVU at age 30–35 y or 5–10 y earlier than earliest onset of ovarian CA in family members.

  –Risk-reducing salpingo-oophorectomy should be strongly considered. (*JAMA*. 2010;304:967)

Source

  –http://www.ahrq.gov/clinic/uspstf/uspsbrgen.htm

Comment

  –**Clinical Issues**

   • Risk factors: age >60 y; low parity; personal history of endometrial, colon, or breast CA; family history of ovarian CA; and hereditary breast/ovarian CA syndrome. Use of oral contraceptives for 5 y decreases the risk of ovarian CA by 50%. (*JAMA*. 2004;291:2705)

   • *Benefit:* There is inadequate evidence to determine whether routine screening for ovarian CA with serum markers such as CA-125 levels, TVU, or pelvic examinations would result in a decrease in mortality from ovarian CA. *Harm.* Problems have been lack of specificity (positive predictive value) and need for invasive procedures to make a diagnosis. Based on solid evidence, routine screening for ovarian CA would result in many diagnostic laparoscopies and laparotomies for each ovarian CA found. (NCI, 2008) (*JAMA.* 2011;305:2295)

- Additionally, cancers found by screening have not consistently been found to be lower stage. (*Lancet Oncol.* 2009;10:327)
- Preliminary results from the Prostate, Lung, Colorectal and Ovarian (PLCO) Cancer Screening Trial: At the time of baseline examination, positive predictive value for invasive cancer was 3.7% for abnormal CA-125 levels, 1% for abnormal TVU results, and 23.5% if both tests showed abnormal results. (*Am J Obstet Gynecol.* 2005;193:1630)
- Large United Kingdom trial assessing multimodal screening strategy (annual CA-125, risk of ovarian Ca algorithm (ROLA), transvaginal ultrasound) versus usual care. 202,639 women recruited (age 50-74) found nonsignificant mortality reduction up to 14 y F/U. (*J Natl Compr Cancer Netw.* 2016; 14:1143. Lancet. 2016; 387:945).

CANCER, PANCREATIC

Population
–Asymptomatic persons.

Recommendation
▶ USPSTF 2010
–**Screening of No Benefit**
Recommends against routine screening.

Source
–http://www.ahrq.gov/clinic/uspstf/uspspanc.htm

Comment
–**Risk Factors – Acquired and Genetic**
- Cigarette smoking has consistently been associated with increased risk of pancreatic CA. *BRCA2* mutation is associated with a 5% lifetime risk of pancreatic CA. Blood group O with lower risk and diabetes with a 2-fold higher risk of pancreatic CA. (*J Natl Cancer Inst.* 2009;101:424) (*J Clin Oncol.* 2009;27:433)
- USPSTF concluded that the harms of screening for pancreatic CA—the very low prevalence, limited accuracy of available screening tests, invasive nature of diagnostic tests, and poor outcomes of treatment—exceed any potential benefits.
- Patients with a strong family history (≥2 first-degree relatives with pancreatic CA) should undergo genetic counseling and

may benefit from interval screening with CA 19–9, CT scan, and magnetic resonance cholangiopancreatography (MRCP). (*Nat Rev Gastroenterol Hepatol.* 2012;9:445-453)

CANCER, PROSTATE

Population
–Men age ≥50 y.[a]

Recommendations
▶ ACS 2010
–Discuss annual prostate-specific antigen (PSA) and digital rectal exam (DRE) if ≥10-y life expectancy.[b]
–Discuss risks and benefits of screening strategy to enable an informed decision.

Source
–http://www.cancer.org

Comment
–**Prevalence of Prostate CA**
  • There are 220,800 new cases of prostate cancer and 27,500 deaths expected in 2017.

Population
–Asymptomatic men.

Recommendation
▶ USPSTF 2012
–**Recent Guidelines**
  • Do not use PSA-based screening for prostate CA. There is convincing evidence that PSA-based screening results in the detection of many cases of asymptomatic prostate CA and that a substantial percentage of men will have a tumor that will progress so slowly that it would remain asymptomatic for the patient's lifetime.
  • Because of the current inability to distinguish tumors that will remain indolent from those destined to be lethal, many men are subjected to the harms of treatment for a prostate CA that would never become symptomatic.

---

[a]Men in high-risk groups (1 or more first-degree relatives diagnosed before age 65 y, African Americans) should begin screening at age 45 y. Men at higher risk because of multiple first-degree relatives affected at an early age could begin testing at age 40 y (http://www.cancer.org/).
[b]Men who ask their doctor to make the decision should be tested. Discouraging testing or not offering testing is inappropriate.

- The benefits of PSA-based screening for prostate CA do not outweigh the harms (this recommendation applies to high-risk patients as well—African American/positive family history[a]). There is ongoing significant criticism of the USPSTF prostate screening recommendations. (*JAMA.* 2011;306:2715) (*JAMA.* 2011;306:2719) (*JAMA.* 2011;306:2721)

  –USPSTF 2017 update prostate cancer - in progress

  –Below age 55 - no screening

  –From 55-69, discuss potential benefits and harms of PSA screening (false postive results) over diagnosis and over treatment and treatment complications vs. small potential benefit of reducing the chance of dying of prostate cancer.

  –USPSTF rrecommends individualized decision making so that each man can understand the potential benefits and harms of screening and make his decision.

  –Men older than age 70 - USPSTF recommends no PSA based screening for this group

  –In high risk patients (African Americans, 1st degree family members with prostate cancer and BRCA 1and 2, the recommendation is to again help the patient weigh benefits and risks. The decision is whether to screen or not is left to the patient. Screening after age 70 is not recommended.

Sources

–http://www.ahrq.gov/clinic/uspstf/uspsprca.htm

–*Ann Intern Med.* 2012; 157:120-134

–*Ann Intern Med.* 2011;155:762-771

–UPDATE 2017

Population

–Asymptomatic men.

Recommendation

▶ ACP 2013

–**Statement of guidance**

- For men between age 50 and 69 y, discuss limited benefits and substantial harm of screening for prostate CA. Do not do PSA testing unless patient expresses a clear preference for screening.
- Do not screen PSA in average-risk men younger than 50 or older than 70 y or in men with a life expectancy of <10 y.

Sources

–*Ann Intern Med.* 2013;159:761-769

–*Ann Intern Med.* 2013;158:145-153

Comment
–Risks and Benefits of Prostate Screening
- There is good evidence that PSA can detect early-stage prostate CA (2-fold increase in organ-confined disease at presentation with PSA screening), but mixed and inconclusive evidence that early detection improves health outcomes or mortality.
- Two long-awaited studies add to the confusion. A U.S. study of 76,000 men showed increased prostate CA in screened group, but no reduction in risk of death from prostate CA. A European study of 80,000 men showed a decreased rate of death from prostate CA by 20% but significant overdiagnosis (there was no difference in overall death rate). To prevent 1 death from prostate CA, 1410 men needed to be screened and 48 cases of prostate CA found. Patients older than age 70 y had an increased death rate in the screened group. (*N Engl J Med.* 2009;360:1310,1320) (*N Engl J Med.* 2012;366:981) (*N Engl J Med.* 2012;366:1047)
- These 2 very large studies set the framework for new PC guidelines. The U.S. study (prostate, lung, colorectal and ovarian cancer screening trial) showed no evidence for overall survival benefit from PSA screening and postulated that many patients with low grade cancers were treated aggressively leading to morbidity and mortality. Subsequent evaluation found that approximately 90% of ptients in the control arm had undergone PSA testing during the course of the trial. This fact makes the trial result uninterpretable. The European study found that PSA screening did reduce prostate specific mortality by 20%. In this trial 781 men needed to be invited to screening to prevent one death. What should be the response to this new data? First we can improve survival by recognizing low risk patients to be followed by active surveillance and not exposed to treatment until evidence of disease progression. Recognized high risk patients (African Americans and men with 1st degree relatives with prostate cancer) should be screened early and frequently. Average risk men can be screened by PSA twice between the ages of 45 and 55 and if the PSA is 0.70 ng/mL their risk of lethal prostate cancer is quite low. Guideline groups are presently workin on new guidelines for PC screening to minimize over treatment of this disease but at the same time screening a higher risk population for aggressive prostate cancer at a stage that can be treated with conservative intent.
- *N Engl J Med.* 2017; 376:1285
- *J Clin Onc.* 2016; 34:3499-3501
- *J Clin Onc.* 2016; 34:3481-3491
- *J Clin Onc.* 2016; 34:2705-2711.

- *Benefit:* Insufficient evidence to establish whether a decrease in mortality from prostate CA occurs with screening by DRE or serum PSA. *Harm:* Based on solid evidence, screening with PSA and/or DRE detects some prostate CAs that would never have caused important clinical problems. Based on solid evidence, current prostate CA treatments result in permanent side effects in many men, including erectile dysfunction and urinary incontinence. (NCI, 2008)
- Men with localized, low-grade prostate CAs (Gleason score 2–4) have a minimal risk of dying from prostate CA during 20 y of follow-up (6 deaths per 1000 person-years) (*JAMA.* 2005;293:2095) (*N Engl J Med.* 2014;370:932)
- Many physicians continue to screen African American men and men with a strong FH of prostate cancer despite the new guidelines. (*J Urol.* 2002; 168:483) (*J Natl Cancer Inst.* 2000; 92:2009) (*JAMA.* 2014; 311:1143)
- Increase in prostate cancer distant metastases at diagnosis in the United States over the last 3 y. (*JAMA Oncol.* 2016; 2:1657).

Population

–Asymptomatic men.

Recommendation

▶ EAU 2010

–There is a lack of evidence to support or disregard widely adopted, population-based screening programs for early detection of prostate CA.

Source

–www.uroweb.org

Comments

–Radical prostatectomy (vs. watchful waiting) reduces disease-specific and overall mortality in patients with early stage prostate CA (*N Engl J Med.* 2011;364:1708). This benefit was seen only in men age >65 y. Active surveillance for low-risk patients (*J Clin Oncol.* 2010;28:126) (*Ann Intern Med.* 2012;156:582) is safe and increasingly used as an alternative to radical prostatectomy. A gene signature profile reflecting virulence and treatment responsiveness in prostate CA is now available. (*J Clin Oncol.* 2008; 26:3930) (*J Natl Compr NNetr.* 2016;14:659)

–PSA velocity (>0.5–0.75 ng/y rise) is predictive for the presence of prostate CA, especially with a PSA of 4–10. (*Eur Urol.* 2009;56:573)

–Multi-parametric MRI scanning is emerging as a tool for more accurate detection of early prostate cancer as well as distinguishing indolent from high-grade cancers. (*J Urol.* 2011;185:815) (*Nat Rev Clin Oncol.* 2014;11:346)

–African American men have double the risk of prostate cancer and a >2-fold risk of prostate cancer–specific death. These patients and those with first-degree relatives <65 y with prostate cancer are at high enough risk to justify PSA screening until a definitive study of this population is available. (*JAMA*. 2014;311:1143)

Population

–Asymptomatic men.

Recommendation

▶ NCCN 2016

–**NCCN GUIDELINES 2016**
- Informed decision making.
- Obtain PSA testing in healthy men age 45–75 y
- PSA <1 ng/mL—DRE normal—repeat testing @ 2–4 y intervals
- PSA 1–3 ng/mL—DRE normal—repeat testing @ 1–2 y intervals
- PSA >3 ng/mL or suspicious DRE—consider biopsy and work-up for benign disease.
- (*J Natl. Compr Canc Netw.* 2015;13:570) (*Mayo Clin Proc.* 2016;91:17)
- After age 70 PSA testing should be individualized and indications for biopsy carefully evaluated.
- Refer patients for prostate biopsy if serum PSA rises >0.9 ng/mL in 1 y.

Sources

–www.cancerscreening.nhs.uk
–NCCN Guidelines 2016

Comments

1. PSA screening is confounded by the morbidity and mortality associated with the treatment of prostate cancer. Molecular profiling that can stratify patients into high-risk and low-risk groups is a critical need for individualized adaptive therapies, which could minimize toxicity and maximize benefit from there in many patients (oncotype, Decipher and Polaris are now available to look at molecular profiling).
2. This NCCN recommendation aims to strike a balance between testing too seldom and testing too often to "maximize benefit and minimize harm."

CANCER, SKIN (MELANOMA)

Recommendations
▶ USPSTF 2016

–Evidence is insufficient to recommend for or against routine screening using a total-body skin examination for early detection of cutaneous melanoma, basal cell carcinoma, or squamous cell skin CA.[a,b] (*JAMA.* 2016;316:429)

–Recommends counseling children, adolescents, and young adults age 10–24 y who have fair skin to minimize exposure to ultraviolet radiation to reduce the risk of skin cancer.

Source
–http://www.ahrq.gov/clinic/uspstf/uspsskca.htm

Comment
–**Benefits and Harms**
  • Benefits: Evidence is inadequate to determine whether visual exam of the skin in asymptomatic individuals would lead to a reduction in mortality from melanoma skin CA. 76,400 U.S. men and women will develop melanoma in 2016 and 10,100 will die from the disease.
  • Harms: Based on fair though unqualified evidence, visual examination of the skin in asymptomatic persons may lead to unavoidable increases in harmful consequences. This includes misdiagnosis, overdiagnosis, and resulting cosmetic adverse effects from biopsy and overtreatment. (*NCI*, 2016)
  • 28 million people in the United States use UV indoor tanning salons, increasing risk of squamous, basal cell cancer, and malignant melanoma. (*J Clin Oncol.* 2012;30:1588)
  • The frequency of melanoma has been increasing for at least 30 y.
  • In the last 5 y the rates of melanoma have plateaued or declined in individuals <50 y/o.
  • Risk of melanoma increases with age. Median age at diagnosis is 63 y and median age at death is 69 y.

[a]Clinicians should remain alert for skin lesions with malignant features when examining patients for other reasons, particularly patients with established risk factors. Risk factors for skin CA include evidence of melanocytic precursors (atypical moles), large numbers of common moles (>50), immunosuppression, any history of radiation, family or personal history of skin CA, substantial cumulative lifetime sun exposure, intermittent intense sun exposure or severe sunburns in childhood, freckles, poor tanning ability, and light skin, hair, and eye color.
[b]Consider educating patients with established risk factors for skin CA (see above) concerning signs and symptoms suggesting skin CA and the possible benefits of periodic self-examination. Alert at-risk patients to significance of asymmetry, border irregularity, color variability, diameter >6 mm, and evolving change in previous stable mole. All suspicious lesions should be biopsied (excisional or punch, not a shave biopsy) (*Ann Intern Med.* 2009;150:188) (USPSTF; ACS; COG).

- Clinical features of increased risk of melanoma (family history, multiple nevi previous melanoma) are linked to sites of subsequent malignant melanoma, this may be helpful in surveillance. *JAMA Dermatol.* 2017; 153:23.
- There are no guidelines for patients with familial syndromes (familial atypical mole and melanoma [FAM-M]), although systematic surveillance is warranted.[c]

[c]Consider dermatologic risk assessment if family history of melanoma in ≥2 blood relatives, presence of multiple atypical moles, or presence of numerous actinic keratoses.

CANCER, TESTICULAR

Population

–Asymptomatic adolescent and adult males.[a]

Recommendations

▶ AAFP 2008, USPSTF 2011

–Recommend against routine screening. Be aware of risk factors for testicular CA—previous testis CA (2%–3% risk of second cancer), cryptorchid testis, family history of testis CA, HIV (increased risk of seminoma), and Klinefelter syndrome.
–There is a 3- to 5-fold increase in testis cancer in white men vs. other ethnicity. (*N Engl J Med.* 2014;371:2005) (*N Engl J Med.* 2007;356:1835)

Sources

–http://www.aafp.org/online/en/home/clinical/exam.html
–http://www.ahrq.gov/clinic/uspstf/uspstest.htm

Population

–Asymptomatic men.

Recommendation

▶ ACS 2004

–Testicular exam by physician as part of routine cancer-related checkup. (*Ann Int Med.* 2011;154:483) If there is any concern on exam, an ultrasound of the testis will be relaiable in discovery of malignancy as small as 1-2 mm in size but benign lesions are also found by ultrasound in this population. (*J Urol.* 2003; 170:1783)

Source

–http://www.cancer.org

[a]Patients with history of cryptorchidism, orchiopexy, family history of testicular CA, or testicular atrophy should be informed of their increased risk for developing testicular CA and counseled about screening. Such patients may then elect to be screened or to perform testicular self-examination. Adolescent and young adult males should be advised to seek prompt medical attention if they notice a scrotal abnormality. (USPSTF)

Population
–High-risk males.[a]

Recommendation

▶ EAU 2008
–Self-physical exam is advisable.

Source
–www.uroweb.org

Comment
–**Benefits and Harms**
  • Benefits: Based on fair evidence, screening would not result in appreciable decrease in mortality, in part because therapy at each stage is so effective.
  • Harms: Based on fair evidence, screening would result in unnecessary diagnostic procedures and occasional removal of a noncancerous testis. (NCI, 2011)
  • In 2016 approximatley 8850 men in the U.S. were diagnosed with testicular cancer but only 400 men died of ths disease. Worldwide there are approximately 72,000 cases and 9000 deaths annually. (*CA Caner J Clin.* 2017; 67:7)

CANCER, THYROID

Population
–Asymptomatic persons.

Recommendations

▶ USPSTF 2017
–Recommends against the use of ultrasound screening in asymptomatic persons.
–Be aware of higher-risk patients: radiation administered in infancy and childhood for benign conditions (thymus enlargement, acne), which results in an increased risk beginning 5 y after radiation and continuing until >20 y later; nuclear fallout exposure; history of goiter; family history of thyroid disease; female gender; Asian race. (*Int J Cancer.* 2001;93:745) (*N Engl J Med.* 2015; 373:2347) (*N Engl J Med.* 2012; 367:705)

Sources
–http://www.aafp.org/online/en/home/clinical/exam.html
–http://www.cancer.org

Comment

- **Clinical Facts**
  - Neck palpation for nodules in asymptomatic individuals has sensitivity of 15%–38% and specificity of 93%–100%. Only a small proportion of nodular thyroid glands are neoplastic, resulting in a high false-positive rate. (USPSTF 2016) *JAMA.* 2017; 317:1882.
  - Fine-needle aspiration (FNA) is the procedure of choice for evaluation of thyroid nodules. (*Otolaryngol Clin North Am.* 2010;43:229-238)

CAROTID ARTERY STENOSIS (CAS) (ASYMPTOMATIC)

Population

- Asymptomatic adults.

Recommendations

▶ **ASN 2007, USPSTF 2014, AHA/ASA 2011, ACCF/ACR/AIUM/ ASE/ASN/ICAVL/SCAI/SCCT/SIR/SVM/SVS 2011, AAFP 2013**

- Screening of the general population or a selected population based on age, gender, or any other variable alone is not recommended.
- Inappropriate to screen asymptomatic adult.

Sources

- *J Neuroimaging.* 2007;17:19-47
- USPSTF. Carotid Artery Stenosis: Screening. 2014.
- *J Am Coll Cardiol.* 2012;60(3):242-276
- Choosing Wisely: American Academy of Family Physicians. 2013.
- *Stroke.* 2011;42(2):e26

Recommendation

▶ **ACR–AIUM–SRU 2016, ACC/AHA/ASA/ACR/SVS 2011**

- Indications for carotid ultrasound: evaluation of patients with a cervical bruit.

Source

- *Stroke.* 2011;42(8):e464-e540
- ACR–AIUM–SPR–SRU Practice Parameter for the Performance of an Ultrasound Examination of the Extracranial Cerebrovascular System. 2016. http://www.acr.org/~/media/ACR/Documents/PGTS/guidelines/US_Extracranial_Cerebro.pdf

Recommendation

▶ **Society of Thoracic Surgeons 2013**

- Recommends against routine evaluation of carotid artery disease prior to cardiac surgery in the absence of symptoms or other high-risk criteria.

Source
   –Choosing Wisely: Society of Thoracic Surgeons. 2013.

Comments
   1. The prevalence of internal CAS of ≥70% varies from 0.5%–8% based on population-based cohort utilizing carotid duplex ultrasound. For population age >65 y estimated prevalence is 1%. No risk stratification tool further distinguishes the importance of CAS. No evidence suggests that screening for asymptomatic CAS reduces fatal or nonfatal strokes.
   2. Carotid duplex ultrasonography to detect CAS ≥60%; sensitivity, 94%; specificity, 92%. (*Ann Intern Med.* 2007;147(12):860)
   3. If true prevalence of CAS is 1%, number needed to screen to prevent 1 stroke over 5 y = 4368; to prevent 1 disabling stroke over 5 y = 8696. (*Ann Intern Med.* 2007;147(12):860)

CELIAC DISEASE

Population
   –Children and adults.

Recommendation
▶ USPSTF 2017, AAFP 2017
   –Insufficient evidence regarding screening of asymptomatic people.

Source
   –AAFP Clinical Recommendation: Screening for Celiac Disease. 2017.
   –*JAMA.* 2017;317(12):1252.

Recommendation
▶ NICE 2015
   –Serologic testing to rule out celiac disease should be performed for any of the following signs, symptoms, or associated conditions: persistent unexplained abdominal or gastrointestinal symptoms, faltering growth, prolonged fatigue, unexpected weight loss, severe or persistent mouth ulcers, unexplained iron, vitamin B12 or folate deficiency, type 1 diabetes, autoimmune thyroid disease, irritable bowel syndrome (in adults).
   –Screen first-degree relatives of people with coeliac disease.
   –General population screening not recommended.

Source
   –NICE. Coeliac disease: recognition, assessment and management. 2015.

Comments

1. Patients must continue a gluten-containing diet during diagnostic testing.
2. IgA tissue transglutaminase (TTG) is the test of choice (>90% sensitivity/specificity), along with total IgA level.
3. IgA endomysial antibody test is indicated if the TTG test is equivocal.
4. Avoid antigliadin antibody testing.
5. Consider serologic testing for any of the following: Addison disease; amenorrhea; autoimmune hepatitis; autoimmune myocarditis; chronic immune thrombocytopenic purpura (ITP); dental enamel defects; depression; bipolar disorder; Down syndrome; Turner syndrome; epilepsy; lymphoma; metabolic bone disease; chronic constipation; polyneuropathy; sarcoidosis; Sjögren syndrome; or unexplained alopecia.

CHLAMYDIA

Population
–Women age ≤25 y who are sexually active.

Recommendation
▶ CDC 2015, AAP 2014
–Screen for chlamydia annually.

Sources
–CDC. Sexually Transmitted Diseases Guidelines, 2015.
–*Pediatrics*. 2014;134(1):e302.

Population
–Women age <25 y who are sexually active

Recommendation
▶ USPSTF 2014
–Screen for chlamydia and gonorrhea. Screening interval to be determined by patient's sexual practices.

Sources
–USPSTF. Chlamydia and Gonorrhea: Screening.

Population
–Young heterosexual men; nonpregnant women >25y without risk factors.

Recommendation
▶ CDC 2015, USPSTF 2014
–Insufficient evidence for or against routine screening.
–Consider screening in high prevalence clinical settings.

Sources
- USPSTF. Chlamydia and Gonorrhea: Screening.
- CDC. Sexually Transmitted Diseases Guidelines, 2015.

Comments

1. *Chlamydia* is a reportable infection to the Public Health Department in every state.

Population

- Men who have sex with men.

Recommendation

▶ CDC 2015
- Annual testing, regardless of condom use.
- Frequency of q 3–6 mo for high risk activity.

Source
- CDC. 2015 Sexually Transmitted Diseases Treatment Guidelines.

Comments

1. Urine nucleic amplification acid test (NAAT) for *Chlamydia* for men who have had insertive intercourse.
2. NAAT of rectal swab for men who have had receptive anal intercourse.

Population

- Pregnant women.

Recommendations

▶ CDC 2015
- Recommends screening for chlamydial infection for all pregnant women <25y old and for older women at increased risk.
- Test at first contact, then re-test in 3rd trimester.

Source
- CDC. 2015 Sexually Transmitted Diseases Treatment Guidelines.

Recommendations

▶ AAP/ACOG 2012
- Screen all women for chlamydial infection at first prenatal visit.
- AAP & ACOG. Guidelines for Perinatal Care, 7th Ed. 2012.

CHOLESTEROL AND LIPID DISORDERS

Population
–Infants, children, adolescents, or young adults (age <20 y).

Recommendations
▶ USPSTF 2016, NLA 2011

–In familial hypercholesterolemia (FH), universal screening at age 9–11 y with a fasting lipid panel or nonfasting non-HDL-C. If non-HDL-C ≥145 m/dL, perform fasting lipid panel.
–Genetic screening for FH is generally not needed for diagnosis or clinical management.
–Cascade screening: testing lipid levels in all first-degree relatives of diagnosed FH patients.
–Insufficient evidence to recommend for or against routine universal lab screening.

Source
–*J Clin Lipidol.* 2011;5:S1-S8
–*JAMA.* 2016;316:625-633.

Recommendation
▶ AHA 2007

–Selective screening: patients age >2 y with a parent age <55 y with coronary artery disease, peripheral artery disease, cerebrovascular disease, or hyperlipidemia should be screened with fasting panel.

Source
–*Circulation.* 2007;115:1947-1967

Comments
1. Childhood drug treatment of dyslipidemia lowers lipid levels but effect on childhood or adult outcomes is uncertain.
2. Lifestyle approach is recommended starting after age 2 y.

Recommendations
▶ National Heart, Lung and Blood Institute Integrated Guidelines 2012

–Selective screening age >2 y: positive family history (FH) of dyslipidemia, presence of dyslipidemia, or the presence of overweight, obesity, hypertension, diabetes, or a smoking history.
–Universal screening in adolescents regardless of FH between age 9 and 11 y and again between age 18 and 21 y.

Source

—NHLBI, Expert Panel on Integrated Guidelines for Cardiovascular Health and Risk Reduction in Children and Adolescents. 2012.

Comments

—Fasting lipid profile is recommended. If within normal limits repeat testing in 3–5 y is recommended.

—Fasting lipid profile or nonfasting non–high-density lipoprotein (HDL) cholesterol level.

Population

—Asymptomatic adults 40–79 y.

Recommendations

▶ ACC/AHA 2013

—Perform 10-y ASCVD Risk Score.

—High-risk categories include:

1. Primary elevation of LDL-C ≥ 190 mg/dL.
2. Diabetes (type 1 or 2) with LDL-C 70–189 mg/dL and without clinical ASCVD.
3. Without clinical ASCVD or diabetes with LDL-C 70–189 mg/dL and estimated 10-y ASCVD risk score ≥7.5%.

Sources

—*Circulation. 2013;2013;01.cir.0000437738.63853.7a*

Comment

—Prior to initiating statin therapy perform lipid panel, ALT, HgbA1c to R/O DM, and baseline CK (if patient is at increased risk for muscle events based on personal or family history of statin intolerance).

Population

—Adults with diabetes.

Recommendations

▶ ADA 2013

—Measure fasting lipids at least annually in adults with diabetes.

—Every 2 y for adults with low-risk lipid values (LDL-C <100 mg/dL, HDL-C >50 mg/dL, TG <150 mg/dL).

Source

—*Diabetes Care. 2013;36(suppl 1):S11–S66*

Population

–Adults >40 y old.

Recommendations

▶ ESC 2016

–Perform SCORE risk assessment tool available at: www.heartscore.org
–Secondary hyperlipidemia should be ruled out.
–Total Cholesterol and LDL-C primary target: goal LDL ≤70 mg/dL in patients with very high CV risk, LDL ≤100 mg/dL in patients with high CV risk.
–Secondary targets are non-HDL-C and ApoB.
–HDL is not recommended as a target for treatment.

Source

–European Society of Cardiology. Dyslipidaemias 2016.

Comment

–No overt CVD: LDL-C goal <100 mg/dL (2.6 mmol/L).

Population

–Adults >20 y.

Recommendations

▶ NLA 2014

–Fasting lipid profile (LDL-C and TG) or nonfasting lipid panel (non-HDL-C and HDL-C) should be measured at least every 5 y.
–Also assess ASCVD risk.
–Non-HDL-C (primary target), ApoB (secondary target) have more predictive power than LDL-C.
–Apolipoprotein B (ApoB) is considered an optional, secondary target for therapy. More predictive power than LDL-C, but not consistently superior to non-HDL-C.
–HDL-C is not recommended as a target therapy.

Sources

–*J Clin Lipidol.* 2014;8:473-488.

Comment

–Non-HDL-C values:
–Desirable <130 mg/dL.
–Above desirable 130–159.
–Borderline high 160–189.
–High 190–219.
–Very high ≥ 220.

Recommendation

▶ NCEP III 2004

–Check fasting lipoprotein panel (if testing opportunity is nonfasting, use nonfasting total cholesterol [TC] and HDL) every 5 y if in desirable range; otherwise, see management algorithm.

Sources
–*Circulation*. 2002;106:3143-3421
–*Circulation*. 2004;110:227-239

Population

–Men ≥ 40 y.
–Women ≥ 50 y or postmenopausal.
–All patients with any of the following conditions, regardless of age: smoking actively, diabetes, HTN, family history CVD or HLD, erectile dysfunction, CKD, inflammatory disease, HIV, COPD, clinical evidence of atherosclerosis or AAA, clinical manifestation of HLD, obesity with BMI > 27.

Recommendations

▶ Canadian Cardiovascular Society CCS 2012

–For all, screening should be performed with history and examination, LDL, HDL, TG, and non-HDL.
–Optional: ApoB (instead of standard lipid panel), urine albumin:creatinine ratio (if eGFR >60, HTN, diabetes).
–If Framingham Risk Score <5%, repeat every 4–5 y.
–If Framingham Risk Score ≥5%, repeat every year.

Source
–*Can J Cardiol*. 2013:29:151-167

CHOLESTEROL GUIDELINES

Source	Recommended Lipoprotein Measurements for Risk Assessment	Recommended Lipoprotein Targets of Therapy	Recommended Risk Assessment Algorithm
National Cholesterol Education Program Adult Treatment Panel III[7,8]	Fasting lipid panel Calculation of non-HDL-C when TG >200 mg/dL	Primary target: LDL-C Secondary target: non-HDL-C	Identify number of CHD risk factors Framingham 10-y absolute CHD risk
International Atherosclerosis Society[16]	Fasting lipid panel with calculation of non-HDL-C	Non-HDL-C LDL-C is considered alternative target of therapy	Lifetimes risk of total ASCVD morbidity/ mortality (by Framingham, CV Lifetime Risk pooling project, or QRisk)
European Society of Cardiology/European Atherosclerosis Society[22]	Fasting lipid panel with calculation of non-HDL-C and TC/HDL-C ratio ApoB or ApoB/ apoA1 ration are considered alternative risk markers	Primary target: LDC-C Secondary targets: non-HDL or ApoB in patients with cardiometabolic risk	10-y risk of total fatal ASCVD by the Systematic Coronary Risk Evaluation (SCORE) system
Canadian Cardiovascular Society[27]	European Society of Cardiology/ European Atherosclerosis Society	Primary target: LDL-C Secondary targets: non-HDL-C and ApoB	10-y risk of total ASCVD events by the Framingham Risk Score
American Association of Clinical Endocrinologists[31]	Fasting lipid panel Calculation of non-HDL-C more accurate risk assessment if TG in between 200 and 500 mg/dL, diabetes, insulin resistance, or established CAD	Primary targets: LDL-C Secondary targets: non-HDL-C in patients with cardiometabolic risk or established CAD ApoB recommended to assess success of LDL-C-lowering therapy	Men: Framingham Risk Score (10-y risk of coronary event) Women: Reynolds Risk Score (10-y risk of coronary event, stroke, or other major heart disease)

CHOLESTEROL GUIDELINES *(Continued)*

Source	Recommended Lipoprotein Measurements for Risk Assessment	Recommended Lipoprotein Targets of Therapy	Recommended Risk Assessment Algorithm
American Diabetes Association/ American Heart Association Statement on Cardiometabolic Risk[38]	Stronger risk discrimination provided by non-HDL-C, ApoB, LDL-P	Strong recommendation for ApoB and non-HDL-C as secondary targets	30-y/lifetime global ASCVD risk
American Diabetes Association: Standards of Medical Care in Diabetes[39]	Fasting lipid panel	LDL-C	Not applicable in setting of diabetes (CHD risk equivalent)
Kidney Disease: Improving Global Outcomes: Clinical Practice Guideline for Lipid Management in Chronic Kidney Disease[41]	Fasting lipid panel to screen for more severe forms of dyslipidemia and secondary causes of dyslipidemia	None: therapy guided by absolute risk of coronary event based on age, and stage of CKD or eGFR	CKD considered CHD risk equivalent Treatment with evidence-based statins/statin doses based on age, and stage of CKD or eGFR
Secondary Prevention of Atherosclerotic Cardiovascular Disease in Older Adults: A Scientific Statement from the American Heart Association[36]	Fasting lipid panel Calculation of non-HDL-C when TG >200 mg/dL	Primary target: LDL-C Secondary target: non-HDL-C	N/A
National Lipid Association: Familial Hypercholesterolemia[40]	Fasting lipid panel	LDL-C	Not applicable due to extremely high lifetime risk
Expert Panel on Integrated Guidelines for Cardiovascular Health and Risk Reduction in Children and Adolescents[34,35]	Fasting lipid panel with calculation of non-HDL-C	Primary target: LDL-C Secondary target: non-HDL-C	No risk algorithm, treatment based on number of ASCVD risk factors

AHA Women's Cardiovascular Disease Prevention Guidelines[17]	Fasting lipid panel Consider hs-CRP in women >60 y and CHD risk >10%	LDL-C	Updated Framingham risk profile (coronary, cerebrovascular, and peripheral arterial disease and heart failure events) Reynolds Risk Score (10-y risk of coronary event, stroke, or other major heart disease)
2013 American College of Cardiology/American Heart Association: Blood Cholesterol Guidelines for ASCVD Prevention[50]	Fasting lipid panel to screen for more severe forms of dyslipidemia and secondary causes of dyslipidemia	LDL-C measured for assessment of therapeutic response and compliance Therapy guided by identification of 40 categories of patients who benefit from high- or moderate-dose statin therapy	CV Risk Calculator based on Pooled Risk Equations (10-y risk of total ASCVD events) Lifetime risk provided for individuals 20–59 y of age

apoA1, apolipoprotein A1; ApoB, apolipoprotein B; ASCVD, atherosclerotic cardiovascular disease; CAD, coronary artery disease; CHD, coronary heart disease; CKD, chronic kidney disease; CV, cardiovascular; eGFR, estimated glomerular filtration rate; HDL-C, high-density lipoprotein cholesterol; hs-CRP, high-sensitivity C-reactive protein; LDL-C, low-density lipoprotein-cholesterol; LDL-P, low-density lipoprotein particle; TC, total cholesterol; TG, triglycerides.

Source: Pamela B, Morris, Christie M, et al. Review of clinical practice guidelines for the management of LDL-related risk. *JACC.* 2014;64(2):196-206.

CHRONIC OBSTRUCTIVE PULMONARY DISEASE

Population
–Adults, asymptomatic.

Recommendation

▶ USPSTF 2016
–Do not screen asymptomatic adults for COPD

Sources
–*JAMA*. 2016;315(13):1372-7.

Comment
–Detection while asymptomatic doesn't alter disease course or improve outcomes.

–Several symptom-based questionnaires have high sensitivity for COPD.

–In symptomatic patients (ie, dyspnea, chronic cough or sputum production with a history of exposure to cigarette smoke or other toxic fumes), diagostic spirometry to measure FEV1/FVC ratio is indicated.

CORONARY ARTERY DISEASE

Population
–Adults at low risk of CHD events[a]

Recommendation

▶ AAFP 2012, USPSTF 2012, American College of Physicians 2012, American Society of Echocardiography 2013, American College of Cardiology 2013
–Do not routinely screening in men and women at low risk for CHD risk.[b] with resting electrocardiogram (ECG), exercise treadmill test (ETT), stress echocardiogram, or electron-beam CT for coronary calcium.

–Do not screen with stress cardiac imaging or advanced non-invasive imaging in the initial evaluation of patients without cardiac symptoms, unless high-risk markers are present

–Do not perform annual stress cardiac imaging or advanced non-invasive imaging as part of routine follow-up in asymptomatic patients.

[a]Increased risk for CHD events: older age, male gender, high BP, smoking, elevated lipid levels, diabetes, obesity, sedentary lifestyle. Risk assessment tool for estimating 10-y risk of developing CHD events available online, http://cvdrisk.nhlbi.nih.gov/calculator.asp or see Appendices VI and VII.
[b]AHA scientific statement (2006): Asymptomatic persons should be assessed for CHD risk. Individuals found to be at low risk (<10% 10-y risk) or at high risk (>20% 10-y risk) do not benefit from coronary calcium assessment. High-risk individuals are already candidates for intensive risk-reducing therapies. In clinically selected, intermediate-risk patients, it may be reasonable to use electron-beam CT or multidetector computed tomography (MDCT) to refine clinical risk prediction and select patients for more aggressive target values for lipid-lowering therapies (*Circulation*. 2006;114:1761-1791).

Sources
–AAFP Clinical Recommendation: Coronary Heart Disease. 2012.
–Choosing Wisely: American College of Physicians, 2012. http://www.choosingwisely.org/societies/american-college-of-physicians/
–Choosing Wisely: American Academy of Family Physicians. 2013. http://www.choosingwisely.org/societies/american-academy-of-family-physicians/
–Choosing Wisely. American Society of Echocardiography. 2012. http://www.choosingwisely.org/societies/american-society-of-echocardiography/
–Choosing Wisely: American College of Cardiology. 2014. http:/www.choosingwisely.org/societies/american-college-of-cardiology/
–*Ann Intern Med.* 2012;157:512-518

Comment
–USPSTF recommends against screening asymptomatic individuals because of the high false-positive results, the low mortality with asymptomatic disease, and the iatrogenic diagnostic and treatment risks.

Populations
–All asymptomatic adults age ≥20 y.
–Risk Score Assessment

Recommendations
▶ ACC/AHA 2013, ESC 2012
–ASCVD Risk Score has replaced the FRS in the United States for patients age 40–79 y.
–Assess 10-y ASCVD risk score every 4–6 y.
–Framingham Risk Score (FRS), including blood pressure (BP) and cholesterol level, should be obtained in asymptomatic adults age ≥20 y.
–The SCORE Risk Score remains the screening choice in Europe.
–No benefit in genetic testing, advanced lipid testing, natriuretic peptide testing, high-sensitivity C-reactive protein (CRP), ankle-brachial index, carotid intima-medial thickness, coronary artery score on electron-beam CT, homocysteine level, lipoprotein (a) level, CT angiogram, MRI, or stress echocardiography regardless of CHD risk.

Sources
–*Circulation.* 2007;115:402-426
–*J Am Coll Cardiol.* 2010;56(25): 2182-2199

Population

–Adults at intermediate risk of CHD events.

Recommendations

▶ ACC/AHA 2013, ESC 2012

–May be reasonable to consider use of coronary artery calcium and high-sensitivity CRP (hsCRP) measurements in patients at intermediate risk.

–hs-CRP is not recommended in low- or high-risk individuals.

Sources

–*Eur Heart J.* 2007;28(19): 2375-2414
–*Eur Heart J.* 2012;33:1635-1701
–*J Am Coll Cardiol.* 2007;49:378-402
–*Circulation.* 2013; 2014;129(25 Suppl 2):S49-73

Comment

–10-y ASCVD risk calculator (The Pooled Cohort Equation) can be found at: http://tools.acc.org/ASCVD-Risk-Estimator/

Population

–Adults at high risk of CHD events.

Recommendations

▶ AAFP 2012, AHA 2007, USPSTF 2012

–Insufficient evidence to recommend for or against routine screening with ECG, ETT.

–In addition, there is insufficient evidence to recommend routine MRI.

Sources

–*Arch Intern Med.* 2011;171(11): 977-982
–*AAFP Clinical Recommendations: Coronary Heart Disease.* 2012.
–*Ann Intern Med.* 2012;157:512-518

Population

–Men and Women with no History of CHD.

Recommendation

▶ USPSTF 2009

–Insufficient evidence to assess the balance of benefits and harms of using the nontraditional risk factors to prevent CHD events (hs-CRP, ankle-brachial index [ABI], leukocyte count, fasting blood glucose level, periodontal disease, carotid intima-media thickness, coronary artery calcification [CAC] score on electron-beam computed tomography, homocysteine level, and lipoprotein[a] level).

Source
  –USPSTF. Coronary Heart Disease: Screening Using Non-Traditional
  Risk Factors. 2009.

Comment
  –10-y ASCVD risk calculator (The Pooled Cohort Equation) can be
  found at: http://tools.acc.org/ASCVD-Risk-Estimator/

Population
  –Women.

Recommendations

▶ **ACCF/AHA 2011**

  –Cardiac risk stratification by the Framingham Risk Score should be
  used. High risk in women should be considered when the risk is ≥10%
  rather than ≥20%.
  –An alternative 10-y risk score to consider is the Reynolds Risk Score,
  although it requires measurement of hs-CRP.

Source
  –*J Am Coll Cardiol.* 2011;57(12):1404-1423

Population
  –Adults with stable CAD.

Recommendations

▶ **CCS 2013**

  –Risk assessment by Framingham Risk Score should be completed
  every 3–5 y for men age 40–75 y and women age 50–75 y. Frequency
  of measurement should increase if history of premature cardiovascular
  disease (CVD) is present. Calculate and discuss a patient's
  "cardiovascular age" to improve the likelihood that the patient will
  reach lipid targets and that poorly controlled hypertension will be
  treated.

Source
  –*Can J Cardiol.* 2013;29:151-167

Recommendation

▶ **AAFP 2009, AHA/APA 2008**

  –All patients with acute myocardial infarction (MI) to be screened for
  depression at regular intervals during and post hospitalization.

Source
  –*Circulation.* 2008;118:1768-1775
  –*Ann Fam Med.* 2009;7(1):71-79

DEMENTIA

Population
 –Adults.

Recommendation

▶ ICSI 2014
 –Insufficient evidence to recommend for or against routine dementia screening.

Source
 –ISCI. Preventive Services for Adults, 20th Ed. 2014.

Population
 –Adults over 65 y.

Recommendation

▶ CTFPHC 2016
 –Do not screen asymptomatic adults for cognitive impairment.

Source
 –*CMAJ.* 2016 Jan 5;188(1):37-46

Recommendation

▶ USPSTF 2014
 –Insufficient evidence to recommend for or against routine dementia screening.

Source
 –*Ann Intern Med.* 2014 Jun 3;160(11):791-7

Comments
 –False positive rate for screening is high, and treatment interventions do not show consistent benefits.

DEPRESSION

Population
 –Children age 7–11 y.

Recommendation

▶ USPSTF 2016
 –Insufficient evidence to recommend for or against routine screening.

Source
 –*Ann Intern Med.* 2016;164(5):360-6

Population

–Adolescents.

Recommendation

▶ USPSTF 2016

–Screen all adolescents age 12–18 y for major depressive disorder (MDD). Systems should be in place to ensure accurate diagnosis, appropriate psychotherapy, and adequate follow-up.

Source

–*Ann Intern Med.* 2016;164(5):360-6

Comments

1. Screen in primary care clinics with the Patient Health Questionnaire for Adolescents (PHQ-A) (73% sensitivity; 94% specificity) or the Beck Depression Inventory-Primary Care (BDI-PC) (91% sensitivity; 91% specificity). See Appendix I.
2. Treatment options include pharmacotherapy (fluoxetine and escitalopram have FDA approval for this age group), psychotherapy, collaborative care, psychosocial support interventions, and CAM approaches.
3. SSRI may increase suicidality in some adolescents, emphasizing the need for close follow-up.

Population

–Adults.

Recommendation

▶ USPSTF 2016, ICSI 2016

–Recommend screening adults for depression, including pregnant and postpartum women. Have staff-assisted support systems in place for accurate diagnosis, effective treatment, and follow-up.

Sources

–*JAMA.* 2016;315(4):380-7
–ISCI. Depression, Adult in Primary Care, 17th Ed. 2016.

Comments

1. PHQ-2 is as sensitive (96%) as longer screening tools:
   a. "Over the past 2 wk, have you felt down, depressed, or hopeless?"
   b. "Over the past 2 wk, have you felt little interest or pleasure in doing things?"
2. Optimal screening interval is unknown.

DEVELOPMENTAL DYSPLASIA OF THE HIP (DDH)

Population
–Infants.

Recommendation
▶ ICSI 2013, AAFP 2010, USPSTF 2006.
  –Evidence is insufficient to recommend routine screening for DDH in infants as a means to prevent adverse outcomes.

Comment
  –There is evidence that screening leads to earlier identification; however, 60%–80% of the hips of newborns identified as abnormal or suspicious for DDH by physical examination, and >90% of those identified by ultrasound in the newborn period, resolve spontaneously, requiring no intervention.
  –The USPSTF was unable to assess the balance of benefits and harms of screening for DDH, but was concerned about the potential harms associated with treatment, both surgical and nonsurgical, of infants identified by routine screening.

Sources
  –ICSI. Preventive Services for Children and Adolescents, 19th Ed. 2013.
  –USPSTF. Developmental Hip Dysplasia: Screening. 2006.

Population
–Infants up to 6 mo.

Recommendations
▶ AAOS 2014
  1. Recommend against universal ultrasound screening of newborns.
  2. Ultrasound recommended for infants before 6 mo for a history of breech presentation, family history, or history of clinical hip instability.
  3. Limited evidence supports brace treatment for hips in infants with a positive instability examination.

Source
  –American Academy of Orthopaedic Surgeons (AAOS). American Academy of Orthopaedic Surgeons clinical practice guideline on detection and nonoperative management of pediatric developmental dysplasia of the hip in infants up to 6 mo of age. Rosemont (IL): American Academy of Orthopaedic Surgeons (AAOS); 2014.

DIABETES MELLITUS, GESTATIONAL (GDM)

Population
–Pregnant women after 24 wk of gestation.

Recommendation
▶ USPSTF 2014
–Recommends screening for gestational diabetes mellitus in asymptomatic pregnant women.

Source
–USPSTF. Gestational Diabetes Mellitus, Screening. 2014.

Recommendations
▶ ACOG 2013
–1-h glucose screening test with 50-g anhydrous glucose load should be performed between 24 and 28 gestational weeks with a cutoff value of either 135 or 140 mg/dL.
–A 3-h glucose tolerance test should be performed if the 1-h glucose screening test is abnormal.
  • May use either the Carpenter and Coustan criteria or the National Diabetes Data Group criteria.
–Screen women with GDM 6–12 wk postpartum for overt diabetes.

Source
–ACOG. Gestational diabetes mellitus. Washington (DC): American College of Obstetricians and Gynecologists (ACOG); 2013 Aug. 11 p. (ACOG practice bulletin; no. 137)

Comment
–Insufficient evidence to support screening for gestational diabetes prior to 24 gestational weeks.

DIABETES MELLITUS (DM), TYPE 2

Population
–Pregnant women.

Recommendations
▶ ADA 2012
1. Screen for undiagnosed DM type 2 at first prenatal visit if age ≥45 y or if risk factors for DM are present.[a]
2. For all other women, screen at 24–28 wk with a 75-g 2-h oral glucose tolerance test (OGTT) in the morning after an overnight fast of at least 8 h.

Source
    –*Diabetes Care* 2012 Jan; 35(Suppl 1): S11-S63.

Population
    –Children at start of puberty or age ≥10 y.

Recommendation

▶ ADA 2012
    –Screen all children at risk for DM type 2.[a]

Source
    –*Diabetes Care* 2012 Jan; 35(Suppl 1): S11-S63.

Comments
    1. Preexisting diabetes if:
        a. Fasting glucose ≥126 mg/dL.
        b. 2-h glucose ≥200 mg/dL after 75-g glucose load.
        c. Random glucose ≥200 mg/dL with classic hyperglycemic symptoms.
        d. Hemoglobin A1c ≥6.5%.
    2. Criteria for GDM by 75-g 2-h OGTT if any of the following are abnormal:
        a. Fasting ≥92 mg/dL (5.1 mmol/L).
        b. 1 h ≥180 mg/dL (10.0 mmol/L).
        c. 2 h ≥153 mg/dL (8.5 mmol/L).

Population
    –Adults.

Recommendation

▶ ADA 2011
    –Screen asymptomatic adults age ≥45 y or if risk factors for DM are present.[b]

Source
    –*Diabetes Care.* 2012; 35(Suppl 1): S11-S63.

---

[a]Test asymptomatic children if BMI >85% for age/gender, weight for height >85th percentile, or weight >120% of ideal for height plus any two of the following: FH of DM in first- or second-degree relative; high-risk ethnic group (eg, Native American, African American, Latino, Asian American, or Pacific Islander); Acanthosis nigricans; HTN; dyslipidemia, polycystic ovary syndrome; small-for-gestational-age birth weight; maternal history of DM or GDM during the child's gestation.
[b]DM risk factors: overweight (BMI ≥25 kg/m2) and an additional risk factor: physical inactivity; first-degree relative with DM; high-risk ethnicity (eg, African American, Latino, Native American, Asian American, Pacific Islander); history of GDM; prior baby with birth weight >9 lb; hypertension (HTN) on therapy or with BP ≥140/90 mm Hg; HDL-C level <35 mg/dL (0.90 mmol/L) and/or a triglyceride level >250 mg/dL (2.82 mmol/L); polycystic ovary syndrome; history of impaired glucose tolerance or HgbA1c ≥5.7%; Acanthosis nigricans; or cardiovascular disease.

Population
–Adults

Recommendation

▶ USPSTF 2015

–Screen as part of cardiovascular risk assessment if age 40–70 y and BMI >25.

Sources
–USPSTF. Abnormal Blood Glucose and Type 2 Diabetes Mellitus: Screening. 2015.

Comment
–Screen at least every 3 y in asymptomatic adults.

FALLS IN THE ELDERLY

Population
–All older persons.

Recommendation

▶ NICE 2013, AAOS 2001, AGS 2010, British Geriatrics Society 2001

–Ask at least yearly about falls.

Sources
–NICE. Falls: assessment and prevention of falls in older people. London (UK): National Institute for Health and Care Excellence (NICE); 2013 Jun. 33 p. (Clinical guideline; no. 161).

–2010 AGS/BGS Clinical Practice Guideline: Prevention of Falls in Older Persons: www.americangeriatrics.org/files/documents/health_care_pros/Falls.Summary.Guide.pdf

Population
–All persons admitted to long-term care facilities.

Recommendation

▶ CTF 2005

–Recommend programs that target the broad range of environmental and resident-specific risk factors to prevent falls and hip fractures.[a]

Source
–http://canadiantaskforce.ca/guidelines/all-guidelines/2005-prevention-of-falls-in-long-term-care-facilities/

[a]Postfall assessments may detect previously unrecognized health concerns

Comments

1. Individuals are at increased risk if they report at least 2 falls in the previous year, or 1 fall with injury. Risk factors: Intrinsic: lower-extremity weakness, poor grip strength, balance disorders, functional and cognitive impairment, visual deficits. Extrinsic: polypharmacy (≥4 prescription medications), environment (poor lighting, loose carpets, lack of bathroom safety equipment).
2. Calcium and vitamin D supplementation reduces falls by 45% over 3 y in women, but no effect is seen in men. (*Arch Intern Med.* 2006;166:424)
3. A fall prevention clinic appears to reduce the number of falls among the elderly. (*Am J Phys Med Rehabil.* 2006;85:882)
4. All who report a single fall should be observed as they stand up from a chair without using their arms, walk several paces, and return (see Appendix II). Those demonstrating no difficulty or unsteadiness need no further assessment. Those who have difficulty or demonstrate unsteadiness, have ≥1 fall, or present for medical attention after a fall should have a fall evaluation.
5. Free "Tip Sheet" for patients from AGS (http://www.healthinaging.org/public_education/falls_tips.php)
6. Of US adults age ≥65 y, 15.9% fell in the preceding 3 mo; of these, 31.3% sustained an injury that resulted in a doctor visit or restricted activity for at least 1 d. (*MMWR Morb Mortal Wkly Rep.* 2008;57(9):225)
7. See also page 126 for Fall Prevention and Appendix II.

FAMILY VIOLENCE AND ABUSE

Population
–Children, women, and older adults.

Recommendation
▶ USPSTF 2013
   –Women of childbearing age should be screened for intimate partner violence.
   –Insufficient evidence to recommend for or against routine screening of parents or guardians for the physical abuse or neglect of children, or of older adults or their caregivers for elder abuse.

Sources
–USPSTF. Intimate Partner Violence and Abuse of Elderly and Vulnerable Adults: Screening. 2013.
–USPSTF. Child Maltreatment: Primary Care Interventions. 2013.

Comments

1. Screening for intimate partner violence in emergency departments and pediatric clinics shows high prevalence (10%–20%) and does not increase harm. (*Ann Emerg Med.* 2008;51:433) (*Pediatrics.* 2008;121:e85)
2. In screening for intimate partner violence, women often prefer self-completed approaches (written or computer-based) over face-to-face questioning. (*JAMA.* 2006;296:530)
3. All providers should be aware of physical and behavioral signs and symptoms associated with abuse and neglect, including burns, bruises, and repeated suspect trauma.
4. CDC publishes a toolkit of assessment instruments: https://www.cdc.gov/violenceprevention/pdf/ipv/ipvandsvscreening.pdf

FETAL ANEUPLOIDY

Population

–Pregnant women.

Recommendations

▶ ACOG 2016

1. All women should be offered screening. The decision should be reached through informed patient choice, including discussion of sensitivity, positive screening and false-positive rates and risks/benefits of diagnostic testing (amniocentesis and chorionic villous sampling).
2. No one screening test is superior.

Comments

–Risk of chromosomal anomaly by maternal age at term:
- 20 y old: 1 in 525.
- 30 y old: 1 in 384.
- 35 y old: 1 in 178.
- 40 y old: 1 in 62.
- 45 y old: 1 in 18

Source
–*Obstet Gynecol.* 2016:127(5);e123-e137

GLAUCOMA

Population
–Adults.

Recommendations

▶ USPSTF 2013
–Insufficient evidence to recommend for or against screening adults for glaucoma.

Sources
–USPSTF. Glaucoma: Screening. 2013.

GONORRHEA

Population
–Women age ≤25 y who are sexually active, and older women at high risk.[a]

Recommendation

▶ CDC 2015, AAP 2014
–Screen for gonorrhea annually.

Source
Pediatrics. 2014;134(1):e302.
CDC. 2015 Sexually Transmitted Diseases Treatment Guidelines.

Population
–Women age <25 y who are sexually active.

Recommendation

▶ USPSTF 2014
–Screen for chlamydia and gonorrhea. Screening interval to be determined by patient's sexual practices.

Source
–USPSTF. Chlamydia and Gonorrhea: Screening. 2014.

---

[a]Women age <25 y are at highest risk for gonorrhea infection. Other risk factors that place women at increased risk include a previous gonorrhea infection, the presence of other sexually transmitted diseases (STDs), new or multiple sex partners, inconsistent condom use, commercial sex work, and drug use.

Population
–Young heterosexual men

Recommendation
▶ CDC 2015, USPSTF 2014
–Insufficient evidence for or against routine screening.
–Consider screening in high prevalence clinical settings.

Sources
–USPSTF. Chlamydia and Gonorrhea: Screening. 2014.
–CDC. 2015 Sexually Transmitted Diseases Treatment Guidelines.

Population
–Men who have sex with men.

Recommendation
▶ CDC 2015
–Annual testing, regardless of condom use.
–Frequency of q 3–6 mo for high risk activity.

Source
–CDC. 2015 Sexually Transmitted Diseases Treatment Guidelines.

Comment
–Gonorrhea is a reportable illness to state Public Health Departments.

GROUP B STREPTOCOCCAL (GBS) DISEASE

Population
–Pregnant women.

Recommendation
▶ CDC 2010, AAFP 2015
–Universal screening of all women at 35–37 gestational weeks for GBS colonization with a vaginal–rectal swab.

Source
–AAFP Clinical Recommendation: Group B Strep. 2015.
–Prevention of Perinatal Group B Streptococcal Disease: Revised Guidelines from CDC, 2010.

Comment
–Women who are colonized with GBS should receive intrapartum antibiotic prophylaxis to prevent neonatal GBS sepsis.

GROWTH ABNORMALITIES, INFANT

Population
–Children 0–59 mo.

Recommendation

▶ CDC 2010

–Use the 2006 World Health Organization (WHO) international growth charts for children age <24 mo.

Source

–Use of World Health Organization and CDC Growth Charts for Children Aged 0-59 Months in the United States. 2010.

Comments
1. The Centers for Disease Control and Prevention (CDC) and American Academy of Pediatricians (AAP) recommend the WHO as opposed to the CDC growth charts for children age <24 mo.
2. The CDC growth charts should still be used for children age 2–19 y.
3. This recommendation recognizes that breast-feeding is the recommended standard of infant feeding, and therefore the standard against which all other infants are compared.

HEARING IMPAIRMENT

Population
–Newborns.

Recommendation

▶ USPSTF 2008, ISCI 2013

–Routine screening of all newborn infants for hearing loss.

Sources

–ISCI. Preventive Services for Children and Adolescents, 19th Ed. 2013.
–USPSTF. Hearing Loss in Newborns: Screening. 2008.

Comments
1. Screening involves either a 1-step or a 2-step process.
2. The 2-step process includes otoacoustic emissions (OAEs) followed by auditory brainstem response (ABR) in those who fail the OAE test.
3. The 1-step process uses either OAE or ABR testing.

Population
–Adults age >50 y.

Recommendation
▶ ICSI 2014, USPSTF 2012

–Insufficient evidence regarding screening the general population.

–Question older adults periodically about hearing impairment, counsel about availability of hearing aid devices, and make referrals for abnormalities when appropriate. See also Appendix II: Functional Assessment Screening in the Elderly.

Sources
–ISCI. Preventive Services for Adults. 2014.
–USPSTF. Hearing Loss in Older Adults: Screening. 2012.

Comments
1. Adults of age >50 y 20%–40%, and >80% of adults age ≥80 y, have some degree of hearing loss.
2. Additional research is required to determine if hearing loss screening can lead to improved health outcomes.
3. No harm from hearing loss screening.
4. No harm related to hearing aid use.

HEMOCHROMATOSIS (HEREDITARY)

Population
–Adults.

Recommendation
▶ AASLD 2011

–**Guidelines**
• Screen people with iron studies and a serum *HFE* mutation analysis if they have first-degree relatives with *HFE*-related hemochromatosis. (*Blood.* 2008;111:3373)

Sources
–http://www.aasld.org/practiceguidelines/Practice%20Guideline%20
Archive/Diagnosis%20and%20Management%20of%20
Hemochromatosis.pdf
–http://www.aafp.org/online/en/home/clinical/exam.html
–http://www.ahrq.gov/clinic/uspstf/uspshemoch.htm

Population

–Asymptomatic adults.

Recommendation

▶ AAFP 2008, USPSTF 2006

–Recommend against routine genetic screening for hemochromatosis in asymptomatic adults. Patients with a family history should be counseled with further testing based on clinical considerations. (*Arch Intern Med.* 2006;166:269) (*Blood.* 2008;111:3373)

Sources

–http://www.aasld.org/practiceguidelines/Practice%20Guideline%20 Archive/Diagnosis%20and%20Management%20of%20 Hemochromatosis.pdf
–http://www.aafp.org/online/en/home/clinical/exam.html
–http://www.ahrq.gov/clinic/uspstf/uspshemoch.htm

Comment

–**Clinical Implications**

- There is fair evidence that clinically significant disease caused by hereditary hemochromatosis is uncommon in the general population. Male homozygotes for *C282Y* gene mutation have a 2-fold increase in the incidence of iron overload-related symptoms, compared with females.
- There is poor evidence that early therapeutic phlebotomy improves morbidity and mortality in screening-detected vs. clinically detected individuals.
- Both men and women who have a heterozygote *C282Y* gene mutation rarely develop iron overload.

Population

–Adults.

Recommendations

▶ ACP 2005

–Insufficient evidence to recommend for or against screening.[a]
–In case-finding for hereditary hemochromatosis, serum ferritin and transferrin saturation tests should be performed initially. (*Ann Int Med.* 2008;149:270) (*Ann Int Med.* 2006;145:200)

Sources

–*Ann Intern Med.* 2005;143:517-521
–http://www.acponline.org/clinical/guidelines/
–*N Engl J Med.* 2004;350:2383

[a]Discuss the risks, benefits, and limitations of genetic testing in patients with a positive FH of hereditary hemochromatosis, or those with elevated serum ferritin levels or transferrin saturation.

Comments

–If testing is performed, cutoff values for serum ferritin levels >200 μg/L in women and >300 μg/L in men and transferrin saturation >45% may be used as criteria for case-finding, but there is no general agreement about diagnostic criteria.

–For clinicians who choose to screen, one-time screening of non-Hispanic white men with serum ferritin level and transferrin saturation has highest yield.

HEMOGLOBINOPATHIES

Population

–Newborns.

Recommendation

▶ AAFP 2010, USPSTF 2007

–Recommend screening all newborns for hemoglobinopathies (including sickle cell disease).

Sources

–http://www.guideline.gov/content.aspx?id=38619
–http://www.uspreventive servicestaskforce.org/uspstf07/sicklecell/sicklers.htm

Comment

–Newborn screen tests for phenylketonuria (PKU), hemoglobinopathies, and hypothyroidism.

HEPATITIS B VIRUS INFECTION

Population

–Adults.

Recommendations

▶ NICE 2013

–Offer transient elastography as the initial test of liver cirrhosis for all adults with HBV infection.

–Liver ultrasound and α-fetoprotein every 6 mo for HBV infection with cirrhosis to screen for hepatocellular carcinoma.

Source

–National Clinical Guideline Centre. Hepatitis B (chronic). Diagnosis and management of chronic hepatitis B in children, young people and adults. London (UK): National Institute for Health and Care Excellence (NICE); 2013 Jun. 45 p. (Clinical guideline; no. 165).

Population

–Pregnant women.

Recommendation

▶ USPSTF 2009, CDC 2015, ACOG 2015, AAP 2012, AAFP 2009

–Screen all women with HBsAg at their first prenatal visit.

Sources

–*Ann Intern Med.* 2009;150(12):874-876.
–ACOG/CDC Screening and Referral Algorithm for Hepatitis B Virus (HBV) Infection among Pregnant Women. 2015.
–AAP/ACOG. Guidelines for Perinatal Care, 7th Ed. 2012.
–AAFP Clinical Recommendation: Hepatitis. 2009.
–CDC. 2015 Sexually Transmitted Diseases Treatment Guidelines.

Population

–Adults and children.

Recommendations

▶ USPSTF 2014, CDC 2008

1. Recommend routine screening for HBV infection of newly arrived immigrants from countries where the HBV prevalence rate is >2%.[a]
2. People with behavioral exposures should be screened (ie, men who have sex with men, intravenous drug users)
3. People receiving cytotoxic or immunosuppressive therapy should be screened.
4. Hepatitis B testing should be part of the workup for unexplained liver disease (ie, elevated alanine transaminase (ALT).
5. To prevent transmission, the following groups should be tested for HBsAg: hemodialysis patients, pregnant women, and persons known or suspected of having been exposed to HBV (ie, infants born to HBV-infected mothers, household contacts and sex partners of infected persons, and persons with known occupational or other exposures to infectious blood or body fluids.

Sources

–USPSTF. Hepatitis B Virus Infection: Screening, 2014.
–Weinbaum, CM; Williams, I; Mast E; et al. CDC MWWR; Recommendations for Identification and Public Health Management of Persons with Chronic Hepatitis B Virus Infection. 2008 / 57(RR08);1-20
–Hepatology. 2016 Jan;63(1):261-83

---

[a]Immigrants from Asia, Africa, South Pacific, Middle East (except Israel), Eastern Europe (except Hungary), the Caribbean, Malta, Spain, Guatemala, and Honduras.

Comments

1. Breast-feeding is not contraindicated in women with chronic HBV infection if the infant has received hepatitis B immunoglobulin (HBIG)-passive prophylaxis and vaccine-active prophylaxis.
2. All pregnant women who are HBsAg-positive should be reported to the local Public Health Department to ensure proper follow-up.
3. Immunoassays for HBsAg have sensitivity and specificity >98% (*MMWR.* 1993;42:707).

HEPATITIS C VIRUS (HCV) INFECTION, CHRONIC

Population

–Pregnant women at increased risk.[a]

Recommendation

▶ ACOG 2012, CDC 2015

–Perform routine counseling and testing at the first prenatal visit.

Sources

–American College of Obstetricians and Gynecologists (ACOG). Viral hepatitis in pregnancy. Washington (DC): ACOG; 2007. (ACOG practice bulletin; no. 86)
–CDC. 2015 Sexually Transmitted Diseases Treatment Guidelines.

Comments

1. Route of delivery has not been shown to influence rate of vertical transmission of HCV infection. Cesarean section should be reserved for obstetric indications only.
2. Breast-feeding is not contraindicated in women with chronic HCV infection.

Populations

–Persons at increased risk for HCV infection.[a]
–Adults born between 1945 and 1965.

Recommendations

▶ AASLD 2014, USPSTF 2013, WHO 2014, CDC 2012

–Recommend HCV antibody testing by enzyme immunoassay in all high-risk adults.
–One-time HCV antibody testing for HCV screening in all adults born between 1945 and 1965.

[a] HCV risk factors: HIV infection; sexual partners of HCV-infected persons; persons seeking evaluation or care for STDs, including HIV; history of injection-drug use; persons who have ever been on hemodialysis; intranasal drug use; history of blood or blood component transfusion or organ transplant prior to 1992; hemophilia; multiple tattoos; children born to HCV-infected mothers; and health care providers who have sustained a needlestick injury.

Sources
  –*Hepatology*. 2015;62(3):932
  –USPSTF. Hepatitis C: Screening. 2013.
  –CDC: Recommendations for the Identification of Chronic Hepatitis C
   Virus Infection Among Persons Born During 1945–1965. MMWR.
   2012;61(4)
  –Guidelines for the screening, care and treatment of persons with hepatitis
   C infection. Geneva, Switzerland: World Health Organization; 2014.

Comments

1. HCV RNA testing should be performed for:
   a. Positive HCV antibody test result in a patient.
   b. When antiviral treatment is being considered.
   c. Unexplained liver disease in an immunocompromised patient with a
      negative HCV antibody test result.
   d. Suspicion of acute HCV infection.
2. HCV genotype should be determined in all HCV-infected persons
   prior to interferon treatment.
3. Seroconversion may take up to 3 mo.
4. Of persons with acute hepatitis C, 15%–25% resolve their infection;
   of the remaining, 10%–20% develop cirrhosis within 20–30 y after
   infection, and 1%–5% develop hepatocellular carcinoma.
5. Patients testing positive for HCV antibody should receive a nucleic
   acid test to confirm active infection. A quantitative HCV RNA test
   and genotype test can provide useful prognostic information prior to
   initiating antiviral therapy. (*JAMA*. 2007;297:724)

HERPES SIMPLEX VIRUS (HSV), GENITAL

Population
  –Adolescents, adults, and pregnant women.

Recommendation

▶ CDC 2015, USPSTF 2016
  –Recommend against routine serologic screening for HSV.

Sources
  –*JAMA*. 2016;316(23):2525-2530.
  –*CDC*. 2015 Sexually Transmitted Diseases Treatment Guidelines.

Comments

1. In women with a history of genital herpes, routine serial cultures for
   HSV are not indicated in the absence of active lesions.
2. Women who develop primary HSV infection during pregnancy have
   the highest risk for transmitting HSV infection to their infants.

HUMAN IMMUNODEFICIENCY VIRUS (HIV)

Population
–Pregnant women.

Recommendations

▶ AAFP 2010, USPSTF 2013
–Clinicians should screen all pregnant women for HIV.

▶ CDC 2015
–Include HIV testing in panel of routine prenatal screening tests.
–Retest high-risk women at 36 wk' gestation.
–Rapid HIV testing of women in labor who have not received prenatal HIV testing.

Sources
–AAFP Clinical Recommendation: HIV Infection, Adolescents and Adults. 2013.
–USPSTF. HIV Infection: Screening. 2013.
–CDC. 2015 Sexually Transmitted Diseases Treatment Guidelines.

Comment
–Rapid HIV antibody testing during labor identified 34 HIV-positive women among 4849 women with no prior HIV testing documented (prevalence: 7 in 1000). Eighty-four percent of women consented to testing. Sensitivity was 100%, specificity was 99.9%, positive predictive value was 90%. (*JAMA*. 2004;292:219).

Population
–Adolescents and adults

Recommendation

▶ AAFP 2013
–Screen everyone age 18–65 y. Consider screening high risk individuals[a] of other ages.

▶ USPSTF 2013
–Screen everyone age 15–65 y old. Consider screening high risk individuals of other ages.

---

[a] Risk factors for HIV: men who have had sex with men after 1975; multiple sexual partners; history of intravenous drug use; prostitution; history of sex with an HIV-infected person; history of sexually transmitted disease; history of blood transfusion between 1978 and 1985; or persons requesting an HIV test.

▶ **CDC 2015**

–Screen everyone age 13 y old to 64 y old. Consider screening high-risk individuals of other ages.

Sources

–AAFP Clinical Recommendations: HIV Infection, Adolescents and Adults
–CDC. 2015 Sexually Transmitted Diseases Treatment Guidelines.
–USPSTF. HIV Infection: Screening. 2013.

Comments

1. HIV testing should be voluntary and must have a verbal consent to test. Patients may "opt out" of testing.
2. Educate and counsel all high-risk patients regarding HIV testing, transmission, risk-reduction behaviors, and implications of infection.
3. If acute HIV is suspected, also use plasma RNA test.
4. False-positive results with electroimmunoassay (EIA): nonspecific reactions in persons with immunologic disturbances (eg, systemic lupus erythematosus or rheumatoid arthritis), multiple transfusions, recent influenza, or rabies vaccination.
5. Confirmatory testing is necessary using Western blot or indirect immunofluorescence assay.
6. Awareness of HIV positively reduces secondary HIV transmission risk and high-risk behavior and viral load if on highly active antiretroviral therapy (HAART). (CDC, 2006)

HYPERTENSION (HTN), CHILDREN AND ADOLESCENTS

Population

–Age 3–20 y[a]

Recommendations

▶ **Pediatrics 2011, NHLBI 2012**

–Children age ≥3 y should have BP measured at each encounter with health care provider.

Sources

–*Pediatrics.* 2011;128:s213.
–*Pediatrics.* 2004;114:555-576

---

[a]In children age <3 y, conditions that warrant BP measurement include: prematurity, very low birth weight, or neonatal complications; congenital heart disease; recurrent urinary tract infections (UTIs), hematuria, or proteinuria; renal disease or urologic malformations; FH of congenital renal disease; solid-organ transplant; malignancy or bone marrow transplant; drugs known to raise BP; systemic illnesses; increased intracranial pressure.

–Expert Panel on Integrated Guidelines for Cardiovascular Health and Risk Reduction in Children and Adolescents. NHLBI. 2012.

–A Pocket Guide to Blood Pressure Management in Children. NHLBI. 2012.

Recommendation

▶ AAFP 2013, USPSTF 2013

–Evidence is insufficient to recommend for or against routine screening.

Sources

–AAFP Clinical Recommendations: Hypertension, Children and Adolescents. 2013.

–USPSTF. Blood Pressure in Children and Adolescents (Hypertension): Screening. 2013.

–*Pediatrics*. 2013;132:1–8.

Comments

1. Hypertension: average systolic blood pressure (SBP) or diastolic blood pressure (DBP) ≥95th percentile for gender, age, and height on 3 or more occasions. See Appendixes.
2. Prehypertension: average SBP or DBP 90th–95th percentile.
3. Adolescents with BP ≥120/80 mm Hg are prehypertensive.
4. Evaluation of hypertensive children: assess for additional risk factors. Follow-up BP: if normal, repeat in 1 y; if prehypertensive, repeat BP in 6 mo; if stage 1, repeat in 2 wk; if symptomatic or stage 2, refer or repeat in 1 wk.
5. Indications for antihypertensive drug therapy in children: symptomatic HTN, secondary HTN, target-organ damage, diabetes, persistent HTN despite nonpharmacologic measures.
6. Screening for hypertension in children and adolescents hasn't been proven to reduce adverse cardiovascular outcomes in adults.

HYPERTENSION (HTN), ADULTS

Population

–Adults age >18 y.

Recommendations

▶ USPSTF 2015, AAFP 2009, CHEP 2015, ESH/ESC 2013, Canadian Task Force on Preventive Health Care 2013

1. Screen for HTN.
2. HTN is >140/90 mm Hg on two or more BP readings.
3. All adults should have their BP assessed at all appropriate clinical visits.

4. Ambulatory BP monitoring (ABPM) is the standard to confirm diagnosis.

5. Annual F/U of patients with high-normal BP (2-y risk of developing HTN is 40%).

Sources
-*Am Fam Physician*. 2009;79(12): 1087-1088
-http://www.aafp.org/online/en/home/clinical/exam.html
-USPSTF: High Blood Pressure in Adults: Screening. 2015.
-Hypertension Canada: http://www.hypertension.ca/en/chep
-*Can Fam Physician*. 2013;59(9): 927-933.
-*J Hypertens*. 2007;25:1105
-*Eur Heart J*. 2013;34:2159–2219

Recommendations

▶ **ESH/ESC 2013**

-In cases of severe BP elevation, especially if associated with end-organ damage, the diagnosis can be based on measurements taken at a single visit.

-In asymptomatic subjects with hypertension but free of CVD, chronic kidney disease (CKD), and diabetes, total cardiovascular risk stratification using the SCORE model is recommended as a minimal requirement.

Sources
-*J Hypertens*. 2007;25:1105
-*Eur Heart J*. 2013;34:2159-2219

Comments

1. Electronic (oscillometric) measurement methods are preferred to manual measurements. Routine auscultatory Office BP Measurements (OBPMs) are 9/6 mm Hg higher than standardized research BPs (primarily using oscillometric devices). (CHEP, 2015)

2. Confirm diagnosis out-of-office before starting treatment.

3. ABPM has better predictive ability than OBPM.

4. Home BP Measurement (HBPM) is recommended if ABPM is not tolerated, not readily available or due to patient preference. 15%–30% of elevations by OBPM will have lower BP at home. (USPSTF, 2015)

5. Assess global cardiovascular risk in all hypertensive patients. Informing patients of their global risk ("vascular age") improves the effectiveness of risk factor modification.

Population

–Age >18 y.

Recommendation

▶ JNC 8 2014

–Treatment thresholds:
  - Age ≥ 60: 150/90.
  - Age <60: 140/90.
  - DM or CKD: 140/90.

Source

–*JAMA*. 2014;311(5):507-520

Comment

–"Hypertension" and "pre-hypertension" are no longer defined.

Population

–Age >65 y.

Recommendation

▶ ACCF/AHA 2011

–Identification and treatment of systolic and diastolic HTN in the very elderly are beneficial in reduction in all-cause mortality and stroke death.

Source

–*J Am Coll Cardiol.* 2011;57(20):2037-2110

Comments

–Increased frequency of systolic HTN compared with younger patients.
–HTN is more likely associated with end-organ damage and more often associated with other risk factors.

ILLICIT DRUG USE

Population

–Adults, adolescents, and pregnant women.

Recommendation

▶ USPSTF 2008, ICSI 2014

–Insufficient evidence to recommend for or against routine screening for illicit drug use.

Sources

–ISCI Preventive Services for Adults, 20th ed. 2014.
–USPSTF. Drug Use, Illicit: Screening. 2008.

KIDNEY DISEASE, CHRONIC (CKD)

Population
    –Adults.

Recommendations

▶ USPSTF 2012

1. Insufficient evidence to recommend for or against routine screening.

Source
    –USPSTF. Chronic Kidney Disease (CKD): Screening. 2012.

▶ ACP 2013, AAFP 2014

1. Do not screen adults unless they have symptoms or risk factors.
2. Adults taking an ACE inhibitor or ARB should not be tested for proteinuria, regardless of diabetes status.

Sources
    –AAFP Clinical Recommendations: Chronic Kidney Disease. 2014.
    –*Ann Intern Med.* 2013;159(12):835

▶ NICE 2014

1. Monitor glomerular filtration rate (GFR) at least annually in people prescribed drugs known to be nephrotoxic.[a]
2. Screen renal function in people at risk for CKD.[b]

Source
    –Early identification and management of chronic kidney disease in adults in primary and secondary care. London (UK): NICE; 2014

[a]Examples: calcineurin inhibitors, lithium, or nonsteroidal anti-inflammatory drugs (NSAIDs).
[b]DM, HTN, CVD, structural renal disease, nephrolithiasis, benign prostatic hyperplasia (BPH), multisystem diseases with potential kidney involvement (eg, systemic lupus erythematosus [SLE]), FH of stage 5 CKD or hereditary kidney disease, or personal history of hematuria or proteinuria.

LEAD POISONING

Population
    –Children age 1–5 y.

Recommendations

▶ AAFP 2006, USPSTF 2006, CDC 2000, AAP 2000

1. Insufficient evidence to recommend for or against routine screening in asymptomatic children at increased risk.[a]

[a]Child suspected by parent, health care provider, or Health Department to be at risk for lead exposure; sibling or playmate with elevated blood lead level; recent immigrant, refugee, or foreign adoptee; child's parent or caregiver works with lead; household member uses traditional folk or ethnic remedies or cosmetics or who routinely eats food imported informally from abroad; residence near a source of high lead levels.

2. Recommends against screening in asymptomatic children at average risk.

Sources

–USPSTF. Lead Levels in Childhood and Pregnancy: Screening. 2006.

–*Pediatrics.* 1998;101(6):1702

–Advisory Committee on Childhood Lead Poisoning Prevention. Recommendations for Blood Lead Screening of Young Children Enrolled in Medicaid: Targeting a Group at High Risk. *CDC MMWR.* 2000;49(RR14);1-13.

–AAFP Clinical Recommendations: Lead Poisoning. 2006.

Comments

1. CDC recommends that children who receive Medicaid benefits should be screened unless high-quality, local data demonstrates the absence of lead exposure among this population.

2. Screen at ages 1 and 2 y, or by age 3 y if a high-risk child has never been screened.

3. As of 2012, the threshold for elevated blood lead level has been lowered to 5 µg/dL (Low Level Lead Exposure Harms Children: A Renewed Call for Primary Prevention. CDC. 2012.

Population

–Pregnant women.

Recommendation

▶ AAFP 2006

–Recommends against screening in asymptomatic pregnant women.

Source

AAFP Clinical Recommendations: Lead Poisoning. 2006.

▶ CDC 2010

–Routine blood lead testing of pregnant women is recommended in clinical settings that serve populations with specific risk factors for lead exposure.[b]

Source

–Guidelines for the Identification and Management of Lead Exposure in Pregnant and Lactating Women. Atlanta: CDC. 2010.

---

[b]Important risk factors for lead exposure in pregnant women include recent immigration, pica practices, occupational exposure, nutritional status, culturally specific practices such as the use of traditional remedies or imported cosmetics, and the use of traditional lead-glazed pottery for cooking and storing food.

Comments

1. Risk assessment should be performed during prenatal visits and continue until age 6 y.
2. CDC personal risk questionnaire:
   a. Does your child live in or regularly visit a house (or other facility, eg, daycare) that was built before 1950?
   b. Does your child live in or regularly visit a house built before 1978 with recent or ongoing renovations or remodeling (within the last 6 mo)?
   c. Does your child have a sibling or playmate who has or did have lead poisoning? (http://www.cdc.gov/nceh/lead/publications/screening.htm)

MOTOR VEHICLE SAFETY

Population

–Children and adolescents.

Recommendation

▶ ICSI 2013

–Recommend that all health care providers ask about
   a. Car seats.
   b. Booster seats.
   c. Seat belt use.
   d. Helmet use while riding motorcycles.

Source

–Preventive Services for Children and Adolescents, 19th Ed. ISCI. 2013.

Comment

–One study demonstrated a 21% reduction in mortality with the use of child restraint systems vs. seat belts in children age 2–6 y involved in motor vehicle collisions. (*Arch Pediatr Adolesc Med.* 2006;160:617-621)

NEWBORN SCREENING

Population

–Newborns

Recommendation

▶ ICSI 2013

–All newborns should receive a newborn metabolic screening test prior to hospital discharge.

Source

–Preventive Services for Children and Adolescents, 19th Ed. ISCI. 2013.

Comment

–The newborn screen should be performed after 24 h of age. Infants who receive their newborn screen before 24 h of age should have it repeated before 2 wk of age.

OBESITY

Population

–Children age ≥6 y.

Recommendation

▶ AAFP 2010, USPSTF 2010

–The AAFP recommends that clinicians screen children age 6 y and older for obesity.

Source

–USPSTF. Obesity in Children and Adolescents: Screening. 2010.

Comment

–Obese children should be offered intensive counseling and behavioral interventions to promote improvement in weight status.

Population

–Children age ≥2 y

Recommendation

▶ ICSI 2013

–Height, weight, and body mass index (BMI) should be recorded annually starting at age 2 y.

Source

–Preventive Services for Children and Adolescents, 19th Ed. ISCI. 2013.

Comments

1. Children with a BMI ≥25 are 5 times more likely to be overweight as adults when compared with their normal-weight counterparts.
2. Overweight children should be counseled about wholesome eating, 30–60 min of daily physical activity, and avoiding soft drinks.

Population

–Adults age >18 y.

Recommendation

▶ AAFP 2012, USPSTF 2012

–Recommends screening all adults and offering intensive counseling and behavioral interventions to promote sustained weight loss in obese adults with BMI ≥30 kg/m².

Source
  –USPSTF. Obesity in Adults: Screening and Management. 2012.

Comment
  –Intensive counseling involves more than one session per month for at least 3 mo.

Recommendation

▶ ICSI 2014
  –Height, weight, and BMI should be measured at least annually.

Source
  –Preventive Services for Adults, 20th Ed. ISCI. 2014.

Comment
  –Intensive intervention to promote weight loss should be offered to all obese adults (BMI ≥30 or waist circumference ≥40 in. [men] or ≥35 in. [women])

Recommendations

▶ VA/DoD 2014
  1. Height, weight, and BMI should be measured at least annually.
  2. Consider annual measurement of waist circumference as well.

Source
  –VA/DoD Clinical Practice Guideline for Screening and Management of Overweight and Obesity, Version 2.0. 2014

Comment
  1. Intensive intervention to promote weight loss should be offered to
     a. Obese adults (BMI ≥30 or waist circumference ≥40 in. [men] or ≥35 in. [women]).
     b. Overweight adults (BMI 25–29.9) with an obesity-associated condition.[a]

OSTEOPOROSIS

Population
  –Women age ≥65y, and younger women at increased risk.

Recommendation

▶ USPSTF 2011, ACPM 2009, ACOG 2012, ISCI 2014, NAMS 2010
  –Routine screening for women using either dual-energy x-ray absorptiometry (DXA) of the hip and lumbar spine, or quantitative ultrasonography of the calcaneus.

[a]HTN, DM type 2, dyslipidemia, obstructive sleep apnea, degenerative joint disease, or metabolic syndrome.

Sources
   −USPSTF. Osteoporosis: Screening. 2011.
   −*Osteoporosis*. Washington (DC): ACOG; 2012. (ACOG practice bulletin; no. 129).
   −*Menopause*. 2010;17(1):23.
   −Preventive Services for Adults, 20th Ed. ISCI. 2014.
   −*Am J Prev Med*. 2009;36(4):366–375

Comments
   1. USPSTF specifically defines 'increased risk' as having a fracture risk equivalent to that of a 65-y white woman.
   2. The optimal screening interval is unclear.
   3. Screening should not be performed more frequently than every 2 y.
   4. ACOG: If FRAX score does not suggest treatment, DEXA should be repeated every 15 y if T-score >=1.5, every 5 y if T-score -1.5 to -1.99, and annually if T-score is -2.0 to -2.49.
   5. Ten-year risk for osteoporotic fractures can be calculated for individuals by using the FRAX tool (http://www.shef.ac.uk/FRAX/).
   6. Quantitative ultrasonography of the calcaneus predicts fractures of the femoral neck, hip, and spine as effectively as does DXA.
   7. The criteria for treatment of osteoporosis rely on DXA measurements.

Population
   −Older men.

Recommendation
▶ USPSTF 2011
   −Insufficient evidence to recommend for or against routine osteoporosis screening.

Source
   −USPSTF. Osteoporosis: Screening. 2011.

Population
   −Men age ≥70 y.

Recommendation
▶ NOF 2008, ACPM 2009
   −Recommend routine screening via bone mineral density (BMD).
   −Consider screening men age 50-69 with risk factors.

Source
   −*Am J Prev Med*. 2009;36(4)

Comment
   −Repeat every 3–5 y if "normal" baseline score; if high risk, then every 1–2 y.

PELVIC EXAMINATIONS

Population
–Asymptomatic, nonpregnant women.

Recommendation
▶ AAFP 2017, ACP 2014
–Do not perform routine screening pelvic examinations.

Source
–AAFP Clinical Recommendation. Screening Pelvic Exam. 2017.
–*Ann Intern Med.* 2014;161(1):67-72.

Recommendation
▶ USPSTF 2017
–Insufficient evidence to recommend for or against screening pelvic examinations.

Source
–*JAMA.* 2017;317(9):947-953

Recommendation
▶ ACOG 2012
–Screen all women age 21+ with annual pelvic exam

Source
–*Obstet Gynecol.* 2012;120:421-4

Comments
–Pelvic examination remains a necessary component of evaluation for many complaints.
–While tradition and patient or physician experience may support an annual exam, outcome data does not (nor does the data clearly refute the exam).
–Potential harms associated with screening include overdiagnosis, fear/anxiety/embarrasment, discomfort, additional diagnostic procedures.

PHENYLKETONURIA (PKU)

Population
–Newborns.

Recommendation
▶ Advisory Committee on Heritable Disorders in Newborns and Children 2015, USPSTF 2008
–Recommend screening all newborns for PKU as part of a uniform screening panel.

Sources
–Advisory Committee on Heritable Disorders in Newborns and Children. 2015.
–USPSTF. Phenylketonuria in Newborns: Screening. 2008.

Comment
–Newborn screen tests for PKU, hemoglobinopathies, hypothyroidism, and several other heritable disorders.

RH (D) INCOMPATIBILITY

Population
–Pregnant women.

Recommendations
▶ AAFP 2010, USPSTF 2007
1. Recommend blood typing and Rh (D) antibody testing for all pregnant women at their first prenatal visit.
2. Repeat Rh (D) antibody testing for all unsensitized Rh (D)-negative women at 24–28 wk' gestation.

Sources
–http://www.guideline.gov/content.aspx?id=38619
–http://www.uspreventiveservicestaskforce.org/3rduspstf/rh/rhrs.htm

Comment
–Rh (D) antibody testing at 24–28 wk can be skipped if the biologic father is known to be Rh (D)-negative.

SCOLIOSIS

Population
–Adolescents.

Recommendation

▶ AAFP 2013, USPSTF 2004

–Recommend against routine screening of asymptomatic adolescents for idiopathic scoliosis.

Sources
–Choosing Wisely: Scoliosis in Adolescents. AAFP, 2013.
–USPSTF. Idiopathic Scoliosis in Adolescents: Screening. 2004.

SLEEP APNEA

Population
–Asymptomatic Adults

Recommendation

▶ USPSTF 2017, AAFP 2017

–Insufficient evidence to recommend for or against routine screening.

Sources
–AAFP. Obstructive Sleep Apnea in Adults: Screening. 2017.
–*JAMA.* 2017;317(4):407-414.

SPEECH AND LANGUAGE DELAY

Population
–Preschool children.

Recommendation

▶ AAFP 2015, USPSTF 2015

–Evidence is insufficient to recommend for or against routine use of brief, formal screening instruments in primary care to detect speech and language delay in children up to age 5 y.

Sources
–AAFP Clinical Recommendation. Speech and Language Delay. 2015.
–*Pediatrics.* 2015;136(2):e474-81

Comments

1. Fair evidence suggests that interventions can improve the results of short-term assessments of speech and language skills; however, no studies have assessed long-term consequences.
2. In a study of 9000 toddlers in the Netherlands, 2-time screening for language delays reduced the number of children who required special education (2.7% vs. 3.7%) and reduced deficient language performance (8.8% vs. 9.7%) at age 8 y. (*Pediatrics.* 2007;120:1317)
3. Studies have not fully addressed the potential harms of screening or interventions for speech and language delays, such as labeling, parental anxiety, or unnecessary evaluation and intervention.
4. Insufficient evidence to recommend a specific test, but parent-administered tools are best (examples: Communicative Development Inventory, Infant-Toddler Checklist, Language Development Survey, Ages and Stages Questionnaire).

SYPHILIS

Population

–Pregnant women.

Recommendation

▶ CDC 2015, AAFP 2009, USPSTF 2009

–Strongly recommend routine screening of all pregnant women at the first prenatal visit.

Sources

–2015 Sexually Transmitted Diseases Treatment Guidelines. CDC.
–USPSTF. Syphilis Infection in Pregnancy: Screening. 2009.

Population

–Persons at increased risk.[a]

Recommendation

▶ USPSTF 2016, AAFP 2016, CDC 2015

–Screen high-risk persons.

Sources

–*JAMA.* 2016;315(21):2321-7
–AAFP Clinical Recommendations. Syphilis. 2016.
–2015 Sexually Transmitted Diseases Treatment Guidelines. CDC.

---

[a]High risk includes commercial sex workers, persons who exchange sex for money or drugs, persons with other STDs (including HIV), sexually active homosexual men, and sexual contacts of persons with syphilis, gonorrhea, *Chlamydia*, or HIV infection.

Comments

1. A nontreponemal test (Venereal Disease Research Laboratory [VDRL] test or rapid plasma reagent [RPR] test) should be used for initial screening.
2. All reactive nontreponemal tests should be confirmed with a fluorescent treponemal antibody absorption (FTA-ABS) test.
3. Women at high risk for syphilis or who are previously untested should be tested again at 28 gestational weeks. Consider testing a third time at the time of delivery.
4. Syphilis is a reportable disease in every state.

THYROID DISEASE

Population
–Adults.

Recommendations

▶ AAFP 2010, ICSI 2010, USPSTF 2015

–Insufficient evidence to recommend for or against routine screening for thyroid disease.

▶ ATA 2012

–ATA recommends screening men and women older than age 35 y for hypothyroidism every 5 y.

▶ AACE 2012

–AACE recommends screening older adults with a thyroid-stimulating hormone (TSH) measurement.

Sources
–Preventive Services for Adults, 20th Ed. ISCI. 2014.
–*Endocr Pract.* 2012;18(6):988
–*Ann Intern Med.* 2015;162(9):641-50

Population
–Newborns.

Recommendation

▶ ICSI 2013, AAFP 2008, USPSTF 2008, AAP 2012, Discretionary Advisory Committee on Heritable Disorders in Newborns and Children 2015.

–Recommend screening for congenital hypothyroidism in newborns.

Sources
- Preventive Services for Children and Adolescents, 19th Ed. ISCI, 2013.
- *Pediatrics.* 2006;119(6):2290
- *Pediatrics.* 2012;129(4):e1103
- AAFP Clinical Recommendations: Thyroid. 2008.
- Advisory Committee on Heritable Disorders in Newborns and Children
- USPSTF. Congenital Hypothyroidism: Screening. 2008.

Comments
- <1% of adults have subclinical hypothyroidism; outcomes data to support treatment are lacking.
- Individuals with symptoms and signs potentially attributable to thyroid dysfunction and those with risk factors for its development may require TSH testing.
- Higher risk individuals are those with an autoimmune disorder, pernicious anemia, history of neck radiation, first-degree relative with a thyroid disorder, and those with psychiatric disorders.

Population
- Women who are pregnant or immediately postpartum.

Recommendation
▶ ATA 2017
- Insufficient evidence to recommend for or against routine screening of all women
- TSH levels should be obtained at confirmation of pregnancy if:
    1. A history or current symptoms of thyroid dysfunction.
    2. Known thyroid antibody positivity or presence of a goiter.
    3. History of head or neck radiation or prior thyroid surgery.
    4. Age >30 y.
    5. Autoimmune disorders.
    6. History of pregnancy loss, preterm delivery, or infertility.
    7. Multiple prior pregnancies.
    8. Family history of thyroid disease.
    9. BMI ≥40 kg/m^2.
    10. Use of amiodarone or lithium, or recent administration of iodinated radiologic contrast.
    11. Residing in an area of known moderate to severe iodine insufficiency.

Source
- *Thyroid.* 2017;27(3):315

TOBACCO USE

Population
–Adults.

Recommendation
▶ AAFP 2015, USPSTF 2015, ICSI 2014
–Recommend screening all adults for tobacco use and provide tobacco cessation interventions for those who use tobacco products.

Population
–Pregnant women.

Recommendation
▶ AAFP 2015, USPSTF 2015, ICSI 2014
–Recommend screening all pregnant women for tobacco use and provide pregnancy-directed counseling and literature for those who smoke.

Sources
–AAFP Clinical Preventive Service Recommendation: Tobacco Use. 2015.
–USPSTF. Tobacco Smoking Cessation in Adults, Including Pregnant Women: Behavioral and Pharmacotherapy Interventions. 2015.
–Preventive Services for Adults, 20th Ed. ISCI. 2014.

Comment
–The "5-A" framework is helpful for smoking cessation counseling:
  a. Ask about tobacco use.
  b. Advise to quit through clear, individualized messages.
  c. Assess willingness to quit.
  d. Assist in quitting.
  e. Arrange follow-up and support sessions.

Population
–Children and adolescents.

Recommendations
▶ AAFP 2013
–Evidence is insufficient to recommend for or against routine screening.
–Counsel school-aged children and adolescents against starting use.
▶ ICSI 2013
–Screen for tobacco use beginning at age 10, and reassess at every opportunity.

Sources
–Preventive Services for Children and Adolescents, 19th Ed. ICSI, 2013.
–AAFP Clinical Recommendations: Tobacco Use. 2013.

Comment
–The avoidance of tobacco products by children and adolescents is desirable. It is uncertain whether advice and counseling by health care professionals in this area is effective.

▼ TUBERCULOSIS, LATENT

Population
–Persons at increased risk of developing tuberculosis (TB).

Recommendation

▶ **USPSTF 2016,CDC 2010**

–Screening by tuberculin skin test (TST) or interferon-gamma release assay (IGRA) is recommended. Frequency of testing is based on likelihood of further exposure to TB and level of confidence in the accuracy of the results.

Sources
–*JAMA*. 2016;316(9):962-9
–*CDC MWWR*. 2010;59(RR-5)

Comments
1. Risk factors include birth or residence in a country with increased TB prevelence and residence in a congregate setting (shelters, correctional facilities).
2. Typically, a TST is used to screen for latent TB.
3. IGRA is preferred if:
   a. Testing persons who have a low likelihood of returning to have their TST read.
   b. Testing persons who have received a bacille Calmette-Guérin (BCG) vaccination.

VISUAL IMPAIRMENT, GLAUCOMA, OR CATARACT

Population
–Older adults.

Recommendation
▶ USPSTF 2016
    –Insufficient evidence to recommend for or against visual acuity screening or glaucoma screening in older adults.

Source
    –*JAMA*. 2016 Mar 1;315(9):908-14

Recommendation
▶ ICSI 2014
    –Objective vision testing (Snellen chart) recommended for adults age ≥65 y.

Source
    –Preventive Services for Adults, 20th Ed. ICSI. 2014.

Population
–Children ≤4 y.

Recommendation
▶ ICSI 2013
    –Vision screening recommended for children age ≤4 y.

Source
    –Preventive Services for Children and Adolescents, 19th Ed. ICSI, 2013.

Comment
    –Screen for amblyopia, strabismus, or decreased visual acuity.

Populations
–Children 3–5 y.
–Children <3 y.

Recommendations
▶ USPSTF 2011
    –Vision screening for all children 3–5 y at least once to detect amblyopia.
    –Insufficient evidence for vision screening in children <3 y of age.

Source
    –USPSTF. Visual Impairment in Children Ages 1-5: Screening. 2011.

Comment
    –May screen with a visual acuity test, a stereoacuity test, a cover–uncover test, and the Hirschberg light reflex test.

VITAMIN D DEFICIENCY

Population
–Nonpregnant adults age 18 y or older.

Recommendations
▶ USPSTF 2015, Endocrine Society 2011
–Insufficient evidence to screen for vitamin D deficiency in asymptomatic adults.
–Serum 25-hydroxyvitamin D level recommended as diagnostic test in patients at risk[a] for deficiency.

Sources
–*J Clin Endocrinol Metab.* 2011;96(7):1911-1930.
–*Ann Intern Med.* 2015;162(2):133-40

[a]Indications for screening include rickets, osteomalacia, osteoporosis, CKD, hepatic failure, malabsorption syndromes, hyperparathyroidism, certain medications (anticonvulsants, glucocorticoids, AIDS drugs, antifungals, cholestyramine), African-American and Hispanic race, pregnancy and lactation, older adults with history of falls or nontraumatic fractures, BMI >30, and granulomatous diseases.

Disease Prevention

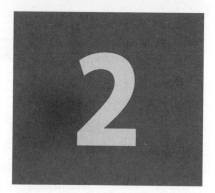

ASTHMA

Population
–Children.

Recommendation
▶Global Initiative for Asthma (GINA) 2017

–Advise pregnant women and parents of young children not to smoke.
–Encourage vaginal delivery.
–Minimize use of acetaminophen and broad spectrum antibiotics during first year of life

Source
–Global Initiative for Asthma. 2017.

Comments
–Environmental exposures such as automobile exhaust and dust mites are associated with higher rates of asthma, while others (household pets and farm animals) may be protective. Avoiding tobacco smoke and air pollution is protective, but allergen avoidance measures have not been shown to be effective primary prevention.
–Public health interventions to reduce childhood obesity, increase fruit and vegetable intake, improve maternal-fetal health, and reduce socioeconomic inequality would address major risk factors. (*Lancet.* 2015;386:1075-85)

BACK PAIN, LOW

Population
  –Adults.

Recommendation
  ▶AAFP 2004, USPSTF 2004
    –Insufficient evidence for or against the use of interventions to prevent low-back pain in adults in primary care settings.

  Sources
    –AAFP Clinical Recommendations: Low Back Pain. 2004.
    –USPSTF. Low Back Pain. 2004.

Comment
    –Insufficient evidence to support back strengthening exercises, mechanical supports, or increased physical activity to prevent low-back pain.

Primary Prevention of Cancer (Ca): NCI Evidence Summary 2017

BREAST CANCER

▶Minimize Known Risk Factor Exposure
  –**Hormone Replacement Therapy**
    • Approximately 26% increased incidence of invasive breast cancer with combination hormone replacement therapy (HRT) (estrogen and progesterone-Prempro).
    • Estrogen alone with mixed evidence—unlikely to increase risk of breast cancer significantly (decreases risk in African Americans).
  –**Ionizing Radiation to Chest and Mediastinum**
    • Increased risk begins approximately 10 y after exposure. Risk depends on dose and age at exposure (woman with radiation from age 15–30 y at highest risk). These patients often have received mediastinal radiation for Hodgkin Lymphoma.
  –**Obesity**
    • In Women's Health Initiative (WHI), relative risk (RR) = 2.85 for breast CA for women >82.2 kg compared with women <58.7 kg only in post menopausal women
  –**Alcohol**
    • RR for intake of 4 alcoholic drinks/day is 1.32.
    • RR increases approximately 7% for each drink per day.

- Family history—risk is doubled if a single first-degree relative develops breast cancer. Five-fold increased risk if 2 first degree relative are diagnosed with breast cancer. (*Breast CA Res Treat.* 2012; 133:1097).

–**Factors of Unproven or Disproven Association**
  - Abortions.
  - Environmental factors.
  - Diet and vitamins.
  - Underarm deodorant/anti-persperpants - no evidence to support increased risk of breast ca. (*J Natl Cancer Inst.* 2002; 94:1578).

–Epidemiologic studies suggest vitamin D may decrease risk of breast cancer and breast cancer recurrence. Randomized controlled trials are needed. (*N Engl J Med.* 2011;364:1385) (*Medicine.* 2013;92:123).
  - Active and passive cigarette smoking.
  - Use of statin drugs.
  - Use of low-dose daily aspirin.

–Population-based studies have shown reduction in breast CA risk with one 81 mg aspirin daily but more data needed. (*J Clin Oncol.* 2010;25:1467) (*Lancet Oncol.* 2012;13:518)
  - Use of bisphosphonates for >1 y with 28% relative reduction in risk for postmenopausal breast CA. (*J Clin Oncol.* 2010;28:3577) (*J Ntl Cancer Inst.* 2011;103:1752)
  - New large study from Kaiser Permanente Northern California shows serum Vitamin D levels independently associated with breast cancer prognostic characteristics and patient prognosis. A randominzed trial is needed. Underarm deoderants/antiperspirants—no evidence to support. (*JAMA Oncol.*2017; 3:351-357) (*J Natl Cancer Inst.* 2002; 94:1578)

▶Therapeutic Approaches to Reduce Breast Cancer Risk

  –**Tamoxifen (Postmenopausal and High-Risk Premenopausal Women)**
    - Treatment with tamoxifen for 5 y reduced breast CA risk by 40%–50%. USPSTF reemphasizes discussion with women at increased risk of breast cancer to strongly consider chemoprevention with selective estrogen receptor modulators (SERMs) or aromatase inhibitors (AIs in post menopausal women only). (*Ann Intern Med.* 2013;159:698-718)
    - Meta-analysis shows RR = 2.4 (95% confidence interval [CI], 1.5–4.0) for endometrial CA and 1.9 (95% CI, 1.4–2.6) for venous thromboembolic events.

- **Raloxifene (Postmenopausal Women)**
  - Similar effect as tamoxifen in reduction of invasive breast CA, but does not reduce the incidence of noninvasive tumors—studied only in postmenopausal women.
  - Similar risks as tamoxifen for venous thrombosis, but no risk of endometrial CA or cataracts. (*Lancet.* 2013;381:1827)
- **Aromatase Inhibitors**
  - Anastrozole reduces the incidence of new primary breast CAs by 50% compared with tamoxifen; similar results have been reported with letrozole and exemestane treatment (*Lancet.* 2014;383:1041). Aromatase inhibitor use as a prevention of breast cancer will reduce the risk of developing breast cancer by 3-5%.
  - There is a 65% reduction in the risk of breast CA occurrence in postmenopausal women treated with exemestane for 5 y (chemoprevention). (*N Engl J Med.* 2011;364:2381)
  - Harmful effects of aromatase inhibitors include decreased bone mineral density and increased risk of fracture, hot flashes, increased falls, decreased cognitive function, fibromyalgia, and carpal tunnel syndrome. There are no life-threatening side effects.
  - Fracture rate for women being treated with anastrozole was 5.9% compared with 3.7% for those being treated with tamoxifen. The use of calcium, vitamin D, biphosphonates and denosumab for patients at bone risk on aromatase inhibitors reduces the risk. (*J Clin Onc.* 2012;30:3665)
- **Prophylactic Bilateral Mastectomy (High-Risk Women)**
  - Reduces risk of breast cancer as much as 90%
  - Approximately 6% of high risk women undergoing bilateral mastectomies were dissatisfied with their decision after 10 y. Regrets about mastectomy were less common among women who opted not to have breast reconstruction.
- **Prophylactic Salpingo-oophorectomy among *BRCA*-Positive Women**
  - Breast CA incidence decreased as much as 50%.
  - Nearly all women experience some sleep disturbances, mood changes, hot flashes, and bone demineralization, but the severity of these symptoms varies greatly.
  - Salpingo-oophorectomy should be done in BRCA 1 patients at 35 y of age and >40 y of age in BRCA 2 patients.
  - In patients who have uterus removed as well, it is safe to give estrogen replacement. (*Eur J Cancer.* 2016;52:138)
- **Exercise**
  - Exercising >120 min/wk results in average risk reduction of developing breast cancer by 30%–40%. There is also a 30%

reduction in breast cancer recurrence in patients who have had breast CA. (*Eur J Cancer*. 2016;52:138)

- The effect may be greatest for premenopausal women of normal or low body weight.

–**Breast-Feeding**

- The RR of breast CA is decreased 4.3% for every 12 mo of breast-feeding, in addition to 7% for each birth.

–**Pregnancy before Age 20 y**

- Approximately 50% decrease in breast CA compared with nulliparous women or those who give birth after age 35 y.

–**Dense Breasts**

- Women have increased risk of breast CA proportionate to breast density. Relative risk 1.79 for 50% density and 4.64 for women with >75% breast density. (*Cancer Epidemiol Biomarkers Prev*. 2006;15:1159) (*Br J Cancer*. 2011;104:871)
- No known interventional method to reduce breast density.
- Adding ultrasound to mammography will improve sensitivity and specificity and is more accurate than tomosynthesis without radiation exposure. (*J Clin Onc*. 2016;34:1882) (*J Clin Onc*. 2016;34:1840)

CERVICAL CANCER

▶Minimize Risk Factor Exposure

–**Human Papillomavirus (HPV) Infection**[a]

- Abstinence from sexual activity; condom and/or spermicide use (RR, 0.4).
- HPV vaccination ideally at age 9–13 y—also given to females age 13–26 y if no previous vaccination.

–**Cigarette Smoke (Active or Passive)**

- Increased risk of high-grade cervical intraepithelial neoplasia (CIN) or invasive cancer 2- to 3-fold among HPV-infected women.

–**High Parity**

- HPV-infected women with 7 or more full-term pregnancies have a 4-fold increased risk of squamous cell CA of the cervix compared with nulliparous women.

–**Long-Term Use of Oral Contraceptives (>5 y)**

- Increases risk by 3-fold.
- Longer use related to even higher risk.

[a]Methods to minimize risk of HPV infection include abstinence from sexual activity and the use of barrier contraceptives and/or spermicidal gel during sexual intercourse.

▶Therapeutic Approaches

–HPV-16/HPV-18 Vaccination[b]

- Reduces incidence and persistent infections with efficacy of 91.6% (95% CI, 64.5–98.0) and 100% (95% CI, 45–100), respectively; duration of efficacy is not yet known; impact on long-term cervical CA rates also unknown but likely to be significant. 2 doses of vaccine if 9–14 y/o, 3 doses if 15-26 y/o. (*Lancet*. 2009;374:1975) (*N Engl J Med*. 2015;372:711) (*N Engl J Med*. 2015;372:775)
- Also will likely decrease risk of other HPV-driven malignancies (oropharynx and anal CA).

–Screening with PAP Smears

- Estimates from population studies suggest that screening may decrease CA incidence and mortality by <80%. Adding screening for HPV after age 30 y increases sensitivity and reduces frequency of screening to every 5 y if both are negative.
- HPV screening only, without a PAP smear, is being studied in developing countries.

[b]On June 8, 2006, the U.S. Food and Drug Administration (FDA) announced approval of Gardasil, the first vaccine developed to prevent cervical CA, precancerous genital lesions, and genital warts caused by HPV types 6,11,16, and 18. The vaccine is approved for use in females age 9–26 y (http://www.fda.gov). A bivalent vaccine, Cervarix, is also FDA approved with activity against HPV subtypes 16 and 18 (*N Engl J Med*. 2006;354:1109-1112).

COLORECTAL[a] CANCER

▶Minimize Risk Factor Exposure

–Risk Factor CRC

- Excessive alcohol use, RR is 1.41 for >45 g/d (>4.5 drinks/d).
- Cigarette smoking—RR for current smokers vs. never smokers- 1.18
- Obesity—RR for woman with a body mass index (BMI) >29 is 1.45. Similar increase seen in colorectal CA (CRC) mortality. (*N Engl J Med*. 2003; 348:1625)

–Preventive Strategy

- Regular physical activity—a meta-analysis of 52 studies showed a 24% reduction in incidence of CRC.
- Increased consumption of fruits and reduction in red meat and processed meat consumption may lower rhe risk of CRC. (*JAMA*. 2005; 293:172) (*Cancer Res*. 2010; 70:2401).
- B6 (pyridoxal-5'-phosphate) levels are inversely associated with risk of colon CA. B6 found in cereals, meat, fish, vegetables, bananas, and avocado. (*JAMA*. 2010;303:1077)

[a]Cereal fiber supplementation and diets low in fat and high in fiber, fruits, and vegetables do not reduce the rate of adenoma recurrence over a 3- to 4-y period.

- If family history of CRC (no genetic abnormality) increase frequency of surveillance. (*Gasterenterology*. 2015; 149:1438).

▶Therapeutic Approaches

- Based on solid evidence, nonsteroidal anti-inflammatory drugs (NSAIDs) reduce the risk of adenomas, but how much this reduces the risk of CRC is uncertain. Harms include upper gastrointestinal (UGI) bleeding (4–5/1000 people/y), chronic kidney disease (CKD), and cardiovascular (CV) events.[b]

- Based on solid evidence, daily aspirin use for at least 5 y reduces CRC incidence and mortality (40%), with an absolute risk reduction from 3.1% to 1.9%. Harm of low-dose aspirin use includes approximately 10 to 30 extra cases of UGI bleeding complications per 1000 users over a 1-y period. Risk increases with age. Benefit shown in other GI cancers as well. (*Lancet*. 2011;377:31) (*JAMA*. 2015;313:1133).

- USPSTF approves use of low-dose aspirin for prevention of colorectal cancer in adults 50–59 y old. Benefits statistically shown after 10 y of daily aspirin use. In 60–69 y old decision to take low-dose aspirin is individualized based on risk factors. Aspirin not recommended in patients <50 or older than 70. (*Ann Intern Med*. 2016;164;836) (*Ann Intern Med*. 2016; 164;777).

–**Postmenopausal Combination Hormone Replacement (Not Estrogen Alone)**

- Based on solid evidence (WHI), 44% reduction seen in CRC incidence among HRT users.

- Based on solid evidence (WHI), combination HRT users have a 26% increased invasive breast CA risk, a 29% increase in coronary heart disease (CHD) events, and a 41% increase in stroke rates. These risks obviate use of HRT for CRC prevention. Estrogen-only HRT does not impact on the incidence or survival of CRC.

–**Polyp Removal**

- Based on fair evidence, removal of adenomatous polyps reduces the risk of CRC, especially polyps >1 cm. (*Ann Intern Med*. 2011;154:22) (*Gastrointest Endosc*. 2014;80:471).

- Based on fair evidence, complications of polyp removal include perforation of the colon and bleeding estimated at 7–9 events per 1000 procedures.

–**Interventions without Benefit**

- Statins do not reduce the incidence or mortality of CRC.

- Data are inadequate to show a reduction in the risk of CRC from calcium or vitamin D supplementation. Fair data that calcium

---

[b]There is solid evidence that NSAIDs reduce the risk of adenomas, but the extent to which this translates into a reduction in CRC is uncertain.

intake >1000 mg/day will increase risk of myocardial infarction (MI). (*Br Med J.* 2010;341:3691) (*J Clin Onc.* 2011; 29:3775).

- Low-fat, high-fiber diet does not reduce the risk of CRC to a significant degree.
- Insufficient evidence to assess benefits and harms of regular use of multivitamins to prevent cancer. (*Ann Intern Med.* 2013;159:824)
- USPSTF recommends against use of beta-carotene or vitamin E supplements. (*Ann Inter Med.* 2014;160:558)

ENDOMETRIAL CANCER

▶Minimize Risk Factor Exposure

–**Unopposed estrogen is a significant risk factor for the development of uterine cancer**

- Unopposed estrogen use in post menopausal women for 5 or more years, more than doubled the risk of endometrial CA compared to women who did not use estrogen. Other significant events include storke (39% relative increase) and pulmonary embolus (34% relative increase). (*Lancet.* 2005; 365:1543) (*JAMA.* 2004; 291:1701).
- Obesity—risk increases 1.59-fold for each 5 kg/m^2 change in body mass.
- Lack of exercise—regular exercise (2 h/wk) with 38%–48% decrease in risk.
- Tamoxifen—used for >2 y has a 2.3- to 7.5-fold increased risk of endometrial CA (usually stage I— 95% cure rate with surgery).
- Nulliparous women have a 35% increased risk of endometrial CA.
- Endometrial hyperplasia and atypia—50% go on to develop uterine cancer. Most often occurs in women over 50 y old. (*Gynecol.* 1995; 5:233).

▶Therapeutic Approaches

–**Oral Contraception (Estrogen and Progesterone Containing)**

- Use of oral contraceptives for 4 y reduces the risk of endometrial CA by 56%; 8 y, by 67%; and 12 y, by 72%, but will increase risk of breast cancer by 26%.

–**Increasing Parity and Lactation**

- 35% reduction vs. nulliparous women-increasing length of breast-feeding with decreasing risk.

–**Weight Loss**

- Insufficient evidence to conclude weight loss is associated with a decreased incidence of endometrial cancer.

ESOPHAGUS CANCER

▶Minimize Risk Factor Exposure

–**Risk Factors**
- Avoidance of tobacco and alcohol abuse would significantly decrease risk of squamous cell CA of esophagus. (*Natl Cancr Inst.* 2003; 95:1404)
- The combined use of alcohol and smoking is associated with a 3- to 7-fold increased risk of esophageal cancer (account for 90% squamous cell esophageal CA).
- Diet high in cruciferous vegetables will decrease risk of esophageal CA.
- Avoid ingestion of coffee or tea at temperatures >149° F. (*Inst J Cancer.* 2009;125:491)
- ASA or NSAID use decreases the risk of developing or dying from esophageal CA by 43%. (*Gastroenterology.* 2003;124:47-56) (*Gastroenterology.* 2012;142:442)

▶Therapeutic Approaches

–**Risk Reduction**
- Randomized controlled trial has shown that radiofrequency ablation of Barrett's esophagus (BE) with moderate or severe dysplasia may lead to eradication of dysplasia and reduced risk of progression to malignancy. (*N Engl J Med.* 2009;360:2277-2288)
- Longstanding GERD associated with BE and increased risk of esophageal CA (*PLOS.* 2014; 9:e103508)
- Uncertain if elimination of GERD by surgical or medical therapy will reduce the risk of esophageal adenocarcinoma although a few trials show benefit. (*Gastroenterology.* 2010; 138:1297).
- No trials in the United States have shown any benefit from the use of chemoprevention with vitamins and/or minerals to prevent esophageal cancer. (*Am J Gastroenterology.* 2014;109:1215) (*Gut.* 2016;65:548)

GASTRIC

▶Minimize Risk Factor Exposure

–**Risk Factors**
- *Helicobacter pylori* eradication with decreased risk of gastric cancer from 1.7% to 1.1%.
- Deficient consumption of fruits/vegetables.
- Avoid salted, smoked, or poorly preserved foods.

- Smoking—relative risk = 1.6. (*Tumor*. 2009;95:13)
- Workers in rubber and coal industry.

▶Therapeutic Approaches

–**Clinical Considerations**

- Anti-*H. pylori* therapy may reduce risk but effect on mortality unclear. A study over 15 y showed a 40% reduction in risk of gastric CA with *H. pylori* eradication. (*Ann Intern Med*. 2009;151:121) (*J Natl Cancer Inst*. 2012;104:488) *H. pylori* eradication will also reduce the risk of mucosa-associated lymphoid tumor (MALT lymphoma).
- Dietary interventions—eating more fruits, vegetables, and less processed foods reduces risk of gastric cancer by 10%–15%.
- Smoking cessation will reduce risk by 20%–30%.
- Patients with hereditary susceptibility (HNPCC, e-cadherin mutation, Li-Fraumeni syndrome), pernicious anemia, atrophic gastritis, partial gastrectomy or gastric polyps should be followed carefully for early cancer symptoms and for upper endoscopy at intervals according to risk.

LIVER CANCER

▶Minimize Risk Factor Exposure

–**Risk Factor**

- Avoidance of cirrhosis (hepatitis B and C, excessive alcohol use, hepatic steatosis (NASH), alpha 1 anti-trypsin deficiency, Wilson's disease, and hemochromatosis).
- Aflatoxins from improperly stored grains and nuts, most prominent in Africa. (*Lancet*. 1992; 339:943)

▶Therapeutic Approaches

–**Hepatitis B Virus (HBV) Vaccination (Newborns of Mothers Infected with HBV)**

- HBV vaccination of newborns of Taiwanese mothers reduced the incidence of hepatocellular carcinoma (HCC) from 0.7 to 0.36 per 100,000 children after about 10 y. (*Clin Cancer Res*. 2005;11:7953)
- New effective anti-viral therapy for hepatitis C. Ledipasvir and Sofobuvir (Harvoni) will very likely decrease the risk for HCC in near future (*N Engl J Med*. 2013;368:1907)
- Irradiation of HCV occurs in over 95% of patients treated with this new anti viral therapy

LUNG CANCER

▶Minimize Risk Factor Exposure
–**Risk Factors for Lung CA**
- Cigarette smoking (20-fold increased risk) and second-hand exposure to tobacco smoke (20% increased risk) both medication and counseling better than either alone in increasing cessation rates.
- Beta-carotene, in pharmacologic doses, actually increases the risk of lung CA, especially in high-intensity smokers.
- Avoid radon gas exposure, severe air pollution (*Am J Respir Crit Care Med*. 2006;173:667)
- Avoid occupational exposures (asbestos, arsenic, nickel, and chromium).
- Air pollution—40% increased risk of lung CA with highest pollution exposure.
- Radiation exposure (*Chest*. 2003; 123:215).

▶Therapeutic Approaches
–**Minimize Risk of Lung CA**
- No evidence that vitamin E/tocopherol, retinoids, vitamin C, or beta-carotene in any dose reduces the risk of lung CA. (*Ann Inter Med*. 2013;159:824)
- Minimize indoor exposure to radon, (can be measured in home), especially if smoker. Avoid occupational exposures (asbestos, arsenic, nickel, chromium, beryilium, and cadmium)
- Stopping tobacco use will lower the risk of lung and other cancers but at 15 y there is still a 2- to 3-fold increased risk of lung cancer.
- At least 2/3 of patients newly diagnosed with lung cancer will die of their disease. Early detection is critical. (*Chest*. 2017; 151:193).

ORAL CANCER

▶Minimize Risk Factor Exposure
–**Risk Factors**
- Tobacco cessation (in any form, including smokeless).
- Alcohol and dietary factors—double the risk for people who drink 3–4 drinks/d vs. nondrinkers (*Cancer Causes Control*. 2011; 22:1217).
- Betel-quid chewing. (*Cancer*. 2014;135:1433)
- Oral HPV infection—found in 6.9% of general population and found in 70%–75% of patients with oropharyngeal squamous cell cancer (*N Engl J Med*. 2007; 356:1944)
- Lip cancer—avoid chronic sun exposure and smokeless tobacco.

▶Therapeutic Approaches

–Clinical Features

- Oropharyngeal squamous cell CAs (tonsil and base of tongue) are related to HPV infection (types 16 and 18) in 75% of patients. This correlates with sexual practices, number of partners, and may be prevented by HPV vaccine. HPV (+), non-smokers haveimproved cure rate by 35%–45%. (*N Engl J Med.* 2010;363:82) (*N Engl J Med.* 2010;363:24) There is inadequate evidence to suggest change in diet will reduce risk of oral cancer

OVARIAN CANCER

▶Minimize Risk Factor Exposure

–Risk Factors

- Postmenopausal use of unopposed estrogen replacement will lead to a 3.2-fold increased risk of OC after >20 y of use.
- Talc exposure and use of fertility drugs have inadequate data to show increased risk of ovarian CA – remains controversial.
- If a woman is newly diagnosed with ovarian cancer she should be tested for BRCA 1 or 2 at any age—if positive, family members should be tested for that specific gene mutation and undergo genetic counseling.

–Obesity and height of OC

- Elevated BMI including during adolescence associated with increased mortality from ovarian CA. (*J Natl Cancer Inst.* 2003;95:1244)
- Taller women with higher risk of OC. RR of OC per 5 cm increase in height is 1.07

▶Therapeutic Approaches

–Risk Reduction

–Oral Contraceptives

- 5%–10% reduction in ovarian CA per year of use, up to 80% maximum risk reduction.
- Increased risk of deep venous thrombosis (DVT) with oral contraceptive pill (OCP). The risk amounts to about 3 events per 10,000 women per year; increased breast CA risk among long-term OCP users of about 1 extra case per 100,000 women per year.
- Tubal ligation decreases the risk of ovarian cancer (30% reduction).
- Breast feeding associated with an 8% decrease in OC with every 5 mo of breast feeding.

–**Prophylactic Salpingo-oophorectomy**—in high-risk women (eg, *BRCA1* or *2* gene mutation).

- Ninety percent reduction in ovarian CA risk and 50% reduction in breast cancer with bilateral salpingo-oophorectomy.
- If prophylactic salpingo-oophorectomy is done prior to menopause, approximately 50% of women experience vasomotor symptoms; there is a 4.5-fold increased risk of heart disease especially in women <40 y old following oophorectomy.
- <40 y old following oophorectomy.

PROSTATE CANCER

▶Minimize Risk Factor Exposure

–Family history of prostate CA in men age <60 y defines risk. One first-degree relative with prostate CA increases the risk 3-fold, 2 first-degree relatives increase the risk 5-fold. The incidence of prostate CA in African Americans is increased by 2-fold, occurs at a younger age and is more virulent with increased death rate compared to caucasion men.

–High dietary fat intake does not increase risk for prostate CA but is associated with more aggressive cancers and shorter survivals.

▶Therapeutic and Preventive Approaches

–**Finasteride**

- Decreased 7-y prostate CA incidence from 25% (placebo) to 18% (finasteride), but no change in mortality.
- Trial participants report reduced ejaculate volume (47%–60%); increased erectile dysfunction (62%–67%); increased loss of libido (60%–65%); increased gynecomastia (3%–4.5%).

–**Dutasteride**

- Absolute risk reduction of 22.8%.
- No difference in prostate CA-specific or overall mortality. Concern raised by mild incease in more aggressive cancers in patients on dutasteride (Gleason score of 7–10). (*N Engl J Med.* 2013;369:603) (*N Engl J Med.* 2010;302:1192).

–**Vitamins and Minerals**

- Vitamin E/alfa-tocopherol—inadequate data—one study showed a 17% increase in prostate CA with vitamin E alone. (*JAMA.* 2011;306:1549)
- Selenium—no study shows benefit in reducing risk of prostate CA.
- Lycopene—largest trials to date show no benefit. (*Am J Epidemiol.* 2010;172:566)

SKIN CANCER

▶Minimize Risk Factor Exposure

–Avoid sunburns and tanning booths,[a] especially severe blistering sunburns at a younger age.

▶Therapeutic Approaches

–Sunscreen, protective clothing, limited time in the sun, avoiding blistering sunburn in adolescence and young adults

–Self exam of skin looking for changes that could possibly be cancer, higher risk patients need to be examined by dermatologist every 6–12 mo.

–Nicotinamide (Vitamin B$_3$) shows promise in preventing skin cancers but further studies are required. (*J Invest Dermatol.* 2012; 132:1498)

–Chemopreventive agents (beta carotene, isoretinoin, selenium and celecoxib) have not shown prevention of new skin cancers in randomized clinical trials. (*Arch Dermatol.* 2000; 136:179)

Source

–http://www.cancer.gov/types/skin/hp/skin-prevention pdq

CATHETER-RELATED BLOODSTREAM INFECTIONS

Population

–Adults and children requiring intravascular catheters.

Recommendations

▶IDSA 2011, CDC 2011

1. Educate staff regarding proper procedures for insertion and maintenance of intravascular catheters.
2. The arm is preferred over the leg for catheter insertion.
3. Use a central venous catheter (CVC) when the duration of IV therapy is likely to exceed 6 d.
4. Avoid the femoral vein for central venous access in adult patients.
5. Subclavian vein is preferred over femoral or internal jugular vein to minimize infection risk for nontunneled CVC.
6. Use ultrasound guidance to place CVCs to minimize mechanical complications.
7. Promptly remove a CVC that is no longer essential.
8. Wash hands before and after catheter insertion, replacement, accessing, or dressing an intravascular catheter.

[a] Twenty-eight million Americans per year use indoor tanning salons—increased risk of squamous cell and basal cell cancers greater than melanoma. Source: http://www.cancer.gov/cancertopics/pdq/prevention.

9. Use maximal sterile barrier precautions including a cap, mask, sterile gown, sterile gloves, and a sterile full-body drape for the insertion of CVCs.
10. Chlorhexidine skin antisepsis preferred over povidone-iodine.
11. Avoid antibiotic ointments on insertion sites.

Sources
–*Clin Infect Dis.* 2011;52(9):e162-e193.
–CDC Intravascular Catheter-related Infection: https://www.cdc.gov/infectioncontrol/guidelines/BSI/index.html

Comment
–Clean gloves should be worn when changing the catheter dressings.

CESAREAN SECTION

Population
–Pregnant women with history of prior cesarean delivery.

Recommendations
▶AAFP 2014, ACOG 2010

1. Attempting a vaginal birth after cesarean (VBAC) is safe and appropriate for most women.
2. Enourage and facilitate planning for VBAC. If necessary, refer to a facility that offers trial of labor after cesarean (TOLAC).

Sources
–AAFP Clinical Recommendation: Vaginal Birth After Cesarean. 2014.
–*Obstet Gynecol.* 2010 Aug;116(2 Pt 1):450

Comments
1. Obtained informed consent for VBAC, including risk to patient, fetus, future fertility, and the capabilities of local delivery setting.
2. Develop facility guidelines to promote access to VBAC and improve quality of care for women who elect TOLAC.
3. A calculator for probability for successful VBAC is available here: https://mfmu.bsc.gwu.edu/PublicBSC/MFMU/VGBirthCalc/vagbirth.html

Population
–Women in labor.

Recommendations
▶ACOG/SMFM/NICHHD 2013

1. Induce labor only for medical indications. If induction performed for nonmedical reasons, ensure that gestational age is >39 weeks and cervix is favorable

2. Do not diagnose failed induction or arrest of labor until sufficient time[a] has passed.
3. Consider intermittent auscultation rather than continuous fetal monitoring if heart rate is normal.

Source
−*Obstet Gynecol.* 2012;120(5):1181.

Comments

1. If fetal heart rate variability is moderate, other factors have little association with fetal neurologic outcomes.
2. Doctors who are salaried have lower cesarean rates than those paid fee-for-service.
3. Informed consent for the first cesarean should include discussion of effect on future pregnancies, including risks of uterine rupture and abnormal implantation of placenta.

COLITIS, *CLOSTRIDIUM DIFFICILE*

Population

−Adults and children taking antibiotics.

Recommendation

▶Cochrane Database of systematic reviews 2013

−Recommend probiotics for prevention of *C. difficile-associated* diarrhea (CDAD) after a course of antibiotics.

Source
−Probiotics for the prevention of Clostridium difficile-associated diarrhea in adults and children. Cochrane Collaboration. 2013.

Population

−Adults and children.

Recommendations

▶ACG 2013

−Hospital-based infection control programs can decrease the spread of CDI.
−Recommend antibiotic stewardship programs.
−Contact precautions should be maintained until the patient no longer has diarrhea.

---

[a]**Failed induction:** inability to generate contractions every 3 min and cervical change after 24 h of oxytocin administration and rupture of membranes, if feasible. **Arrest of labor, first stage:** 6 cm dilation, membrane rupture, and 4 h of adequate contractions or 6 h of inadequate contractions without cervical change. **Arrest of labor, second stage:** no descent or rotation for 4 h (nulliparous woman with epidural), 3 h (nulliparous woman without epidural or multiparous woman with epidural), or 2 h (multiparous woman without epidural).

–Patients with CDI should be treated in a private room.

–Hand hygiene and barrier precautions, including gloves and gowns, should be used by all health care workers and visitors entering the room of any patient with known or suspected CDI.

–Single-use disposable equipment should be used for prevention of CDI transmission. Nondisposable medical equipment should be dedicated to the patient's room and other equipment should be thoroughly cleaned after use in a patient with CDI.

–Disinfection of environmental surfaces is recommended using an Environmental Protective Agency (EPA)–registered disinfectant with *C. difficile* sporicidal label claim or 5000 ppm. Chlorine-containing cleaning agents in areas of potential contamination by *C. difficile*.

–Although there is moderate evidence that 2 probiotics (*Lactobacillus rhamnosus* GG and *Saccharomyces boulardii*) decrease the incidence of antibiotic associated diarrhea, there is insufficient evidence that probiotics prevent *C. difficile* infection.

Source
–*Am J Gastroenterol.* 2013;108(4):478

Comment
–Probiotics lower the incidence of CDAD by about 65% after a course of antibiotics.

CONCUSSION

Population
–Children and young adults.

Recommendations
▶AAN 2013

–School-based professionals should be educated by licensed healthcare professionals to understand the risks of a concussion.

–Licensed health care professionals should educate athletes about concussion risks.

–Athletes with a concussion should be prohibited from returning to play or practice in contact sports until a licensed healthcare provider has cleared them to return.

–Licensed healthcare providers should recommend retirement for any athlete with repeated concussions who has chronic, persistent neurologic or cognitive deficits.

Source
–*Neurology.* 2013;80(24):2250

COPD EXACERBATION

Population
–Adults with COPD.

Recommendations

▶GOLD 2017
–Recommend smoking cessation. Support with pharmacotherapy and nicotine replacement.
–Give influenza and pneumococcal vaccines.
–Pulmonary rehabilitation improves symptoms and quality of life.
–Pharamcotherapy reduces exacerbations.
–If no h/o hospitalzation and <2 lifetime exacerbations:
–Rare symtpoms: SABA
–Persistent symptoms: LAMA, LABA, or both
–If h/o hospitalization and 2+ lifetime exacerbation:
–Rare symtpoms: LAMA; add LABA or ICS if further exacerbations
–Persistent symptoms: LAMA & LABA & ICS

Source
–Global Strategy for the Diagnosis, Management, and Prevention of COPD. 2017.

▶ACCP 2015
–Recommend annual flu vaccine, smoking cessation counseling, monthly follow-up visit, and written action plans.
–If recent exacerbation, pulmonary rehabilitation.
–If moderate to severe disease, inhaled maintenance therapy.
–First line: ICS + LABA.
–Second line: LAMA+LABA or LAMA alone.

Source
–*Chest.* 2015;147:894-942.

Comments
–LABA: Long-acting beta agonist.
–LAMA: Long-acting muscarinic agonist.
–ICS: Inhaled corticosteroid.
–SABA: Short-acting beta agonist
–See Chapter 3, page 229 for specifics of COPD management.

DENTAL CARIES

Population
–Infants and children up to age 5 y.

Recommendations

▶USPSTF 2014, AAP 2014, AAFP 2014.

1. Recommends application of fluoride varnish to the primary teeth of all infants and children starting at the age of primary teeth eruption.
2. Recommends oral fluoride supplementation starting at age 6 mo for children whose water supply is fluoride deficient (<0.7 mg/L).

Source
  –AAFP Clinical Recommendation 2014
  –*Pediatrics*. 2014;133(5):s1-s10.

Comments

- Fluoride mouthwash used regularly by children under 16 reduces risk of dental caries by >25%. (*Cochrane Database Syst Rev*. 2016;7:CD002284)
- The CDC's My Water's Fluoride resource provides county-level information on content of fluoride in the water system.

CLINICAL RECOMMENDATIONS FOR USE OF PROFESSIONALLY APPLIED OR PRESCRIPTION-STRENGTH, HOME-USE TOPICAL FLUORIDE AGENTS FOR CARIES PREVENTION IN PATIENTS AT ELEVATED RISK OF DEVELOPING CARIES		
Age Group or Dentition Affected	Professionally Applied Topical Fluoride Agent	Prescription-Strength, Home-Use Topical Fluoride Agent
Younger than 6 y	2.26% fluoride varnish at least every 3 to 6 mo (**In Favor**)	
6–18 y	2.26% fluoride varnish at least every 3 to 6 mo (**In Favor**) or 1.23% fluoride (acidulated phosphate fluoride [APF]) gel for 4 min at least every 3 to 6 mo (**In Favor**)	0.09% fluoride mouthrinse at least weekly (**In Favor**) or 0.5% fluoride gel or paste twice daily (**Expert Opinion For**)
Older than 18 y	2.26% fluoride varnish at least every 3 to 6 mo (**Expert Opinion For**) or 1.23% fluoride (APF) gel for at least 4 min every 3 to 6 mo (**Expert Opinion For**)	0.09% fluoride mouthrinse at least weekly (**Expert Opinion For**) or 0.5% fluoride gel or paste twice daily (**Expert Opinion For**)
Adult Root Caries	2.26% fluoride varnish at least every 3 to 6 mo (**Expert Opinion For**) or 1.23% fluoride (APF) gel for 4 min at least every 3 to 6 mo (**Expert Opinion For**)	0.09% fluoride mouthrinse daily (**Expert Opinion For**) or 0.5% fluoride gel or paste twice daily (**Expert Opinion For**)

CLINICAL RECOMMENDATIONS FOR USE OF PROFESSIONALLY APPLIED OR PRESCRIPTION-STRENGTH, HOME-USE TOPICAL FLUORIDE AGENTS FOR CARIES PREVENTION IN PATIENTS AT ELEVATED RISK OF DEVELOPING CARIES   (*Continued*)

Additional Information:

- 0.1% fluoride varnish, 1.23% fluoride (APF) foam, or prophylaxis pastes are not recommended for preventing coronal caries in all age groups (**Expert Opinion Against**). See American Dental Association (ADA) publication for recommendation strength by age group. The full report, which includes more details, is available at ebd.ada.org.
- No prescription-strength or professionally applied topical fluoride agents except 2.26% fluoride varnish are recommended for children younger than 6 y (**Expert Opinion Against**), but practitioners may consider the use of these other agents on the basis of their assessment of individual patient factors that alter the benefit to harm relationship.
- Prophylaxis before 1.23% fluoride (APF) gel application is not necessary for coronal caries prevention in all age groups (**Expert Opinion Against**). See ADA publication for recommendation strength by age group. No recommendation can be made for prophylaxis prior to application of other topical fluoride agents. The full report, which includes more details, is available at the ebd.ada.org.
- **Patients at low risk of developing caries may not need additional topical fluorides other than over-the-counter fluoridated toothpaste and fluoridated water.**

Source: Weyant RJ, et al. Topical fluoride for caries prevention. Chicago, IL: American Dental Association; 2013. http://www.guideline.gov/content.aspx?id=47553.

DIABETES MELLITUS (DM), TYPE 2

Population

–Persons with impaired glucose tolerance (IGT).[a]

Recommendations

▶ADA 2017

1. Intensive lifestyle modification with a goal of sustained 7% weight loss.
2. Moderate physical activity such as brisk walking at least 150 min/week.
3. Consider initiation of metformin for patients at highest risk for developing diabetes (eg, BMI 35 kg/m^2 or greater, those age 60 y or younger, and those with prior gestational diabetes mellitus [GDM]).

Source

–*Diabetes Care.* 2017;40:S6-S135.

[a]IGT if fasting glucose 110-125 mg/dL, 2-h glucose after 75-g anhydrous glucose load 140-199 mg/dL, or HgbA1c 5.7%-6.4%.

Comments

1. Recommendations for disease prevention:
   a. Annual influenza vaccine.
   b. Pneumococcal polysaccharide vaccine if 2 y or older with one-time revaccination when over 64 y.
   c. Hepatitis B vaccine series if unvaccinated and 19–59 y of age.
   d. Aspirin 81 mg daily for primary prevention if 10-y risk of significant CAD is at least 10% (by Framingham Risk Score); includes most men over 50 y and most women over 60 y.

Population

–Persons with abnormal blood glucose or BMI >25.

Recommendation

▶USPSTF 2016

–Intensive behavioral intervention to promote healthy diet and physical activity.

Source

–*Ann Intern Med.* 2015;163(11):861-8.

DOMESTIC VIOLENCE

Population

–Adolescents and adult women.

Recommendation

▶WHO 2010

–Recommend school-based programs that emphasize preventing dating violence.

Source

–World Health Organization. Preventing intimate partner and sexual violence against women. 2010.

Comments

–Interventions of possible, but not proven, efficacy include:

1. School-based programs that teach children to recognize and avoid sexually abusive situations.
2. Empowerment and relationship skills training for women.
3. Programs that change social and cultural gender norms.

DRIVING RISK

Population

–Adults with dementia.

Recommendations

▶AAN 2010

  –Assess patients with dementia for the following characteristics that place them at increased risk for unsafe driving:
  1. Caregiver's assessment that the patient's driving ability is marginal or unsafe.
  2. History of traffic citations.
  3. History of motor vehicle collisions.
  4. Reduced driving mileage.
  5. Self-reported situational avoidance.
  6. Mini-Mental Status Exam score <24.
  7. Aggressive or impulsive personality.

Source
  –*Neurology.* 2010;74(16):1316

ENDOCARDITIS

Populations

  –Endocarditis is more likely a result of random exposure to bacteremia rather than associated with procedures.
  –Certain persons are at highest risk for adverse sequelae from endocarditis.[a]

Recommendations

▶AHA 2007, ESC 2015

  1. Dental procedures: give prophylaxis[b] for certain procedures,[c] give prophylaxis for highest-risk patients.[d]

---

[a]Patients with prosthetic valves; previous endocarditis; selected patients with congenital heart disease (unrepaired cyanotic congenital heart disease; completely repaired congenital heart defect with prosthetic material or device during first 6 mo after procedure; repaired cyanotic CHD with residual defects at or near-repair site); and cardiac transplant recipients who develop valvulopathy.
[b]Standard prophylaxis regimen: amoxicillin (adults 2 g; children 50 mg/kg orally 1 h before procedure). If unable to take oral medications, give ampicillin (adults 2.0 g IM or IV; children 50 mg/kg IM or IV within 30 min of procedure). If penicillin-allergic, give clindamycin (adults 600 mg; children 20 mg/kg orally 1 h before procedure) or azithromycin or clarithromycin (adults 500 mg; children 15 mg/kg orally 1 h before procedure). If penicillin-allergic and unable to take oral medications, give clindamycin (adults 600 mg; children 20 mg/kg IV within 30 min before procedure). If allergy to penicillin is not anaphylaxis, angioedema, or urticaria, options for nonoral treatment also include cefazolin (1 g IM or IV for adults, 50 mg/kg IM or IV for children); and for penicillin-allergic, oral therapy includes cephalexin 2 g PO for adults or 50 mg/kg PO for children (IM, intramuscular; IV, intravenous; PO, by mouth, orally).
[c]Such procedures include treatment of respiratory tract infections, gastrointestinal or genitourinary infections, skin and soft tissue infections, and implantation of cardiac valve, graft, or pacemakers.
[d]Highest risk patients are those with prosthetic valve, history of cardiac repair with prosthetic material, previous episode of IE, or congenital heart disease.

2. Other procedures: consider prophlaxis for highest-risk patients for invasive procedures through infected tissue.[e]

3. Antibiotic prophylaxis is no longer indicated for native valvular heart disease unless previous endocarditis is present.

Sources

–*Eur Heart J.* 2015;36(44):3075-3128.

–*Circulation.* 2007;116:1736

–*Circulation.* 2008;52:676-685

Comments

1. Emphasis is on providing prophylaxis to patients at greatest risk of endocarditis.

2. General consensus suggests few cases of infective endocarditis can be prevented by preprocedure prophylaxis with antibiotics.

FALLS IN THE ELDERLY

Population

–Older adults.

Recommendations

▶USPSTF 2012, Cochrane Database of Systematic Reviews 2012

1. Recommend vitamin D supplementation (800 international units [IU] orally daily).

2. Recommend home-hazard modification (eg, adding nonslip tape to rugs and steps, provision of grab bars, etc.) for all homes of persons age >65 y.

3. Recommend exercise or physical therapy interventions targeting gait and balance training.

4. Insufficient evidence to recommend a multifactorial assessment and management approach for all elderly persons (65 y and older).

5. Recommend vitamin D supplementation to elderly patients in care facilities. This reduces the rate of falls by 37%.

Sources

–USPSTF. Falls Prevention in Older Adults: Counseling and Preventive Medication. 2012

–Interventions for preventing falls in older people in care facilities and hospitals. Cochrane Collaborative. 2012.

---

[e]Consider prophylaxis for procedures involving manipulation of gingival or periapical region or perforation of oral mucosa. Do not give prophylaxis for superficial caries, suture removal, placement of appliances, etc.

Comments

1. 30%–40% of all community-dwelling persons age >65 y fall at least once a year.
2. Falls are the leading cause of fatal and nonfatal injuries among persons age >65 y.
3. A review and modification of chronic medications, including psychotropic medications, is important although not proven to reduce falls. Please see appendix for Beers List of potentially problematic medications.

FRACTURES

Population
–Noninstitutionalized postmenopausal women.

Recommendation
▶USPSTF 2013

–Recommends against daily supplementation with ≤400 IU Vitamin D and ≤1000 mg calcium for primary prevention of fractures.

Source
–*Ann Intern Med.* 2013;158(9):691

Comment
–Insufficient evidence for vitamin D and calcium supplementation in anyone for the primary prevention of fractures.

GONORRHEA, OPHTHALMIA NEONATORUM

Population
–Newborns.

Recommendation
▶USPSTF 2011

–Recommend prophylactic ocular topical medication against gonococcal ophthalmia neonatorum for all newborns.

Source
–USPSTF: Ocular Prophylaxis for Gonococcal Optthalmia Neonatorum. 2011

Comments

–Erythromycin 0.5% ointment is only agent available in U.S. for this application.

–Canadian Paediatric Society now recommends against universal prophylaxis given incomplete efficacy of erythromycin, rarity of the condition, and disruption in maternal-infant bonding. Instead, they recommend screening mothers for gonorrhea and chlamydia infection and, if infected with gonorrhea at the time of delivery, treating the infant with ceftriaxone (*Paediatr Child Health.* 2015;20:93-96).

GOUT

Population

–Adults.

Recommendations

▶American College of Rheumatology 2012

–Recommend a urate-lowering diet and lifestyle measures for patients with gout to prevent exacerbations.

–Urate-lowering medications[a] are indicated for gout with Stage 2–5 CKD or recurrent gout attacks and hyperuricemia (uric acid >6 mg/dL)

–Anti-inflammatory prophylaxis[b] indicated for 6 mo after an attack and for 3 mo after uric acid level falls <6 mg/dL

Source

–*Arthritis Care Res.* 2012;64(1):1431-1446.

Comments

–Minimize or avoid alcohol and purine-rich meat and seafood.

–Limit consumption of high-fructose corn syrup-sweetened soft drinks and energy drinks.

–Increase low-fat dairy products and vegetable intake.

[a]Colchicine 0.6 mg daily-bid; naproxen 250mg bid is second-line; low-dose prednisone is third-line.
[b]Allopurinol, febuxostat, probenecid; goal uric acid level <6 mg/dl

GROUP B STREPTOCOCCAL (GBS) INFECTION

Population
–Pregnant women.

Recommendations

▶CDC 2010

1. Intrapartum antibiotic prophylaxis (IAP) to prevent early-onset invasive GBS disease in newborns is indicated for high-risk pregnancies.[a]
2. IAP is **not** indicated for GBS colonization or GBS bacteriuria **during a previous pregnancy**, negative vaginal-rectal GBS culture, or if a cesarean delivery is performed with intact membranes and before the onset of labor (regardless of GBS screening culture status).

Source
–*CDC MWWR. 2010;59(RR10);1-32*

Comments

1. Penicillin G is the agent of choice for IAP.
2. Ampicillin is an acceptable alternative to penicillin G.
3. Cefazolin may be used if the patient has a penicillin allergy that does not cause anaphylaxis, angioedema, urticaria, or respiratory distress.
4. Clindamycin or erythromycin may be used if the patient has a penicillin allergy that causes anaphylaxis, angioedema, urticaria, or respiratory distress.

HORMONE REPLACEMENT THERAPY

Population
–Postmenopausal women.

Recommendation

▶AAFP 2012, USPSTF 2012

–Recommend against the use of combined estrogen and progestin for the prevention of chronic conditions (eg, osteoporosis).

Source
–USPSTF. Menopausal Hormone Therapy: Preventive Medication. 2012.

---

[a]Indications for IAP: previous infant with invasive GBS disease; history of GBS bacteriuria during current pregnancy; positive GBS vaginal-rectal screening culture within 5 wk of delivery; unknown GBS status with any of the following: preterm labor at <37 gestational weeks, amniotic membrane rupture ≥18 h, intrapartum fever ≥100.4°F (≥38°C); intrapartum nucleic acid amplification test positive for GBS.

Population

–Postmenopausal women who have had a hysterectomy.

Recommendation

▶AAFP 2012, USPSTF 2012

–Recommend against the use of estrogen for the prevention of chronic conditions (eg, osteoporosis).

Source

–USPSTF. Menopausal Hormone Therapy: Preventive Medication. 2012.

Comment

–This recommendation does not apply to women under the age of 50 y who have undergone a surgical menopause and require estrogen for hot flashes and vasomotor symptoms.

HUMAN IMMUNODEFICIENCY VIRUS (HIV), OPPORTUNISTIC INFECTIONS

Population

–HIV-infected adults and adolescents.

Recommendation

▶CDC 2009

–See the following table (from the clinical practice guidelines at *CDC MMWR.* 2009;58(RR04);1-198).

Source

–*CDC MMWR.* 2009;58(RR04);1-198

Population

–HIV-infected children.

Recommendation

▶CDC 2009

–See table below (from the clinical practice guidelines at *CDC MMWR.* 2009;58(RR04);1-198).

Source

–*CDC MMWR.* 2009;58(RR04);1-198

Comment

–This recommendation does not apply to women under the age of 50 who have undergone a surgical menopause and require estrogen for hot flashes and vasomotor symptoms.

PROPHYLAXIS TO PREVENT FIRST EPISODE OF OPPORTUNISTIC DISEASE AMONG HIV-INFECTED ADULTS

Pathogen	Indication	First Choice	Alternative
Pneumocystis carinii pneumonia (PCP)	CD4+ count <200 cells/µL (AII) or oropharyngeal candidiasis (AII) CD4+ <14% or history of AIDS-defining illness (BII) CD4+ count >200 but <250 cells/µL if monitoring CD4+ count every 1–3 mo is not possible (BIII)	Trimethoprim-sulfamethoxazole (TMP-SMX), 1 DS PO daily (AII): or 1SS daily (AII)	• TMP-SMX 1DSPOTIW(BI); or • Dapsone 100 mg PO daily or 50 mg PO bid (BI); or • Dapsone 50 mg PO daily + pyrimethamine 50 PO weekly + leucovorin 25 mg PO weekly (BI); or • Aerosolized pentamidine 300 mg via Respirgard III nebulized every month (BI); or • Atovaquone 1500 mg PO daily (BI); or • Atovaquone 1500 mg + pyrimethamine 25 mg + leucovorin 10 mg PO daily (CIII)
Toxoplasma gondii encephalitis	*Toxoplasma* IgG-positive patients with CD4+ count <100 cells/µL (AII) Seronegative patients receiving PCP prophylaxis not active against toxoplasmosis should have toxoplasma serology retested if CD4+ count declines to <100 cells/µL (CIII) Prophylaxis should be initiated if seroconversion occurred (AII)	TMP-SMX 1 DS PO daily (AII)	• TMP-SMX 1DSOITIW (BIII); or • TMP-SMX 1 SS PO daily (BIII); • Dapsone 50 mg PO daily + pyrimethamine 50 mg PO weekly + leucovorin 25 mg PO weekly (BI); or • (Dapsone 200 mg + pyrimethamine 75 mg + leucovorin 25 mg) PO weekly (BIII); • (Atovaquone 1500 mg ± pyrimethamine 25 mg + leucovorin 10 mg) PO daily (CIII)
Mycobacterium tuberculosis infection (TB) (treatment of latent TB infection [LTBI]	(+) diagnostic test for LTBI, no evidence of active TB, and no prior history of treatment for active or latent TB (AII)	Isoniazid (INH) 300 mg PO daily (AII) or 900 mg PO biw (BII) for 9 mo—both plus pyridoxine 50 mg PO daily (BII)	• Rifampin (RIF) 600 mg PO daily × 4 mo (BIII); or • Isoniazid (INH) for 6 mo; or • Isoniazid (INH) 900 mg and Rifapentene (RPT) 900 mg weekly × 3 mo

	Indication	Preferred Therapy	Comment
	(–) diagnostic test for LTBI and no evidence of active TB, but close contact with a person with infectious pulmonary TB (AII) A history of untreated or inadequately treated healed TB (ie, old fibrotic lesions) regardless of diagnostic tests for LTBI and no evidence of active TB (AII)	For persons exposed to drug-resistant TB, selection of drugs after consultation with public health authorities (AII)	• RFB 300 mg PO daily (BI) (dosage adjustment based on drug–drug interactions with ART); rule out active TB before starting RFB
Disseminated *Mycobacterium avium* complex (NAC) disease	CD4+ count <50 cells/µL—after ruling out active MAC infection (AI)	Azithromycin 1200 mg PO once weekly (AI); or Clarithromycin 500 mg PO bid (AI); or azithromycin 600 mg PO twice weekly (BIII)	
Streptococcus pneumoniae infection	CD4+ count >200 cells/µL and no receipt of pneumococcal vaccine in the last 5 y (AII) CD4+ count <200 cells/µL—vaccination can be offered (CIII) In patients who received polysaccharide pneumococcal vaccination (PPV) when CD4+ count <200 cells/µL but has increased to >200 cells/µL in response to ART (CIII)	23-valent PPV 0.5 mL IM × 1 (BII) Revaccination every 5 y may be considered (CIII)	
Influenza A and B virus infection	All HIV-infected patients (AII)	Inactivated influenza vaccine 0.5 mL IM annually (AIII)	

PROPHYLAXIS TO PREVENT FIRST EPISODE OF OPPORTUNISTIC DISEASE AMONG HIV-INFECTED ADULTS (Continued)

Pathogen	Indication	First Choice	Alternative
Histoplasma capsulatum infection	CD4+ count >150 cells/μL and at high risk because of occupational exposure or live in a community with a hyperendemic rate of histoplasmosis (>10 cases/100 patient-y) (CI)	Itraconazole 200 mg PO daily (CI)	
Coccidioidomycosis	Positive IgM or IgG serologic test in a patient from a disease-endemic area, and CD4+ count <250 cells/μL (CIII)	Fluconazole 400 mg PO daily (CIII) Itraconazole 200 mg PO bid (CIII)	
Varicella-zoster virus (VZV) infection	*Preexposure prevention:* Patient with CD4+ count >200 cells/μL who have not been vaccinated, have no history of varicella or herpes zoster, or who are seronegative for VZV (CIII) Note: Routine VZV serologic testing in HIV-infected adults is not recommended *Postexposure, close contact with a person who has active varicella or herpes zoster:* For susceptible patients (those who have no history of vaccination or infection with either condition, or are known to be VZV seronegative [AIII])	*Preexposure prevention:* Primary varicella vaccination (Varivax), 2 doses (0.5 mL SQ) administered 3 mo apart (CIII) If vaccination results in disease because of vaccine virus, treatment with acyclovir is recommended (AIII) *Postexposure therapy:* Varicella-zoster immune globulin (VZIG) 125 IU per 10 kg (maximum of 625 IU) IM, administered within 96 h after exposure to a person with active varicella or herpes zoster (AIII)	• VZV-susceptible household contacts of susceptible HIV-infected persons should be vaccinated to prevent potential transmission of VZV to their HIV-infected contacts (BIII) *Alternative postexposure therapy:* • Postexposure varicella vaccine (Varivax) 0.5 mL SQ × 2 doses, 3 mo apart if CD4+ count >200 cells/μL (CIII); or • Preemptive acyclovir 800 mg PO 5×/d for 5 d (CIII) • These two alternatives have not been studied in the HIV population

		Note: As of June 2007, VZIG can be obtained only under a treatment IND (1-800-843-7477, FFF Enterprises)	
Human papillomavirus (HPV) infection	Women age 15–26 y (CIII)	HPV quadrivalent vaccine 0.5 mL IM months 0, 2, and 6 (CIII)	
Hepatitis A virus (HAV) infection	HAV-susceptible patients with chronic liver disease, or who are injection-drug users, or men who have sex with men (AII). Certain specialists might delay vaccination until CD4+ count >200 cells/µL (CIII)	Hepatitis A vaccine 1 mL IM × 2 doses—at 0 and 6–12 mo (AII) IgG antibody response should be assessed 1 mo after vaccination; nonresponders should be revaccinated (BIII)	
Hepatitis B virus (HBV) infection	All HIV patients without evidence of prior exposure to HBV should be vaccinated with HBV vaccine, including patients with CD4+ count <200 cells/µL (AII) *Patients with isolated anti-HBc:* (BIII) (consider screening for HBV DNA before vaccination to rule out occult chronic HBV infection)	Hepatitis B vaccine IM (Engerix-B 20 µg/mL or Recombivax HB 10 µg/mL) at 0, 1, and 6 mo (AII) Anti-HBs should be obtained 1 mo after receipt of the vaccine series (BIII)	Some experts recommend vaccinating with 40-µg doses of either vaccine (CIII)

PROPHYLAXIS TO PREVENT FIRST EPISODE OF OPPORTUNISTIC DISEASE AMONG HIV-INFECTED ADULTS (Continued)

Pathogen	Indication	First Choice	Alternative
	Vaccine nonresponders: Defined as anti-HBs <10 IU/mL 1 mo after a vaccination series For patients with low CD4+ count at the time of first vaccination series, certain specialists might delay revaccination until after a sustained increase in CD4+ count with ART	Revaccinate with a second vaccine series (BIII)	Some experts recommend revaccinating with 40 µg doses of either vaccine (CIII)
Malaria	Travel to disease-endemic area	Recommendations are the same for HIV-infected and noninfected patients. One of the following three drugs is usually recommended, depending on location: atovaquone/proguanil, doxycycline, or mefloquine. Refer to the following website for the most recent recommendations based on region and drug susceptibility: http://www.cdc.gov/malaria/ (AII)	

BID, twice daily; BIW, two times weekly; DS, double strength; IM, intramuscular; PO, by mouth; SS, single strength; SQ, subcutaneous; TIW, three times weekly.

PROPHYLAXIS TO PREVENT FIRST EPISODE OF OPPORTUNISTIC INFECTIONS AMONG HIV-EXPOSED AND HIV-INFECTED INFANTS AND CHILDREN, UNITED STATES[a,b]

Pathogen	Indication	Preventive Regimen	
		First Choice	Alternative
		STRONGLY RECOMMENDED AS STANDARD OF CARE	
Pneumocystis pneumoniae[c]	HIV-infected or HIV-indeterminate infants age 1–12 mo; HIV-infected children age 1–5 y with CD4 count of <500 cells/mm^3 or CD4 percentage of <15%; HIV-infected children age 6–12 y with CD4 count of <200 cells/mm^3 or CD4 percentage of <15%	• TMP-SMX 150/750 mg/m^2 body surface area per day (max: 320/1600 mg) orally divided into 2 doses daily and administered 3 times weekly on consecutive days (AI) • Acceptable alternative dosage schedules for the same dose (AI): single dose orally 3 times weekly on consecutive days; 2 divided doses orally daily; or 2 divided doses orally 3 times weekly on alternate days	• Dapsone: children age >1 mo, 2 mg/kg body weight (max 100 mg) orally daily; or 4 mg/kg body weight (max 200 mg) orally weekly (BI) • Atovaquone: children age 1–3 mo and >24 mo, 30 mg/kg body weight orally daily; children age 4–24 mo, 45 mg/kg body weight orally daily (BI) • Aerosolized pentamidine: children age >5 y, 300 mg every month by Respirgard II (Marquest, Englewood, CO) nebulizer (BI) • Doxycycline 100 mg orally daily for children >8 y (2.2 mg/kg/d)
Malaria	Travel to area in which malaria is endemic	• Recommendations are the same for HIV-infected and HIV-uninfected children. Refer to http://www.cdc.gov/malaria/ for the most recent recommendations based on region and drug susceptibility • Mefloquine 5 mg/kg body weight orally 1 time weekly (max 250 mg)	• Chloroquine base 5 mg/kg base orally up to 300 mg weekly for sensitive regions only (7.5 mg/kg chloroquine phosphate)

PROPHYLAXIS TO PREVENT FIRST EPISODE OF OPPORTUNISTIC INFECTIONS AMONG HIV-EXPOSED AND HIV-INFECTED INFANTS AND CHILDREN, UNITED STATES[a,b]   (Continued)

Pathogen	Indication	Preventive Regimen	
		First Choice	Alternative
		STRONGLY RECOMMENDED AS STANDARD OF CARE	
		• Atovaquone/proguanil (Malarone) 1 time daily • 11–20 kg = 1 pediatric tablet (62.5 mg/25 mg) • 21–30 kg = 2 pediatric tablets (125 mg/50 mg) • 31–40 kg = 3 pediatric tablets (187.5 mg/75 mg) • >40 kg = 1 adult tablet (250 mg/100 mg)	
Mycobacterium tuberculosis	Tuberculin skin test (TST) reaction >5 mm or prior positive TST result without treatment, regardless of current TST result	• Isoniazid 10–15 mg/kg body weight (max 300 mg) orally daily for 9 mo (AII); or 20–30 mg/kg body weight (max 900 mg) orally 2 times weekly for 9 mo (BII)	• Rifampin 10–20 mg/kg body weight (max 600 mg) orally daily for 4–6 mo (BIII)
Isoniazid-sensitive	TST result and previous treatment, close contact with any person who has Contagious TB. TB disease must be excluded before start of treatment		
Isoniazid-resistant	Same as previous pathogen; increased probability of exposure to isoniazid-resistant TB	• Rifampin 10–20 mg/kg body weight (max 600 mg) orally daily for 4–6 mo (BIII)	• Uncertain

Pathogen	Indication	First Choice	Alternative
Multidrug-resistant isoniazid and rifampin	Same as previous pathogen; increased probability of exposure to multidrug-resistant TB	• Choice of drugs requires consultation with public health authorities and depends on susceptibility of isolate from source patient	
Mycobacterium avium complex[d]	For children age >6 y with CD4 count of <50 cells/mm³; age 2–5 y with CD4 count of <75 cells/mm³; age 1–2 y with CD4 count of <500 cells/mm³; age <1 y with CD4 count of <750 cells/mm³	• Clarithromycin 7.5 mg/kg body weight (max 500 mg) orally 2 times daily (AII), or azithromycin 20 mg/kg body weight (max 1200 mg) orally weekly (AII)	• Azithromycin 5 mg/kg body weight (max 250 mg) orally daily (AII); children age >6 y, rifabutin 300 mg orally daily (BI)
Varicella-zoster virus[e]	Substantial exposure to varicella or shingles with no history of varicella or zoster or seronegative status for VZV by a sensitive, specific antibody assay or lack of evidence for age-appropriate vaccination	• VZIG 125 IU per 10 kg (max 625 IU) IM, administered within 96 h after exposure[f] (AIII)	• If VZIG is not available or >96 h have passed since exposure, some experts recommend prophylaxis with acyclovir 20 mg/kg body weight (max 800 mg) per dose orally 4 times a day for 5–7 d. Another alternative to VZIG is intravenous immune globulin (IVIG), 400 mg/kg, administered once. IVIG should be administered within 96 h after exposure (CIII)
Vaccine-preventable pathogens	Standard recommendations for HIV-exposed and HIV-infected children	Routine vaccinations	
Toxoplasma gondii[g]	Immunoglobulin G (IgG) antibody to *Toxoplasma* and severe immunosuppression: HIV-infected children age <6 y with CD4 <15%; HIV-infected children age >6 y with CD4 <100 cells/mm³ (BIII)	• TMP-SMX, 150/750 mg/m² body surface area daily orally in 2 divided doses (BIII) • Acceptable alternative dosage schedules for same dosage (AI): single dose orally 3 times weekly on consecutive days; 2 divided doses orally daily; or 2 divided doses orally 3 times weekly on alternate days	• Dapsone (children age >1 mo) 2 mg/kg body weight or 15 mg/m² body surface area (max 25 mg) orally daily; *plus* pyrimethamine 1 mg/kg body weight (max 25 mg) orally daily; *plus* leucovorin 5 mg orally every 3 d (BI) • Atovaquone (children age 1–3 mo and >24 mo, 30 mg/kg body weight orally daily; children age 4–24 mo, 45 mg/kg body weight orally daily) with or without pyrimethamine 1 mg/kg body weight or 15 mg/m² body surface area (max 25 mg) orally daily; *plus* leucovorin 5 mg orally every 3 d (CIII)

PROPHYLAXIS TO PREVENT FIRST EPISODE OF OPPORTUNISTIC INFECTIONS AMONG HIV-EXPOSED AND HIV-INFECTED INFANTS AND CHILDREN, UNITED STATES [a,b] (Continued)

Pathogen	Indication	Preventive Regimen	
		First Choice	Alternative
		STRONGLY RECOMMENDED AS STANDARD OF CARE	
Invasive bacterial infection	Hypogammaglobulinemia (ie, IgG <400 mg/dL)	• IVIG (400 mg/kg body weight every 2–4 wk) (AI)	
Cytomegalovirus (CMV)	CMV antibody positivity and severe immunosuppression (CD4 <50 cells/mm³)	• Valganciclovir 900 mg orally 1 time daily with food for older children who can receive adult dosing (CIII)	

[a] Abbreviations: CMV, cytomegalovirus; FDA, Food and Drug Administration; HIV, human immunodeficiency virus; IgG, immunoglobulin G; IM, intramuscularly; IVIG, intravenous immune globulin; PCP, *Pneumocystis pneumoniae*; TB, tuberculosis; TMP-SMX, trimethoprim-sulfamethoxazole; TST, tuberculin skin test; VZV, varicella-zoster virus.

[b] Information in these guidelines might not represent FDA approval or FDA-approved labeling for products or indications. Specifically, the terms "safe" and "effective" might not be synonymous with the FDA-defined legal standards for product approval. Letters and roman numerals in parentheses after regimens indicate the strength of the recommendation and the quality of the evidence supporting it.

[c] Daily trimethoprim-sulfamethoxazole (TMP-SMX) reduces the frequency of certain bacterial infections. TMP-SMX, dapsone-pyrimethamine, and possibly atovaquone (with or without pyrimethamine) protect against toxoplasmosis; however, data have not been prospectively collected. Compared with weekly dapsone, daily dapsone is associated with lower incidence of PCP but higher hematologic toxicity and mortality. Patients receiving therapy for toxoplasmosis with sulfadiazine-pyrimethamine are protected against PCP and do not need TMP-SMX.

[d] Substantial drug interactions can occur between rifamycins (ie, rifampin and rifabutin) and protease inhibitors and nonnucleoside reverse transcriptase inhibitors. A specialist should be consulted.

[e] Children routinely being administered IVIG should receive VZIG if the last dose of IVIG was administered >21 d before exposure.

[f] As of 2007, VZIG can be obtained only under a treatment Investigational New Drug protocol.

[g] Protection against toxoplasmosis is provided by the preferred *anti-Pneumocystis* regimens and possibly by atovaquone.

HYPERTENSION (HTN)

Population
  –Persons at risk for developing HTN. [a]

Recommendations

▶CHEP[b] 2015, JNC 8, 2014, ICSI 15th Ed 2014, ESC 2013

  –Recommend weight loss, reduced sodium intake, moderate alcohol consumption, increased physical activity, potassium supplementation, and modification of eating patterns.

  –Above the normal replacement levels, supplementation of K, Ca, and Mg is not recommended for the prevention or treatment of HTN.

Sources
  –Hypertension Canada
  –*JAMA*. 2014;311(5):507-520
  –Kenning I, Kerandi H, Luehr D, et al. Institute for Clinical Systems Improvement. Hypertension Diagnosis and Treatment. 2014.
  –*Eur Heart J*. 2013;34:2159-2219

Population
  –Patients age >65 y.

Recommendation

▶ACCF/AHA 2011

  –Lifestyle management is effective in all ages.

Source
  –*J Am Coll Cardiol*. 2011;57(20): 2037-2114

Comments

1. A 5 mm Hg reduction in systolic blood pressure in the population would result in a 14% overall reduction in mortality from stroke, a 9% reduction in mortality from CHD, and a 7% decrease in all-cause mortality.

2. Weight loss of as little as 10 lb (4.5 kg) reduces blood pressure and/or prevents HTN in a large proportion of overweight patients.

---

[a]Family history of HTN; African American (black race) ancestry; overweight or obesity; sedentary lifestyle; excess intake of dietary sodium; insufficient intake of fruits, vegetables, and potassium; excess consumption of alcohol.
[b]Canadian Hypertension Education Program

LIFESTYLE MODIFICATIONS FOR PREVENTION OF HYPERTENSION

- Maintain a healthy body weight for adults (BMI, 18.5–24.9 kg/m^2; waist circumference <102 cm for men and <88 cm for women).
- Reduce dietary sodium intake to no more than 100 mmol/d (approximately 6 g of sodium chloride or 2.4 g of sodium/d). Per CHEP 2015: adequate intake 2000 mg daily (all >19 y old) (80% in processed foods; 10% at the table or in cooking). 2000 mg sodium (Na) = 87 mmol sodium (Na)= 5 g of salt (NaCl) ~1 teaspoon of table salt.
- Engage in regular aerobic physical activity, such as brisk walking, jogging, cycling, or swimming (30–60 min per session, 4 –7 d/wk), in addition to the routine activities of daily living. Higher intensities of exercise are not more effective. Weight training exercise does not adversely influence BP.
- Limit alcohol consumption to no more than 2 drinks (eg, 24 oz [720 mL] of beer, 10 oz [300 mL] of wine, or 3 oz [90 mL] of 100-proof whiskey) per day in most men and to no more than one drink per day in women and lighter-weight persons.
- Maintain adequate intake of dietary potassium (>90 mmol [3500 mg]/d). Above the normal replacement levels, supplementation of potassium, calcium, and magnesium is not recommended for prevention or treatment of hypertension.
- Daily K dietary intake > 80 mmol
- Consume a diet that is rich in fruits and vegetables and in low-fat dairy products with a reduced content of saturated and total fat (Dietary Approaches to Stop Hypertension [DASH] eating plan).
- Advice in combination with pharmacotherapy (varenicline, bupropion, nicotine replacement therapy) should be offered to all smokers with a goal of smoking cessation.
- Stress management should be considered as an intervention in hypertensive patients in whom stress may be contributing to BP elevation.

Sources: CHEP 2015: http://guidelines.hypertension.ca. *Hypertension*. 2003;42:1206-1252. *ASH 2009: J Clin Hypertens*. 2009;11:358-368.
2013 ACC/AHA Guideline on lifestyle management to reduce CV risk: a report of the American College of Cardiology/American Heart Association Task Force on Practice Guidelines. *Circulation*. 2013;01. cir.0000437740.48606.d1.

IMMUNIZATIONS, ADULTS

Population
–Adults.

Recommendation
▶CDC 2013

–Recommends immunizing adults according to the Centers for Disease Control and Prevention (CDC) recommendations unless contraindicated (see Appendix IX).

Source
–CDC: Adult Immunization Schedule

IMMUNIZATIONS, INFANTS AND CHILDREN

Population
–Infants and children age 0–18 y.

Recommendation
▶CDC 2013

–Recommends immunizing infants and children according to the CDC recommendations unless contraindicated (see Appendix IX).

Sources
–CDC: Child and Adolescent Schedule
–CDC: Catch-Up Immunization Schedule

INFLUENZA, CHEMOPROPHYLAXIS

Population
–Children and adults.

Recommendation
▶AAP 2016

The following situations warrant chemoprophylaxis
1. Children at high risk for complications who cannot receive vaccine, or within 2 wk of receiving vaccine.
2. Family members or health care providers who are unimmunizad and likely to have ongoing exposure to high-risk or unimmunized children younger than 24 mo of age.
3. Unimmunized staff and children in an institutional setting during an outbreak.
4. Supplement vaccination in high-risk immunocompromised children.

5. Post-exposure prophylaxis for close contacts of infected person who are at high risk of complications.
6. Children at high risk and their close contacts if circulating viral strains are not well matched by vaccine.

▶IDSA 2009, CDC 2011, AAP 2016

1. Consider antiviral chemoprophylaxis for adults and children age >1 y at high risk of influenza complications (see the Influenza, Vaccination section) when any of the following conditions are present:
   a. Influenza vaccination is contraindicated (anaphylactic hypersensitivity to eggs, acute febrile illness, history of Guillain-Barré syndrome within 6 wk of a previous influenza vaccination.)
   b. Unvaccinated adults or children when influenza activity has been detected in the community. Vaccinate simultaneously.
   c. Unvaccinated adults and children in close contact with people diagnosed with influenza.
   d. Residents of extended-care facilities with an influenza outbreak.

Sources
–CID 2009;48:1003-32
–CDC: https://www.cdc.gov/flu/professionals/antivirals/summary-clinicians.htm

Comments

1. Influenza vaccination is the best way to prevent influenza.
2. Antiviral chemoprophylaxis is not a substitute for influenza vaccination.
3. Agents for chemoprophylaxis of influenza A (H1N1) and B: zanamivir or oseltamivir.
4. Children at high risk of complications include those with chronic diseases such as asthma, diabetes, cardiac disease, immune suppression and neurodevelopmental disorders.

INFLUENZA, VACCINATION

Population
–All persons age >6 mo.

Recommendations

▶CDC 2016, AAP 2016

1. All persons age >6 mo should receive the seasonal influenza vaccine annually.
2. All children age 6 mo to 8 y should receive 2 doses of the vaccine (>4 wk apart) during their first season of vaccination.
3. The live attenuated influenza vaccine (Flumist quadrivalent) should not be used due to low efficacy.

Sources
–*Pediatrics.* 2016;138(4):e20162527.
–CDC: https://www.cdc.gov/vaccines/hcp/acip-recs/vacc-specific/flu.html

Comment

1. Highest-risk groups for influenza complications are:
   –Pregnant women.
   –Children age 6 mo to 5 y.
   –Adults age >50 y.
   –Persons with chronic medical conditions.[a]
   –Residents of extended-care facilities.
   –Morbidly obese (BMI >40) persons.
   –Health care personnel.
   –Household contacts of persons with high-risk medical conditions or caregivers of children age <5 y or adults age >50 y.
   –Children and adolescents receiving long-term aspirin therapy.
   –American Indians or Alaska Natives.

KIDNEY INJURY, ACUTE

Population

–Adults and children.

Recommendations

▶NICE 2013, VA/DoD 2014

–Recommend volume expansion to at risk adults who will receive intravenous iodinated contrast.
  • CKD with eGFR <40 mL/min.
  • CHF.
  • Renal transplant.
  • 75 y or over.
–Consult a pharmacist to assist with drug dosing in adults or children at risk for AKI.

Sources
–Acute kidney injury. Prevention, detection and management of acute kidney injury up to the point of renal replacement therapy. London (UK): National Institute for Health and Care Excellence (NICE); 2013.
–VA/DoD clinical practice guideline for the management of chronic kidney disease in primary care. Washington (DC): Department of Veterans Affairs, Department of Defense; 2014.

[a]Chronic heart, lung, renal, liver, hematologic, cancer, neuromuscular, or seizure disorders, severe cognitive dysfunction, diabetes, HIV infection, or immunosuppression.

Comment

–Inconsistent evidence for *N*-acetylcysteine use to prevent contrast-induced nephropathy.

MOTOR VEHICLE INJURY

Population

–Infants, children, and adolescents.

Recommendations

▶ICSI 2013

1. Providers should ask the family about the use of car seats, booster seats, and seat belts.
2. Ask children and adolescents about helmet use in recreational activities.

Source

–ISCI: Preventive Services for Children and Adolescents, 19th Ed. 2013.

Comments

1. Head injury rates are reduced by approximately 75% in motorcyclists who wear helmets compared with those who do not.
2. Properly used child restraint systems can reduce mortality up to 21% compared with seat belt usage in children age 2–6 y.

Population

–Elderly.

Recommendation

▶EAST 2015

–Screen for risk factors for MVC-related injury (alcohol abuse, frailty, DM, hearing impairment, visual impairment, CAD).

Source

–*J Trauma Acute Care Surg.* 2015;79(1):152

Comment

–Behavioral interventions (ie, seat-belt reminder signs near senior centers) improve safety practices.

MYOCARDIAL INFARCTION (MI), ASPIRIN THERAPY

Population

–Asymptomatic adults.

Recommendations

▶ACCP 2012, USPSTF 2016

–Age 50–59 y: Initiate aspirin if 10-y CVD risk is >10%, life expectancy is >10 y, and willing to take low-dose aspirin consistently for 10 y.

–Age 60–69 y: "Consider" aspirin if 10-y CVD risk is >10%, especially if at low risk for bleeding, have life expectancy > 10 y, and are willing to take aspirin consistently for 10 y (fewer MIs are prevented and more GI bleeds are provoked compared to the 50–59 y age group).

–Age <50 y: evidence insufficient, benefit likely less because CVD risk is likely lower.

–Age >70 y: evidence insufficient, risk of bleeding increases significantly.

▶FDA 2016

–Data do not support the general use of aspirin for primary prevention of a heart attack or stroke. Aspirin is associated with "serious risks," including increased risk of intracerebral and GI bleeding.

Sources

–USPSTF: Aspirin Use to Prevent Cardiovascular Disease and Colorectal Cancer : Preventive Medication. 2016.

–*Chest.* 2012;141(2 Suppl):e637S-68S.

–FDA: Use of Aspirin for Primary Prevention of Heart Attack and Stroke. 2016.

Comments

–ACC/AHA "ABCS" of primary prevention presents risk reduction for ASCVD for mainstays of primary prevention: Aspirin therapy in appropriate patients (RR 0.90), Blood pressure control (RR 0.84 for CHD, 0.64 for Stroke), Cholesterol management (RR 0.75) and Smoking cessation (RR 0.73). *JACC.* 2017;69(12):1617-1636.

–Risks of aspirin therapy: hemorrhagic stroke and GI bleeding (risk factors include age, male sex, GI ulcers, upper GI pain, concurrent NSAID/anticoagulant use, and uncontrolled hypertension).

–Establish risk factors by the ACC/AHA pooled cohort equation in all adults.

–In a report showing a 50% reduction in the population's CHD mortality rate, 81% was attributable to primary prevention of CHD through tobacco cessation and lipid- and blood pressure-lowering activities. Only 19% of CHD mortality reduction occurred in patients with existing CHD (secondary prevention). *BMJ.* 2005;331:614.

MYOCARDIAL INFARCTION (MI), DIETARY THERAPY

Population
–All adults.

Recommendations
▶AHA/ACC 2013, ESC 2012, AHA/ACCF 2011

–*Dietary guidelines*: (1) Balance calorie intake and physical activity to achieve or maintain a healthy body weight. (2) Consume diet rich in vegetables and fruits. (3) Choose whole grain, high-fiber foods. (4) Consume fish, especially oily fish, at least twice a week. (5) Limit intake of saturated fats to <7% energy, trans fats to <1% energy, and cholesterol to <300 mg/d by:
  • Choosing lean meats and vegetable alternatives.
  • Selecting fat-free (skim), 1% fat, and low-fat dairy products.
  • Minimizing intake of partially hydrogenated fats. (6) Minimize intake of beverages and foods with added sugars. (7) Choose and prepare foods with little or no salt. (8) If you consume alcohol, do so in moderation. (9) Follow these recommendations for food consumed/prepared inside *and* outside of the home.
–Recommended diets: DASH, USDA Food Pattern, or AHA Diet. *Avoid use of and exposure to tobacco products.*

▶CCS 2012

–The Mediterranean, Portfolio, or DASH diets are recommended to improve lipid profiles or decrease cardiovascular disease (CVD) risk.

Sources
–Eckel RH, Jakicic JM, Ard JD, et al. 2013 ACC/AHA Guideline on lifestyle management to reduce CV risk: a report of the American College of Cardiology/American Heart Association Task Force on Practice Guidelines.
–*Can J Cardiol.* 2013;29(2):151-167.

MYOCARDIAL INFARCTION (MI), STATIN THERAPY

Population
–Asymptomatic adults.

Recommendations

▶ACC/AHA 2013
–10-y ASCVD risk score (updated ATP III guidelines): 3 high-risk groups identified, based on ASCVD score and LDL-C levels.
–Lifestyle management and drug therapy recommended in all three categories.
–Statin drugs remain the treatment of choice based upon outcome data.
–For therapy see Chapter 3 (page 258).

Source
–Stone NJ, Robinson JG, Lichtenstein AH, et al. 2013 ACC/AHA Guideline on the Treatment of Blood Cholesterol to Reduce Atherosclerotic Cardiovascular Disease Risk in Adults: a report of the American College of Cardiology/American Heart Association Task Force on Practice Guidelines. Circulation. 2014:24;129(25 Suppl 2):S1-45.

▶Cochrane 2011
–Statin therapy should be employed in primary prevention only in high-risk patients (Framingham risk >20%).
–Restraint should be exercised in patients at low or intermediate 10-y risk (<10%; 10%–20%).
–If low or intermediate 10-y risk, calculate *lifetime risk* to better assess benefit of statin therapy.

Sources
–*Cochrane Database Syst Rev.* 2011;(1):CD004816
–*Am J Med.* 2012;125:440-446
–*Circulation.* 2006;113:791-798
–*N Engl J Med.* 2012;366:321-329

▶ACP 2004

–Statins should be used for primary prevention of macrovascular complications if patient has type 2 DM and other CV risk factors (age >55 y, left ventricular hypertrophy, previous cerebrovascular disease, peripheral arterial disease, smoking, or HTN).

Comments

1. Short-term reduction in low-density lipoprotein (LDL) using dietary counseling by dietitians is superior to that achieved by physicians. (*Am J Med*. 2000;109:549)
2. Statin therapy can safely reduce the 5-y incidence of major CVD events (coronary revascularization, stroke) by about one-fifth per mmol/L reduction in LDL cholesterol. (*Lancet*. 2005;366(9493):1267-1278)

▶CCS 2013

–An increased risk of new-onset type 2 diabetes might apply to statin therapy. A recent review of the existing data suggest that potential mechanisms include increased insulin levels, reduced insulin sensitivity, and selection bias. However, the overall data strongly suggest that the reduction in CVD events outweighs the minor effect on glucose homeostasis.

Source

–*Can J Cardiol*. 2013;29(2):151-167.

▶Society of General Internal Medicine 2015

–Statin use was associated with an increased likelihood of new diagnoses of DM, diabetic complications, and overweight/obesity in healthy people taking statin for primary prevention.

Source

–Mansi I, Frei CR, Wang CP, Mortensen EM. Statins and new-onset diabetes mellitus and diabetic complications: a retrospective cohort study of US healthy adults. *J Gen Intern Med*. 2015;30:1599.

▶FDA Warning 2012, CCS 2013

–Statins may cause nonserious reversible cognitive side effects as well as increased blood sugar and HbA1c levels.

Sources

–*N Engl J Med*. 2012;366:321-329
–*Ann Intern Med*. 2004;140(8):644-649.

Population
    –History of CVA.
Recommendation
▶AHA/ASA 2012
    –Large-vessel ischemic stroke is a CHD risk. Small-vessel disease, may
    be considered CHD risk equivalent.
Source
        –*Stroke.* 2012;43(7):1998-2027.
Comment
    –Meta-analysis concludes ASA prophylaxis reduces ischemic stroke risk
    in women (–17%) and MI events in men (–32%). No mortality benefit
    is seen in either group. Risk of bleeding is increased in both groups to
    a similar degree as the event rate reduction. Initiation of therapy based
    on a case by case basis. (*JAMA.* 2006;295:306-313) (*Arch Intern Med.*
    2012;172:209-216)

MYOCARDIAL INFARCTION (MI), SPECIAL POPULATIONS

Population
    –Adults with HTN.
Recommendations
▶JNC 8, 2013
    –See Chapter 3, page 360 for JNC 8 treatment algorithms.
Source
    –*JAMA.* 2014;311(5):507-520
▶AHA/ACCF 2012, ACP 2007, AHA/ACC/ASH 2015
    –Goal: blood pressure (BP) <140/90 mm Hg for population with
    stable CAD.
    –BP target <140/90 mm Hg is reasonable for the secondary prevention
    of CV events in patients with HTN and CAD. Class IIa, level of
    evidence, B.
    –BP target <130/80 mm Hg may be appropriate in some individuals with
    CAD, previous MI, stroke or TIA, or CAD risk equivalents (carotid
    artery disease, PAD, abdominal aortic aneurysm). Class IIb, level of
    evidence, B.
    –In patients with an elevated DBP and CAD with evidence of myocardial
    ischemia, BP should be lowered slowly, and caution is advised in
    inducing decreases in DBP <60 mm Hg in any patients with DM or

who is >60 y. In older hypertensive patients with wide pulse pressures, lowering SBP may cause very low DBP values <60 mm Hg. This should alert clinicians to assess carefully any untoward signs or symptoms, especially those resulting from myocardial ischemia. Class IIa, level of evidence, C.

–If ventricular dysfunction is present, lowering the goal to 120/80 mm Hg may be considered.

Sources
–*Circulation*. 2007;115:2761-2788
–*Circulation*. 2012;26:3097-3137
–Rosendorff C, Lackland DT, Allison M, et al. Treatment of HTN in patients with CAD. *J Am Coll Cardiol*. 2015;65(18):1998-2038.

▶CHEP 2015, ESC 2014
–Recommends low-dose ASA for vascular protection, in hypertensive patients ≥ 50 y; caution should be exercised if BP is not controlled.
–Low-dose ASA for hypertensives with h/o CV events; consider in hypertensives without prior history who are at higher risk

Sources
–Hypertension Canada: https://guidelines.hypertension.ca
–*Eur Heart J*. 2012;33(13):1635

▶ESC/ECH 2013
–<130/80 mm Hg goal in diabetics and other high-risk patients has not been supported by trials. No benefit and possible harm is suggested with SBP <130 mm Hg.
–Elderly patients' SBP goal is <160 mm Hg.

Source
–*J Hypertens*. 2013;31:1281-1357

Population
–Diabetes mellitus.

Recommendation
▶ADA 2014
–Lipid Goals: Normal fasting glucose (≤130 mg/dL) and HbA1c (<7.5%), BP <140/80 mm Hg; low-density-lipoprotein cholesterol (LDL-C) <100 mg/dL (or <70 for high risk), high-density-lipoprotein cholesterol (HDL-C) >50 mg/dL and triglycerides <150 mg/dL.
–Consider ASA (75–162 mg/d) if at increased CV risk (10-y > 10% based on Framingham risk score (see Chapter 4, pages 536–539), and in men age >50 y or women age >60 y with one additional risk factor.

Sources
  -*N Engl J Med.* 2008;358:2545-2559
  -*N Engl J Med.* 2008;358:2560-2572
  -*Diabetes Care.* 2014;37(s1): S14-S80.

Population
  -Smoking.

Recommendation
▶AHA 2006, ADA 2014
  -Advise all patients not to smoke.

Sources
  -*Diabetes Care.* 2014;37(1)
  -*Circulation. 2006;114:82-96*

Comments
1. Intensive glucose lowering should be avoided in patients with a history of hypoglycemic spells, advanced microvascular or macrovascular complications, long-standing DM, or if extensive comorbid conditions are present.
2. DM with BP readings of 130–139/80–89 mm Hg that persist after lifestyle and behavioral therapy should be treated with angiotensin-converting enzyme (ACE) inhibitor or angiotensin receptor blocker (ARB) agents. Multiple agents are often needed. *Administer at least one agent at bedtime.*
3. No advantage of combining ACE inhibitor and ARB in HTN Rx (ONTARGET Trial). (*N Engl J Med.* 2008;358:1547-1559)

Recommendation
▶ESC 2012
  -Avoid passive smoking.

Source
  -*Eur Heart J.* 2012;33:1635-1701

Comment
  -New evidence on the health effects of passive smoking strengthens the recommendation on passive smoking. Smoking bans in public places, by law, lead to a decrease in incidence of myocardial infarction.

Population

–Women.

Recommendations

▶AHA 2011

–Standard CVD lifestyle recommendations, *plus:*

–Waist circumference <35 in.

–Omega-3 fatty acids if high risk (EPA 1800 mg/d).[a]

–BP <120/80 mm Hg.

–Lipids: LDL-C <100 mg/dL, HDL-C >50 mg/dL, triglycerides <150 mg/dL.

–ASA (75–325 mg/d) indicated only in high-risk women.[a]

–In women age >65 y, *consider* ASA (81 mg daily or 100 mg every other day) if BP is controlled and the benefit of ischemic stroke and MI prevention is likely to outweigh the risk of a GI bleed and hemorrhagic stroke.

Source

–*J Am Coll Cardiol.* 2011;57(12):1404-1423

Comments

1. Estrogen plus progestin hormone therapy should not be used or continued.
2. Antioxidants (vitamins E and C, and β-carotene), folic acid, and B_{12} supplementation are not recommended to prevent CHD.
3. ASA is not indicated to prevent MI in low-risk women age <65 y.

Population

–Adults at risk of CV disease.

Recommendations

▶ESC 2007, ESC 2012

–Smoking cessation.

–Weight reduction if BMI >25 kg/m^2 or waist circumference >88 cm in women and >102 cm in men.

–No further weight gain if waist circumference 80–88 cm in women and 94–102 cm in men.

–Thirty minutes of moderately vigorous exercise on most days of the week.

–Healthy diet.

–Antihypertensives when BP >140/90 mm Hg. Statins when total cholesterol >190 mg/dL or LDL >115 mg/dL.

–In patients with known CV disease: ASA and statins.

–In patients with DM: glucose-lowering drugs.

---

[a]High risk: CHD or risk equivalent or 10-y absolute CHD risk >20% based on Framingham risk score (see Appendix VI, pages 536–539).

–Psychosocial risk factor.

–Low socioeconomic status, lack of social support, stress at work and in family life, depression, anxiety, hostility, and the type D personality contribute both to the risk of developing CVD and the worsening of clinical course and prognosis of CVD. These factors act as barriers to treatment adherence and efforts to improve lifestyle, as well as to promoting health and well-being in patients and populations. In addition, distinct psychobiologic mechanisms have been identified, which are directly involved in the pathogenesis of CVD.

–Psychological interventions can counteract psychosocial stress and promote healthy behaviors and lifestyle.

–Cognitive-behavioral methods are effective in supporting persons in adopting a healthy lifestyle.

–More evidence on the impact of total diet/dietary patterns such as the Mediterranean type of diet has gained interest in recent years.

–Antihypertensive treatment is beneficial in patients age >80 y.

–Aspirin is no longer recommended for primary prevention in people with diabetes.

–Nurse-coordinated prevention programs are effective across a variety of practice settings.

Sources
–*Eur Heart J.* 2007;28:2375
–*Eur Heart J.* 2012;33:1635-1701

Comment
–European Society of Cardiology recommends using the SCORE Risk System to estimate risk of atherosclerotic CV disease.

NEURAL TUBE DEFECTS

Population
–Women of childbearing age.

Recommendation
▶USPSTF 2016, AAFP 2016, ACOG 2016
–Women should take a daily supplement containing 400–800 µg of folic acid if planning or capable of pregnancy.

Sources
–*JAMA.* 2017;317(2):183-189
–*Int J Gynaecol Obstet.* 2003;83(1):123-33.
–AAFP Clinical Recommendation: http://www.aafp.org/patient-care/clinical-recommendations/all/neural-tube-defects.html

Comments

1. Folic acid supplementation should start at least 1 mo before conception and continue through the first 2–3 mo of pregnancy.
2. The CDC, ACOG, AAFP and AAP recommend 4 mg/d folic acid for women with a history of a child affected by a neural tube defect.

OBESITY

Population

–Adolescents and adults.

Recommendations

▶ICSI 2013

1. Recommends a team approach for weight management in all persons of normal weight (BMI 18.5–24.9) or overweight (BMI 25–29.9) including:
   a. Nutrition.
   b. Physical activity.
   c. Lifestyle changes.
   d. Screen for depression.
   e. Screen for eating disorders.
   f. Review medication list and assess if any medications can interfere with weight loss.
2. Recommends regular follow-up to reinforce principles of weight management.

Source

–Fitch A, Everling L, Fox C et al. Prevention and management of obesity fo radults. Bloomington (MN): ISCI;2013.

Comments

1. Recommend 30–60 min of moderate physical activity on most days of the week.
2. Nutrition education focused on decreased caloric intake, encouraging healthy food choices, and managing restaurant and social eating situations.
3. Weekly weight checks.
4. Encourage nonfood rewards for positive reinforcement.
5. Stress management techniques.
6. 5–10% weight loss can produce a clinically significant reduction in heart disease risk.

Population

–Children.

Recommendations

▶Endocrine Society 2017

1. Educate children and parents about healthy diets and the importance of regular physical activity.
2. Encourage school systems to promote healthy eating habits and provide health education courses.
3. Foster healthy sleep patterns.
4. Balance screen time with opportunities for physical activity.
5. Clinicians should help educate families and communities about healthy dietary and activity habits.

Source

–*J Clin Endocrinol Metab.* 2017;102(3):709-757.

Comments

1. Avoid the consumption of calorie-dense, nutrient-poor foods (eg, juices, soft drinks, "fast food" items, and calorie-dense snacks). Consume whole fruits rather than juices.
2. Control calorie intake by portion control.
3. Reduce saturated dietary fat intake for children age >2 y.
4. Increase dietary fiber, fruits, and vegetables.
5. Eat regular, scheduled meals and avoid snacking.
6. Limit television, video games, and computer time to 2 h daily.

OSTEOPOROTIC HIP FRACTURES

Population

–Postmenopausal women.

Recommendation

▶USPSTF 2012

–Recommends against the routine use of combined estrogen and progestin for the prevention of osteoporotic fractures.

Population

–Postmenopausal women who have had a hysterectomy.

Recommendation

▶USPSTF 2012

–Recommends against the routine use of estrogen for the prevention of osteoporotic fractures in postmenopausal women who have had a hysterectomy

Source
  –USPSTF. Menopausal Hormone Therapy: Preventive Medication. 2012.

Comment
  –The results of studies including the WHI and the Heart and Estrogen/
  Progestin Replacement Study reveal that HRT probably reduces
  osteoporotic hip and vertebral fractures and may decrease the risk of
  colon CA; however, HRT may lead to an increased risk of breast CA,
  stroke, cholecystitis, dementia, and venous thromboembolism. HRT
  does not decrease the risk of coronary artery disease (CAD).

OTITIS MEDIA

Population
  –Children 6 mo to 12 y.

Recommendations
▶AAP 2013
  –Do not use prophylactic antibiotics to reduce the frequency of episodes
  of AOM in children with recurrent AOM.
  –Exclusive breast-feeding for at least the first 6 mo of life.
  –Vaccines recommended for all children to prevent bacterial AOM:
  • Pneumococcal vaccine.
  • Influenza vaccine.
  • Avoid tobacco exposure.

Source
  –*Pediatrics*. 2013;131(3):e964-99

POSTPARTUM HEMORRHAGE

Population
  –Pregnant women.

Recommendations
▶WHO 2012
  –Uterotonic medications should be given to all women during the third
  stage of labor.
  • Oxytocin10 IU, IV, or IM is first choice.
  • Methylergometrine or oral/rectal misoprostol is the alternative.
  –Controlled cord traction is recommended for removal of the placenta.

Source
  –WHO recommendations for the prevention and treatment of postpartum hemorrhage. Geneva (Switzerland): World Health Organization; 2012.

PREECLAMPSIA

Population
  –Pregnant women at increased risk of preeclampsia.

Recommendation
▶USPSTF 2014
  –Use of aspirin 81 mg/d after 12th wk of gestation in women with ≥ 1 major risk factor for preeclampsia.

Source
  –*Ann Intern Med.* 2014;161:819-826

Comment
  –Major risk factors: personal history of preecclampsia, multifetal gestation, chronic hypertension, DM, renal disease, autoimmune disease.

PRETERM BIRTH

Population
  –Pregnant women.

Recommendations
▶ACOG 2012
  –Advise against the use of maintenance tocolytics to prevent preterm birth.
  –Avoid antibiotics for the purpose of prolonging gestation or improving neonatal outcome in preterm labor and intact membranes.
  –In women with prior spontaneous preterm delivery, progesterone therapy should be started between 16–24 wk gestation.

Source
  –*Obstet Gynecol.* 2012;120(4):964-973.

Comments
  –No evidence to support the use of prolonged tocolytics for women with preterm labor.
  –No evidence to support strict bed rest for the prevention of preterm birth.
  –The positive predictive value of a positive fetal fibronectin test or a short cervix for preterm birth is poor in isolation.

PRESSURE ULCERS

Population
–Adults or children with impaired mobility.

Recommendations
▶NICE 2014, ACP 2015

1. Recommend a risk assessment of all persons in both outpatient and inpatient settings (eg, the Braden Scale in adults and Braden Q Scale in children).
2. Recommend education of patient, family, and caregivers regarding the causes and risk factors of pressure ulcers.
3. Recommend caution when using compression stockings with lower-extremity arterial disease.
4. Avoid thigh-high stockings when compression stockings are used.
    a. Avoid dragging patient when moving.
    b. Pad skin-to-skin contact.
    c. Lubricate or powder bed pans prior to placing under patient.
    d. Keep skin moisturized.
5. Recommend minimizing pressure on skin, especially areas with bony prominences.
    a. Turn patient side-to-side every 2 h.
    b. Pad areas over bony prominences.
    c. Use heel protectors or place pillows under calves.
    d. Consider a bariatric bed for patients weighing over 300 lb.
    e. Consider high-specification foam (not air) mattress for high-risk patients admitted to secondary care or who are undergoing surgery.
6. Recommend managing moisture.
    a. Moisture barrier protectant on skin.
    b. Frequent diaper changes.
    c. Scheduled toileting.
    d. Treat candidiasis if present.
    e. Consider a rectal tube for stool incontinence with diarrhea.
7. Recommend maintaining adequate nutrition and hydration.
8. Recommend keeping the head of the bed at or <30° elevation.

Sources
–National Clinical Guideline Centre. Pressure ulcers: prevention and management of pressure ulcers. London (UK): National Institute for Health and Care Excellence; 2014
–*Ann Intern Med.* 2015;162(5):359-69.

Comment

1. Outpatient risk assessment for pressure ulcers:
   a. Is the patient bed or wheel chair bound?
   b. Does the patient require assistance for transfers?
   c. Is the patient incontinent of urine or stool?
   d. Any history of pressure ulcers?
   e. Does the patient have a clinical condition placing the patient at risk for pressure ulcers?
      i. DM.
      ii. Peripheral vascular disease.
      iii. Stroke.
      iv. Polytrauma.
      v. Musculoskeletal disorders (fractures or contractures).
      vi. Spinal cord injury.
      vii. Guillain-Barré syndrome.
      viii. Multiple sclerosis.
      ix. CA.
      x. Chronic obstructive pulmonary disease.
      xi. Coronary heart failure.
      xii. Dementia.
      xiii. Preterm neonate.
      xiv. Cerebral palsy.
   f. Does the patient appear malnourished?
   g. Is equipment in use that could contribute to ulcer development (eg, oxygen tubing, prosthetic devices, urinary catheter)?

SEXUALLY TRANSMITTED INFECTIONS (STIS)

Population
–Sexually active adolescents and high-risk adults.

Recommendation

▶USPSTF 2014

–Recommend high-intensity behavioral counseling to prevent STIs for all sexually active adolescents and for adults at increased risk for STIs. Include basic information about STIs, condom use, communication about safe sex, problem solving, and goal setting.

Source
–USPSTF: Sexually Transmitted Infections. 2014.

STROKE

Population
–Adults.

Recommendations

▶AHA/ASA 2011
–Treat known CV risk factors.[a]

▶FDA 2014
–FDA does not support the general use of aspirin for primary prevention of strokes or heart attacks, given risk of cerebral and gastroenteral bleeding.

Sources
–FDA Consumer Updates 2014: https://www.fda.gov/Drugs/ResourcesForYou/Consumers/ucm390574.htm
–*Stroke*. 2011;42:517-584

STROKE, ATRIAL FIBRILLATION

Population
–Atrial fibrillation.

Recommendations

▶AHA/ACC 2014, 2015

1. Prioritize rate control; consider rhythm control if this is the first event, and if it occurs in a young patient with minimal heart disease or if symptomatic.
2. Rate control goal is <110 beats/min in patients with stable ventricular function (ejection fraction [EF] >40%).
3. Antithrombotic therapy is required. Anticoagulation or antiplatelet therapy is determined by ACC/AHA or CHA_2DS_2VASc (nonvalvular atrial fibrillation) guidelines.
4. For patients with AF who have mechanical valves, warfarin is recommended with an INR target of 2–3 or 2.5–3.5, depending on the type and location of prosthesis.
5. For patients with non-valvular AF with a history of stroke, TIA or $CHA_2DS_2VASc \geq 2$, oral anticoagulation is recommended: warfarin (INR: 2–3) or DOACs (novel oral anticoagulation agents)—see treatment.

[a]Major modifiable risk factors: hypertension, cigarette smoke exposure, diabetes, atrial fibrillation, dyslipidemia, carotid artery stenosis, sickle cell disease, postmenopausal hormone therapy, poor diet, physical inactivity, obesity.

6. In patients treated with warfarin, INR should be performed weekly until INR is stable and at least monthly when INR is in range and stable.

7. Renal function should be evaluated prior to initiation of direct thrombin or factor Xa inhibitors and should be reevaluated when clinically indicated and at least annually.

8. Initially clinicians should identify low-risk AF patients who do not require antithrombotic therapy (CHA_2DS_2VASc score, 0 for men, 1 for women). Patients with at least 1 risk factor (except when the only risk is being a woman) should be offered OAC. The patient's individual risk of bleeding should be addressed (BP control, discontinuing unnecessary medications such as ASA or non-steroidal anti-inflammatory drugs).

9. In non-valvular AF with $CHA_2DS_2VASc = 0$ no antithrombotic therapy or treatment with ASA or an OAC may be considered.

10. Following coronary revascularization (PCI or surgical) in patients with $CHA_2DS_2VASc \geq 2$, may be reasonable to use Clopidogrel with OAC but without ASA.

Sources
–*Circulation.* 2014;130(23):e199-267.
–*JAMA.* 2015;313(19):1950-1962.

Comments

1. Strokes and nonfatal strokes are reduced in diabetic patients by lower BP targets (<130/80 mm Hg). In the absence of harm, this benefit appears to justify the lower BP goal.

2. Average stroke rate in patients with risk factors is approximately 5% per year.

3. Adjusted-dose warfarin and antiplatelet agents reduce absolute risk of stroke.

4. Women have a higher prevalence of stroke than men.

5. Women have unique risk factors for stroke, such as pregnancy, hormone therapy, and higher prevalence of hypertension in older ages.

Population
–Atrial fibrillation.

Recommendations

▶ECS 2010, 2012

–ESC recommends the CHA_2DS_2VASc score as more predictive for stroke risk, especially with a low $CHADS_2$ score. DOACs offer better efficacy, safety, and convenience compared with OAC with VKAs.

–In high-risk patient unsuitable for anticoagulation, dual antiplatelet therapy (ASA plus clopidogrel) is reasonable.

Sources
   –*Eur Heart J.* 2010;31:2369-2429
   –*Eur Heart J. 2012;33:2719-2747*

Comments

1. Absolute cerebrovascular accident (CVA) risk reduction with dual antiplatelet Rx is 0.8% per year balanced by increased bleeding risk 0.7% ACTIVE Trial.
2. In high-risk patients with history of TIA/minor ischemic stroke, dual antiplatelet therapy (ASA+Plavix), started in the first 24 h, is superior to ASA alone in preventing stroke in the first 90 d, without having increased risk of hemorrhage.

Population

–Atrial fibrillation.

Recommendations

▶FDA Warning 2011

–Dronedarone should not be used in patients who have chronic AF with associated severe HF or LV systolic dysfunction.
–See Management Algorithm. For therapy, see Chapter 3, page 194 pharmacologic and antithrombotic recommendations.
–Dronedarone is contraindicated in patients with NYHA Class IV heart failure or NYHA Class II–III heart failure with a recent decompensation requiring hospitalization or referral to a specialized heart failure clinic.
–Dronedarone reduces the incidence of AF recurrences, hospitalization, and death in patients with paroxysmal or persistent AF. However, dronedarone should not be used in high-risk patients with permanent AF or patients with unstable chronic heart failure (HF) due to safety concerns. *J Clin Pharm Ther.* 2014;39(2):112-117.

Sources
   –http://www.fda.gov/Drugs/DrugSafety/ucm240011.htm

Comment

–Dronedarone doubles rate of CV death, stroke, and heart failure in patients with chronic atrial fibrillation.

Population

–Atrial fibrillation.

Recommendations

▶HRS 2014, 2015

–Given the impact of AF on stroke and the association of AF with cognitive dysfunction, brain imaging may improve the care of AF patients by helping to stratify stroke risk in AF patients. Presence of subclinical brain infarcts is robustly associated with the subsequent risk of stroke. Short-term risk of stroke after transient ischemic attack (TIA) was 3-fold higher in patients with a brain infarct on MRI compared to those without.

–Compared to warfarin, DOACs offer relative efficacy, safety, and convenience. Warfarin efficacy and safety depend on the quality of anticoagulation control, as reflected by the average time in therapeutic range (TTR). Due to the difficulty of achieving therapeutic international normalized ratios (INRs) quickly after starting warfarin, an increased risk of stroke has been observed in the 30 d after initiation of warfarin.

–In patients with nonvalvular atrial fibrillation, a high SAMe-TT2R2 score (reflecting poor anticoagulation control with poor time in therapeutic range) was associated with more bleeding, adverse cardiovascular events, and mortality during follow-up.

Sources
–*Heart Rhythm.* 2015;12(1):e5-e25.
–*Am J Med.* 2014;127(11):1083-1088.

Population
–Atrial fibrillation.

Recommendations
▶CCS 2012

–All patients should be stratified using $CHADS_2$ and HASBLED risk scores. Patients with $CHADS_2$ = 0 should have $CHADS_2$-VaSc score calculated. All patients with $CHADS_2$ = 2 and most of the ones with $CHADS_2$ = 1 should have OAC therapy.

–When OAC therapy is recommended, dabigatran and rivaroxaban are preferred over warfarin. Rate control goal is <100 beats/min. In stable CAD, ASA (75–325 mg) for $CHADS_2$ = 0, OAC for most $CHADS_2$ = 1. In high-risk patients with ACS, ASA + clopidogrel + OAC might be required (with adequate assessment of risk of stroke, recurrent CAD events, and hemorrhage).

Source
–*Can J Cardiol.* 2012;28:125-136

STROKE,ᵃ SPECIAL POPULATIONS

Population
- –HTN.

Recommendations

▶JNC 8
- –Treat to goal SBP <140 mm Hg.
- –If age ≥60 y, treat to <150/90.
- –If comorbid diabetes or chronic kidney disease, treat to <140/90 mm Hg.

▶AHA/ASA 2011
- –Treat to goal <140/90 mmHg.
- –If HTN with diabetes or renal disease, treat to <130/80 mm Hg.

Comments
- –See Chapter 3 (page 360) for JNC-8 treatment algorithms.

Sources
- –*JAMA*. 2014;311(5):507-520.
- –*Stroke*. 2011;42:517-584

Population
- –DM.

Recommendations

▶AHA/ASA 2011
1. Six-fold increase of stroke.
2. Short-term glycemic control does not lower macro vascular events.
3. HgA1c goal is <6.5%.
4. Goal is <130/80 mm Hg.
5. Statin therapy.
6. Consider ACE inhibitor or ARB therapy for further stroke risk reduction.

Source
- –*Stroke*. 2011;42:517-584

Population
- –Asymptomatic CAS.

Recommendations

▶USPSTF 2014, AHA/ASA 2011
1. No indication for general screening for CAS with ultrasonography.
2. Screen for other stroke risk factors and treat aggressively.

ᵃAssess risk of stroke in all patients. See Appendix VII, pages 540–543 for risk assessment tool.

3. ASA unless contraindicated.

4. Prophylactic carotid endarterectomy (CEA) for patients with high-grade (>70%) CAS by ultrasonography when performed by surgeons with low (<3%) morbidity/mortality rates may be useful in selected cases depending on life expectancy, age, sex, and comorbidities.

5. However, recent studies have demonstrated that "best" medical therapy results in a stroke rate <1%.

6. The number needed to treat (NNT) in published trials to prevent one stroke in 1 y in this asymptomatic group varies from 84 up to 2000. (*J Am Coll Cardiol.* 2011;57(8):e16-e94)

Sources

1. USPSTF: Carotid Artery Stenosis: https://www.uspreventiveservice staskforce.org/Page/Document/RecommendationStatementFinal/ carotid-artery-stenosis-screening

2. *Neurology.* 2011;77:751-758

3. *Neurology.* 2011;77:744-750

4. *Stroke.* 2011;42:517-584

Population

–Symptomatic CAS.

Recommendations

▶ASA/ACCF/AHA/AANN/AANS/ACR/CNS 2011

–Optimal timing for CEA is within 2 wk of posttransient ischemic attack.

–CEA plus medical therapy is effective within 6 mo of symptom onset with >70% CAS.

–Intense medical therapy alone is indicated if the occlusion is <50%.

–Intensive medical therapy plus CEA may be considered with obstruction 50%–69%.

–Surgery should be *limited* to male patients with a low perioperative stroke/death rate (<6%) and should have a life expectancy of at least 5 y.

Sources

–*J Am Coll Cardiol.* 2011;57(8):1002-1038

–*Neurology.* 2005;65(6):794-801

–*Arch Intern Med.*2011;171(20):1794-1795

–*Stroke.* 2011;42:517-584

–*Stroke.* 2011;42:227-276

Comments

–Medical treatment of asymptomatic CAS should be aggressive.

–Surgical intervention should be individualized, guided by comparing comorbid medical conditions and life expectancy to the surgical morbidity and mortality.

–Atherosclerotic intracranial stenosis: ASA should be used in preference to warfarin.

–Warfarin—significantly higher rates of adverse events with no benefit over ASA. (*N Engl J Med.* 2005;352(13):1305-1316)

–Qualitative findings (embolic signals and plaque ulceration) may identify patients who would benefit from asymptomatic CEA.

Populations

–Cryptogenic CVA.

–Hyperlipidemia.

Recommendations

▶ASA/ACCF/AHA/AANN/AANS/ACR/CNS 2011

–Carotid artery stenting is associated with increased nonfatal stroke frequency but this is offset by decreased risk of MI post-CEA.

–Cryptogenic CVA with patent foramen ovale should receive ASA 81 mg/d.

Sources

–*J Am Coll Cardol.* 2011;57(8):1002-1044.

–*J Am Coll Cardiol.*2009;53(21):2014-2018

–*N Engl J Med.* 2012;366:991-999

–*N Engl J Med.* 2013;368:1083-1091

Comments

–Consider referral to tertiary center for enrollment in randomized trial to determine optimal Rx.

–Closure I trial demonstrated no benefit at 2 y of patent foramen ovale (PFO) closure device over medical therapy.

–In 2013, the PC Trial also failed to demonstrate significant benefit in reducing recurrent embolic events in patients undergoing PFO closure compared to medical therapy, at 4 y follow-up.

Population

–Sickle cell disease.

Recommendations

▶ASA/ACCF/AHA/AANN/AANS/ACR/CNS 2011

–Transfusion therapy (target reduction of hemoglobin S from a baseline of >90% to <30%) is effective for reducing stroke risk in those children at elevated stroke risk (*Class I; level of evidence, B*).

–Begin screening with transcranial Doppler (TCD) at age 2 y.

–Transfusion therapy is recommended for patients at high-stroke risk per TCD (high cerebral blood flow velocity >200 cm/s).

–Frequency of screening not determined.

Sources
−*J Am Coll Cardol.* 2011;57(8):1002-1044.
−*ASH Education Book.* 2013;2013(1):439-446.

Population
−Primary prevention in women.

Recommendations

▶ACC/ASA 2014

−Higher lifetime risk, third leading cause of death in women, 53.5% of new recurrent strokes occur in women.
−Sex-specific risk factors: pregnancy, preeclampsia, gestational diabetes, oral contraceptive use, postmenopausal hormone use, changes in hormonal status.
−Risk factors with a stronger prevalence in women: migraine with aura, atrial fibrillation, diabetes, hypertension, depression, psychosocial stress.

Source
−*Circulation.* 2011;123:1243-1262

Population
−Oral contraceptives/menopause, postmenopausal hormone therapy.

Recommendations

▶ACC/ASA 2014

−Stroke risk with low-dose OC users is about 1.4–2 times that of non-OC users.
−Measurement of BP is recommended prior to initiation of hormonal contraception therapy.
−Routine screening for prothrombotic mutations prior to initiation of hormonal contraception is not useful.
−Among OC users, aggressive therapy of stroke risk factors may be reasonable.
−Hormone therapy (conjugated equine estrogen with or without medroxyprogesterone) should not be used for primary or secondary prevention of stroke in postmenopausal women.
−Selective estrogen receptor modulators, such as raloxifene, tamoxifen, or tibolone, should not be used for primary prevention of stroke.

Source
−*Stroke.* 2014;45:1545-1588

SAM$_E$TT$_2$R$_2$ SCORE	
Sex (female)	1
Age > 60	1
Medical history (> 2 comorbidities: HTN, DM, CAD/MI, PAD, CHF, history of stroke, pulmonary disease, hepatic or renal disease)	1
Treatment (rhythm control strategy) (interacting medications, eg, beta-blocker, verapamil, amiodarone)	1
Tobacco use (within 2 y)	2
Race (non-white)	2
Maximum points	8
Interpretation	Score > 2 = DOAC Score 0–2 = VKA with TTR > 65%–70%

Source: Fauchier L, Angoulvant D, Lip GY. The SAMe-TT$_2$R$_2$ score and quality of anticoagulation in atrial fibrillation: a simple aid to decision-making on who is suitable (or not) for vitamin K antagonists. doi: http://dx.doi.org/10.1093/europace/euv088.

SUDDEN INFANT DEATH SYNDROME (SIDS)

Population
–Newborns and infants.

Recommendation
▶AAP 2016
–Place their infants to sleep on their backs
–Use a firm sleep surface without soft objects or loose bedding.
–Breastfeed.
–For the first 6–12 m, infants should sleep in parents' room (but not in parents' bed).
–Avoid smoke exposure, alcohol and illicit drug use, overheating.

Source
–*Pediatrics*. 2016;138(5):e20162938

Comments
–Stomach and side sleeping have been identified as major risk factors for SIDS.
–Pacifiers may be protective.

SURGICAL SITE INFECTIONS (SSI)

Population
-Women undergoing cesarean sections.

Recommendations

▶Cochrane Database of Systematic Reviews 2014
-Recommend a vaginal preparation with povidone-iodine solution immediately prior to cesarean delivery.
-Recommend administration of prophylactic IV antibiotics preoperatively within 60 min of skin incision as opposed to administration after cord clamping.

Source
-http://www.cochrane.org/CD007892/PREG_vaginal-cleansing-before-cesarean-delivery-to-reduce-post-cesarean-infections

Comments
-A vaginal prep prior to cesarean section reduces the incidence of postpartum endometritis. This benefit was especially true for women in active labor or with rupture membranes.
-The incidence of maternal infectious morbidity is decreased (RR 0.54) when prophylactic antibiotics are administered preoperatively as opposed to after cord clamping.

TOBACCO USE

Population
-School-aged children and adolescents.

Recommendation

▶AAFP/USPSTF 2013
-Recommends that primary care clinicians provide interventions including education or brief counseling to prevent the initiation of tobacco use.

Comment
-The efficacy of counseling to prevent tobacco use in children and adolescents is uncertain.

Source
-USPSTF: Tobacco Use in Children and Adolescents: Primary Care Interventions. 2013.

VENOUS THROMBOEMBOLISM (VTE) PROPHYLAXIS IN NONSURGICAL PATIENTS

Populations
–Medical patients with low risk (**Padua Prediction score—see Table I**).
–Medical patients with high risk (*JAMA*. 2012;307:306)(**Padua Prediction score—see Table I**).

Recommendations
▶ACCP 2016, ACP 2011
–Recommend against the use of pharmacologic prophylaxis or mechanical prophylaxis in low risk patients.
–Recommend anticoagulant in high risk patients
  • Thromboprophylaxis with low-molecular-weight heparin (LMWH)—equivalent of enoxaparin 40 mg SQ daily; fondaparinux 2.5 mg SQ daily. Low-dose unfractionated heparin (UFH) 5000 units bid or tid should be used only in patients with significant renal diseae. UFH has a 10-fold increased risk of heparin induced thrombocytopenia (HIT). Women are 2.5 times likely to develop HIT compared to men.
  • If patient bleeding or high risk of bleeding (see Table II), mechanical prophylaxis with graduated compression stockings (GCS) or intermittent pneumatic compression (IPC) recommended.
  • When bleeding risk decreases, substitute pharmacologic thromboprophylaxis for mechanical prophylaxis.
  • Continue thromboprophylaxis for duration of hospital stay.
  • Extended prophylaxis after discharge not recommended for medical patients but should be considered if patient has underlying thrombotic risk (See Table III).

Sources
–*Ann Intern Med.*2011;155:625-632.
–*Chest 2016; 149: 315-352*
–http://www.uwhealth.org/files/uwheath/docs/anticoagulation/VTE

Comments
–**Clinical Perspective**
  • Routine ultrasound screening for DVT is not recommended in any group.
  • 150–200,000 deaths from VTE in the United States per year. Hospitalized patients have a VTE risk which is 130-fold greater than that of community residents. (*Mayo Clin Proc.* 2001;76:1102)
  • Neither heparin nor warfarin is recommended prophylactically for patients with central venous catheters.

- In higher risk long-distance travelers, frequent ambulation, calf muscle exercises, aisle seat, and below-the-knee graduated compression stockings (GCS) are recommended over aspirin or anticoagulants.
- Hospitalized Inpatients with solid tumors without additional risk factors for VTE (history of DVT, thrombophilic drugs, immobilization), should be treated with prophylactic dose LMWH.
- Be cautious in patients with Ccr <20 to 30 mL/min—UFH or dalteparin (half dose) preferred.
- Consider adjusted LMWH dose in patients <50 kg or >110 kg in weight. Monitor with heparin anti 10a activity testing.
- Inferior vena cava (IVC) filter indicated in patients with diagnosed DVT with or without pulmonary embolism (PE) who cannot be anticoagulated because of bleeding. There are no other situations where a filter has been proven to be beneficial.
- IVC filter should not be used prophylactically.
- Although several studies have shown survival benefit for VTE prophylaxis in surgical patients, this has not been proven in medical patients. (*N Engl J Med.* 2011;365:2463) (*N Engl J Med.* 2007;356:1438)
- In patients with cancer and VTE use LMWH. The new oral anticoagulants are being tested and will probably have a role in cancer related VTE in the near future. Warfarin is inferior to LMWH. (*Lancet Oncol.* 2008;9:577) (*Thromb Res.* 2012;130:853)
- In patients with mechanical heart valves use warfarin for anticoagulation. The direct oral anticoagulants(DOACs) are inferior. (*N Engl J Med.* 2013;369:1206)

TABLE I

RISK FACTORS FOR VTE IN HOSPITALIZED MEDICAL PATIENTS—PADUA PREDICTIVE SCALE	
Risk Factor	**Points**
Active cancer[a]	3
Previous VTE	3
Reduced mobility[b]	3
Underlying thrombophilic disorder[c]	3
Recent (<1 mo) trauma or surgery	2
Age (>70 y)	1
Congestive heart failure (CHF) or respiratory failure	1

RISK FACTORS FOR VTE IN HOSPITALIZED MEDICAL PATIENTS—PADUA PREDICTIVE SCALE   (*Continued*)

Risk Factor	Points
Acute MI or stroke	1
Acute infection or inflammatory disorder	1
Obesity (BMI > 30)	1
Thrombophilic drugs (hormones, tamoxifen, erythroid stimulating agents, lenalidomide, bevacizumab)	1
High risk: >4 points—11% risk of VTE without prophylaxis	
Low risk: <3 points—0.3% risk of VTE without prophylaxis	

[a]Local or distant metastasis, chemotherapy or radiation within last 6 mo.
[b]Bed rest for >3 d.
[c]Hereditary thrombophilia (see **Table III**) and antiphospholipid antibody syndrome, nephrotic syndrome, hemolytic anemia.

TABLE II

RISK FACTORS FOR BLEEDING (*CHEST*. 2011;139:69-79)

Risk Factor[c,d]	N = 10,866% of Patients	Overall Risk
Active gastroduodenal ulcer	2.2	4.15
GI bleed <3 mo previous	2.2	3.64
Platelet count <50 K	1.7	3.37
Age ≥85 y (vs. 40 y)	10	2.96
Hepatic failure (INR[a] >1.5)	2	2.18
Renal failure (GFR[b] <30 mL/min)	11	2.14
ICU admission	8.5	2.10
Current cancer	10.7	1.78
Male sex	49.4	1.48

[a]International normalized ratio.
[b]Glomerular filtration rate.
[c]Although not studied in medical patients, antiplatelet therapy would be expected to increase risk of bleeding.
[d]Go to www.outcomes-umassmed.org/IMPROVE/risk_score/vte/index.html to calculate the risk of bleeding for individual patients.

TABLE III

HEREDITARY THROMBOPHILIC DISORDERS		
Disorder	% of U.S. Population	Increase in Lifetime of Risk of Clot
Resistance to activated protein C (factor V Leiden mutation)	5–6	3×
Prothrombin gene mutation	2–3	2.5×
Elevated factor 8 (>175% activity)	6–8	2–3×
Elevated homocysteine	10–15	1.5–2×
Protein C deficiency	0.37	10×
Protein S deficiency	0.5	10×
Antithrombin deficiency	0.1	25×
Homozygous factor V Leiden	0.3	60×

VENOUS THROMBOEMBOLISM (VTE) IN SURGICAL PATIENTS

Populations
- **Risk Stratification**
- **SURGICAL**
  - Low risk—<40 y, minor surgery, no risk factor, Caprini score <2 (see Table IV).
  - Intermediate risk—minor surgery plus risk factors, age 40–60 y, major surgery with no risk factors;[a, b] Caprini score 3–4.
  - High risk—major surgery plus risk factors,[a, b] high-risk medical patient, major trauma, spinal cord injury, craniotomy, total hip or knee arthroplasty (THA, TKA) thoracic, abdominal, pelvic cancer surgery.

Recommendation
▶ACCP 2016

- **Preventive Measures**
  - Early ambulation—consider mechanical prophylaxis and intermittent pneumatic compression, graduated compression stocking (IPC or GCS).
  - UFH 5000 U SQ q 8-12 h should ONLY be used in patients with renal disease with a Ccr <20 to 30 mL/min.

[a]Eye, ear, laparoscopy, cystoscopy, and arthroscopic operations.
[b]Prior VTE, cancer, stroke, obesity, congestive heart failure pregnancy, thrombophilic medications (tamoxifen, raloxifene, lenalidomide, thalidomide, erythroid-stimulating agents).

- LMWH equivalent to enoxaparin 40 mg SQ 2 h before surgery then daily or 30 mg q12h SQ starting 8–12 h postop.
- Fondaparinux 2.5 mg SQ daily starting 8–12 h postop.
- LMWH—equivalent to enoxaparin 40 mg SQ 2 h preoperative then daily or 30 mg SQ q12h starting 8–12 h postop and also use mechanical prophylaxis with IPC or GCS.
- Extend prophylaxis for as long as 28–35 d in high-risk patients. In THA, TKA ortho patients, acceptable VTE prophylaxis also includes rivaroxaban 10 mg/d, dabigatran 225 mg/d, adjusted dose warfarin, and aspirin, although LMWH is preferred. DOACs are likely to play a larger role in the future as trials continue to show superiority over warfarin. (*Ann Int Med.* 2013;159:275) (*Thromb Haemot.* 2011;105:444)
- If high risk of bleeding, use IPC alone. (*Ann Intern Med.* 2012;156:710) (*Ann Intern Med.* 2012;156:720) (*JAMA.* 2012;307:294)
- Do not use UFH for prophylaxis if Ccr is >20 cc/min. There is a 10 fold increased risk of HIT compared to LMWH.

Source
  –*Chest.* 2016;149:315

Comment

–**Clinical Points**

- 75%–90% of surgical bleeding is structural. VTE prophylaxis adds minimally to risk of bleeding.
- With creatinine clearance <20 to 30 cc/min UFH with partial thromboplastin time (PTT) monitoring is preferred (decrease dose if PTT prolonged). In all other situations LMWH or DOACs are preferred to reduce the risk HIT.
- Patients with liver disease and prolonged INR are still at risk for clot. Risk-to-benefit ratio of VTE prophylaxis should be individualized.
- Epidural anesthesia— to place catheter wait 18 h after daily prophylactic dose of LMWH, and 24 h after prophylactic dose of fondaparinux. For patients on BID therapeutic LMWH anticoagulation or once daily LMWH wait more than 24 hrs before placing epidural catheter. Patients on DOACs should hold their anticoagulation for 3-5 days. After placing or removing an epidural catheter hold on starting anticoagulation for 6 to 8 h.
- Prophylactic IVC filter for high-risk surgery is *not* recommended.
- For cranial and spinal surgery patients at low risk for VTE use mechanical prophylaxis—high-risk patients should have pharmacologic prophylaxis added to mechanical prophylaxis once hemostasis is established and bleeding risk decreased.

- Patients at high risk of bleeding[c] with major surgery should have mechanical prophylaxis (IPC, GCS)— initiate anticoagulant prophylaxis if risk lowered.
- Surgical patients receive indicated prophylaxis 60% of the time compared to 40% in medical patients.

–http://www.fda.gov/Drugs/ResourcesForYou/Consumers/ucm390574.htm

TABLE IV

CAPRINI RISK STRATIFICATION MODEL			
1 Point	**2 Points**	**3 Points**	**5 Points**
• Age 41–60 y • Minor surgery • BMI >251 g/m² • Swollen legs • Varicose veins • Pregnancy or postpartum • History of recurrent spontaneous abortion • Sepsis (<1 mo) • Lung disease • History of acute MI • Congestive heart failure (CHF) (<1 mo) • History of inflammatory bowel disease • Medical patient at bed rest	• Age 61–74 y • Arthroscopic surgery • Major open surgery >45 min • Laparoscopic surgery • Malignancy • Confined to bed • Immobilizing cast • Central venous catheter	• Age >75 y • History VTE • Family history of VTE • Factor V Leiden • Prothrombin gene mutation • Lupus anticoagulant • Elevated homocysteine • Other congenital or acquired thrombophilia	• Stroke (<1 mo) • Elective arthroplasty; hip, pelvis, or leg fracture • Acute spinal cord injury (<1 mo)
		Caprini Score <3: low risk Caprini Score 3–4: intermediate risk Caprini Score >5: high risk	

[c]SELECTED FACTORS IN THE RISING RISK OF MAJOR BLEEDING COMPLICATIONS
General Risk Factors
Active bleeding, previous major bleed, known untreated bleeding disorder, renal or liver failure, thrombocytopenia, acute stroke, uncontrolled high BP, concomitant use of anticoagulants, or antiplatelet therapy
Procedure-Specific Risk Factors
Major abdominal surgery—extensive cancer surgery, pancreatic-duodenectomy, hepatic resection, cardiac surgery, thoracic surgery (pneumonectomy or extended resection). Procedures where bleeding complications have especially severe consequences: craniotomy, spinal surgery, spinal trauma.

Disease Management

3

ABDOMINAL AORTIC ANEURYSM (AAA)

▶ Risk Factors of Developing AAA

- –Age >60 y. About 1 person in 1000 develops an abdominal aortic aneurysm between the ages of 60 and 65. Screening studies have shown that abdominal aortic aneurysms occur in 2% to 13% of men and 6% of women >65 y.
- –Smoking markedly increases risk for AAA. The risk is directly related to number of years smoking and decreases in the years following smoking cessation.
- –Men develop AAA 4–5 times more often than women.
- –AAA is more common in white population compared to other ethnicities.
- –History of CHD, PAD, HTN, and hypercholesterolemia.
- –Family history of AAA increases the risk of developing the condition and accentuates the risks associated with age and gender. The risk of developing an aneurysm among brothers of a person with a known aneurysm who are >60 y of age is as high as 18%.

▶ Risk of Expansion

- –Age >70 y, cardiac or renal transplant, previous stroke, severe cardiac disease, tobacco use.

▶ Risk of AAA Rupture

- –The evidence suggests that aneurysms expand at an average rate of 0.3–0.4 cm y.
- –The annual risk of rupture based upon aneurysm size is estimated as follows:
  - <4.0 cm in diameter = <0.5%.
  - Between 4.0 and 4.9 cm in diameter = 0.5%–5%.
  - Between 5.0 and 5.9 cm in diameter = 3%–15%.

- Between 6.0 and 6.9 cm in diameter = 10%–20%.
- Between 7.0 and 7.9 cm in diameter = 20%–40%.
- ≥8.0 cm in diameter = 30%–50%.

–Aneurysms that expand rapidly (>0.5 cm over 6 mo) are at high risk of rupture.

–Growth tends to be more rapid in smokers and less rapid in patients with peripheral artery disease or diabetes mellitus.

–The risk of rupture of large aneurysms (≥5.0 cm) is significantly greater in women (18%) than in men (12%).

–Other risk factors for rupture: cardiac or renal transplant, decreased forced expiratory volume in 1 s, higher mean BP, larger initial AAA diameter, current tobacco use—length of time smoking is more significant than amount smoked.

▶ ACCF/AHA 2005/2011 Recommendations

Pharmacologic Therapy

–All patients with AAA should have BP and fasting serum lipids monitored and controlled as recommended for patients with atherosclerotic disease (Class I, LOE C).

–Smoking cessation: Counseling and medications should be provided to all patients with AAA or family history of AAA.

–Patients with infrarenal or juxtarenal AAA 4.0–5.4 cm in diameter should be monitored by ultrasounds or CT scans every 6–12 mo to detect expansion (Class I, LOE A).

–In patients with AAA <4.0 cm in diameter, monitoring by ultrasound every 2–3 y is reasonable (Class IIa, LOE B).

–Perioperative administration of β-adrenergic blocking agents, in the absence of contraindications, is indicated to reduce the risk of adverse cardiac events and mortality in patients with coronary artery disease undergoing surgical repair of atherosclerotic aortic aneurysms (Class I, LOE A).

Surgical Therapy

–Patients with infrarenal or juxtarenal AAAs ≥5.5 cm in diameter should undergo repair to eliminate risk of rupture (Class I, LOE B).

–Repair is probably indicated in patients with suprarenal or type IV thoracoabdominal aortic aneurysm >5.5–6.0 cm in diameter (Class IIa, LOE B).

–Intervention is not indicated for asymptomatic infrarenal or juxtarenal AAA if <5.0 cm in diameter in men or <4.5 cm in diameter in women (Class III, LOE A).

–In patients with clinical triad of abdominal and/or back pain, a pulsatile abdominal mass, and hypotension, immediate surgical evaluation is indicated (Class I, LOE B).

–In patients with symptomatic AAA, repair is indicated regardless of diameter (Class I, LOE C).

–Open or endovascular repair of infrarenal AAAs and/or common iliac aneurysms is indicated in patients who are good surgical candidates (Class I, LOE A).

–Periodic long-term surveillance imaging should be performed to monitor for vascular leak, document shrinkage/stability of the excluded aneurysm sac, confirm graft position, and determine the need for further intervention in patients who have undergone endovascular repair of infrarenal aortic and/or iliac aneurysms (Class I, LOE A).

–Open aneurysm repair is reasonable to perform in patients who are good surgical candidates but who cannot comply with the periodic long-term surveillance required after endovascular repair (Class IIa, LOE C).

–Endovascular repair of infrarenal aortic aneurysm in patients who are at high surgical or anesthetic risk (presence of coexisting severe cardiac, pulmonary, and/or renal disease) is of uncertain effectiveness (Class IIb, LOE B).

▶ ESC 2014 Recommendations

Pharmacologic Therapy

–Smoking cessation is recommended to slow the growth of the AAA.

–Patients with HTN and AAA should be treated with β-blockers as a first-line treatment.

–ACEI and statins should be considered in patients with AAA to reduce risk of cardiovascular risk.

–Enlargement of AAA is usually associated with the development of an intraluminal mural thrombus. Overall data on the benefits of ASA in reducing AAA growth are contradictory; however, given the strong association between AAA and other atherosclerotic diseases, the use of ASA may be considered according to the presence of other cardiovascular comorbidities.

–Surveillance is indicated and safe in patients with AAA with a maximum diameter <5.5 cm and slow growth <1 cm/y.

–In patients with small AAA, imaging should be considered:
  • Every 4 y for AAA 2.5–2.9 cm diameter.
  • Every 3 y for AAA 3.0–3.9 cm diameter.
  • Every 2 y for AAA 4.0–4.4 cm diameter.
  • Every year for AAA >4.5 cm diameter.

Surgical Therapy

–AAA repair is indicated if:
  • AAA >5.5 cm in diameter.
  • Aneurysm growth >1 cm/y.

–If a large aneurysm is anatomically suitable for EVAR,[a] either open or endovascular repair is recommended in patients with acceptable surgical risk.

–If a large aneurysm is anatomically unsuitable for EVAR, open aortic repair is recommended.

–In patients with asymptomatic AAA, who are unfit for open repair, EVAR, along with best medical, treatment may be considered.

–In patients with suspected rupture of AAA, immediate abdominal ultrasound or CT is recommended.

–In case of ruptured AAA, emergency repair is indicated.

–In case of symptoms but nonruptured AAA, urgent repair is indicated.

–In case of symptomatic AAA anatomically suitable for EVAR, either open or endovascular aortic repair is recommended.

Sources: Adapted from http://www.uptodate.com/contents/abdominal-aortic-aneurysm-beyond-the-basics. Hirsch AT, Haskal ZJ, Hertzer NR, et al. ACC/AHA guidelines for the management of patients with peripheral arterial disease (lower extremity, renal, mesenteric, and abdominal aortic).*J Vasc Inter Radiol.* 2006;17:1383-1398.
Rooke TW, Hirsch AT, Misra S, et al. 2011 ACCF/AHA focused update of the guideline for the management of patients with peripheral artery disease (updating the 2005 guideline). *JACC.* 2011 Nov 1;58(19):2020-2045.
Erbel R, Aboyans V, Boileau C, et al. 2014 ESC guidelines on the diagnosis and treatment of aortic diseases. Document covering acute and chronic aortic diseases of the thoracic and abdominal aorta of the adult. The Task Force for the diagnosis and treatment of aortic disease of the European Society of Cardiology (ESC). *Eur Heart J.* 2014;35:2873-2926. doi:10.1093/eurheartj/ehu281.

[a]EVAR, endovascular aortic repair.

ABNORMAL LIVER CHEMISTRIES

Recommendations
▶ American College of Gastroenterology 2017

ALGORITHM FOR EVALUTION OF ASPARTATE AMINOTRANSFERASE (AST) AND/OR ALANINE AMINOTRANSFERASE (ALT) LEVEL

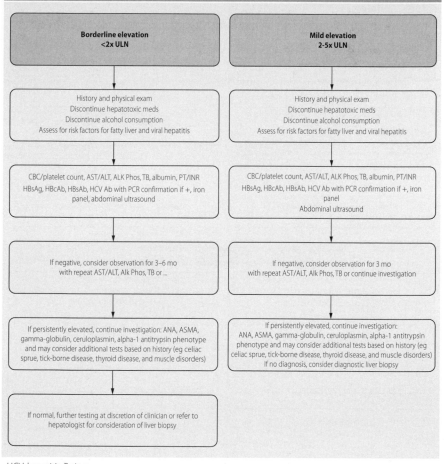

Borderline elevation <2x ULN	Mild elevation 2-5x ULN
History and physical exam Discontinue hepatotoxic meds Discontinue alcohol consumption Assess for risk factors for fatty liver and viral hepatitis	History and physical exam Discontinue hepatotoxic meds Discontinue alcohol consumption Assess for risk factors for fatty liver and viral hepatitis
CBC/platelet count, AST/ALT, ALK Phos, TB, albumin, PT/INR HBsAg, HBcAb, HBsAb, HCV Ab with PCR confirmation if +, iron panel, abdominal ultrasound	CBC/platelet count, AST/ALT, ALK Phos, TB, albumin, PT/INR HBsAg, HBcAb, HBsAb, HCV Ab with PCR confirmation if +, iron panel Abdominal ultrasound
If negative, consider observation for 3–6 mo with repeat AST/ALT, Alk Phos, TB or ...	If negative, consider observation for 3 mo with repeat AST/ALT, Alk Phos, TB or continue investigation
If persistently elevated, continue investigation: ANA, ASMA, gamma-globulin, ceruloplasmin, alpha-1 antitrypsin phenotype and may consider additional tests based on history (eg celiac sprue, tick-borne disease, thyroid disease, and muscle disorders)	If persistently elevated, continue investigation: ANA, ASMA, gamma-globulin, ceruloplasmin, alpha-1 antitrypsin phenotype and may consider additional tests based on history (eg celiac sprue, tick-borne disease, thyroid disease, and muscle disorders) If no diagnosis, consider diagnostic liver biopsy
If normal, further testing at discretion of clinician or refer to hepatologist for consideration of liver biopsy	

HCV, hepatitis C virus.

ALGORITHM FOR EVALUTION OF ELEVATED SERUM ALKALINE PHOSPHATASE

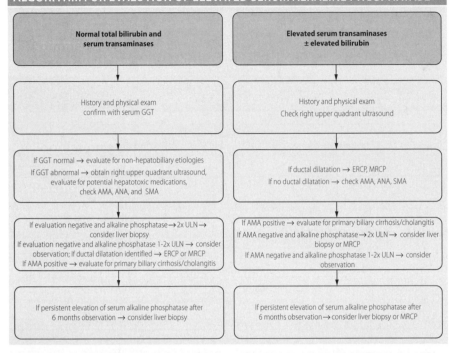

Normal total bilirubin and serum transaminases

History and physical exam
confirm with serum GGT

If GGT normal → evaluate for non-hepatobiliary etiologies
If GGT abnormal → obtain right upper quadrant ultrasound,
evaluate for potential hepatotoxic medications,
check AMA, ANA, and SMA

If evaluation negative and alkaline phosphatase → 2x ULN →
consider liver biopsy
If evaluation negative and alkaline phosphatase 1-2x ULN → consider
observation; If ductal dilatation identified → ERCP or MRCP
If AMA positive → evaluate for primary biliary cirrhosis/cholangitis

If persistent elevation of serum alkaline phosphatase after
6 months observation → consider liver biopsy

Elevated serum transaminases ± elevated bilirubin

History and physical exam
Check right upper quadrant ultrasound

If ductal dilatation → ERCP, MRCP
If no ductal dilatation → check AMA, ANA, SMA

If AMA positive → evaluate for primary biliary cirrhosis/cholangitis
If AMA negative and alkaline phosphatase → 2x ULN → consider liver
biopsy or MRCP
If AMA negative and alkaline phosphatase 1-2x ULN → consider
observation

If persistent elevation of serum alkaline phosphatase after
6 months observation → consider liver biopsy or MRCP

ALGORITHM FOR EVALUTION OF ELEVATED SERUM TOTAL BILIRUBIN

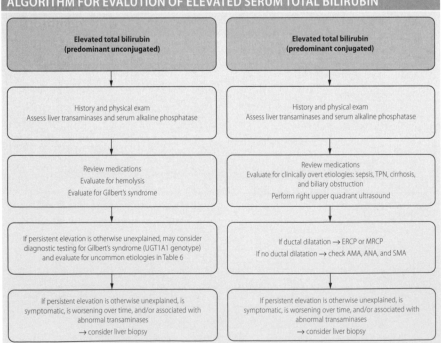

Elevated total bilirubin (predominant unconjugated)

History and physical exam
Assess liver transaminases and serum alkaline phosphatase

Review medications
Evaluate for hemolysis
Evaluate for Gilbert's syndrome

If persistent elevation is otherwise unexplained, may consider
diagnostic testing for Gilbert's syndrome (UGT1A1 genotype)
and evaluate for uncommon etiologies in Table 6

If persistent elevation is otherwise unexplained, is
symptomatic, is worsening over time, and/or associated with
abnormal transaminases
→ consider liver biopsy

Elevated total bilirubin (predominant conjugated)

History and physical exam
Assess liver transaminases and serum alkaline phosphatase

Review medications
Evaluate for clinically overt etiologies: sepsis, TPN, cirrhosis,
and biliary obstruction
Perform right upper quadrant ultrasound

If ductal dilatation → ERCP or MRCP
If no ductal dilatation → check AMA, ANA, and SMA

If persistent elevation is otherwise unexplained, is
symptomatic, is worsening over time, and/or associated with
abnormal transaminases
→ consider liver biopsy

Source
  –ACG Clinical Guideline: evaluation of abnormal liver chemistries. *Am J Gastroenterol.* 2017;112:18–35.

ACTIVE SURVEILLANCE (AS) FOR THE MANAGEMENT OF LOCALIZED PROSTATE CANCER

Population
  –Men with early clinically localized prostate cancer (Stages T_1 and T_2 and Gleason score less than or equal to 7).

Recommendations
▶ CCO 2016, ASCO 2016

  –For most patients with low-risk (Gleason score of 6 or less) localized prostate cancer with a PSA < 10, active surveillance (AS) is the recommended disease management strategy.
  –Younger age, high-volume Gleason 6 cancer, patient preference, and/or African American ethnicity should be taken into account since definitive therapy may be warranted for select patients.
  –For patients with limited life expectancy (<5 y) and low-risk cancer watchful waiting may be more appropriate than active surveillance.
  –Active treatment (radical prostatectomy (RP) or radiation therapy (RT)) is recommended for most patients with intermediate-risk (Gleason score 7) localized prostate cancer. For select patients with low volume, intermediate-risk (Gleason score 3 + 4 =7) localized prostate cancer, AS may be offered.
  –The AS protocol should include the following tests:
   • A PSA test every 3–6 mo.
   • Direct rectal exam at least once a year.
   • At least a 12 core confirmatory transrectal ultrasound-guided biopsy (including anterior directed cores) within 6 to 12 mo and then serial biopsy every 2 to 5 y thereafter or more frequently if clinically warranted. Men with limited life expectancy may transition to watchful waiting and avoid further biopsies.
  –For patients undergoing AS who are reclassified to a high-risk category (Gleason score now 7 or greater and/or significant increase in volume of Gleason 6 tumor consideration should be given to active therapy (RP or RT).

Comments

1. There are other ancillary tests that may make a difference in deciding when definitive therapy is indicated. The multiparametric MRI (mpMRI) and genomic testing of the malignant prostate cancer may reveal larger tumor size or unfavorable mutations that put the patient in a higher risk category which will need definitive therapy.
2. Data at 10-y follow-up from both observational and randomized trials show a very similar survival, although patients on surveillance had an increase in frequency of metastatic disease and clinical progression. (*N Engl J Med.* 2016;375:1415)
3. This approach is especially beneficial to patients older than 65 who after have comorbidities and higher risk of complications. Active surveillance also significantly avoids over-treatment and therapy-related morbidity. A recent 10-y follow-up comparing monitoring, surgery, and radiation therapy treatment outcomes resulted in very similar overall survival.

Sources
–ASCO *J Clin Oncol.* 2016;34:2182-2190
–*N Engl J Med.* 2016;375:1415
–*N Engl J Med.* 2014;370:932
–*Eur Urol.* 2015;67:233

ADRENAL INCIDENTALOMAS

Population
–Adults.

Recommendations

▶ AACE 2009

–Recommends clinical, biochemical, and radiographic evaluation for evidence of hypercortisolism, aldosteronism, the presence of pheochromocytoma, or a malignant tumor.
–Patients who will be managed expectantly should have reevaluation at 3–6 mo and then annually for 1–2 y.

Source
–https://www.aace.com/files/adrenal-guidelines.pdf

Comments

1. A 1-mg overnight dexamethasone suppression test can be used to screen for hypercortisolism.
2. Measure plasma-fractionated metanephrines and normetanephrines to screen for pheochromocytoma.
3. Measure plasma renin activity and aldosterone concentration to assess for primary or secondary aldosteronism.

ADULT PSYCHIATRIC PATIENTS IN THE EMERGENCY DEPARTMENT

Populations
–Adult patients presenting to ED with psychiatric symptoms.
–Adults with abnormal liver chemistries.

Recommendations
–No role for routine laboratory testing. Medical history, examination, and previous psychiatric diagnoses should guide testing.
–No role for routine neuroimaging studies in the absence of focal neurological deficits.
–Risk assessment tools should not be used in isolation to identify low-risk adults who are safe for ED discharge if they presented with suicidal ideations.
–Ketamine is one option for immediate sedation in severely agitated adults who may be violent or aggressive.

Source
–Nazarian DJ, Broder JS, Thiessen ME, Wilson MP, Zun LS, Brown MD; American College of Emergency Physicians. Clinical policy: critical issues in the diagnosis and management of the adult psychiatric patient in the emergency department. *Ann Emerg Med.* 2017 Apr;69(4):480-498.

ALCOHOL USE DISORDERS

Population
–Adults.

Recommendations
▶ ICSI 2010, NICE 2010, VA/DoD 2009
–For patients identified with alcohol dependence, schedule a referral to a substance use disorders specialist before the patient has left the office.
–Refer all patients with alcohol abstinence syndrome to a hospital for admission.
–Recommend prophylactic thiamine for all harmful alcohol use or alcohol dependence.
–Refer suitable patients with decompensated cirrhosis for consideration of liver transplantation once they have been sober from alcohol for ≥3 mo.
–Recommend pancreatic enzyme supplementation for chronic alcoholic pancreatitis with steatorrhea and malnutrition.

Sources
   –https://www.icsi.org/_asset/gtjr9h/PrevServAdults.pdf
   –http://www.guidelines.gov/content.aspx?id=23784
   –http://www.guidelines.gov/content.aspx?id=15676

Comments
   1. Assess all patients for a coexisting psychiatric disorder (dual diagnosis).
   2. Addiction-focused psychosocial intervention is helpful for patients with alcohol dependence.
   3. Consider adjunctive pharmacotherapy under close supervision for alcohol dependence:
      a. Naltrexone.
      b. Acamprosate.

ANAPHYLAXIS

Population
   –Children and adults.

Recommendations
▶ NICE 2011, EACCI 2014
   –Blood samples for mast cell tryptase testing should be obtained at onset and after 1–2 h.
   –All people ≥16 y suspected of having an anaphylactic reaction should be observed for at least 6–12 h before discharge.
   –All children younger than age 16 y suspected of having an anaphylactic reaction should be admitted for observation.
   –Patients treated for an anaphylactic reaction should be referred to an allergy specialist.
   –Treat anaphylaxis with epinephrine (1:1000) 0.01 mg/kg (maximum 0.5 mg) SC; may repeat as necessary IM every 15 min.
   –Patients should be prescribed an epinephrine injector (eg, EpiPen).
   –Patients with circulatory instability should be placed supine with lower extremities raised and given intravenous saline 20 mL/kg bolus.
   –Recommend inhaled β-2 agonists and glucocorticoids for wheezing or signs of bronchoconstriction.
   –H_1- and H_2-blockers can be added for cutaneous signs of anaphylaxis.

Sources
   –http://www.nice.org.uk/nicemedia/live/13626/57474/57474.pdf
   –http://www.guideline.gov/content.aspx?id=48690

Comment

–Anaphylaxis is defined as a severe, life-threatening, generalized hypersensitivity reaction. It is characterized by the rapid development of:
- Airway edema.
- Bronchospasm.
- Circulatory dysfunction.

ANDROGEN DEFICIENCY SYNDROME

Population

–Adult men.

Recommendations

▶ Endocrine Society 2010

1. Recommends an AM total testosterone level for men with symptoms and signs of androgen deficiency.[a]
2. Measure a serum luteinizing hormone (LH) and follicular stimulating hormone (FSH) in all men with testosterone deficiency.
3. Recommends a dual-energy x-ray absorptiometry scan for all men with testosterone deficiency.
4. Testosterone therapy indicated for androgen deficiency syndromes unless contraindications exist.[b]

Source

–http://www.guidelines.gov/content.aspx?id=16326

Comment

1. Testosterone therapy options:
   a. Testosterone enanthate or cypionate 150–200 mg IM every 2 wk.
   b. Testosterone patch 5–10 mg qhs.
   c. 1% testosterone gel 5–10 g daily.
   d. Testosterone 30 mg to buccal mucosa q12h.

[a]Lethargy, easy fatigue, lack of stamina or endurance, reduced libido, mood changes, irritability, and loss of libido and motivation.
[b]Breast cancer (CA), prostate CA, hematocrit >50%, untreated severe obstructive sleep apnea, severe obstructive urinary symptoms, or uncontrolled heart failure.

ANEMIA–USE OF ERYTHROPOIETIC AGENTS

Population
–Adult patients with cancer and anemia.

Recommendation

▶ American Society of Hematology/American Society of Clinical Oncology (ASH/ASCO) 2010

–**Approach to Anemic Cancer Patients**
- History, physical exam, and diagnostic studies to exclude other causes of anemia aside from chemotherapy or malignant marrow infiltration.
- The FDA label now limits the use of Erythrocyte Stimulating Agents (ESA) ONLY to anemic cancer patients receiving chemotherapy with palliative intent. (*N Engl J Med*. 2007;356:2448) ESA is NOT to be used in patients with curable malignancies or in patients with cancer not on chemotherapy. Side effects of thrombosis and potentially increased cancer growth should be discussed with the patient. (*J Natl Cancer Inst*. 2013;105:1018)
- Epoetin and darbepoetin are equal in efficacy.
- ESA should not be used if hemoglobin >10 g/dL. The main benefit of ESA is to reduce transfusion need. (*Br J Cancer*. 2010;102:301)
- FDA-approved starting dose of epoetin is 150 U/kg 3 times/wk or 40,000 U weekly. For darbepoetin the dose is 2.25 µg/kg weekly or 500 µg every 3 wk subcutaneously.
- Stop ESAs at 6–8 wk if no evidence of a response. Check for underlying tumor progression, iron deficiency, or other causes of anemia.
- Dose of ESAs should be lowest concentration needed to avoid transfusion. Keep hemoglobin <12.
- Periodic monitoring of ferritin and iron studies is recommended since ESAs will not improve hemoglobin if the patient is iron deficient.
- Use of ESAs in lower-risk myelodysplastic syndrome to decrease transfusions is approved if erythropoietin level is <500 mµ/mL. The use of low dose filgrastrin (100 µg once or twice/wk) will increase responsiveness to ESAs.

Source
–ASH/ASCO guidelines update on use of epoetin and darbepoetin. *Blood*. 2010;116:4045-4059.

Comment

-**Important Facts about ESAs**
  • Early studies raising hemoglobin level to >12 g/dL resulted in significant increased risk of venous thromboembolus.
  • Beware of clot risk when using ESAs with other thrombophilic drugs (tamoxifen, BCP, lenalidomide).
  • The molecular structure of darbepoetin increases its half-life, allowing for less frequent injections.
  • 50% of cancers will have erythropoietin receptors on the cell surface. It has NOT been proven that ESAs interaction with cell surface receptors leads to cellular proliferation.
  • When patients stop chemotherapy for whatever reason, ESAs must be stopped and transfusion therapy substituted according to FDA guidelines.
  • The addition of intravenous iron to ESAs will increase hemoglobin more rapidly since iron is sequestered in the reticuloendothelial system in the cancer-associated anemia of chronic disease. (*N Engl J Med.* 2005; 352:1011)
  • ESAs widely used in chronic renal insufficiency, reducing need for transfusion significantly. Iron often given to these patients to keep ferritin level between 100 and 500 ng/mL and transferrin saturation 20%–50%. (*N Engl J Med.* 2010;362:3).

ANKYLOSING SPONDYLITIS AND SPONDYLOARTHRITIS

Population

-Adults with ankylosing spondylitis (AS) or nonradiographic spondyloarthritis.

Recommendations

▶ ACR/Spondylitis Association of America/Spondyloarthritis Research and Treatment Network 2015

-**Recommendations for treatment of ankylosing spondylitis**
  • Scheduled NSAIDs.
  • Tumor necrosis factor inhibitor (TNFi) therapy.
  • Recommends addition of slow-acting anti-rheumatic drugs when TNFi medications contraindicated.
  • Local parenteral corticosteroids for active sacroiliitis, active enthesitis, or peripheral arthritis for symptoms refractory to NSAIDs.
  • Avoid systemic corticosteroid use.
  • Refer to an ophthalmologist for concomitant iritis.

- Recommend TNFi monoclonal antibody therapy for AS with inflammatory bowel disease.
- Physical therapy program.
- Screen for fall risk, osteoporosis.

−**Recommendations for treatment of nonradiographic axial spondyloarthritis**
  - NSAIDs.
  - Tumor Necrosis Factor inhibitor (TNFi) therapy.

Source
−Ward MM, Deodhar A, Akl EA, et al. American College of Rheumatology/Spondylitis Association of America/Spondyloarthritis Research and Treatment Network 2015 Recommendations for the treatment of ankylosing spondylitis and nonradiographic axial spondyloarthritis. *Arthritis Rheumatol.* 2016 Feb;68(2):282-298.

ANXIETY

Population
−Adults.

Recommendations

▶ NICE 2011

−Recommends cognitive behavioral therapy for generalized anxiety disorder (GAD).
−Recommends sertraline if drug treatment is needed.
−If sertraline is ineffective, recommend a different selective serotonin reuptake inhibitor (SSRI) or selective noradrenergic reuptake inhibitor (SNRI).
−Avoid long-term benzodiazepine use or antipsychotic therapy for GAD.

Source
−http://www.nice.org.uk/nicemedia/live/13314/52599/52599.pdf

APNEA, CENTRAL SLEEP (CSAS)

Population
−Adults.

Recommendations

▶ American Academy of Sleep Medicine 2012

−**Primary CSAS**
  - Positive airway pressure therapy may be used to treat primary CSAS.

- Limited evidence to support the use of acetazolamide for CSAS.
- Zolpidem or triazolam may be used to treat CSAS if patients are not at high risk for respiratory depression.

–**CSAS related to CHF**
- Nocturnal oxygen therapy.
- CPAP therapy targeted to normalize the apnea-hypopnea index.

–**CSAS related to ESRD**
- Options for therapy include CPAP, nocturnal oxygen, and bicarbonate buffer use during dialysis.

Source
- http://www.guideline.gov/content.aspx?id=35175

APNEA, OBSTRUCTIVE SLEEP (OSA)

Population
- Adults.

Recommendations

▶ AASM 2017

- Recommends that diagnostic testing for OSA be performed in conjunction with a comprehensive sleep evaluation.
- Recommends that a polysomnogram, or home sleep apnea testing with a technically adequate device, be used for the diagnosis of OSA in uncomplicated adult patients presenting with signs and symptoms that indicate an increased risk of moderate to severe OSA.
- Recommends that a polysomnogram, rather than home sleep apnea testing, be used for the diagnosis of OSA in patients with significant cardiorespiratory disease, potential respiratory muscle weakness due to neuromuscular condition, awake hypoventilation or suspicion of sleep related hypoventilation, chronic opioid medication use, and history of stroke or severe insomnia.
- Recommends that if a single home sleep apnea testing is negative, inconclusive, or technically inadequate, a polysomnogram be performed for the diagnosis or exclusion of OSA.

Sources
- http://guidelines.gov/summaries/summary/50887/
- Kapur VK, Auckley DH, Chowdhuri S, et al. Clinical practice guideline for diagnostic testing for adult obstructive sleep apnea: an American Academy of Sleep Medicine clinical practice guideline. *J Clin Sleep Med.* 2017 Mar 15;13(3):479-504.

▶ **ACP 2013**
- –All overweight adults diagnosed with OSA should lose weight.
- –Recommends nocturnal CPAP (continuous positive airway pressure) therapy as first-line therapy for OSA.
- –Option to use mandibular advancement devices for those patients intolerant of CPAP.

Source
- –http://www.guideline.gov/content.aspx?id=47136

ASCITES, DUE TO CIRRHOSIS

Population
- –Adults with cirrhosis.

Recommendations
▶ **AASLD 2013**
- –Diagnostic paracentesis is recommended for all patients with new-onset ascites.
- –The routine use of platelets or fresh frozen plasma prior to a paracentesis is not recommended.
- –Ascitic fluid analysis:
  - Cell count with differential.
  - Albumin.
  - Protein.
  - Bedside inoculation of aerobic and anaerobic culture bottles.
- –Management of cirrhotic ascites:
  - Alcohol cessation.
  - <2 g sodium/d.
  - Oral furosemide and spironolactone in a 2:5 ratio.
  - Fluid restriction not necessary unless serum sodium <125 mmol/L.
  - All patients with cirrhosis and ascites should be considered for liver transplantation.
  - Avoid NSAIDs.
  - Cautious use of ACEI or ARB.
- –Management of refractory cirrhotic ascites
  - Avoid propranolol.
  - Avoid ACEI or ARB.
  - Consider use of oral midodrine.
  - Serial therapeutic paracentesis is a treatment option.

- Transjugular intrahepatic portosystemic shunt (TIPSS) is a therapeutic option in carefully selected patients.
- Albumin 6–8 g/L ascitic fluid removed indicated for large volume paracentesis >5 L.

–Management of spontaneous bacterial peritonitis (SBP)
  - Recommend cefotaxime 2 g IV q8h.
  - Alternative is ofloxacin 400 mg PO bid.
  - Add albumin 1.5 g/kg/d on day 1 and 1 g/kg/d on day 3 if creatinine >1 mg/dL, BUN >30 mg/dL, or bilirubin >4 mg/dL.

–SBP prophylaxis
  - Cefotaxime or oral norfloxacin for 7 d in patients admitted for upper gastrointestinal bleed.
  - Long-term oral trimethoprim-sulfamethoxazole or norfloxacin for any patient with a history of SBP.
  - Consider SBP prophylaxis if ascitic fluid protein <1.5 g/dL in association with creatinine >1.2 mg/dL or sodium <130 mmol/L or bilirubin >3 mg/dL.

–Hepatorenal syndrome options for treatment
  - Midodrine + SQ Octreotide + albumin.
  - Norepinephrine infusion + albumin.
  - Referral for liver transplantation.

–Hepatic hydrothorax
  - Chest tube is contraindicated.
  - Dietary sodium restriction and diuretics is first-line therapy.
  - TIPSS is an option for refractory cases.

–Avoid percutaneous gastrotomy tube placement in patients with ascites.

Source
  –http://www.guideline.gov/content.aspx?id=45103

ASTHMA

Population
  –Children age >5 y, adolescents, and adults.

Recommendations
▶ GINA 2017

1. Diagnosis of asthma by history: typical symptoms are a combination of shortness of breath, cough, wheezing, and chest tightness; variability over time and in intensity; frequent triggers; FEV1 and FEV1/FVC ratio are reduced and increase by more than 12% after a bronchodilator challenge.

2. Recommend classification of asthma by level of symptom control.
3. Recommend a chest radiograph at the initial visit to exclude alternative diagnoses.
4. Recommend assessing for tobacco use and strongly advise smokers to quit.
5. Recommend spirometry with bronchodilators to determine the severity of airflow limitation and its reversibility.
   a. Repeat spirometry at least every 1–2 y for asthma monitoring.
6. Consider allergy testing for history of atopy, rhinitis, rhinorrhea, and seasonal variation or specific extrinsic triggers.
7. Recommend an asthma action plan based on peak expiratory flow (PEF) monitoring for all patients.
8. Recommend allergen and environmental or occupational trigger avoidance.
9. Physicians should help educate patients, assist them in self-management, develop goals of treatment, create an asthma action plan, and regularly monitor asthma control.

STEPWISE APPROACH TO ASTHMA MANAGEMENT

Stepwise approach to asthma treatment

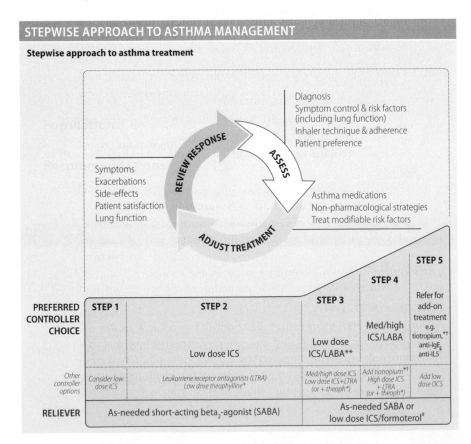

1. Asthma exacerbations should be treated with:
   a. Corticosteroids.
      –Prednisolone 1 mg/kg PO daily (up to 50 mg) or equivalent × 7 d for mild-to-moderate exacerbations.
      –Methylprednisolone 1 mg/kg IV q6h initially for severe exacerbations.
   b. Magnesium sulfate 2 g IV.
   c. Oxygen to keep SpO_2 >90%.
   d. Rapid-acting β-agonists (4–10 puffs albuterol pMDI with spacer or 2.5-5 mg nebulized every 20 min for 1 h).
   e. Ipratropium bromide stepwise approach.
   f. Consider bilevel positive airway pressure (Bi-PAP) for acute asthma exacerbations.
   g. No role for routine antibiotics. Use antibiotics only for definite bacterial infections.
2. Develop a chronic medication regimen for patients adjusted based on their asthma action plan.

Source
   –*2017 Global Initiative for Asthma* (http://www.ginasthma.org)

Comments
1. Controlled asthma defined by:
   a. Daytime symptoms ≤2×/wk.
   b. No limitations of daily activities.
   c. No nocturnal symptoms.
   d. Need for reliever medicines ≤2×/wk.
   e. Normal or near-normal lung function.
   f. No exacerbations.
2. Partially controlled asthma if:
   a. Daytime symptoms >2×/wk.
   b. Any limitations of daily activities or any nocturnal symptoms.
   c. Need for reliever medicines ≤2×/wk.
   d. <80% predicted PEF or forced expiratory volume at 1 s (FEV_1).
   e. Any exacerbations.
3. Uncontrolled asthma if there are ≥3 features of partially controlled asthma in any week.
4. Risk factors for adverse asthma events:
   a. Poor clinical control.
   b. Frequent asthma exacerbations.
   c. History of ICU admission for asthma exacerbation.
   d. FEV_1 <60% predicted.
   e. Exposure to cigarette smoke.
   f. Need for high-dose medications.

5. Recommend an inhaled corticosteroid for partially controlled or uncontrolled asthma.
6. Add a long-acting β-agonist or leukotriene inhibitor for incomplete control with inhaled corticosteroid alone.
7. Short-acting β_2-agonists should be used as needed for relief of acute asthma symptoms or 20 min prior to planned exercise in exercise-induced asthma. Alternatives for exercise-induced asthma include a leukotriene inhibitor or cromolyn.
8. For difficult-to-control asthma:
   a. Treat potentially aggravating conditions: rhinitis, gastroesophageal reflux disease (GERD), nasal polyps.
   b. Consider alternative diagnoses: chronic obstructive pulmonary disease (COPD) or vocal cord dysfunction.

ASYMPTOMATIC BACTERIURIA

Population
–Nonpregnant women.

Recommendation
▶ IDSA 2015
–Do not treat asymptomatic bacteriuria with antibiotics.

Source
–http://www.choosingwisely.org/societies/infectious-diseases-society-of-america/

ATOPIC DERMATITIS (AD)

Population
–Adults and children.

Recommendations
▶ AAD 2014
–Generous application of skin moisturizers after bathing.
–Recommend limited use of hypoallergenic non-soap cleansers.
–Consider wet-wrap therapy with topical corticosteroids for moderate-to-severe AD during flares.
–Twice-daily topical corticosteroids are the first-line therapy for AD.
–Topical calcineurin inhibitors (tacrolimus or pimecrolimus) can be used for maintenance AD therapy.
–Recommend against topical antihistamine therapy for AD.

–Phototherapy is second-line treatment for refractory cases.

–Consider systemic immunomodulating agents for severe cases refractory to topical agents and phototherapy.

Sources

–http://www.guideline.gov/content.aspx?id=48409

–http://www.guideline.gov/content.aspx?id=48410

Comment

–Systemic immunomodulating agents that have been studied in AD are azathioprine, cyclosporine, or methotrexate.

ATRIAL FIBRILLATION

ATRIAL FIBRILLATION: MANAGEMENT OVERVIEW HEART RATE CONTROL

Classification of Atrial Fibrillation (AF)
Paroxysmal = Self-terminating
Recurrent = Two or more episodes
Persistent = Lasts >7 days
Silent = Detected by monitor
Lone = Unassociated with/heart disease

Initiate Treatment
Slow the ventricular rate
Establish anticoagulation
Consider rhythm conversion

Determine Etiology
Hypertension/coronary artery disease
Cardiomyopathy/heart valve disease
Pulmonary disease/hyperthyroidism
Sinus node disease

–Expected ventricular heart rate (HR) in untreated AF is between 110 and 210 beats/min.
  • If HR <110 beats/min, atrioventricular (AV) node disease present.
  • If HR >220 beats/min, preexcitation syndrome (WPW) present.
–Initial choice of AV nodal slowing agent to be determined by:
  • Ventricular rate/blood pressure (BP).
  • Presence of heart failure (HF) or asthma.
  • Associated cardiovascular (CV) symptoms (chest pain/shortness of breath [SOB]).

–**Urgent electrical cardioversion** should be considered if hemodynamic instability or persistent symptoms of ischemia, HF, or if inadequate HR control with optimal medications.

ATRIAL FIBRILLATION: MANAGEMENT OVERVIEW HEART RATE CONTROL   (Continued)

–**Resting HR goal and exercise HR goal** should be determined. Holter monitor best measures the adequacy of the chronic HR control. In acute medical conditions when the patient has noncardiac illness (ie, pneumonia), the resting HR may be allowed to increase to simulate physiologic demands (mimic HR if sinus rhythm was present).

Lenient Target	**Aggressive Target**
Resting HR <110 beats/min May be considered in younger or patients without CV symptoms.	Resting HR <80 beats/min exercise HR <110 beats/min treatment choice if decreased ejection fraction (EF) <40% if symptoms at higher rates.

(ESC recommends HR target <110 beats/min; CCS recommends <100 beats/min; ACCF/AHA/HRS recommends HR target <110 beats/min only if EF >40%.)

–**Consider AV nodal ablation** when chronic HR target cannot be achieved with maximal medical therapy with placement of ventricular pacemaker.

ACCF, American College of Cardiology Foundation; AHA, American Heart Association; CCS, Canadian CV Society; ESC, European Society of Cardiology; HRS, Heart Rhythm Society.

Sources: ACC/AHA/ESC 2006 Guidelines. *J Am Coll Cardiol.* 2006;48:858-906. ACCF/AHA/HRS. *J Am Coll Cardiol.* 2011;57:223-242. ACC/AHA. *Circulation.* 2008;117:1101-1120. ESC 2010 Guidelines. *Eur Heart J.* 2010;31:2369-2429. Comparing the 2010 NA and European AF Guidelines. *Can J Cardiol.* 2011;27:7-13. January CT, Wann LS, Alpert JS, et al. 2014 AHA/ACC/HRS Guideline for the management of patients with atrial fibrillation. *Circulation.* 2014. http://circ.ahajournals.org/content/early/2014/04/10/CIR.0000000000000041.

Data suggest that stopping anticoagulation with warfarin prior to the ablation (even if patients are bridged with low-molecular-weight heparin) is associated with an increased risk of complications compared with an uninterrupted anticoagulation approach. In COMPARE study, patients with CHADS$_2$ score of >1 undergoing catheter ablation for nonvalvular AF, bridged with low-molecular-weight heparin, had a >10-fold increased risk of ischemic stroke or transient ischemic attack in the 48 h after ablation compared with those on uninterrupted warfarin. Patients with atrial fibrillation frequently stop oral anticoagulation therapy following radiofrequency catheter ablation despite an increased risk for stroke, transient ischemic attack, or systemic embolism in the first 3 mo after the procedure, according to the results of a new analysis. If the patient is at a lower risk for stroke, the type of patient that might not need to be anticoagulated to begin with, then the medication can be stopped after 3 mo. Everybody else should remain on oral anticoagulation for at least 12 mo after the ablation. At that point, physicians can reassess a patient's risk factors to determine whether the oral anticoagulation should continue.

Source: O'Riordan M. Stopping anticoagulation after ablation increases stroke risk in first 3 mo. May 21, 2015. (http://www.medscape.com/viewarticle/845106?src=confwrap&uac=91737BX)

For patients undergoing catheter ablation for nonvalvular atrial fibrillation, continuing with uninterrupted rivaroxaban appears to be as safe as uninterrupted oral anticoagulant therapy with warfarin.

Source: O'Riordan M. Uninterrupted rivaroxaban feasible for patients undergoing AF ablation. VENTURE-AF Study. (http://www.medscape.com/viewarticle/845168?src=confwrap&uac=91737BX)

Choosing Wisely American Society of Echocardiography (2013) recommends against transesophageal echocardiography to detect cardiac sources of embolization if a source has been identified and patient management will not change.

Source: http://www.choosingwisely.org/sourcessocieties/american-society-of-echocardiography/.

2014 AHA/ACC/HRS GUIDELINES FOR PREVENTION OF THROMBOEMBOLISM IN PATIENTS WITH AF

- Antithrombotic therapy based on shared decision making, discussion of risks of stroke and bleeding, and patient's preferences.
- Antithrombotic therapy selection based on risk of thromboembolism.
- CHA_2DS_2-VASc score recommended to assess stroke risk.
- Warfarin recommended with mechanical heart valves. Target INR intensity should be based on the type and location of prosthesis.
- With prior stroke, TIA, or CHA_2DS_2-VASc score ≥2, oral anticoagulants are recommended. Options include warfarin or DOACs: dabigatran, rivaroxaban, or apixaban.
- With warfarin, determine INR at least weekly during initiation and monthly when stable.
- Direct thrombin or factor Xa inhibitor recommended over warfarin for nonvalvular AFib.
- Apixiban, rivaroxaban, and dabigatran all are equally efficacious for ischemic stroke and systemic embolism prevention; however, apixiban has decreased incidence of major bleeding and GI bleeding compared to other DOACs.
- Reevaluate the need for anticoagulation at periodic intervals.
- Bridging therapy with LMWH or UFH recommended with a mechanical heart valve or with mitral stenosis if warfarin is interrupted. Bridging therapy should balance risks of stroke and bleeding.
- Without a mechanical heart valve, bridging therapy decisions should balance stroke and bleeding risks against the duration of time patient will not be anticoagulated.
- Evaluate renal function prior to initiation of direct thrombin or factor Xa inhibitors, and reevaluate when clinically indicated and at least annually.
- For atrial flutter, antithrombotic therapy is recommended as for AF.

Sources: Adapted from January CT, Wann LS, Alpert JS, et al. 2014. AHA/ACC/HRS guideline for the management of patients with atrial fibrillation. *Circulation.* 2014. http://circ.ahajournals.org/content/early/2014/04/10/CIR.0000000000000041. *Chest.* 2016;150(6):1302-1312. *Gastroenterology.* 2017;152: 1014-1022. *Brit Med J.* 2016;353:3189.

ATRIAL FIBRILLATION: NONVALVULAR NEW ORAL ANTICOAGULATION AGENTS (EUROPEAN HEART RHYTHM EXECUTIVE SUMMARY 2013, EUROPEAN SOCIETY OF CARDIOLOGY 2012, AMERICAN HEART ASSOCIATION AND AMERICAN STROKE ASSOCIATION 2012)

- New oral anticoagulation agents (DOACs) are alternative agents to the use of warfarin.
- *Quantitative* indicators of the function **are not clinically available** for direct thrombin inhibitors (DTIs) or factor X inhibitors (FXa).
- *Qualitative* indicators of the *presence* of DTI agent (dabigatran) and FXa inhibitors (rivaroxaban and apixaban) are available.
  ◦ Activated partial thromboplastin time (aPTT) is a measure of DTI presence.
  ◦ Prothrombin time (PT) is a measure of FXa inhibitor presence.
- Drug interactions with DOAC agents are generally less than with warfarin but still need to be considered.
- Rivaroxaban should be taken with food to optimize absorption and bioavailability. No other DOAC agents are influenced to food ingestion.
- No interaction is noted between DOAC agents and proton pump inhibitor (PPI) agents and H_2 blockers exist.
- All DOAC agents require dose reduction with renal dysfunction.
- DOAC agents have a short action of duration of 12–24 h and therefore should be avoided in patients with poor medicine adherence.
- No specific antidotes for DOAC agents exist.
  ◦ If no bleeding, hold subsequent doses and observe.
  ◦ If clinical bleeding noted, expert opinion suggests the use of prothrombin complex concentrates (PCCs) 50 U/kg is recommended.
- Preoperatively with normal renal function should hold DOAC agent >=24h before surgery with low bleeding risk and CrCl>80 ml/min; hold DOAC 48-72 hours before surgery with high bleeding risk and CrCl>80 ml/min.

Sources: Heidbuchel H, Verhamme P, Alings M, et al. EHRA practice guide on the use of new oral anticoagulants in patients with nonvalvular atrial fibrillation: executive summary. *Eur Heart J.* 2013;34:2094-2106. Furie KL, Goldstein LB, Albers GW, et al; American Heart Association Stroke Council; Council on Quality of Care and Outcomes Research; Council on Cardiovascular Nursing; Council on Clinical Cardiology; Council on Peripheral Vascular Disease. Oral antithrombotic agents for the prevention of stroke in nonvalvular atrial fibrillation: a science advisory for healthcare professionals from the American Heart Association/American Stroke Association. *Stroke.* 2012;43:3442-3453. Gonsalves WI, Pruthi RK, Patnaik MM. The new oral anticoagulants in clinical practice. *Mayo Clin Proc.* 2013; 88: 495-511. Camm AJ, Lip GY, De Caterina R, et al; ESC Committee for Practice Guidelines, et al. 2012 focused update of the ESC Guidelines for the management of atrial fibrillation: an update of the 2010 ESC Guidelines for the management of atrial fibrillation. Developed with the special contribution of the European Heart Rhythm Association. *Eur Heart J.* 2012;33:2719-2747. *Chest.* 2016;150(6):1302-1312. *Gastroenterology.* 2017;152:1014-1022. *Brit Med J.* 2016;353:3189. *Thrombosis J.* 2017;15:14. *JACC.* Periprocedural Anticoagulation Pathway 2017;69(7): 8 7 1-8 9 8.

DIRECT ORAL ANTICOAGULANTS (DOACS)
DABIGATRAN ETEXILATE (PRADAXA®)

- Direct thrombin inhibitor.
- Dosage:
  - 150 mg 1 tab bid (ClCr >50 mL/min).
  - 75 mg 1 tab bid (ClCr 15–30 mL/min).
  - Not recommended in end-stage CKD on or not on dialysis.
- Pharmacokinetics/pharmacodynamics: Cytochrome P450 metabolism: none; half-life: 12–14 h; renal elimination: 80%.
- ACC/AHA recommends it as a useful alternative to warfarin in patients who have nonvalvular AF and do not have severe renal and liver disease.
- ESC recommends it in patients with nonvalvular AF with at least one moderate risk factor.
- RE-LY Trial (150 mg bid)—similar reduction in stroke and systemic embolism vs. warfarin (2.07% vs. 2.78% per year). Increased GI bleeds compared to warfarin, especially in patients ≥75 y old.
- By FDA 12/2012, risk of bleeding did not appear to be higher in patients with new use of dabigatran compared to new use of warfarin.
- **Switching patients from warfarin to dabigatran:** Discontinue warfarin and start dabigatran when the INR is <2.0.
- **Switching patients from dabigatran to warfarin:** Adjust the starting time of warfarin based on creatinine clearance as follows:
  - For CrCl ≥50 mL/min, start warfarin 3 d before discontinuing dabigatran.
  - For CrCl 30–50 mL/min, start warfarin 2 d before discontinuing dabigatran.
  - For CrCl 15–30 mL/min, start warfarin 1 d before discontinuing dabigatran.
- **Converting from/to parenteral anticoagulants**
  - For patients currently receiving a parenteral anticoagulant, start dabigatran 0–2 h before the time that the next dose of parenteral drug was to be administered or at the time of discontinuation of a continuously administered parenteral drug (eg, intravenous unfractionated heparin).
  - For patients currently taking dabigatran, wait 12 h (CrCl ≥30 mL/min) or 24 h (CrCl <30 mL/min) after the last dose of dabigatran, before initiating treatment with a parenteral anticoagulant.
- If possible, **discontinue dabigatran 1–2 d (CrCl ≥50 mL/min) or 3–5 d (CrCl <50 mL/min) before invasive or surgical procedures.** Consider longer times for patients undergoing major surgery, spinal puncture, or placement of a spinal or epidural catheter or port, in whom complete hemostasis may be required. Restart as soon as possible.
- Discontinuation on Pradaxa without adequate continuous anticoagulation increases the risk of stroke.
- To measure adherence for dabigatran, measure thrombin level. If low, the patient is not taking the medicine.
- Idarucizumab is now approved by the FDA and rapidly reverses direct thrombin inhibition.

Source: Wood S: Dabigatran antidote gets FDA okay for faster review. *Medscape.* June 26, 2014 (http://www.medscape.com/viewarticle/827433).

+ (XARELTO®)

- Direct factor X_a inhibitor.
- FDA indication: Nonvalvular AF, DVT, PE.
- Dosage in nonvalvular AF:
  - ◦ 20 mg 1 tab qhs with meal (CrCl >50 mL/min).
  - ◦ 15 mg 1 tab qhs with meal (CrCl 15–50 mL/min).
  - ◦ Not recommended in end-stage CKD on or not on dialysis.
- Pharmacokinetics/pharmacodynamics: cytochrome P450 metabolism: 32%; half-life: 9–13 h; renal elimination: 33%.
- ROCKET AF trial: Noninferior to warfarin regarding prevention of stroke and systemic embolism. No reduction in rates of mortality or ischemic stroke, but a significant reduction in hemorrhagic stroke and intracranial hemorrhage. Compared to warfarin it was nonsignificantly different in nonmajor bleeding; had significant reduction in fatal bleeding and increased GI bleeding and bleeds requiring transfusion).
- 5 phase III trials of dabigatran vs. warfarin: Patients with major bleeding on dabigatran required more red cell transfusions but received less plasma, required a shorter stay in ICU, and had a trend to lower mortality compared with those who had major bleeding on warfarin.
- Switching from warfarin to rivaroxaban: Discontinue warfarin and start XARELTO as soon as INR <3.
- **Switching from rivaroxaban to warfarin:** No clinical trial data are available to guide converting patients. Company recommends to discontinue rivaroxaban and begin both a parenteral anticoagulant and warfarin at the time the next dose of rivaroxaban would be taken.
- **Rivaroxaban should be stopped at least 24 h before surgeries** or other invasive procedures and should be resumed as soon as possible. If oral medication cannot be taken, consider administering a parenteral anticoagulant.
- Premature discontinuation of rivaroxaban increases the risk of stroke.
- To measure adherence for rivaroxaban, measure factor Xa activity. If low, the patient is not taking the medicine.

Andexanet alfa, an antidote to the factor Xa inhibitor, ANNEXA-R trial, awaiting results of phase 3 summer 2015.

Source: http://www.annalsoflongtermcare.com/content/rivaroxaban-reversal-agent-safe-and-effective-trial-finds-potential-universal-antidote.

APIXABAN (ELIQUIS®)

- Direct factor X_a inhibitor.
- Indication: Nonvalvular AF, DVT prophylaxis after hip or knee replacement surgery.
- Dosage:
  - 5 mg 1 tab bid.
  - 2.5 mg 1 tab bid on patients ≥80 y old, weight ≤60 kg, Cr ≥1.5 mg/dL or patients taking P450 and P-glycoprotein inhibitors.
  - Not recommended in severe CKD or end-stage CKD on or not on dialysis.
  - Avoid concomitant use of rivaroxaban with strong CYP3A4 inhibitors and combined P-gp.
- Pharmacokinetics/pharmacodynamics: Cytochrome P450 metabolism: 15%; half-life: 8–15 h; renal elimination: 40%.
- AVERROES trial: Apixaban was superior in preventing stroke vs. ASA in patients who could not tolerate or were intolerant to warfarin.
- ARISTOTLE trial: Apixaban was superior to warfarin in reducing stroke or systemic embolism by 21%. Also 31% reduction in major bleeding and 11% reduction in all-cause mortality (not CV). Rates of hemorrhagic stroke and ISH (but not ischemic stroke) were lower in apixaban group. GI bleeding was similar in both groups. Apixaban was better tolerated than warfarin with slightly fewer discontinuations.
- **Switching from warfarin to apixaban:** Warfarin should be discontinued and apixaban started when INR <2.
- **Switching from apixaban to warfarin:** Discontinue apixaban and begin both a parenteral anticoagulant and warfarin at the time the next dose of apixaban would have been taken, discontinuing the parenteral anticoagulant when INR reaches an acceptable range.
- **Discontinue apixaban at least 48 h prior to elective surgeries** or invasive procedures with high risk of bleeding and 24 h prior to invasive procedures with low risk of bleeding. Bridging is not generally required. Resume it after surgery as soon as possible.
- Premature discontinuation of apixaban has increased risk of thrombotic events.
- To measure adherence for apixaban, measure factor Xa activity. If low, the patient is not taking the medicine.

Andexanet alfa, an antidote to the factor Xa inhibitor, ANNEXA-A Study, currently seeking approval to FDA. (http://www.medscape.com/viewarticle/832648)
Sources: January CT, Wann LS, Alpert JS, et al. 2014 AHA/ACC/HRS Guideline for the Management of Patients With Atrial Fibrillation. *Circulation.* 2014. http://circ.ahajournals.org/content/early/2014/04/10/CIR.0000000000000041. Ruff CR, Giugliano RP. *Hot Topics Cardiol.* 2010;4:7-14. Ericksson BI, et al. *Clin Pharmacokinet.* 2009;48:1-22. Ruff CR, et al. *Am Heart J.* 2010;160:635-641.
–http://www.pradaxa.com
–http://www.xarelto-us.com
–http://www.eliquis.com

EDOXABAN (SAVAYSA®)

- Factor X_a inhibitor.
- FDA indication: nonvalvular AF, DVT, PE.
- Dosage in nonvalvular AF:
  ◦ 60 mg once daily in patients with CrCl >50 to ≤95 mL/min (CrCl with Cockcroft–Gault equation).
  ◦ 30 mg daily in patients with CrCl 15–50 mL/min.
  ◦ Do not use in patients with CrCl >95 mL/min because of increased risk of ischemic stroke compared to warfarin.
  ◦ Not recommended in patients with moderate or severe hepatic impairment (Child–Pugh B and C).
- Contraindications: active pathological bleeding.
- There is no established way to reverse the anticoagulant effects of edoxaban, which can be expected to persist for approximately 24 h after the last dose. The anticoagulant effect of edoxaban cannot be reliably monitored with standard laboratory testing. Hemodialysis does not significantly contribute to edoxaban clearance.
- Epidural or spinal hematomas may occur in patients treated with edoxaban who are receiving neuroaxial anesthesia or undergoing spinal puncture.
- Concomitant use of drugs affecting hemostasis may increase the risk of bleeding. These include aspirin and other antiplatelet agents, other anti-thrombotic agents, fibrinolytic therapy, and chronic use of nonsteroidal anti-inflammatory drugs.
- Pharmacokinetics/pharmacodynamics: peak plasma concentration: 1–2 h, half-life: 10–14 h; renal elimination: 50%. Steady-state concentrations are achieved in 3 d.
- **The ENGAGE AF-TIMI 48 study:** The median study drug exposure for the edoxaban and warfarin treatment groups was 2.5 y. Bleeding led to treatment discontinuation in 3.9% and 4.1% of patients in the edoxaban 60 mg and warfarin treatment groups, respectively. Treatment arms of edoxaban were noninferior to warfarin for the primary efficacy endpoint of stroke or systemic embolism. However, the 30 mg (15 mg dose-reduced) treatment arm was numerically less effective than warfarin for the primary endpoint, and was also markedly inferior in reducing the rate of ischemic stroke. Approximately half of the edoxaban dose is eliminated by the kidney, and edoxaban blood levels are lower in patients with better renal function, averaging about 30% less in patients with CrCl of >80 mL/min, and 40% less in patients with CrCl >95 mL/min when compared to patients with a CrCl of >50 to ≤80 mL/min. Given the clear relationship of dose and blood levels to effectiveness in the ENGAGE AF-TIMI 48 study, it could be anticipated that patients with better renal function would show a smaller effect of edoxaban compared to warfarin than would patients with mildly impaired renal function, and this was in fact observed.
- **Switching to edoxaban**
  ◦ **Switching patients from warfarin to edoxaban:** Discontinue warfarin and start edoxaban when INR ≤2.5.
  ◦ **Switching patients from OAC other than warfarin or other VKA:** Discontinue the current oral anticoagulant and start edoxaban at the time of the next scheduled dose of the other oral anticoagulant.

- **Switching patients from LMWH to edoxaban:** Discontinue LMWH and start edoxaban at the time of the next scheduled administration of LMWH.
- **Switching patients from unfractionated heparin to edoxaban:** Discontinue the infusion and start edoxaban 4 h later.
- **Switching from edoxaban**
- **Switching patients from edoxaban to warfarin**
- ORAL: For patients taking 60 mg of edoxaban, reduce the dose to 30 mg and begin warfarin concomitantly. For patients receiving 30 mg of edoxaban, reduce the dose to 15 mg and begin warfarin concomitantly. INR must be measured at least weekly and just prior to the daily dose of edoxaban to minimize the influence of edoxaban on INR measurements. Once a stable INR ≥2.0 is achieved, edoxaban should be discontinued and the warfarin continued.
  PARENTERAL: Discontinue edoxaban and administer a parenteral anticoagulant and warfarin at the time of the next scheduled edoxaban dose. Once a stable INR ≥2.0 is achieved the parenteral anticoagulant should be discontinued and the warfarin continued.
- **Switching patients from edoxaban to non-VKA anticoagulants:** Discontinue edoxaban and start the other oral anticoagulant at the time of the next dose of edoxaban.
- **Switching patients from edoxaban to parenteral anticoagulants:** Discontinue edoxaban and start the parenteral anticoagulant at the time of the next dose of edoxaban.
- If possible, discontinue edoxaban at least 24 h before invasive or surgical procedures because of the risk of bleeding. It can be restarted after the surgical or other procedure as soon as adequate hemostasis has been established noting that the time to onset of pharmacodynamic effect is 1–2 h. Administer a parenteral anticoagulant and then switch to oral edoxaban, if oral medication cannot be taken during or after surgical intervention.
- Discontinuation of edoxaban without adequate continuous anticoagulation increases the risk of stroke.

Source: http://www.savaysa.com/.

DOAC COMPARISON CHART

	Warfarin	Dabigatran	Rivaroxaban	Apixaban	Edoxaban
Molecular target	Vitamin-dependent clotting factor	Thrombin	Factor X_a	Factor X_a	Factor X_a
Dosing in AF	Once daily	Twice daily	Once daily	Twice daily	Once daily
Time to peak plasma concentration (min)	240	85–150	30–180	30–120	30–60
Time to peak effect (h)	96–120	2	2–3	1–2	1–2
Half-life (h)	40	14–17	5–9 (increased to 11–13 in elderly)	8–15	9–11
Renal clearance	<1%	80%	33%	25%	35%
Hepatic excretion		20%	66%	75% (hepatic-biliary-intestinal)	65%
Food and drug interactions	Foods rich in vitamin K, substrates of CYP2C9, CYP3A4, and CYP1A2	Strong P-gp inhibitors and inducers	Strong CYP3A4 inducers, strong inhibitors of both CYP3A4 and P-gp	Strong inhibitors and inducers of CYP3A4 and P-gp	Strong P-gp inhibitors
Creatinine clearance below which drug is contraindicated	n/a	<30 mL/min	<15 mL/min	<15 mL/min	<30 mL/min (Japan)

Sources: Lip et al. *J Intern Med.* 2015.
Shields AM, Lip GY. Which drug should we use for stroke prevention in atrial fibrillation? *Curr Opin Cardiol.* 2014 Jul;29(4):293-300.

ANTITHROMBOTIC STRATEGIES FOLLOWING CORONARY ARTERY STENTING IN PATIENTS WITH AF AT MODERATE TO HIGH THROMBOEMBOLIC RISK (IN WHOM ORAL ANTICOAGULATION THERAPY IS REQUIRED)

Hemorrhagic Risk	Clinical Setting	Stent Implanted	Anticoagulation Regimen
Low or intermediate (eg, HAS-BLED score 0–2)	Elective	Bare metal	1 mo: triple therapy of VKA (INR 2.0–2.5) + aspirin ≤100 mg/d + clopidogrel 75 mg/d Up to 12th mo: combination of VKA (INR 2.0–2.5) + clopidogrel 75 mg/d (or aspirin 100 mg/d) Lifelong: VKA (INR 2.0–3.0) alone
	Elective	Drug eluting	3 (–olimus[a] group) to 6 (paclitaxel) mo: triple therapy of VKA (INR 2.0–2.5) + aspirin ≤100 mg/d + clopidogrel 75 mg/d Up to 12th mo: combination of VKA (INR 2.0–2.5) + clopidogrel 75 mg/d (or aspirin 100 mg/d) Lifelong: VKA (INR 2.0–3.0) alone
	ACS	Bare metal/drug eluting	6 mo: triple therapy of VKA (INR 2.0–2.5) + aspirin ≤100 mg/d + clopidogrel 75 mg/d Up to 12th mo: combination of VKA (INR 2.0–2.5) + clopidogrel 75 mg/d (or aspirin 100 mg/d) Lifelong: VKA (INR 2.0–3.0) alone
High (eg, HAS-BLED score ≥3)	Elective	Bare metal[b]	2–4 wk: triple therapy of VKA (INR 2.0–2.5) + aspirin ≤100 mg/d + clopidogrel 75 mg/d Lifelong: VKA (INR 2.0–3.0) alone
	ACS	Bare metal[b]	4 wk: triple therapy of VKA (INR 2.0–2.5) + aspirin ≤100 mg/d + clopidogrel 75 mg/d Up to 12th mo: combination of VKA (INR 2.0–2.5) + clopidogrel 75 mg/d[c] (or aspirin 100 mg/d) Lifelong: VKA (INR 2.0–3.0) alone

ACS, acute coronary syndrome; AF, atrial fibrillation; INR, international normalized ratio; VKA, vitamin K antagonis; Gastric protection with a proton pump inhibitor (PPI) should be considered where necessary.

[a]Sirolimus, everolimus, and tacrolimus.

[b]Drug-eluting stents should be avoided as far as possible, but, if used, consideration of more prolonged (3–6 mo) triple antithrombotic therapy is necessary.

[c]Combination of VKA (INR 2.0–3.0) + aspirin ≤100 mg/d (with PPI, if indicated) may be considered as an alternative.

Source: Adapted from Lip GY, Huber K, Andreotti F, et al. European Society of Cardiology Working Group on Thrombosis. Management of antithrombotic therapy in atrial fibrillation patients presenting with acute coronary syndrome and/or undergoing percutaneous coronary intervention/stent. Thromb Haemost. 2010;103:13-28.

ATRIAL FIBRILLATION: MANAGEMENT OF RHYTHM CONTROL DRUG AND NONPHARMACOLOGIC THERAPY

- **AFFIRM, RACE, PIAF,** and **STAF** trials found no difference in quality of life between rate and rhythm control in atrial fibrillation (AF). The AFFIRM and RACE trials demonstrated no difference in stroke rate or mortality between rate and rhythm control in AF.

Favors Rate Control		Favors Rhythm Control
Asymptomatic in AF		Continued symptoms in AF
∘ Older patients	VS	∘ Younger patients
∘ Advanced heart disease		∘ LONE or minimal heart disease
∘ Comorbid conditions		∘ Few comorbid conditions
∘ Persistent AF		∘ Recent onset/paroxysmal AF

- **Rhythm control:**
Fifty percent of patients with new-onset AF spontaneously convert to sinus in 48 h.
- **2, 3, 4 Cardioversion rule**
  - ∘ New-onset AF <**2 d** in duration—may be considered for acute electrical or drug conversion to sinus rhythm while on heparin.
  - ∘ Onset of AF >**2 d** or of unknown duration—requires either **3 wk** of therapeutic oral anticoagulation (INR 2–3) or a negative transesophageal echocardiogram (TEE) to exclude clot before conversion while on heparin.
  - ∘ In either approach to conversion, oral anticoagulation (OAC) must be continued at least **4 wk** postconversion because of the possibility of delayed return of atrial contraction and clot release. In high-risk patients, lifelong OAC should be considered.
- FDA Warning 2011: Dronedarone should not be used in chronic atrial fibrillation; it doubles rate of cardiovascular (CV) death, stroke, and HF.
- **Nonpharmacologic approach**
  - ∘ AF catheter ablation/MAZE procedure (open surgical approach):
  Consider if antiarrhythmic drug therapy fails or if AF coexists with preexcitation pathway. AF ablation is more effective in younger patients with paroxysmal AF; catheter ablation maintains sinus rhythm approximately 80% as opposed to approximately 40% with drugs at 5 y. May require repeat procedures (average: 1.8 procedures). Long-term anticoagulation should be continued even after successful ablation in patients at high risk for thromboembolism. In low-embolic-risk patients, warfarin may be converted to aspirin (ASA) therapy after 3 mo. (*J Am Coll Cardiol.* 2010;55:735-743)
  - ∘ Consider MAZE procedure if performing open heart surgery for other reasons or if vascular or cardiac anatomy prevents the less invasive catheter approach.
  - ∘ Consider implantable atrial defibrillators: least commonly used treatment.
- **Prevention of atrial remodeling**
  - ∘ Calcium channel blockers.
  - ∘ Angiotensin-converting enzyme (ACE) inhibitors.
  - ∘ Angiotensin receptor blocker (ARB) agents.
  - ∘ Statins.

Sources: ACC/AHA/ESC 2006 Guidelines. *J Am Coll Cardiol.* 2006;48:858-906. ACCF/AHA/HRS. *J Am Coll Cardiol.* 2011;57:223-242. ACC/AHA. *Circulation.* 2008;117:1101-1120. ESC 2010 Guidelines. *Eur Heart J.* 2010;31: 2369-2429. *Circulation.* 2009;119:606-618. January CT, Wann LS, Alpert JS, et al. 2014 AHA/ACC/HRS Guideline for the management of patients with atrial fibrillation. *Circulation.* 2014. (http://circ.ahajournals.org/content/early/2014/04/10/CIR.0000000000000041).

STRATEGIES FOR RHYTHM CONTROL IN PATIENTS WITH PAROXYSMAL[a] AND PERSISTENT AF[b] FROM 2014 AHA/ACC/HRS GUIDELINE FOR THE MANAGEMENT OF PATIENTS WITH ATRIAL FIBRILLATION

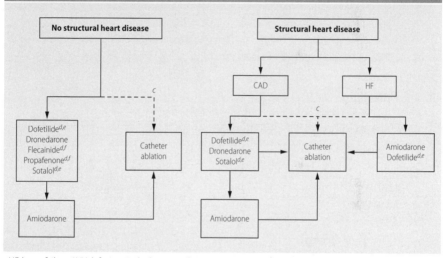

HF, heart failure; LVH, left ventricular hypertrophy.
[a]Catheter ablation is only recommended as first-line therapy for patients with paroxysmal AF (Class IIa recommendation).
[b]Drugs are listed alphabetically.
[c]Depending on patient preference when performed in experienced centers.
[d]Not recommended with severe LVH (wall thickness >1.5 cm).
[e]Should be used with caution in patients at risk for torsades de pointes ventricular tachycardia.
[f]Should be combined with AV nodal blocking agents. AF indicates atrial fibrillation; CAD, coronary artery disease.
Source: January CT, Wann LS, Alpert JS, et al. *J Am Coll Cardiol.* 2014 Dec 2;64(21):e1-76.

Recommendation

▶ Heart Rhythm Society 2014

–Recommends against use of Class Ic antiarrhythmic drugs (Vaughan–Williams) as a first-line agent for the maintenance of sinus rhythm in patients with ischemic heart disease who have experienced prior MI.

Source

–http://www.choosingwisely.org/societies/heart-rhythm-society/

HAS-BLED BLEEDING RISK SCORE FOR WARFARIN THERAPY

Letter	Clinical Characteristics	Points Awarded
H	**Hypertension** (systolic blood pressure [SBP] >160 mm Hg)	1
A	**Abnormal renal function** (presence of chronic dialysis or renal transplantation or serum creatinine ≥2.6 mg/dL) and abnormal liver function (chronic hepatic disease or biochemical evidence of significant hepatic derangement (bilirubin >2× upper limit of normal, in association with glutamic-oxaloacetic transaminase [GOT]/glutamic-pyruvic transaminase [GPT] >3× upper limit normal) *1 point each*	1 or 2
S	**Stroke**	1
B	**Bleeding** (previous bleeding history and/or predisposition to bleeding, eg, bleeding diathesis, anemia)	1
L	**Labile INRs** (unstable/high INRs or poor time in therapeutic range, eg, <60%)	1
E	**Elderly** (age >65 y)	1
D	**Drugs or alcohol** (concomitant use of drugs such as antiplatelet agents, nonsteroidal anti-inflammatory drugs, or alcohol abuse) *1 point each*	1 or 2
		Maximum 9 points

Interpretation

The risk of (spontaneous) major bleeding (intracranial, hospitalization, hemoglobin decrease 2 g/L, and/or transfusion) within 1 y in patients with atrial fibrillation enrolled in the Euro Heart Survey expressed as bleeds per 100 patient-years:

- Score 0:1.13
- Score 2:1.88
- Score 4:8.70
- Score 1:1.02
- Score 3:3.74
- Score 5:12.50
- Score 6–9: insufficient data to quantify risk

Sources:
−2010 Guidelines for the management of atrial fibrillation. *Eur Heart J.* 2010;31:2369-2429; Table 10.
   Pisters R, Lane DA, Nieuwlaat R, de Vos CB, Crijns HJ, Lip GY. A novel user-friendly score (HAS-BLED) to assess 1-y risk of major bleeding in atrial fibrillation patients: the Euro Heart Survey. *Chest.* 2010;138:1093-1100; Table 5.

THROMBOEMBOLIC RISK SCORES IN NONVALVULAR ATRIAL FIBRILLATION				
	CHADS$_2$	**Points**	**CHA$_2$DS$_2$-VASc**	**Points**
C	Congestive heart failure	1	Congestive heart failure **(or *left ventricular systolic dysfunction [LVEF] ≤40%*)**	1
H	Hypertension (blood pressure [BP] consistently >140/90 mm Hg or treated hypertension [HTN] on medication)	1	Hypertension (BP consistently >140/90 mm Hg or treated HTN on medication)	1
A	Age ≥75 y	1	Age ≥75 y	2
D	Diabetes mellitus	1	Diabetes mellitus	1
S$_2$	Prior stroke or transient ischemic attack (TIA)	2	Prior stroke or TIA or ***thromboembolism***	2
V			***Vascular disease (eg, coronary artery disease, peripheral artery disease, myocardial infarction [MI], aortic plaque)***	1
A			***Age 65–74 y***	1
Sc			***Sex category (ie, female gender)***	1
Max.		6		9

STROKE RISK STRATIFICATION WITH THE CHADS$_2$ AND CHA$_2$DS$_2$-VASC SCORES	
	Adjusted Stroke Rate (% per year)
CHADS$_2$ score acronym[a]	
0	1.9
1	2.8
2	4.0
3	5.9
4	8.5
5	12.5
6	18.2

STROKE RISK STRATIFICATION WITH THE CHADS$_2$ AND CHA$_2$DS$_2$-VASC SCORES *(Continued)*

CHADS$_2$-VAS$_c$ score acronym[b]	Adjusted Stroke Rate (% per year)
0	0
1	1.3
2	2.2
3	3.2
4	4.0
5	6.7
6	9.8
7	9.6
8	6.7
9	15.20

[a]C, CHF; H, hypertension; A, age >75 y; D, diabetes mellitus; S, history of stroke or TIA.
[b]C, CHF; H, hypertension; A, age 65–74 y; D, diabetes mellitus; S, history of stroke or TIA; V, vascular disease; A, age 75 y or older; S, female sex.

RISK FACTORS FOR STROKE AND THROMBOEMBOLISM IN NONVALVULAR AF

"Major" Risk Factors	"Clinically Relevant Nonmajor" Risk Factors
Previous • Stroke • TIA • Systemic embolism • Age ≥75 y	• Heart failure or moderate-to-severe left ventricular (LV) systolic dysfunction (LVEF ≤40%) • Hypertension • Diabetes mellitus • Female sex • Age 65–74 y • Vascular disease

Sources: 2010 Guidelines for the management of atrial fibrillation. *Eur Heart J.* 2010;31:2369-2429; Tables 8(a) and (b). Gage BF, Waterman AD, Shannon W, Boechler M, Rich MW, Radford MJ. Validation of clinical classification schemes for predicting stroke. Results from the National Registry of Atrial Fibrillation. *JAMA.* 2001;285:2864-2870.

ATTENTION-DEFICIT HYPERACTIVITY DISORDER (ADHD)

Population
–Children 4–18 y old.

Recommendations
▶ AAP 2011

–Initiate an evaluation for ADHD in any child who presents with academic or behavioral problems and symptoms of inattention, hyperactivity, or impulsivity.

–Consider children with ADHD as children with special health care needs.

–For children age 4–5 y, parent- or teacher-administered behavior therapy is the treatment of choice.

–Methylphenidate is reserved for severe refractory cases.

–For children age 6–18 y, first-line treatment is with FDA-approved medications for ADHD ± behavior therapy.

Source

–http://pediatrics.aappublications.org/content/early/2011/10/14/peds.2011-2654.full.pdf

Population

–Children, young adults, and adults.

Recommendations

▶ NICE 2013

–Health care and education professionals require training to better address the needs of people with ADHD.

–Recommends against universal screening for ADHD in nursery, primary, and secondary schools.

–A diagnosis of ADHD should only be made by a specialist psychiatrist, pediatrician, or other appropriately qualified health care professional with training and expertise in the diagnosis of ADHD.

–Health care professionals should stress the value of a balanced diet, good nutrition, and regular exercise for children, young people, and adults with ADHD.

–Drug treatment is not recommended for preschool children with ADHD.

–Drug treatment is not indicated as the first-line treatment for all school-age children and young people with ADHD. It should be reserved for those with severe symptoms and impairment or for those with moderate levels of impairment who have refused nondrug interventions.

–Where drug treatment is considered appropriate, methylphenidate, atomoxetine, and dexamfetamine are recommended, within their licensed indications, as options for the management of ADHD in children and adolescents.

–For adults with ADHD, drug treatment should be the first-line treatment.

- Following a decision to start drug treatment in adults with ADHD, methylphenidate should normally be tried first.
- Atomoxetine or dexamfetamine should be considered in adults unresponsive or intolerant to an adequate trial of methylphenidate

Source
   –http://www.guideline.gov/content.aspx?id=14325

Comments
   1. Essential to assess any child with ADHD for concomitant emotional, behavioral, developmental, or physical conditions (eg, mood disorders, tic disorders, seizures, sleep disorders, learning disabilities, or disruptive behavioral disorders).
   2. For children 6–18 y, evidence is best to support stimulant medications and less strong to support atomoxetine, ER guanfacine, and ER clonidine for ADHD.

AUTISM

Population
   –Children and young adults.

Recommendations
▶ NICE 2011
   –Consider autism for regression in language or social skills in children <3 y.
   –Clinical signs of possible autism have to be seen in the context of a child's overall development, and cultural variation may pertain.
   –An autism evaluation by a specialist is indicated for any of the following signs of possible autism:
   • Language delay.
   • Regression in speech.
   • Echolalia.
   • Unusual vocalizations or intonations.
   • Reduced social smiling.
   • Rejection of cuddles by family.
   • Reduced response to name being called.
   • Intolerance of others entering into their personal space.
   • Reduced social interest in people or social play.
   • Reduced eye contact.
   • Reduced imagination.
   • Repetitive movements like body rocking.
   • Desire for unchanged routines.
   • Immature social and emotional development.

Source
   –http://www.nice.org.uk/nicemedia/live/13572/56428/56428.pdf

▶ Cochrane Database of Systematic Reviews 2014
  –Recommends against chelation therapy for autism spectrum disorders.

Source
  –http://www.cochrane.org/CD010766/BEHAV_chelation-for-autism-spectrum-disorder-asd

Comment
  –Differential diagnosis of autism includes:
  • Neurodevelopmental disorders.
  • Mood disorders.
  • ADHD.
  • Oppositional defiant disorder.
  • Conduct disorder.
  • Obsessive-compulsive disorder (OCD).
  • Rett syndrome.
  • Hearing or vision impairment.
  • Selective mutism.

AUTISM SPECTRUM DISORDERS (ASDS)

Population
  –Children with ASDs.

Recommendations
▶ American College of Medical Genetics and Genomics 2013
  –Every child with an ASD should have a medical home.
  –A genetic consultation should be offered to all patients with an ASD and their families.
  –Three-generation family history with pedigree analysis.
  –Initial evaluation to identify known syndromes or associated conditions.
  • Examination with special attention to dysmorphic features.
  • If specific syndromic diagnosis is suspected, proceed with targeted testing.
  • If appropriate clinical indicators present, perform metabolic and/or mitochondrial testing (alternatively, consider a referral to a metabolic specialist).
  • Chromosomal microarray: oligonucleotide array-comparative genomic hybridization or single-nucleotide polymorphism array.

- Deoxyribonucleic acid (DNA) testing for fragile X (to be performed routinely for male patients only).
  –*Methyl-CPG-binding protein 2* (*MECP2*) sequencing to be performed for all females with autism spectrum disorders (ASDs).
  –*MECP2* duplication testing in males, if phenotype is suggestive.
  –*Phosphatase and tensin homolog* (*PTEN*) testing only if the head circumference is >2.5 standard deviation (SD) above the mean.

Source
  –http://www.guideline.gov/content.aspx?id=47137

BACK PAIN, LOW

Population
  –Adults.

Recommendations

▶ ACP 2017
  –Consider nonpharmacologic treatments for acute or subacute low-back pain including superficial heat, massage, acupuncture, or spinal manipulation.
  –If pharmacologic treatments needed, start with NSAIDs or skeletal muscle relaxants.
  –For chronic low back pain, start a trial of nonpharmacologic treatments including exercise, multidisciplinary rehabilitation, acupuncture, mindfulness-based stress reduction, tai chi, yoga, biofeedback, cognitive behavioral therapy, or spinal manipulation.
  –For persistent chronic low-back pain, pharmacologic therapy with NSAIDs as first-line therapy and tramadol or duloxetine as second-line therapy.
  –Use opiates for chronic low-back pain only if patients have failed all other therapies and only if the potential benefits outweigh the risks of dependency, addiction, overdose, and misuse.

Sources
  –http://guidelines.gov/summaries/summary/50781/
    noninvasive-treatments-for-acute-subacute-and-chronic-low-
    back-pain-a-clinical-practice-guideline-from-the-american-college-of-
    physicians?q=back+pain

–Qaseem A, Wilt TJ, McLean RM, Forciea MA, Clinical Guidelines Committee of the American College of Physicians. Noninvasive treatments for acute, subacute, and chronic low back pain: a clinical practice guideline from the American College of Physicians. *Ann Intern Med.* 2017 Apr 4;166(7):514-530.

▶ NICE 2009

1. Educate patients and promote self-management of low-back pain.
2. Recommends offering one of the following treatment options:
   a. Structure exercise program.
   b. Manual therapy.[a]
   c. Acupuncture.
3. Consider a psychology referral for patients with a high disability and/or who experience significant psychological distress from their low-back pain.
4. Recommends against routine lumbar spine x-rays.
5. Recommends an MRI scan of lumbar spine only if spinal fusion is under consideration.
6. Consider a referral for surgery in patients with refractory, severe non-specific low-back pain who have completed the programs above and would consider spinal fusion.

Source

–http://www.nice.org.uk/nicemedia/live/11887/44343/44343.pdf

▶ ICSI 2010

–See table.

Source

–https://www.icsi.org/health_initiatives/other_initiatives/low_back_pain/

Comment

1. Analgesic ladder for low-back pain
   a. Recommend scheduled acetaminophen.
   b. Add NSAIDs and/or weak opioids.
   c. Consider adding a tricyclic antidepressant.
   d. Consider a strong opioid for short-term use for people in severe pain.
   e. Refer for specialist assessment for people who may require prolonged use of strong opioids.

[a] Manual therapy includes spinal manipulation, spinal mobilization, and massage.

EVALUATION AND MANAGEMENT OF ACUTE LOW-BACK PAIN

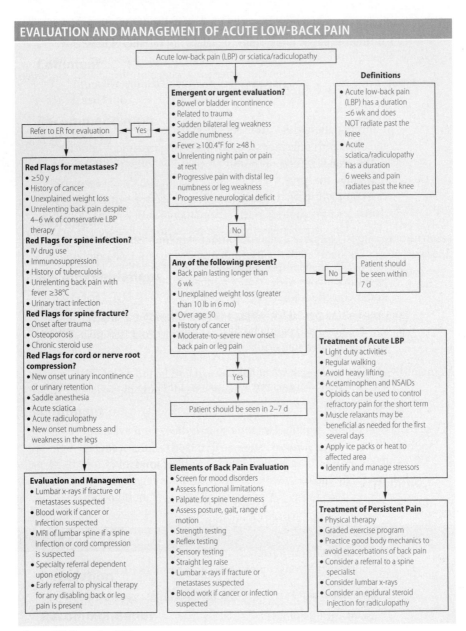

Acute low-back pain (LBP) or sciatica/radiculopathy

Definitions
- Acute low-back pain (LBP) has a duration ≤6 wk and does NOT radiate past the knee
- Acute sciatica/radiculopathy has a duration 6 weeks and pain radiates past the knee

Emergent or urgent evaluation?
- Bowel or bladder incontinence
- Related to trauma
- Sudden bilateral leg weakness
- Saddle numbness
- Fever ≥100.4°F for ≥48 h
- Unrelenting night pain or pain at rest
- Progressive pain with distal leg numbness or leg weakness
- Progressive neurological deficit

Yes → Refer to ER for evaluation

No

Red Flags for metastases?
- ≥50 y
- History of cancer
- Unexplained weight loss
- Unrelenting back pain despite 4–6 wk of conservative LBP therapy

Red Flags for spine infection?
- IV drug use
- Immunosuppression
- History of tuberculosis
- Unrelenting back pain with fever ≥38°C
- Urinary tract infection

Red Flags for spine fracture?
- Onset after trauma
- Osteoporosis
- Chronic steroid use

Red Flags for cord or nerve root compression?
- New onset urinary incontinence or urinary retention
- Saddle anesthesia
- Acute sciatica
- Acute radiculopathy
- New onset numbness and weakness in the legs

Any of the following present?
- Back pain lasting longer than 6 wk
- Unexplained weight loss (greater than 10 lb in 6 mo)
- Over age 50
- History of cancer
- Moderate-to-severe new onset back pain or leg pain

No → Patient should be seen within 7 d

Yes

Patient should be seen in 2–7 d

Treatment of Acute LBP
- Light duty activities
- Regular walking
- Avoid heavy lifting
- Acetaminophen and NSAIDs
- Opioids can be used to control refractory pain for the short term
- Muscle relaxants may be beneficial as needed for the first several days
- Apply ice packs or heat to affected area
- Identify and manage stressors

Evaluation and Management
- Lumbar x-rays if fracture or metastases suspected
- Blood work if cancer or infection suspected
- MRI of lumbar spine if a spine infection or cord compression is suspected
- Specialty referral dependent upon etiology
- Early referral to physical therapy for any disabling back or leg pain is present

Elements of Back Pain Evaluation
- Screen for mood disorders
- Assess functional limitations
- Palpate for spine tenderness
- Assess posture, gait, range of motion
- Strength testing
- Reflex testing
- Sensory testing
- Straight leg raise
- Lumbar x-rays if fracture or metastases suspected
- Blood work if cancer or infection suspected

Treatment of Persistent Pain
- Physical therapy
- Graded exercise program
- Practice good body mechanics to avoid exacerbations of back pain
- Consider a referral to a spine specialist
- Consider lumbar x-rays
- Consider an epidural steroid injection for radiculopathy

Source: ICSI, November 2010.

BARRETT ESOPHAGUS

Population
–Patients with biopsy diagnosis of Barrett esophagus (metaplastic columnar epithelium in distal esophagus).

Recommendations
▶ AGA 2011
  –**No dysplasia**
    Endoscopic surveillance (ES) every 3–5 y.
  –**Low-grade dysplasia**
    • ES every 6–12 mo—consider radiofrequency ablation (RFA)—90% complete eradication of dysplasia.
  –**High-grade dysplasia**
    • ES every 3 mo if no eradication therapy.
  –**Eradication therapy**
    • RFA, photodynamic therapy (PDT), or endoscopic mucosal resection (EMR) is preferred over ES in high-grade dysplasia (strong recommendation).

Sources
–*Gastrointestinal Endoscopy.* 2012;76:1087.
–*Gastroenterology.* 2011;140:1084.
–*N Engl J Med.* 2014;371:836.
–*N Engl J Med.* 2014;371:2499.
–*JAMA.* 2013; 310:627

Comment
–**Clinical Facts**
  • In patients with Barrett esophagus without dysplasia, 0.12% develop esophageal cancer per year compared to 0.5% with low-grade dysplasia.
  • Progression from high-grade dysplasia to cancer is 6% per year. (*N Engl J Med.* 2011;365:1375)
  • Esophagectomy for high-grade dysplasia is an option, but less morbidity with ablation therapy. (*N Engl J Med.* 2009;360:2277)
  • 40% of patients with Barrett esophagus and esophageal cancer have no history of chronic GERD symptoms.
  • Long-term high-dose PPIs or antireflux therapy have been shown to decrease risk of neoplastic progression in patients with Barrett esophagus. (*Clin Gastroenteral Hepatol.* 2013;11:382)
  • Risk of developing cancer is higher among men, older patients (>65 y old) and patients with long segments of Barrett's mucosa or dysplasia. (*Am J Gastroenterol.* 2011;106:1231) (*Gat.* 2016;65:196)

BELL'S PALSY

Population

–Adults with Bell's palsy.

Recommendation

▶ AAN 2012

–For patients with recent-onset Bell's palsy (<72 h of symptoms)
- Steroids are recommended to increase the probability of facial nerve recovery.
  ◦ Prednisone 1 mg/kg PO daily × 7 d.
- Antivirals (eg, acyclovir or valacyclovir) × 7 d given with steroids marginally improves outcomes compared with steroid monotherapy.

Source

–www.guideline.gov/content.aspx?id=38700

Comment

–Antivirals are thought to have a marginal effect at best of facial nerve recovery when added to steroids. The benefit is <7%.

Population

–Adult and children with Bell's palsy.

Recommendations

▶ AAO 2013, Cochrane Database of Systematic Reviews 2015

–No routine lab studies needed for unequivocal Bell's palsy.
–Recommend against routine diagnostic imaging for straightforward Bell's palsy.
–Recommend oral steroids for Bell's palsy with or without antiviral medications if initiated within 72 h of symptom onset in patients 16 y and older.
–Recommend against antiviral monotherapy for Bell's palsy.
–Recommend eye protection for patients with incomplete eye closure.
–Inadequate evidence to support surgical decompression with Bell's palsy.
–Recommend against electrodiagnostic testing for Bell's palsy with incomplete facial paralysis.
–Recommend against physical therapy or acupuncture for Bell's palsy.

Sources

–http://www.guideline.gov/content.aspx?id=47483
–http://www.cochrane.org/CD001869/NEUROMUSC_antiviral-treatment-for-bells-palsy

Comment

–Cochrane analysis found no benefit of adding antivirals to corticosteroids vs. corticosteroid monotherapy.

BENIGN PROSTATIC HYPERPLASIA (BPH)

Population

–Adult men.

Recommendations

▶ AUA 2010

1. Routine measurement of serum creatinine is not indicated in men with BPH.
2. Do not recommend dietary supplements or phytotherapeutic agents for lower urinary tract symptoms (LUTS) management.
3. Patients with LUTS with no signs of bladder outlet obstruction by flow study should be treated for detrusor overactivity.
   a. Alter fluid intake.
   b. Behavioral modification.
   c. Anticholinergic medications.
4. Options for moderate-to-severe LUTS from BPH (AUA symptom index score ≥8).
   a. Watchful waiting.
   b. Medical therapies.
      i. α-blockers.[a]
      ii. 5-Alfa-reductase inhibitors.[b]
      iii. Anticholinergic agents.
      iv. Combination therapy.
   c. Transurethral needle ablation.
   d. Transurethral microwave thermotherapy.
   e. Transurethral laser ablation or enucleation of the prostate.
   f. Transurethral incision of the prostate.
   g. Transurethral vaporization of the prostate.
   h. Transurethral resection of the prostate.
   i. Laser resection of the prostate.
   j. Photoselective vaporization of the prostate.
   k. Prostatectomy.
5. Surgery is recommended for BPH causing renal insufficiency, recurrent urinary tract infections (UTIs), bladder stones, gross hematuria, or refractory LUTS.

---

[a]Alfa-blockers: alfuzosin, doxazosin, tamsulosin, and terazosin. All have equal clinical effectiveness.
[b]5-Alfa-reductase inhibitors: dutasteride and finasteride.

Source

–http://www.guidelines.gov/content.aspx?id=25635&search=aua+2010+bph

Comments

1. Combination therapy with alfa-blocker and 5-alfa-reductase inhibitor is effective for moderate-to-severe LUTS with significant prostate enlargement.
2. Men with planned cataract surgery should have cataract surgery before initiating alfa-blockers.
3. 5-Alfa-reductase inhibitors should not be used for men with LUTS from BPH without prostate enlargement.
4. Anticholinergic agents are appropriate for LUTS that are primarily irritative symptoms and patient does not have an elevated postvoid residual (>250 mL).
5. The choice of surgical method should be based on the patient's presentation, anatomy, surgeon's experience, and patient's preference.

BREAST CANCER FOLLOW-UP CARE

Population

–Early-stage women with curable breast cancer.

Recommendation

▶ American Society of Clinical Oncology (ASCO) 2013

–**Mode of Surveillance**

- Careful history and physical examination every 3–6 mo for first 3 y after primary therapy (with or without adjuvant treatment), then every 6–12 mo for next 2 y and then annually.
- Counsel patients about symptoms of recurrence including new lumps, bone pain, chest pain, dyspnea, abdominal pain, or persistent headaches.
- High-risk women for familial breast CA syndromes should be referred for genetic counseling—high-risk criteria include Ashkenazi Jewish heritage, history of ovarian CA at any age in the patient or any first-degree relatives; any first-degree relative with breast CA before age 50; two or more first- or second-degree relatives diagnosed with breast CA at any age; patient or relative with bilateral breast CA; and history of breast CA in male relative.
- All women should be counseled to perform monthly self-breast examinations.
- Mammography—women treated with breast-conserving therapy should have first posttreatment mammogram no earlier than 6 mo after radiation. Subsequent mammograms every 6–12 mo for surveillance (yearly preferred if stability of mammogram achieved).

- Regular gynecology follow-up with pelvic examination. Tamoxifen increases risk of uterine cancer and patients should be advised to report any vaginal bleeding if they are taking tamoxifen.
- Coordination of care: Risk of recurrence continues through more than 15 y (especially in woman who are hormone receptor positive). Continuity of care by physicians experienced in surveillance of patients and in breast examination is recommended. Follow-up by a primary care physician (PCP) leads to the same outcome as specialist follow-up. If the patient desires transfer of care to PCP, 1 y after definitive therapy is appropriate.

Sources
  −*NCCN Guidelines*. 2015;BINV-16:27
  −*J Clin Oncol*. 2013;31:961-965

Comments

1. **Reduce Routine Investigative Testing**
   - The following routine studies are NOT recommended for routine breast cancer surveillance:
     a. CBC and automated chemistry studies.
     b. Routine chest x-ray.
     c. Bone scans.
     d. Liver ultrasound.
     e. Routine CT scanning.
     f. Routine FDG-PET scanning.
     g. Breast MRI (unless patient has $BRCA_1$ or $BRCA_2$ mutation or previous mediastinal radiation at young age).
     h. Tumor markers including CA27.29, CA15-3, or CEA are not recommended for routine surveillance. (*JAMA*. 1994;27: 1587-1592)

2. Although studies have shown no survival benefit for routine surveillance testing, many oncologists will do routine blood studies including tumor markers especially in higher risk women. The most important follow-up strategy is to make certain patients know and report early signs or symptoms that may reflect recurrent disease.

3. There is a significant difference in the behavior of hormone receptor (HR) positive vs. hormone receptor negative disease. HR-negative disease tends to recur earlier (2–3 y) than HR-positive breast cancer (>50% of relapses occur after 5 y).

4. There is also a 3- to 4-fold increase in risk of brain metastasis in HR-negative women vs. HR-positive women.

5. Overexpression of Her2 is found in 20% of breast cancer patients and targeted therapy in this group has significantly improved prognosis. Her2 overexpressed patients, however, are also at increased risk for brain metastasis.

6. HR-positive patients have a 4-fold increased risk of bone metastasis compared to HR-negative patients in whom metastases to liver, lung, and brain are more common. (*N Engl J Med.* 2007;357:39)

BRONCHITIS, ACUTE

Population
–Adults age ≥18 y.

Recommendations
▶ Michigan Quality Improvement Consortium 2010
1. Recommends against a chest x-ray if all the following are present:
   a. Heart rate <100 beats/min.
   b. Respiratory rate <24 breaths/min.
   c. Temperature <100.4°F (38°C).
2. Recommends against antibiotics.

Source
–http://www.guideline.gov/content.aspx?id=38688

Comments
1. Consider antitussive agents for short-term relief of coughing.
2. β_2 agonists or mucolytic agents should not be used routinely to alleviate cough.

CARBON MONOXIDE POISONING

Population
–Adults presenting to ED with suspected or known carbon monoxide poisoning.

Recommendations
1. Do not use noninvasive carbon monoxide measurements to diagnose carbon monoxide poisoning.
2. Use hyperbaric oxygen or high-flow oxygen therapy for acute carbon monoxide poisoning.
3. Recommend obtaining an EKG and cardiac biomarkers to identify acute myocardial injury in patients with moderate-to-severe carbon monoxide poisoning.

Source
–Wolf SJ, Maloney GE, Shih RD, Shy BD, Brown MD; American College of Emergency Physicians. Clinical policy: critical issues in the evaluation and management of adult patients presenting to the emergency department with acute carbon monoxide poisoning. *Ann Emerg Med.* 2017 Jan;69(1):98-107.e6.

CAROTID ARTERY DISEASE

CAROTID ARTERY STENOSIS

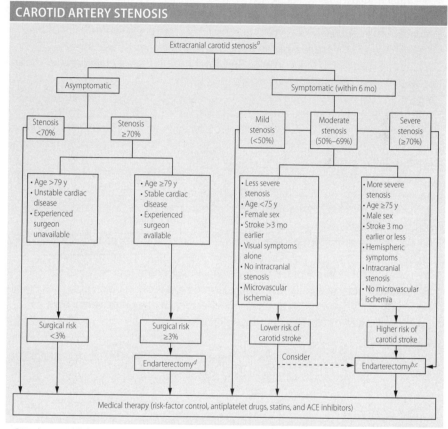

[a]Critical stenosis defined as >70% by noninvasive imaging or >50% by catheter angiography.

[b]Carotid endarterectomy (CEA) in symptomatic patients with average or low surgical risk should generally be reserved for patients with >5 y expectancy, and perioperative stroke/death rate <6%. When CEA is indicated, it should be performed within 2 wk after an ischemic central nervous system (CNS) event.

[c]Carotid artery stenting (CAS) with an embolic protection device is an alternative to CEA in symptomatic patients with average or low surgical risk when >70% obstruction is present, and the periprocedural stroke and mortality rate is <6%. CAS may be chosen over CEA if the neck anatomy is surgically unfavorable or if comorbid conditions make CEA a very high risk.

[d]The annual rate of stroke in asymptomatic patients treated with optimal medical therapy for carotid artery stenosis has decreased to <1%. Therefore, the benefit of CEA or CAS remains controversial in asymptomatic patients. (*Stroke*. 2010;41:975-979)

Source: AHA/ASA 2005 Guidelines. *Circulation*. 2006;113:e872. *Stroke*. 2006;37:577. ASA/ACCF/AHA/AANN/AANS/ACR/ASNR/CNS/SAIP/SCAI/SIR/SNIS/SVM/SVS 2011 Guidelines. *J Am Coll Cardiol*. 2011;57:e16-e94. ACCF/SCAI/SVMB/SIR/ASITN 2007 Consensus. *J Am Coll Cardiol*. 2007;49(1):126-168.

CAROTID ARTERY STENOSIS SURGICAL MANAGEMENT POST-CVA OR STROKE—2014

- CAS (carotid artery stenting) is indicated as an alternative to CEA (carotid endarterectomy) for symptomatic patients at average or low risk of complications associated with endovascular intervention when the diameter of the lumen of the internal carotid artery is reduced by >70% by noninvasive imaging or >50% by catheter-based imaging or noninvasive imaging with corroboration, and the anticipated rate of periprocedural stroke or death is <6% (Class IIa; Level of Evidence (LOE) B).
- It is reasonable to consider patient's age in choosing between CAS and CEA. For older patients (≥70 y), CEA may be associated with improved outcome compared with CAS, particularly when arterial anatomy is unfavorable for endovascular intervention. For younger patients, CAS is equivalent to CEA in terms of risk for periprocedural complication (ie, stroke, MI, or death) and long-term risk for ipsilateral stroke (Class IIa; LOE B).
- CAS and CEA in the above settings should be performed by operators with established periprocedural stroke and mortality rates of <6% for symptomatic patients, similar to that observed in trials comparing CEA to medical therapy and more recent observational studies (Class I; LOE B).
- Routine, long-term follow-up imaging of the extracranial carotid circulation with carotid duplex ultrasonography is not recommended (Class III; Level of Evidence B).
- For patients with recurrent or progressive ischemic symptoms ipsilateral to a stenosis or occlusion of a distal (surgically inaccessible) carotid artery, or occlusion of a midcervical carotid artery after institution of optimal medical therapy, the usefulness of EC/IC bypass is considered investigational (Class IIB; LOE C).

Women only:
- For women with recent TIA or IS and ipsilateral moderate (50%–69%) carotid stenosis, CEA is recommended depending on patient-specific factors, such as age and comorbidities, if the perioperative morbidity and mortality risk is estimated to be <6%.
- In women who are to undergo CEA, aspirin is recommended unless contraindicated, because aspirin was used in every major trial that demonstrated efficacy of CEA.
- For women with recent TIA or IS within the past 6 mo and ipsilateral severe (70%–99%) carotid artery stenosis, CEA is recommended if the perioperative morbidity and mortality risk is estimated to be <6%.
- If a high-risk female patient (ie, 10-y predicted CVD risk ≥10%) has an indication for aspirin but is intolerant to it, the patient should be placed on clopidogrel.
- Aspirin therapy (75–325 mg/d is reasonable in women with diabetes mellitus unless contraindicated.
- When CEA is indicated for women with TIA or stroke, surgery within 2 w is reasonable rather than delaying surgery if there are no contraindications to early revascularization.
- Aspirin therapy can be useful in women >65 y of age (81 mg daily or 100 mg every other day) if blood pressure is controlled and benefit for ischemic and myocardial infarction prevention is likely to outweigh risk of gastrointestinal bleeding and hemorrhagic stroke (Class IIa; Level of Evidence B) and may be reasonable for women <65 y of age for ischemic stroke prevention.

Sources: Guidelines for the Prevention of Stroke in Patients with Stroke and Transient Ischemic Attack: A guideline for healthcare professionals from the American Heart Association/American Stroke Association. *Stroke.* 2014;45. Bushnell C, McCullough LD, Awad IA, et al. Guidelines for the Prevention of Stroke in Women: a Statement for Healthcare Professionals from the American Heart Association/American Stroke Association. *Stroke.* 2014;45. doi: 10.1161/01.str.0000442009.06663.48.

CATARACT

CATARACT IN ADULTS: EVALUATION AND MANAGEMENT ALGORITHM

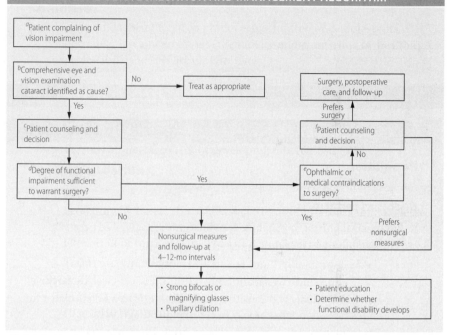

[a]Begin evaluation only when patients complain of a vision problem or impairment.

Identifying impairment in visual function during routine history and physical examination constitutes sound medical practice.

[b]Essential elements of the comprehensive eye and vision exam:

- *Patient history:* Consider cataract if acute or gradual onset of vision loss; vision problems under special conditions (eg, low contrast, glare); difficulties performing various visual tasks. Ask about refractive history, previous ocular disease, amblyopia, eye surgery, trauma, general health history, medications, and allergies. It is critical to describe the actual impact of the cataract on the person's function and quality of life. There are several instruments available for assessing functional impairment related to cataract, including VF-14, Activities of Daily Vision Scale, and Visual Activities Questionnaire.
- *Ocular examination* includes Snellen acuity and refraction; measurement of intraocular pressure; assessment of pupillary function; external exam; slit-lamp exam; and dilated exam of fundus.
- *Supplemental testing:* May be necessary to assess and document the extent of the functional disability and to determine whether other diseases may limit preoperative or postoperative vision. Most elderly patients presenting with visual problems do not have a cataract that causes functional impairment. Refractive error, macular degeneration, and glaucoma are common alternative etiologies for visual impairment.

[c]Once cataract has been identified as the cause of visual disability, patients should be counseled concerning the nature of the problem, its natural history, and the existence of both surgical and nonsurgical approaches to management. The principal factor that should guide decision making with regard to surgery is *the extent to which the cataract impairs the ability to function in daily life.*

The findings of the physical examination should corroborate that the cataract is the major contributing cause of the functional impairment, and that there is a reasonable expectation that managing the cataract will positively impact the patient's functional activity. Preoperative visual acuity is a poor predictor of postoperative functional improvement:

The decision to recommend cataract surgery should not be made solely on the basis of visual acuity.

[d]Patients who complain of mild-to-moderate limitation in activities due to a visual problem, those whose corrected acuities are near 20/40, and those who do not yet wish to undergo surgery may be offered nonsurgical measures for improving visual function. Treatment with nutritional supplements is not recommended. Smoking cessation retards cataract progression.

Indications for surgery: Cataract-impaired vision no longer meets the patient's needs; evidence of lens-induced disease (eg, phacomorphic glaucoma, phacolytic glaucoma); necessary to visualize the fundus in an eye that has the potential for sight (eg, diabetic patient at risk of diabetic retinopathy).

CATARACT IN ADULTS: EVALUATION AND MANAGEMENT ALGORITHM   *(Continued)*

ᵉContraindications to surgery: The patient does not desire surgery; glasses or vision aids provide satisfactory functional vision; surgery will not improve visual function; the patient's quality of life is not compromised; the patient is unable to undergo surgery because of coexisting medical or ocular conditions; a legal consent cannot be obtained; or the patient is unable to obtain adequate postoperative care. Routine preoperative medical testing (12-lead EKG, CBC, measurement of serum electrolytes, BUN, creatinine, and glucose), while commonly performed in patients scheduled to undergo cataract surgery, does not appear to measurably increase the safety of the surgery.
*ᶠ*Patients with significant functional and visual impairment due to cataract who have no contraindications to surgery should be counseled regarding the expected risks and benefits and alternatives to surgery.
Sources: American Academy of Ophthalmology Preferred Practice Pattern: Cataract in the Adult Eye. (2006).
(http://www.aao.org); American Optometric Association Consensus Panel on Care of the Adult Patient with Cataract. Optometric Clinical Practice Guideline: Care of the Adult Patient with Cataract. (2004). (http://www.aoa.org).

CELIAC DISEASE

Population
–Children and adults with celiac disease.

Recommendations

▶ NICE 2015

–Serological testing for suspected celiac disease:
- Test for total IgA and IgA tissue transglutaminase (tTG).
- Use IgA endomysial antibody test if IgA tTG is weakly positive.

–Refer individuals with positive serological tests to a GI specialist for endoscopic duodenal biopsy to confirm the diagnosis.

–For refractory celiac disease despite strict adherence to gluten-free diet:
- Review certainty of diagnosis.
- Consider coexisting conditions such as irritable bowel syndrome, lactose intolerance, microscopic colitis, or inflammatory bowel disease.

Source
–https://guidelines.gov/summaries/summary/49592

CERUMEN IMPACTION

Population
–Children and adults.

Recommendations

▶ AAO-HNS 2008

1. Strongly recommended treating cerumen impaction when it is symptomatic or prevents a needed clinical examination.

2. Clinicians should treat the patient with cerumen impaction with an appropriate intervention:
   a. Ceruminolytic agents.
   b. Irrigation.
   c. Manual removal.

Source

–http://www.entnet.org/practice/cerumenimpaction.cfm

Comment

–Ceruminolytic agents include Cerumenex, addax, Debrox, or dilute solutions of acetic acid, hydrogen peroxide, or sodium bicarbonate.

CHRONIC OBSTRUCTIVE PULMONARY DISEASE (COPD), EXACERBATIONS

Population

–Adults.

Recommendations

▶ ERS/ATS 2017

ERS/ATS RECOMMENDATIONS FOR COPD EXACERBATIONS

TABLE 1 Recommendations for the treatment of chronic obstructive pulmonary disease (COPD) exacerbations

	Recommendation	Strength	Quality of evidence
1	For ambulatory patients with an exacerbation of COPD, we suggest a short course (≤14 days) of oral corticosteroids	Conditional	Very low
2	For ambulatory patients with an exacerbation of COPD, we suggest the administration of antibiotics	Conditional	Moderate
3	For patients who are hospitalised with a COPD exacerbation, we suggest the administration of oral corticosteroids rather than intravenous corticosteroids if gastrointestinal access and function are intact	Conditional	Low
4	For patients who are hospitalised with a COPD exacerbation associated with acute or acute-on-chronic respiratory failure, we recommend the use of noninvasive mechanical ventilation	Strong	Low
5	For patients with a COPD exacerbation who present to the emergency department or hospital, we suggest a home-based management programme (hospital-at-home)	Conditional	Moderate
6	For patients who are hospitalised with a COPD exacerbation, we suggest the initiation of pulmonary rehabilitation within 3 weeks after hospital discharge	Conditional	Very low
7	For patients who are hospitalised with a COPD exacerbation, we suggest not initiating pulmonary rehabilitation during hospitalisation	Conditional	Very low

Source

–Management of COPD exacerbations: a European Respiratory Society/ American Thoracic Society guideline. *Eur Respir J.* 2017;49(3):1600791. doi: 10.1183/13993003.00791-2016. © ERS 2017.

▶ NICE 2010, GOLD 2017

–Recommend noninvasive positive pressure ventilation for moderate-to-severe hypercapnic respiratory failure.

–Prednisolone 30–40 mg orally, or its equivalent IV, should be prescribed for 5-7 d.

–Recommend antibiotics for 5–7 d for COPD exacerbations associated with more purulent sputum or need for mechanical ventilation.

–Bronchodilators can be delivered by either nebulizers or meter-dosed inhalers depending on the patient's ability to use the device during a COPD exacerbation. Bilevel positive airway pressure (Bi-PAP) is indicated for moderate-to-severe COPD exacerbations.

–Bi-PAP decreases mortality, need for mechanical ventilation, infectious complications, and hospital length of stay.

–Subcutaneous heparin or low-molecular-weight heparin for DVT prophylaxis.

–Monitor fluid balance.

–Methylxanthines are not recommended due to its side effect profile.

Sources

–*GOLD 2017 Global Strategy for the Diagnosis, Management and Prevention of COPD,* available at http://goldcopd.org.

–http://www.nice.org.uk/nicemedia/live/13029/49397/49397.pdf

▶ Cochrane Database of Systematic Reviews 2014

–Short-course corticosteroids (7 d or less) is sufficient treatment for adults with a COPD exacerbation.

Source

–http://www.cochrane.org/CD006897/AIRWAYS_are-shorter-courses-of-systemic-steroids-as-effective-as-conventional-longer-courses-in-the-treatment-of-patients-with-flare-ups-of-copd

Comment

–Initial empiric antibiotics should be an aminopenicillin, macrolide, or a tetracycline and should be given for 5–10 d.

CHRONIC OBSTRUCTIVE PULMONARY DISEASE (COPD), STABLE

▶ NICE 2010, GOLD 2017

Population

–Adults.

Recommendations

–Recommends confirming all suspected COPD with postbronchodilator spirometry.

–Recommends spirometry in all persons age >35 y who are current or ex-smokers and have a chronic cough to evaluate for early-stage COPD.

–Recommends smoking cessation counseling.

–GOLD initiative assesses severity of COPD by GOLD Grades 1-4 based on spirometry and GOLD Stages A-D based on symptoms and exacerbation history.

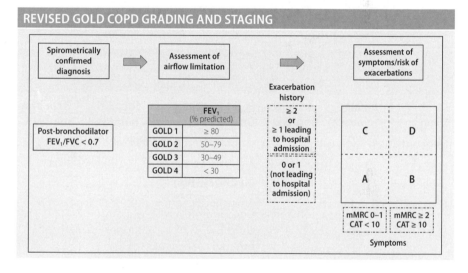

REVISED GOLD COPD GRADING AND STAGING

1. Stepwise medication approach:[a]
   a. Short-acting β-agonist (SABA) and short-acting muscarinic agonist (SAMA) as needed (PRN).
   b. If persistent symptoms, add:
      i. FEV_1 ≥50% of predicted, add either a long-acting β-agonist (LABA) or long-acting muscarinic agonist (LAMA).
      ii. FEV_1 <50% of predicted, add either LABA + inhaled corticosteroid (ICS), or LAMA.
   c. If persistent symptoms, add:
      i. LAMA to LABA + ICS.
      ii. Roflumilast, a phosphodiesterase-4 inhibitor, improves lung function and reduces moderate-to-severe exacerbations for patients with severe COPD.
      iii. Consider azithromycin 250 mg/d for severe COPD with frequent exacerbations.

[a]ICS: beclomethasone, budesonide, ciclesonide, flunisolide, fluticasone, mometasone, and triamcinolone; LABA: arformoterol, formoterol, or salmeterol; LAMA: tiotropium; SABA: albuterol, fenoterol, levalbuterol, metaproterenol, pirbuterol, and terbutaline.

2. Recommend pulmonary rehabilitation for symptomatic patients with moderate-to-severe COPD (FEV$_1$ <50% of predicted).
3. Continuous oxygen therapy should be prescribed for COPD patients with room air hypoxemia (PaO$_2$ ≤55 mm Hg or SpO$_2$ ≤88%).
4. All patients should have a pneumococcal vaccine and annual influenza vaccines.
5. Recommend screening COPD patients for osteoporosis and depression.
6. Recommend against regular mucolytic therapy.
7. Nutritional support indicated for patients with severe COPD with malnutrition.
8. Recommend calculating the BODE index (BMI, airflow obstruction, dyspnea, and exercise capacity on a 6-min walk test) to calculate the risk of death in severe COPD.[b]

COMMON MEDICATIONS FOR THE MANAGEMENT OF COPD

Drug	Inhaler (µg/dose)	Nebulizer (mg/mL)	Drug	Inhaler (µg/dose)	Nebulizer (mg/mL)
Short-acting β$_2$-agonists			**Combination β$_2$-agonist-anticholinergics**		
Albuterol	100–200[M/D]	5	Albuterol-ipratropium	100/20[SMI]	1 vial
Levalbuterol	45–90M	0.21,0.42	**Methylxanthines**		
Long-acting β$_2$-agonists			Aminophylline	200–600 mg pill PO	
Arformoterol		0.0075	Theophylline SR	100–600 mg pill PO	
Formoterol	4.5–12[M/D]	0.01	**Inhaled corticosteroids**		
Indacaterol	75–300[D]		Beclomethasone	50–400[M/D]	0.2–0.4
Salmeterol	25–50[M/D]		Budesonide	100,200,400[D]	0.2,0.25,0.5
Short-acting anticholinergics			Fluticasone	50–500[M/D]	
Ipratropium bromide	20, 40[M]	0.25–0.5	**Combination β$_2$-agonist-corticosteroids**		
Long-acting anticholinergics			Formoterol-budesonide	4.5/160[M]; 9/320[D]	
Aclidinium bromide	322[D]		Formoterol-mometasone	10/200 [M] or 10/400 [M]	
Tiotropium	18[D], 5[SMI]		Salmeterol-fluticasone	50/100, 50/250, 50/500[D] 25/50, 25/125, 25/250[M]	
Phosphodiesterase-4 inhibitors			Vilanterol-fluticasone	25/100[D]	
Roflumilast	500 µg PO daily				

M = metered dose inhalers
D = dry powder inhalers
SMI = Soft mist inhalers
[b]See http://www.nejm.org/doi/full/10.1056/NEJMoa021322#t=article.
Source: Data from *GOLD Guide to COPD Diagnosis, Management and Prevention*. (http://goldcopd.org)

Sources
> –*GOLD 2017 Global Strategy for the Diagnosis, Management and Prevention of COPD,* available at http://goldcopd.org
> –http://www.nice.org.uk/nicemedia/live/13029/49397/49397.pdf

Comments

1. $FEV_1/FVC < 0.7$ confirms the presence of airflow obstruction and COPD.
2. Classification of COPD by spirometry:
   a. Mild COPD = FEV_1 ≥80% of predicted.
   b. Moderate COPD = FEV_1 50–79% of predicted.
   c. Severe COPD = FEV_1 30–49% of predicted.
   d. Very severe COPD = FEV_1 <30% of predicted.
3. Can consider lung volume reduction surgery in patients with severe upper lobe emphysema and low post-pulmonary rehab exercise capacity.
4. Consider roflumilast, a phosphodiesterase-4 inhibitor, to reduce exacerbations for patients with severe chronic bronchitis with frequent exacerbations.

COBALAMIN (B_{12}) DEFICIENCY

Population
> –Adults ≥19 y of age.

Recommendations

▶ British Colombia Medical Services Commission 2012

1. **Who to test:**
   a. Unexplained neurologic symptoms including paresthesias, numbness, poor motor coordination, and cognitive and personality changes.
   b. Macrocytic anemia with oval macrocytes, hypersegmented neutrophils, or pancytopenia.
   c. Elderly (≥75 y old), history of inflammatory bowel disease, gastric or small bowel resection, prolonged vegan diet and specific medications (histamine receptor antagonist, proton pump inhibitors, and metformin).
2. **How to test:**
   a. Perform a complete blood count, peripheral blood smear, and serum B_{12} level.
   b. <220 pmol/L is most recognized cut-off with increasing probability of clinical deficiency. If B_{12} <75 Pmol/L, clinical signs and symptoms are highly likely. In borderline patients with normal renal function, methylmalonic acid levels will be elevated in B_{12} deficient patients.
   c. Elevated LDH, indirect bilirubin, and low haptoglobin are common findings.

3. Treatment—Early

a. Therapy of cobalamin deficiency is important because neurologic symptoms may be irreversible if treatment delayed.

b. Oral crystalline cyanocobalamin is as effective as parenteral B_{12}. 1000 μg/d is the recommended dose but parenteral administration (1000 μg/d for 5–10 d) should be given to patients with neurological symptoms.

c. In these patients 1000–2000 μg/d given orally should follow parenteral administration.

d. Retest serum cobalamin levels after 2–4 mo to ensure they are in the normal range.

Sources

–Medical Services Commission. Cobalamine (vitamin B_{12}) deficiency investigation and management. Victoria British Colombia: Medical Services Commission; January 1, 2012.

–*Blood.* 2008;112:2214-2221.

–*Blood.* 2017;129:2603.

Comments

1. Pernicious anemia (the most common cause of B_{12} deficiency) is an autoimmune illness with antibodies to parietal cells and intrinsic factor resulting in gastric atrophy and malabsorption of food-derived B_{12}.

2. Cobalamin is found exclusively in animal products such as meat, seafood, dairy products, and eggs. Consider supplemental oral B_{12} in patients who are long-term vegans.

3. No matter what the cause of B_{12} deficiency, oral B_{12} (1000–2000 μ) daily will correct lower B_{12} levels.

4. With pure B_{12} deficiency the mean corpuscular volume (MCV) is usually >110. If iron deficiency is also present due to bleed or a trophic gastritis the MCV can be <100.

5. Patients with elevated MCV who are folate deficient must have B_{12} deficiency ruled out since treatment with folate in patients with B_{12} deficiency will accelerate peripheral neuropathy.

6. The incidence of B_{12} deficiency in the elderly (>70 y old) is 5%–10%.

7. Less frequent causes of B_{12} deficiency include *Helicobacter pylori* infection, *Diphyllobothrium latum* infection, nitrous oxide exposure, alcoholism, Zollinger-Ellison syndrome, small bowel diverticulum, and following gastric bypass surgery.

8. Drugs that can cause folate deficiency include trimethoprim, pyrimethamine, methotrexate, and phenytoin.

9. When treating B_{12} and folate deficiency, the MCV may become decreased due to acquired iron deficiency as iron is incorporated into red cell precursors in response to B_{12} and/or folate therapy.

COLITIS, *CLOSTRIDIUM DIFFICILE*

Population
–Adults.

Recommendation

▶ IDSA SHEA 2010

–Treatment of *C. difficile* infection.
- Discontinue antibiotics as soon as possible.
- Avoid antiperistaltic agents.
- Mild-to-moderate *C. difficile* infection: metronidazole 500 mg PO tid × 10–14 d.
- Severe *C. difficile* infection: vancomycin 125 mg PO qid × 10–14 d.
- Severe complicated *C. difficile* infection taking POs: vancomycin 500 mg PO qid ± metronidazole 500 mg IV q8h.
- Severe complicated *C. difficile* infection and NPO: 500 mg in 100 mL normal saline enema per rectum qid ± metronidazole 500 mg IV q8h.
- Administer vancomycin as a tapered regimen for recurrent *C. difficile* infection.

Source
–http://www.doh.state.fl.us/disease_ctrl/epi/HAI/SHEA_IDSA_Clinical_Practice_Cdiff_Guideline.pdf

Comments

1. Testing for *C. difficile* or its toxins should be performed only on diarrheal stool.
2. Testing of stool on asymptomatic patients should be avoided.
3. Enzyme immunoassay (EIA) testing for *C. difficile* toxins A and B is rapid but is less sensitive than the cell cytotoxin assay.
4. Stool for *C. difficile* toxins by polymerase chain reaction (PCR) is rapid and very sensitive and specific.

Population
–Adults and children.

Recommendations

▶ ACG 2013

–Only diarrheal stools should be tested for *C. difficile*.
–Nucleic acid amplification tests (NAAT) for *C. difficile* toxin genes such as polymerase chain reaction (PCR) are superior to toxins A+B enzyme immunoassay (EIA) testing as a standard diagnostic test for *C. difficile* infection (CDI).
–Do not perform repeat testing.
–Avoid testing for cure.

–Management of mild-to-moderate *C. difficile* infection (CDI)
- Stop all unnecessary antibiotics.
- Recommend empiric therapy of CDI regardless of test results if high pretest probability of CDI.
- First-line therapy.
- Metronidazole 500 mg PO tid × 10 d.
- Second-line therapy.
- Vancomycin 125 mg PO qid × 10 d.
- Indicated for intolerance of metronidazole, lack of improvement after 5–7 d on metronidazole, pregnancy, or breast-feeding.
- Avoid antiperistaltic meds.

–Severe or complicated CDI
- Vancomycin 125 mg PO qid AND metronidazole 500 mg IV q8h × 10 d.
- If ileus or severe abdominal distension, use vancomycin 500 mg PO qid AND 500 mg enema PR qid AND metronidazole 500 mg IV q8h × 10 d.
- IV hydration.
- Electrolyte repletion.
- DVT prophylaxis.
- Surgical consult for all patients with complicated CDI.

–Recurrent CDI
- Consider fetal microbiota transplant after third recurrence.

Source
–http://www.guideline.gov/content.aspx?id=45139

Comments

1. Limited evidence that probiotics decrease risk of recurrent CDI.
2. The following patients should be tested for CDI:
   - IBD patients with a flare.
   - IBD patients with a surgically created pouch who develop abdominal pain.
3. Immunosuppressed patients with an acute diarrheal illness.
4. Pregnant patients who develop diarrhea.

Population

–Adult patients with *C. difficile*–associated disease.

Recommendations

▶ EAST 2014

–If surgery is indicated, recommend a subtotal or total colectomy.
–For severe CDAD, patients should undergo surgery prior to the development of shock and need for vasopressors.

Source
–http://www.guideline.gov/content.aspx?id=48870

COLORECTAL CANCER FOLLOW-UP CARE

Population
–Adults with nonmetastatic colorectal cancer (Stages II and III).

Recommendation
▶ American Society of Clinical Oncology Cancer Care Ontario (CCO) 2013
–**Follow-up for Recurrence**
- Surveillance guided by risk of recurrence and functional status of the patient. Early detection of relapse would lead to treatment including surgery for possible cure.
- Highest risk of recurrence during first 4 y after diagnosis. 95% of relapses occur in first 5 y.
- Medical history, physical exam, and CEA testing every 3–6 mo for 5 y. The higher the risk, the more frequent the follow-up.
- Abdominal and chest CT scan is recommended annually for 3 y. Highest risk patients (Stage III, >4 nodes+) should consider imaging every 4–6 mo.
- Routine PET scan not recommended for surveillance.
- Patients with rectal cancer should also have pelvic CT annually for 3–5 y.
- A surveillance colonoscopy should be performed 1 y after initial surgery. If normal, repeat colonoscopy every 5 y. If complete colonoscopy not performed before diagnosis perform it as soon as the patient recovers from adjuvant therapy.
  a. Any new or persistent worsening of symptoms warrant consideration of recurrence.

Source
–*J Clin Oncol.* 2013;31:4465–4470

Comment
–**Clinical Correlation**
- Stage I colon cancer with very low risk of recurrence. Colonoscopy follow-up every 5 y but CEA and imaging not needed.
- Colon cancer with >90% to liver as the first site of metastasis. In rectal cancer, 50% of first metastasis is to lung and 50% to liver. (*CA Cancer J Clin.* 2015;65:5)
- Patients found to have resectable metastatic disease (liver, lungs) or local recurrence who are rendered disease free by surgical or radiofrequency

ablation (RFA) should be followed with frequent surveillance. 10-y
survival is in 30%–40% range. (*J Clin Onc.* 2010;28:2300)

- *BRAF* mutation prognostic for early relapse and chemotherapy
  resistance with shortened survival. (*PloS One.* 2013;8:eb5995)
- Patients with CRC younger than 50 y old or with significant family
  history should be evaluated for Lynch syndrome with microsatellite
  instability and immune histochemistry testing. (*N Engl J Med.*
  2009;361:2449)
- Patients with Stage II CRC with microsatellite instability will have
  a shorter survival if given adjuvant 5-fluorouracil compared to
  placebo. (*Clin Genet.* 2009;76:1)
- Uncertainty remains regarding use of cyclooxygenase inhibitor to
  reduce risk of recurrence but aspirin is now approved to decrease
  risk of CRC.
- Exercise (>150 min/wk), weight loss for high BMI, smoking
  cessation, and healthy diet advised—evidence suggests a decrease
  in disease recurrence.

COMMON COLD

Population
–Children and adults.

Recommendation
▶ Cochrane Database of Systematic Reviews 2013
  –Recommends zinc at a dose of at least 75 mg/d started within 24 h of
  the onset of a common cold.

Source
–http://onlinelibrary.wiley.com/doi/10.1002/14651858.CD001364.pub4/
abstract

Comment
–Zinc at this dose reduces the duration of the common cold by about
1 d, but did not affect the severity of symptoms.

CONCUSSIONS

Population
–Children and young adults.

Recommendations
▶ AAN 2013
  –Standardized sideline assessment tools should be used to assess athletes
  with suspected concussions.

–Teams should immediately remove from play any athlete with a suspected concussion.

–Teams should not permit an athlete to return to play until he/she has been cleared to play by a licensed health care professional.

Source

–http://www.guideline.gov/content.aspx?id=43947

CONSTIPATION, IDIOPATHIC

Population

–Children age ≤18 y.

Recommendations

▶ NICE 2010

–Assess all children for fecal impaction.

–Recommends polyethylene glycol (PEG) as first-line agent for oral disimpaction.

–Add a stimulant laxative if PEG therapy is ineffective after 2 wk.

–Recommends sodium citrate enemas for disimpaction only if all oral medications have failed.

–Recommends a maintenance regimen with PEG for several months after a regular bowel pattern has been established.

–Recommends gradually tapering maintenance dose over several months as bowel pattern allows.

–Recommends adequate fluid intake.

Source

–http://www.nice.org.uk/nicemedia/live/12993/48741/48741.pdf

Comment

–Minimal fluid intake for age

Age (y)	Volume (mL)
1–3	1300
4–8	1700
9–13	2200
14–18	2500

Population

–Adults.

Recommendations

▶ AGA 2013

–Digital examination to evaluate resting sphincter tone.

–Discontinue all medications that can cause constipation.

–Assess for hypercalcemia, hypothyroidism.

–Trial of laxatives and fiber

- Bisacodyl.
- Milk of magnesia.
- Polyethylene glycol.
- Senna.

–Refractory constipation may require biofeedback or pelvic floor retraining.

- Severe cases of refractory slow transit constipation may require a total colectomy with ileorectal anastomosis.

Source

–http://www.gastrojournal.org/article/S0016-5085%2812%2901545-4/fulltext

CONTRACEPTION

PERCENTAGE OF WOMEN EXPERIENCING AN UNINTENDED PREGNANCY WITHIN THE FIRST YEAR OF TYPICAL USE AND THE FIRST YEAR OF PERFECT USE AND THE PERCENTAGE CONTINUING USE AT THE END OF THE FIRST YEAR: UNITED STATES*

% of Women Experiencing an Unintended Pregnancy Within the First Year of Use

Method	Typical Use[a]	Perfect Use[b]	Women Continuing Use at 1 Y[c]
R16 No method[d]	85	85	
R15 Spermicides[e]	28	18	42
R12 Withdrawal	22	4	46
R13 Fertility awareness-based methods	24		47
Standard Days method[f]		5	
Two-Day method[f]		4	
Ovulation method[f]		3	
Symptothermal method[f]	0.4		
Sponge			
R11 Parous women	24	20	
Nulliparous women	12	9	
R9 Diaphragm	12	6	57
Condom[h]			
R10 Female (fc)	21	5	41
Male	18	2	43
R8 Combined pill and Progestin-only pill	9	0.3	67
R7 Evra patch*	9	0.3	67

R6 NuvaRing*	9	0.3	67
R5 Depo-Provera	6	0.2	56
Intrauterine contraceptives			
R4 ParaGard (copper T)	0.8	0.6	78
Mirena (LNg)	0.2	0.2	80
R3 Implanon	0.05	0.05	84
R2 Female sterilization	0.5	0.5	100
R1 Male sterilization	0.15	0.10	100

Emergency Contraceptive Pills: Treatment with COCs initiated within 120 h after unprotected intercourse reduces the risk of pregnancy by at least 60–75%[i]. Pregnancy rates lower if initiated in first 12 h. Progestin-only EC reduces pregnancy risk by 89%.

Lactational Amenorrhea Method: LAM is a highly effective, temporary method of contraception.[j]

[a]Among typical couples who initiate use of a method (not necessarily for the first time), the percentage who experience an accidental pregnancy during the first year if they do not stop use for any other reason. Estimates of the probability of pregnancy during the first year of typical use for spermicides, withdrawal, fertility awareness-based methods, the diaphragm, the male condom the oral contraceptive pill, and Depo-Provera are taken from the 1995 National Survey of Family Growth corrected for underreporting of abortion; see the text for the derivation of estimates for the other methods.

[b]Among couples who initiate use of a method (not necessarily for the first time) and who use it perfectly (both consistently and correctly), the percentage who experience an accidental pregnancy during the first year if they do not stop use for any other reason. See the text for the derivation of the estimate for each method.

[c]Among couples attempting to avoid pregnancy, the percentage who continue to use a method for 1 y.

[d]The percentages becoming pregnant in columns (2) and (3) are based on data from populations where contraception is not used and from women who cease using contraception in order to become pregnant. Among such populations, about 89% become pregnant within 1 y. This estimate was lowered slightly (to 85%) to represent the percentage who would become pregnant within 1 y among women now relying on reversible methods of contraception if they abandoned contraception altogether.

[e]Foams, creams, gels, vaginal suppositories, and vaginal film.

[f]The Ovulation and Two-Day methods are based on evaluation of cervical mucus. The Standard-Days method avoids intercourse on cycle days 8 through 19. The Symptothermal method is a double-check method based on evaluation of cervical mucus to determine the first fertile day and evaluation of cervical mucus and temperature to determine the last fertile day.

[g]Without spermicides.

[h]With spermicidal cream or jelly.

[i]ella, Plan B One-Step and Next Choice are the only dedicated products specifically marketed for emergency contraception. The label for Plan B One-Step (one dose is 1 white pill) says to take the pill within 72 h after unprotected intercourse. Research has shown that all of the brands listed here are effective when used within 120 h after unprotected sex. The label for Next Choice (one dose is 1 peach pill) says to take 1 pill within 72 h after unprotected intercourse and another pill 12 h later. Research has shown that both pills can be taken at the same time with no decrease in efficacy or increase in side effects and that they are effective when used within 120 h after unprotected sex. The Food and Drug Administration has in addition declared the following 19 brands of oral contraceptives to be safe and effective for emergency contraception: Ogestrel (1 dose is 2 white pills), Nordette (1 dose is 4 light-orange pills), Cryselle, Levora, Low-Ogestrel, Lo/Ovral, or Quasence (1 dose is 4 white pills), Jolessa, Portia, Seasonale or Trivora (1 dose is 4 pink pills), Seasonique (1 dose is 4 light-blue-green pills), Enpresse (one dose is 4 orange pills), Lessina (1 dose is 5 pink pills), Aviane or LoSeasonique (one dose is 5 orange pills), Lutera or Sronyx (one dose is 5 white pills), and Lybrel (one dose is 6 yellow pills).

[j]However, to maintain effective protection against pregnancy, another method of contraception must be used as soon as menstruation resumes, the frequency or duration of breastfeeds is reduced, bottle feeds are introduced, or the baby reaches 6 mo of age.

Source: Hatcher RA, Zieman M, Allen AZ, Lathrop E, Haddad L, *Managing Contraception 2017-2018*. Tiger, Georgia: Bridging the Gap Foundation, 2017.

SUMMARY OF CHANGES IN CLASSIFICATIONS FROM WHO MEDICAL ELIGIBILITY CRITERIA FOR CONTRACEPTIVE USE, 4TH EDITION[a,b]

Condition	Sub-Condition	Cu-IUD		LNG-IUD		Implant		DMPA		POP		CHC	
		I	C	I	C	I	C	I	C	I	C	I	C
Age		Menarche to <20 yrs:**2** ≥20 yrs:**1**		Menarche to <20 yrs:**2** ≥20 yrs:**1**		Menarche to <18 yrs:**1** 18-45 yrs:**1** >45 yrs:**1**		Menarche to <18 yrs:**2** 18-45 yrs:**1** >45 yrs:**2**		Menarche to <18 yrs:**1** 18-45 yrs:**1** >45 yrs:**1**		Menarche to <40 yrs:**1** ≥40 yrs:**2**	
Anatomical abnormalities	a) Distorted uterine cavity	4		4									
	b) Other abnormalities	2		2									
Anemias	a) Thalassemia	2		1		1		1		1		1	
	b) Sickle cell disease[3]	2		1		1		1		1		2	
	c) Iron-deficiency anemia	2		1		1		1		1		1	
Benign ovarian tumors	(including cysts)	1		1		1		1		1		1	
Breast disease	a) Undiagnosed mass	1		2		2*		2*		2*		2*	
	b) Benign breast disease	1		1		1		1		1		1	
	c) Family history of cancer	1		1		1		1		1		1	
	d) Breast cancer[3]												
	i) Current	1		4		4		4		4		4	
	ii) Past and no evidence of current disease for 5 years	1		3		3		3		3		3	
Breastfeeding	a) <21 days postpartum					2*		2*		2*		4*	
	b) 21 to <30 days postpartum												
	i) With other risk factors for VTE					2*		2*		2*		3*	
	ii) Without other risk factors for VTE					2*		2*		2*		3*	
	c) 30-42 days postpartum												
	i) With other risk factors for VTE					1*		1*		1*		3*	
	ii) Without other risk factors for VTE					1*		1*		1*		2*	
	d) >42 days postpartum					1*		1*		1*		2*	
Cervical cancer	Awaiting treatment	4	2	4	2	2		2		1		2	
Cervical ectropion		1		1		1		1		1		1	
Cervical intraepithelial neoplasia		1		2		2		2		1		2	
Cirrhosis	a) Mild (compensated)	1		1		1		1		1		1	
	b) Severe[3] (decompensated)	1		3		3		3		3		4	
Cystic fibrosis[3]		1*		1*		1*		2*		1*		1*	
Deep venous thrombosis (DVT)/Pulmonary embolism (PE)	a) History of DVT/PE, not receiving anticoagulant therapy												
	i) Higher risk for recurrent DVT/PE	1		2		2		2		2		4	
	ii) Lower risk for recurrent DVT/PE	1		2		2		2		2		3	
	b) Acute DVT/PE	2		2		2		2		2		4	
	c) DVT/PE and established anticoagulant therapy for at least 3 months												
	i) Higher risk for recurrent DVT/PE	2		2		2		2		2		4*	
	ii) Lower risk for recurrent DVT/PE	2		2		2		2		2		3*	
	d) Family history (first-degree relatives)	1		1		1		1		1		2	
	e) Major surgery												
	i) With prolonged immobilization	1		2		2		2		2		4	
	ii) Without prolonged immobilization	1		1		1		1		1		2	
	f) Minor surgery without immobilization	1		1		1		1		1		1	
Depressive disorders		1*		1*		1*		1*		1*		1*	

Key:

1	No restriction (method can be used)	3	Theoretical or proven risks usually outweigh the advantages
2	Advantages generally outweigh theoretical or proven risks	4	Unacceptable health risk (method not to be used)

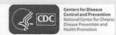

Centers for Disease Control and Prevention
National Center for Chronic Disease Prevention and Health Promotion

Condition	Sub-Condition	Cu-IUD		LNG-IUD		Implant		DMPA		POP		CHC	
		I	C	I	C	I	C	I	C	I	C	I	C
Diabetes	a) History of gestational disease	1		1		1		1		1		1	
	b) Nonvascular disease												
	i) Non-insulin dependent	1		2		2		2		2		2	
	ii) Insulin dependent	1		2		2		2		2		2	
	c) Nephropathy/retinopathy/neuropathy[‡]	1		2		2		3		2		3/4*	
	d) Other vascular disease or diabetes of >20 years' duration[‡]	1		2		2		3		2		3/4*	
Dysmenorrhea	Severe	2		1		1		1		1		1	
Endometrial cancer[‡]		4	2	4	2	1		1		1		1	
Endometrial hyperplasia		1		1		1		1		1		1	
Endometriosis		2		1		1		1		1		1	
Epilepsy[‡]	(see also Drug Interactions)	1		1		1*		1*		1*		1*	
Gallbladder disease	a) Symptomatic												
	i) Treated by cholecystectomy	1		2		2		2		2		2	
	ii) Medically treated	1		2		2		2		2		3	
	iii) Current	1		2		2		2		2		3	
	b) Asymptomatic	1		2		2		2		2		2	
Gestational trophoblastic disease[‡]	a) Suspected GTD (immediate postevacuation)												
	i) Uterine size first trimester	1*		1*		1*		1*		1*		1*	
	ii) Uterine size second trimester	2*		2*		1*		1*		1*		1*	
	b) Confirmed GTD												
	i) Undetectable/non-pregnant ß-hCG levels	1*	1*	1*	1*	1*		1*		1*		1*	
	ii) Decreasing ß-hCG levels	2*	1*	2*	1*	1*		1*		1*		1*	
	iii) Persistently elevated ß-hCG levels or malignant disease, with no evidence or suspicion of intrauterine disease	2*	1*	2*	1*	1*		1*		1*		1*	
	iv) Persistently elevated ß-hCG levels or malignant disease, with evidence or suspicion of intrauterine disease	4*	2*	4*	2*	1*		1*		1*		1*	
Headaches	a) Nonmigraine (mild or severe)	1		1		1		1		1		1*	
	b) Migraine												
	i) Without aura (includes menstrual migraine)	1		1		1		1		1		2*	
	ii) With aura	1		1		1		1		1		4*	
History of bariatric surgery[‡]	a) Restrictive procedures	1		1		1		1		1		1	
	b) Malabsorptive procedures	1		1		1		1		3		COCs: 3 P/R: 1	
History of cholestasis	a) Pregnancy related	1		1		1		1		1		2	
	b) Past COC related	1		2		2		2		2		3	
History of high blood pressure during pregnancy		1		1		1		1		1		2	
History of Pelvic surgery		1		1		1		1		1		1	
HIV	a) High risk for HIV	2	2	2	2	1		1*		1		1	
	b) HIV infection					1*		1*		1*		1*	
	i) Clinically well receiving ARV therapy	1	1	1	1	If on treatment, see Drug Interactions							
	ii) Not clinically well or not receiving ARV therapy[‡]	2	1	2	1	If on treatment, see Drug Interactions							

Abbreviations: C=continuation of contraceptive method; CHC=combined hormonal contraception (pill, patch, and, ring); COC=combined oral contraceptive; Cu-IUD=copper-containing intrauterine device; DMPA = depot medroxyprogesterone acetate; I=initiation of contraceptive method; LNG-IUD=levonorgestrel-releasing intrauterine device; NA=not applicable; POP=progestin-only pill; P/R=patch/ring ‡ Condition that exposes a woman to increased risk as a result of pregnancy. *Please see the complete guidance for a clarification to this classification: www.cdc.gov/reproductivehealth/unintendedpregnancy/USMEC.htm.

SUMMARY OF CHANGES IN CLASSIFICATIONS FROM WHO MEDICAL ELIGIBILITY CRITERIA FOR CONTRACEPTIVE USE, 4TH EDITION [a,b]   (Continued)

Condition	Sub-Condition	Cu-IUD I	Cu-IUD C	LNG-IUD I	LNG-IUD C	Implant I	Implant C	DMPA I	DMPA C	POP I	POP C	CHC I	CHC C
Hypertension	a) Adequately controlled hypertension	1*	1*	1*	1*	1*	1*	2*	2*	1*	1*	3*	3*
	b) Elevated blood pressure levels (properly taken measurements)												
	i) Systolic 140-159 or diastolic 90-99	1*	1*	1*	1*	1*	1*	2*	2*	1*	1*	3*	3*
	ii) Systolic ≥160 or diastolic ≥100‡	1*	1*	2*	2*	2*	2*	3*	3*	2*	2*	4*	4*
	c) Vascular disease	1*	1*	2*	2*	2*	2*	3*	3*	2*	2*	4*	4*
Inflammatory bowel disease‡	(Ulcerative colitis, Crohn's disease)	1	1	1	1	1	1	2	2	2	2	2/3*	2/3*
Ischemic heart disease‡	Current and history of	1	1	2	3	2	3	3	3	2	3	4	4
Known thrombogenic mutations‡		1*	1*	2*	2*	2*	2*	2*	2*	2*	2*	4*	4*
Liver tumors	a) Benign												
	i) Focal nodular hyperplasia	1	1	2	2	2	2	2	2	2	2	2	2
	ii) Hepatocellular adenoma‡	1	1	3	3	3	3	3	3	3	3	4	4
	b) Malignant‡ (hepatoma)	1	1	3	3	3	3	3	3	3	3	4	4
Malaria		1	1	1	1	1	1	1	1	1	1	1	1
Multiple risk factors for atherosclerotic cardiovascular disease	(e.g., older age, smoking, diabetes, hypertension, low HDL, high LDL, or high triglyceride levels)	1	1	2	2	2*	2*	3*	3*	2*	2*	3/4*	3/4*
Multiple sclerosis	a) With prolonged immobility	1	1	1	1	1	1	2	2	1	1	3	3
	b) Without prolonged immobility	1	1	1	1	1	1	2	2	1	1	1	1
Obesity	a) Body mass index (BMI) ≥30 kg/m²	1	1	1	1	1	1	1	1	1	1	2	2
	b) Menarche to <18 years and BMI ≥ 30 kg/m²	1	1	1	1	1	1	2	2	1	1	2	2
Ovarian cancer‡		1	1	1	1	1	1	1	1	1	1	1	1
Parity	a) Nulliparous	2	2	2	2	1	1	1	1	1	1	1	1
	b) Parous	1	1	1	1	1	1	1	1	1	1	1	1
Past ectopic pregnancy		1	1	1	1	1	1	1	1	2	2	1	1
Pelvic inflammatory disease	a) Past												
	i) With subsequent pregnancy	1	1	1	1	1	1	1	1	1	1	1	1
	ii) Without subsequent pregnancy	2	2	2	2	1	1	1	1	1	1	1	1
	b) Current	4	2*	4	2*	1	1	1	1	1	1	1	1
Peripartum cardiomyopathy‡	a) Normal or mildly impaired cardiac function												
	i) <6 months	2	2	2	2	1	1	1	1	1	1	4	4
	ii) ≥6 months	2	2	2	2	1	1	1	1	1	1	3	3
	b) Moderately or severely impaired cardiac function	2	2	2	2	2	2	2	2	2	2	4	4
Postabortion	a) First trimester	1*	1*	1*	1*	1*	1*	1*	1*	1*	1*	1*	1*
	b) Second trimester	2*	2*	2*	2*	1*	1*	1*	1*	1*	1*	1*	1*
	c) Immediate postseptic abortion	4	4	4	4	1*	1*	1*	1*	1*	1*	1*	1*
Postpartum (nonbreastfeeding women)	a) <21 days							1	1	1	1	4	4
	b) 21 days to 42 days												
	i) With other risk factors for VTE					1	1	1	1	1	1	3*	3*
	ii) Without other risk factors for VTE					1	1	1	1	1	1	2	2
	c) >42 days					1	1	1	1	1	1	1	1
Postpartum (in breastfeeding or non-breastfeeding women, including cesarean delivery)	a) <10 minutes after delivery of the placenta												
	i) Breastfeeding	1*	1*	2*	2*								
	ii) Nonbreastfeeding	1*	1*	1*	1*								
	b) 10 minutes after delivery of the placenta to <4 weeks	2*	2*	2*	2*								
	c) ≥4 weeks	1*	1*	1*	1*								
	d) Postpartum sepsis	4	4	4	4								

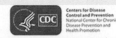

Centers for Disease Control and Prevention
National Center for Chronic Disease Prevention and Health Promotion

Condition	Sub-Condition	Cu-IUD		LNG-IUD		Implant		DMPA		POP		CHC	
		I	C	I	C	I	C	I	C	I	C	I	C
Pregnancy		4*		4*		NA*		NA*		NA*		NA*	
Rheumatoid arthritis	a) On immunosuppressive therapy	2	1	2	1	1		2/3*		1		2	
	b) Not on immunosuppressive therapy	1		1		1		2		1		2	
Schistosomiasis	a) Uncomplicated	1		1		1		1		1		1	
	b) Fibrosis of the liver[§]	1		1		1		1		1		1	
Sexually transmitted diseases (STDs)	a) Current purulent cervicitis or chlamydial infection or gonococcal infection	4	2*	4	2*	1		1		1		1	
	b) Vaginitis (including trichomonas vaginalis and bacterial vaginosis)	2	2	2	2	1		1		1		1	
	c) Other factors relating to STDs	2*	2	2*	2	1		1		1		1	
Smoking	a) Age <35	1		1		1		1		1		2	
	b) Age ≥35, <15 cigarettes/day	1		1		1		1		1		3	
	c) Age ≥35, ≥15 cigarettes/day	1		1		1		1		1		4	
Solid organ transplantation[§]	a) Complicated	3	2	3	2	2		2		2		4	
	b) Uncomplicated	2		2		2		2		2		2*	
Stroke[§]	History of cerebrovascular accident	1		2		2	3	3		2	3	4	
Superficial venous disorders	a) Varicose veins	1		1		1		1		1		1	
	b) Superficial venous thrombosis (acute or history)	1		1		1		1		1		3*	
Systemic lupus erythematosus[§]	a) Positive (or unknown) antiphospholipid antibodies	1*	1*	3*		3*		3*	3*	3*		4*	
	b) Severe thrombocytopenia	3*	2*	2*		2*		3*	2*	2*		2*	
	c) Immunosuppressive therapy	2*	1*	2*		2*		2*	2*	2*		2*	
	d) None of the above	1*	1*	2*		2*		2*	2*	2*		2*	
Thyroid disorders	Simple goiter/ hyperthyroid/hypothyroid	1		1		1		1		1		1	
Tuberculosis[§] (see also Drug Interactions)	a) Nonpelvic	1	1	1	1	1*		1*		1*		1*	
	b) Pelvic	4	3	4	3	1*		1*		1*		1*	
Unexplained vaginal bleeding	(suspicious for serious condition) before evaluation	4*	2*	4*	2*	3*		3*		2*		2*	
Uterine fibroids		2		2		1		1		1		1	
Valvular heart disease	a) Uncomplicated	1		1		1		1		1		2	
	b) Complicated[§]	1		1		1		1		1		4	
Vaginal bleeding patterns	a) Irregular pattern without heavy bleeding	1		1	1	2		2		2		1	
	b) Heavy or prolonged bleeding	2*		1*	2*	2*		2*		2*		1*	
Viral hepatitis	a) Acute or flare	1		1		1		1		1		3/4*	2
	b) Carrier/Chronic	1		1		1		1		1		1	1
Drug Interactions													
Antiretroviral therapy All other ARV's are 1 or 2 for all methods.	Fosamprenavir (FPV)	1/2*	1*	1/2*	1*	2*		2*		2*		3*	
Anticonvulsant therapy	a) Certain anticonvulsants (phenytoin, carbamazepine, barbiturates, primidone, topiramate, oxcarbazepine)	1		1		2*		1*		3*		3*	
	b) Lamotrigine	1		1		1		1		1		3*	
Antimicrobial therapy	a) Broad spectrum antibiotics	1		1		1		1		1		1	
	b) Antifungals	1		1		1		1		1		1	
	c) Antiparasitics	1		1		1		1		1		1	
	d) Rifampin or rifabutin therapy	1		1		2*		1*		3*		3*	
SSRIs		1		1		1		1		1		1	
St. John's wort		1		1		2		1		2		2	

Updated July 2016. This summary sheet only contains a subset of the recommendations from the U.S. MEC. For complete guidance, see: http://www.cdc.gov/reproductivehealth/unintendedpregnancy/USMEC.htm. Most contraceptive methods do not protect against sexually transmitted diseases (STDs). Consistent and correct use of the male latex condom reduces the risk of STDs and HIV.

CS266008-A

SUMMARY OF CHANGES IN CLASSIFICATIONS FROM WHO MEDICAL ELIGIBILITY CRITERIA FOR CONTRACEPTIVE USE, 4TH EDITION[a,b] *(Continued)*

Condition	COC/P/R	POP	DMPA	Implants	LNG-IUD	Cu-IUD	Clarification
Breast-feeding							The U.S. Department of Health and Human Services recommends that infants be exclusively breast-fed during the first 4–6 mo of life, preferably for a full 6 mo. Ideally, breast-feeding should continue through the first year of life (1). {Not included in WHO MEC}
a. <1 mo postpartum {WHO: <6 wk postpartum}	3[b] {4}	2[b] {3}	2[b] {3}	2[b] {3}			
b. 1 mo to <6 mo {WHO: ≥6 wk to <6 mo postpartum}	2[b] {3}						
Postpartum (in breast-feeding or non-breast-feeding women), including postcesarean section							
a. <10 min after delivery of the placenta {WHO: <48 h, including insertion immediately after delivery of the placenta}					2 {1 if not breast-feeding and 3 if breast-feeding}	2 {3}	
b. 10 min after delivery of the placenta to <4 wk {WHO: ≥48 h to <4 wk}					2 {3}		

Deep venous thrombosis (DVT)/pulmonary embolism (PE)						Comments
a. History of DVT/PE, not on anticoagulant therapy						Women on anticoagulant therapy are at risk for gynecologic complications of therapy such as hemorrhagic ovarian cysts and severe menorrhagia. Hormonal contraceptive methods can be of benefit in preventing or treating these complications. When a contraceptive method is used as a therapy, rather than solely to prevent pregnancy, the risk/benefit ratio may be different and should be considered on a case-by-case basis. [Not included in WHO MEC]
i. Lower risk for recurrent DVT/PE (no risk factors)	3 {4}	2 {3}	2 {3}	2 {3}	2 {1}	
b. Acute DVT/PE						
c. DVT/PE and established on anticoagulant therapy for at least 3 mo						
i. Higher risk for recurrent DVT/PE (≥1 risk factors)						
• Known thrombophilia, including antiphospholipid syndrome						
• Active cancer (metastatic, on therapy, or within 6 mo after clinical remission), excluding nonmelanoma skin cancer						
• History of recurrent DVT/PE						
ii. Lower risk for recurrent DVT/PE (no risk factors)	3b {4}				2 {1}	

SUMMARY OF CHANGES IN CLASSIFICATIONS FROM WHO MEDICAL ELIGIBILITY CRITERIA FOR CONTRACEPTIVE USE, 4TH EDITION[a,b] (Continued)

Condition	COC/P/R	POP	DMPA	Implants	LNG-IUD	Cu-IUD	Clarification
Valvular heart disease							
a. Complicated (pulmonary hypertension, risk for atrial fibrillation, history of subacute bacterial endocarditis)						1 {2}	1 {2}
Ovarian cancer[c]						1 {Initiation = 3, Continuation = 2}	1 {Initiation = 3, Continuation = 2}
Uterine fibroids						2 {1 if no uterine distortion and 4 if uterine distortion is present}	2 {1 if no uterine distortion and 4 if uterine distortion is present}

COC, combined oral contraceptive; Cu-IUD, copper intrauterine device; DMPA, depot medroxyprogesterone acetate; DVT, deep venous thrombosis; LNG-IUD, levonorgestrel-releasing intrauterine device; P, combined hormonal contraceptive patch; PE, pulmonary embolism; POP, progestin-only pill; R, combined hormonal vaginal ring; VTE, venous thromboembolism; WHO, World Health Organization.

[a]For conditions for which classification changed for ≥1 methods or the condition description underwent a major modification, WHO conditions and recommendations appear in curly brackets.

[b]Consult the clarification column for this classification.

[c]Condition that exposes a women to increased risk as a result of unintended pregnancy.

SUMMARY OF RECOMMENDATIONS FOR MEDICAL CONDITIONS ADDED TO THE U.S. MEDICAL ELIGIBILITY CRITERIA FOR CONTRACEPTIVE USE[a]

Condition	COC/P/R	POP	DMPA	Implants	LNG-IUD	Cu-IUD	Clarification
History of bariatric surgery[b]							
a. Restrictive procedures: decrease storage capacity of the stomach (vertical banded gastroplasty, laparoscopic adjustable gastric band, laparoscopic sleeve gastrectomy)	1	1	1	1	1	1	
b. Malabsorptive procedures: decrease absorption of nutrients and calories by shortening the functional length of the small intestine (Roux-en-Y gastric bypass, biliopancreatic diversion)	COCs: 3 P/R: 1	3	1	1	1	1	

SUMMARY OF RECOMMENDATIONS FOR MEDICAL CONDITIONS ADDED TO THE U.S. MEDICAL ELIGIBILITY CRITERIA FOR CONTRACEPTIVE USE[A] *(Continued)*

Condition	COC/P/R	POP	DMPA	Implants	LNG-IUD	Cu-IUD	Clarification
Peripartum cardiomyopathy[c]							
a. Normal or mildly impaired cardiac function (New York Heart Association Functional Class I or II: patients with no limitation of activities or patients with slight, mild limitation of activity) (2)							
i. <6 mo	4	1	1	1	2	2	
ii. ≥6 mo	3	1	1	1	2	2	
b. Moderately or severely impaired cardiac function (New York Heart Association Functional Class III or IV: patients with marked limitation of activity or patients who should be at complete rest) (2)	4	2	2	2	2	2	

Condition	Cu-IUD Initiation	Cu-IUD Continuation	LNG-IUD Initiation	LNG-IUD Continuation	Implant	DMPA	POP	COC/P/R	Comments
Rheumatoid arthritis									
a. On immunosuppressive therapy	2	1	2	1	1	2/3[d]	1	2	DMPA use among women on long-term corticosteroid therapy with a history of, or risk factors for, nontraumatic fractures is classified as Category 3. Otherwise, DMPA use for women with rheumatoid arthritis is classified as Category 2.
b. Not on immunosuppressive therapy	1	1	1	1	1	2	1	2	
Endometrial hyperplasia	1	1	1	1	1	1	1	1	
Inflammatory bowel disease (IBD) (ulcerative colitis, Crohn disease)	1	1	1	1	1	2	2	2/3[d]	For women with mild IBD, with no other risk factors for VTE, the benefits of COC/P/R use generally outweigh the risks (Category 2). However, for women with IBD with increased risk for VTE (eg, those with active or extensive disease, surgery, immobilization, corticosteroid use, vitamin deficiencies, fluid depletion), the risks for COC/P/R use generally outweigh the benefits (Category 3).

SUMMARY OF RECOMMENDATIONS FOR MEDICAL CONDITIONS ADDED TO THE U.S. MEDICAL ELIGIBILITY CRITERIA FOR CONTRACEPTIVE USE^a (Continued)

Condition	COC/P/R	POP	DMPA	Implants	LNG-IUD Initiation	LNG-IUD Continuation	Cu-IUD Initiation	Cu-IUD Continuation	Clarification
Solid organ transplantation^b									
a. Complicated: graft failure (acute or chronic), rejection, cardiac allograft vasculopathy	4	2	2	2	3	2	3	2	
b. Uncomplicated	2^e	2	2	2	2		2		Women with Budd-Chiari syndrome should not use COC/P/R because of the increased risk for thrombosis.

^aCOC, combined oral contraceptive; Cu-IUD, copper intrauterine device; DMPA, depot medroxyprogesterone acetate; IBD, inflammatory bowel disease; LNG-IUD, levonorgestrel-releasing intrauterine device; P, combined hormonal contraceptive patch; POP, progestin-only pill; R, combined hormonal vaginal ring; VTE, venous thromboembolism.

^bHistory of bariatric surgery. *Contraception.* 2010;82(1):86–94.

^cCondition that exposes a woman to increased risk as a result of unintended pregnancy.

^dConsult the clarification column for this classification.

^eHistory of solid organ transplantation. *Transplantation.* 2013;95(10):1183–1186.

SUMMARY OF ADDITIONAL CHANGES TO THE U.S. MEDICAL ELIGIBILITY CRITERIA FOR CONTRACEPTIVE USE

Condition/Contraceptive Method	Change
Emergency contraceptive pills	History of bariatric surgery, rheumatoid arthritis, inflammatory bowel disease, and solid organ transplantation was given a Category 1.
Barrier methods	For six conditions—history of bariatric surgery, peripartum cardiomyopathy, rheumatoid arthritis, endometrial hyperplasia, IBD, and solid organ transplantation—the barrier methods are classified as Category 1.
Sterilization	In general, no medical conditions would absolutely restrict a person's eligibility for sterilization. Recommendations from the WHO Medical Eligibility Criteria for Contraceptive Use about specific settings and surgical procedures for sterilization are not included here. The guidance has been replaced with general text on sterilization.
Other deleted items	Guidance for combined injectables, levonorgestrel implants, and norethisterone enanthate has been removed because these methods are not currently available in the United States. Guidance for "blood pressure measurement unavailable" and "history of hypertension, where blood pressure *cannot* be evaluated (including hypertension in pregnancy)" has been removed.
Unintended pregnancy and increased health risk	The following conditions have been added to the WHO list of conditions that expose a woman to increased risk as a result of unintended pregnancy: history of bariatric surgery within the past 2 y, peripartum cardiomyopathy, and receiving a solid organ transplant within 2 y.

CONTRACEPTION, EMERGENCY

Population

–Women of childbearing age who had unprotected or inadequately protected sexual intercourse within the last 5 d and who do not desire pregnancy.

Recommendations

▶ ACOG 2010

–The levonorgestrel-only regimen is more effective and is associated with less nausea and vomiting compared with the combined estrogen-progestin regimen.

–The two 0.75-mg doses of the levonorgestrel-only regimen are equally effective if taken 12–24 h apart.

–The single-dose 1.5-mg levonorgestrel-only regimen is as effective as the 2-dose regimen.

–Recommend an antiemetic agent 1 h before the first dose of the combined estrogen-progestin regimen to reduce nausea.

–Treatment with emergency contraception should be initiated as soon as possible after unprotected or inadequately protected intercourse.

–Emergency contraception should be made available to patients who request it up to 5 d after unprotected intercourse.

Source

–http://www.guidelines.gov/content.aspx?id=15718&search=emergency+contraception

Comments

1. No clinician examination or pregnancy testing is necessary before provision or prescription of emergency contraception.
2. The copper intrauterine device (IUD) is appropriate for use as emergency contraception for women who desire long-acting contraception.
3. Information regarding effective long-term contraceptive methods should be made available whenever a woman requests emergency contraception.

CORONARY ARTERY DISEASE (CAD)

CAD with Chronic Stable Angina

Population

–Patients with chronic stable angina, with CAD, in sinus rhythm, with resting HR ≥70 bpm, that are either treated with optimal tolerated dose of β-blocker or cannot tolerate/have contraindication to β-blockers.

Recommendation

▶ EMA Review 2014

–Ivabradine (Corlentor®, Procoralan®) is used to treat symptoms of long-term stable angina.

Source

–http://www.ema.europa.eu/ema/index.jsp?curl=pages/medicines/human/referrals/Corlentor_and_Procoralan/human_referral_prac_000044.jsp&mid=WC0b01ac05805c516f

Comments

1. 2014 EMA review based on SIGNIFY study showed that ivabradine has not been shown to provide benefits such as reducing the risk of heart attack or cardiovascular death; therefore, the medicine should only be used to alleviate symptoms of angina. Doctors should consider stopping the treatment if there is no improvement in angina symptoms after 3 mo or if the improvement is only limited.
2. Should not be used in combination with verapamil or diltiazem.
3. The risk of AF is increased in the patient treated with ivabradine and doctors should monitor patients for AF.
4. If during treatment HR <50 bpm at rest and patients are symptomatic, the dose should be decreased to 2.5 mg 1 tab bid.

STABLE CORONARY DISEASE ACCF/AHA/ACP/AATS/PCNA/SCAI/STS GUIDELINES 2012, 2014

- Patients presenting with angina pectoris should be classified as *stable* or *unstable*.
- *Acute coronary syndrome* (ACS) includes high-risk unstable angina, non-ST-segment elevation myocardial infarction (NSTEMI) or ST-segment elevation myocardial infarction (STEMI).
- Resting ECG testing is recommended with all symptoms of chest pain (typical or atypical in nature).
- Exercise treadmill is the preferred initial test to be employed if the baseline is normal, the patient can exercise, and the pretest likelihood of coronary disease is intermediate (10%–90%).
- If unable to perform an exercise treadmill, then either a nuclear myocardial perfusion imaging study (MPI) or exercise echocardiogram should be employed if the pretest likelihood is >10%.
- Exercise and imaging studies should be repeated when there is a *change in clinical status* or if needed for exercise prescription.
- *Coronary computed tomography angiogram* (CTA) is a reasonable alternative in patients with an intermediate pretest probability of CAD (FRS) in whom symptoms persist despite prior normal testing, with equivocal stress tests, or in patients who cannot be studied otherwise. CTA in not indicated with known moderate or severe coronary calcification or in the presence of prior stents.
- An echocardiogram is recommended to assess resting LV function and valve disease in patients with suspected CAD, pathological Q waves, presence of heart failure, or ventricular arrhythmias.
- Patients with stable coronary disease should receive:
  ○ Lifestyle guidance (diet, weight loss, smoking cessation, and exercise education): *BP threshold of <140/90 mm Hg* is projected to be the new JCN 8 goal.
  ○ Associated risk factor assessment: Presence of *chronic kidney disease* and *psychosocial factors* such as depression, anxiety, and poor social support have been added to the classic risk factors.
  ○ Appropriate medicine prescription: (ASA 75–162 mg daily, moderate statin dosage, BP control and diabetic control, β-blocker therapy, and sublingual NTG).

STABLE CORONARY DISEASE ACCF/AHA/ACP/AATS/PCNA/SCAI/STS GUIDELINES 2012, 2014 *(Continued)*

- Coronary angiography should be considered in patients surviving sudden cardiac death, with *high-risk noninvasive test results* (large areas of silent ischemia often associated with malignant ventricular arrhythmias) and in patients in whom the *anginal symptoms cannot be controlled* with optimal medical therapy.[a]
- Coronary bypass grafting surgery (CABG) is preferred to angioplasty in diabetic patients with multivessel disease (FREEDOM trial 2012).[b]

(exclusive of stress testing) indicate a high likelihood of severe IHD and who are amenable to, and candidates for, coronary revascularization. Coronary angiography is reasonable in patients with suspected symptomatic SIHD who cannot undergo diagnostic stress testing, or have indeterminate or nondiagnostic stress tests, when there is a high likelihood that the findings will result in important changes to therapy. Coronary angiography might be considered in patients with stress test results of acceptable quality that do not suggest the presence of CAD when clinical suspicion of CAD remains high and there is a high likelihood that the findings will result in important changes to therapy.

[b]A Heart Team approach to revascularization is recommended in patients with diabetes mellitus and complex multivessel CAD. CABG is generally recommended in preference to PCI to improve survival in patients with diabetes mellitus and multivessel CAD for which revascularization is likely to improve survival (3-vessel CAD or complex 2-vessel CAD involving the proximal LAD), particularly if a LIMA graft can be anastomosed to the LAD artery, provided the patient is a good candidate for surgery.

Source: Fihn SD, Blankenship JC, Alexander KP, et al. 2014 ACC/AHA/AATS/PCNA/SCAI/STS focused update of the guideline for the diagnosis and management of patients with stable ischemic heart disease. *J Am Coll Cardiol.* 2014. doi:10.1016/j.jacc.2014.07.017.

CORONARY ARTERY DISEASE: SEXUAL FUNCTION—AHA AND PRINCETON CONSENSUS PANEL RECOMMENDATIONS 2013

- Erectile dysfunction (ED) is associated with CAD and often precedes the diagnosis of CAD.
- ED was associated with an increased risk for CV events and all-cause mortality.
- Angina pectoris during sexual activity represents <5% of all angina attacks.
- Patients with CAD with angina pectoris should undergo full medical evaluation prior to partaking in sexual activity.
- Patients should be able to perform 3–5 metabolic equivalents (METs) on a treadmill or climb 2 flights of stairs or walk briskly without angina before engaging in sexual activity.
- Post-uncomplicated MI if no symptoms on mild-to-moderate activity exist >1 wk, patient may resume sexual activity.
- Post-angioplasty within 1-wk sexual activity is reasonable if the radial groin site is healed.

[a]Coronary angiography is useful in patients with presumed SIHD who have unacceptable ischemic symptoms revascularization. Coronary angiography is reasonable to define the extent and severity of coronary artery disease (CAD) in patients with suspected SIHD whose clinical characteristics and results of noninvasive testing

- Sexual activity is reasonable after 6–8 wk post coronary bypass, being limited by the sterna healing or pain.
- If residual coronary lesions persist post revascularization, exercise stress testing is recommended to evaluate for significant ischemia.
- Sexual activity is contraindicated in patients with angina at low effort, refractory angina or unstable angina.
- Nitrate therapy is contraindicated with phosphodiesterase 5 (PDE5) inhibitor therapy.
- Following sildenafil (Viagra) or vardenafil (Levitra) at least 24 h must elapse before nitrates can be started; ≥48 h if tadalafil (Cialis) is used.
- Beta-blockers, calcium channel blockers, and Ranolazine are not contraindicated; however, they may impair erectile dysfunction.

Sources: Schwartz BG, Kloner RA. Clinical cardiology: physician update: erectile dysfunction and cardiovascular disease. *Circulation.* 2011;123:98-101. Nehra A, Jackson G, Martin Miner, et al. The Princeton III consensus recommendations for the management of erectile dysfunction and cardiovascular disease. *Mayo Clin Proc.* 2012;87:766-778. Kloner RA, Henderson L. Sexual function in patients with chronic angina pectoris. *Am J Cardiol.* 2013;111:1671-1676.

CORONARY ARTERY DISEASE: THERAPY FOR UNSTABLE ANGINA—NSTEMI ACCF/AHA 2012 CLASS I RECOMMENDATIONS

- Aspirin (ASA) 325 mg should be administered promptly to all patients unless contraindicated.
- Clopidogrel 300–600 mg bolus or prasugrel 60 mg should be administered to all ASA-allergic patients.
- Risk stratification to initial invasive or conservative therapy is required. Early invasive treatment is indicated with refractory angina, hemodynamic or electrical instability. Most procedures are performed within 2–24 h, depending on the stability of the patient. TIMI and GRACE scores are often employed to select invasive vs. conservative therapy.
- Dual antiplatelet ASA + (clopidogrel or ticagrelor) therapy is indicated upstream (before percutaneous coronary intervention) in the invasive group as well as in the conservative group.
- A *loading dose* of clopidogrel 600 mg, prasugrel 60 mg, or ticagrelor 180 mg should be given prior to PCI.
- *Maintenance therapy* of clopidogrel 75 mg daily, prasugrel 10 mg daily, or ticagrelor 90 mg twice daily should be *continued up to 12 mo*.
- If a history of gastrointestinal (GI) bleeding is noted, a PPI agent or H_2 blocker should be added to the dual antiplatelet therapy.
- PPI agents may be safely used with clopidogrel or pantoprazole. No interaction exists between PPIs and prasugrel, ticagrelor, or factor Xa inhibitors or dabigatran.
- In the conservative therapy group if recurrent ischemia, heart failure, or serious arrhythmias occur, coronary angiogram is indicated.

CORONARY ARTERY DISEASE: THERAPY FOR UNSTABLE ANGINA— NSTEMI ACCF/AHA 2012 CLASS I RECOMMENDATIONS (*Continued*)

- Nasal oxygen is indicated if arterial saturation is <90%, if respiratory distress is present, or other high-risk features for hypoxemia.
- Sublingual and intravenous nitroglycerin (NTG) are indicated for clinical angina.
- Oral β-blockers should be administered within the first 24 h unless contraindicated. Intravenous beta-blocker if chest pain is ongoing.
- ACE inhibitors should be administered within 24 h in patients with clinical heart failure (HF) with decreased ejection fraction (≤40%), if not contraindicated.
- Consider percutaneous coronary intervention (PCI) of the culprit coronary vessel with staged PCIs for other significant but less critical lesions. Consider CABG for significant left main lesion, double- or triple-vessel disease with decreased ejection fraction. The SYNTAX score may have predictive value in selecting PCI vs. CABG.
- *Myocardial perfusion imaging (MPI)* is indicated prior to discharge if conservative therapy is chosen.
- Dual antiplatelet (ASA 81 mg and clopidogrel 75 mg daily, prasugrel 10 mg daily, or ticagrelor 90 mg twice daily) is indicated for *at least 12 mo*. ASA should be continued lifelong.
- If warfarin is indicated postcoronary stent, see Anticoagulation with Stent section.
- Postdischarge medications include ASA, clopidogrel 75 mg, β-blocker dose to control heart rate, statin agent, and possible ACE inhibitor if decreased ejection fraction or clinical heart failure, diabetes, or hypertension is present.

Sources: 2012 Writing Committee Members, Jneid H, Anderson JL, Wright RS, et al; American College of Cardiology Foundation; American Heart Association Task Force on Practice Guidelines. 2012 ACCF/AHA focused update of the guidelines for the management of patients with unstable angina/non-ST elevation myocardial infarction (updated the 2007 guideline and replacing the 2011 focus update): a report of the American College of Cardiology Foundation/American Heart Association Task Force on Practice Guidelines. *Circulation.* 2012;126:875-910. ACC/AHA 2007 Guidelines. *J Am Coll Cardiol.* 2007;50(7):652-726. Wright RS, Anderson JL, Adams CD, et al. 2011 ACCF/AHA focused update of the Guidelines for the Management of Patients with Unstable Angina/Non-ST-Elevation Myocardial Infarction (updating the 2007 guideline): a report of the American College of Cardiology Foundation/American Heart Association Task Force on Practice Guidelines developed in collaboration with the American College of Emergency Physicians, Society for Cardiovascular Angiography and Interventions, and Society of Thoracic Surgeons. *J Am Coll Cardiol.* 2011;57:1920-1959. ESC 2011. ECS Guidelines. http://eurheartj.oxfordjournals.org/. Palmerini T, Genereux P, Caixeta A, et al. Prognostic value of the SYNTAX score in patients with acute coronary syndromes undergoing percutaneous coronary intervention: analysis from the ACUITY (Acute Catheterization and Urgent Intervention Triage StrategY) trial. *J Am Coll Cardiol.* 2011;57:2389-2397. Patel MR, Dehmer GJ, Hirshfeld JW, Smith PK, Spertus JA. ACCF/SCAI/STS/AATS/AHA/ASNC/HFSA/SCCT 2012. Appropriate use criteria for coronary revascularization focused update: a report of the American College of Cardiology Foundation Appropriate Use Criteria Task Force, Society for Cardiovascular Angiography and Interventions, Society of Thoracic Surgeons, American Association for Thoracic Surgery, American Heart Association, American Society of Nuclear Cardiology, and the Society of Cardiovascular Computed Tomography. *J Am Coll Cardiol.* 2012;59:857-876.

CORONARY ARTERY DISEASE: MANAGEMENT FOR ST-ELEVATION MYOCARDIAL INFARCTION—ACCF/AHA 2013 CLASS I RECOMMENDATIONS

- Patients with ST-elevation myocardial infarction with ischemic symptoms within 12 h should be treated by PCI.
- Primary PCI should be performed within **90 min** from initial medical contact by an experienced catheterization cardiologist.
- Emergency transport to PCI-capable hospital is recommended. The term "Code STEMI" is often used to confer the time urgency of the transfer. In-ambulance ECG monitoring should be used to identify ST-segment elevation.
- Emergency transfer from a non-PCI capable to a PCI-capable hospital should be considered if transfer to catheterization laboratory is capable within **120 min**.
- Fibrinolytic therapy should be considered if PCI is not capable within the optimal time frame. If fibrinolytic therapy is considered, it should be started with 30 min of hospital arrival.
- ASA 162–325 mg should be administered before primary PCI and continued indefinitely at 81 mg daily.
- $P2Y_{12}$ receptor inhibitor should be given *upstream* or *during* primary PCI and should be *continued for 1 y* with either bare metal stent or drug-eluting stents. Options include clopidogrel, prasugrel, and ticagrelor. $P2Y_{12}$ receptor inhibitors: clopidogrel 75 mg daily, prasgruel 10 mg daily (5 mg daily—in patients <60 kg or ≥75 y old), ticagrelor 90 mg bid. Prasugrel should not be administered to patients with a history of prior stroke or TIA.
- Anticoagulation therapy with unfractionated heparin and bivalirudin should be discussed with the invasive cardiologist.
- Urgent PCI of the infarct artery should be addressed urgently with stent placement. Noninfarct artery occlusions should be evaluated postinfarction to evaluate ischemia requiring subsequent PCI.
- Urgent coronary artery bypass surgery is indicated if the coronary anatomy is not amenable to PCI.
- Therapy with statin agents, β-blockers, and ACE inhibitors are indicated as with NSTEMIs.

Source: American College of Emergency Physicians, Society for Cardiovascular Angiography and Interventions, O'Gara PT, Kushner FG, Ascheim DD, et al. 2013 ACCF/AHA guideline for the management of ST-elevation myocardial infarction: executive summary: a report of the American College of Cardiology Foundation/ American Heart Association Task Force on Practice Guidelines. *J Am Coll Cardiol.* 2013;61(4):485-510.

CORONARY ARTERY DISEASE: ELEVATED TROPONIN LEVEL—AMERICAN COLLEGE OF CARDIOLOGY FOUNDATION TASK FORCE 2012

- Elevated troponin levels are an *imperfect diagnostic test* and are dependent upon the probability of underlying CAD. New high-sensitivity troponin assays require further testing.
- Establishing **high pretest probability** and **global risk scores** (TIMI, GRACE, PERSUIT) are often needed to determine the significance of elevated troponin levels.
- Clinical factors that establish a high pretest probability include a history of typical angina, typical ECG changes consistent with ischemia (ST-segment changes), history of established coronary risk factors, or the history of known CAD.
- Elevated troponin levels in patients with *high pretest probability of CAD* (typical chest pain and ECG changes of ischemia) have a predictive accuracy of ≥95% to establish acute coronary syndrome.
- Elevated troponin levels in patients with *low pretest probability of CAD* (atypical chest pain and nonspecific ECG changes) have a predictive accuracy of only 50% to establish ACS.
- *Global risk scores* should be employed to further establish the role of early conservative vs. early invasive therapy in patients with elevated troponin levels and a high pretest probability.
- Cardiac causes for elevated troponin levels are ACS, coronary spasm or embolism, cocaine or methamphetamine use, stress cardiomyopathy, congestive heart failure, myocarditis or pericarditis, trauma, infiltrative diseases, postprocedure (ablation, electric shock, coronary bypass surgery, and post-coronary angioplasty).
- Noncardiac causes for elevated troponin levels are pulmonary embolus, renal failure, stroke, sepsis, drug toxicity (anthracycline), and hypoxia.

Source: Newby LK, Jesse RL, Babb JD, et al. ACCF 2012 expert consensus document of practical clinical considerations in the interpretation of troponin elevations: a report of the American College of Cardiology Foundation task force on Clinical Expert Consensus Documents. *J Am Coll Cardiol.* 2012;60:2427-2463.

CORONARY ARTERY DISEASE: LONG-TERM ANTIPLATELET THERAPY— AMERICAN COLLEGE OF CHEST PHYSICIANS 2012

- ASA is recommended for persons ≥50 y old *without symptomatic* CVD at 75–100 mg daily.
- Mono antiplatelet therapy with ASA 75–100 mg or clopidogrel 75 mg is recommended with *established CAD.*
- Dual antiplatelet therapy (ticagrelor 90 mg twice daily plus ASA 81 mg or clopidogrel 75 mg plus ASA 75–100 mg daily) for 1-y post-ACS with PCI with or without stent placement.
- Dual antiplatelet therapy with *elective PCI without stent* should receive clopidogrel 75 mg or ASA 75–100 mg daily for 1 mo, then long-term ASA therapy is recommended.
- Dual antiplatelet therapy with *elective PCI and bare metal stent (BMS) is recommended for at least 1 mo and for drug eluting stent (DES)* is recommended for at least 6 mo.
- No antiplatelet or OAC is recommended with systolic dysfunction without thrombus. If LV thrombus is present, OAC is recommended for 3 mo.

Sources: Vandvik PO, Lincoff AM, Gore JM, et al; American College of Chest Physicians. Primary and secondary prevention of cardiovascular disease: Antithrombotic Therapy and Prevention of Thrombosis, 9th ed: American College of Chest Physician Evidence-Based Clinical Practice Guidelines. *Chest.* 2012;141:e637S-e668S. 2016 ACC/AHA Guideline Focused Update on Duration of Dual Antiplatelet Therapy in Patients with Coronary Artery Disease: a report of the American College of Cardiology/American Heart Association Task Force on Clinical Practice Guidelines. *Circulation.* 2016;134:e123–e155.

CORONARY ARTERY DISEASE: STENT THERAPY USE OF TRIPLE ANTICOAGULATION TREATMENT—AMERICAN COLLEGE OF CARDIOLOGY/ AMERICAN HEART ASSOCIATION/EUROPEAN SOCIETY OF CARDIOLOGY

The prudent use of triple anticoagulation therapy with aspirin, clopidogrel, and warfarin in AF patients at high risk of thromboembolism and recent coronary stent placement remains a *matter of clinical judgment,* balancing the risk of thrombotic vs. bleeding events.

Facts:
- Bare-metal stents are the stents of choice if TAT is required.
- Drug-eluting stents should be reserved for high-risk clinical or anatomic situations (diabetic patients or if the coronary lesions are unusually long, totally occlusive, or in small blood vessels) if TAT is required.
- Dual antiplatelet therapy with clopidogrel (75 mg/d) and ASA (81 mg/d) is the most effective therapy to *prevent coronary stent thrombosis.*
- Warfarin anticoagulation is the most effective therapy to *prevent thromboembolism* in high-risk AF patients as defined by the $CHA_2DS_2\text{-}VAS_c$ risk score (≥2).
- In nonvalvular AF okay to consider NOACs. Following coronary revascularization, in high-risk patients with AF it may be reasonable to use clopidogrel 75 mg daily concurrently with OAC but without ASA.
- TAT is the most effective therapy to *prevent* both *coronary stent thrombosis* and the *occurrence* of embolic strokes in high-risk patients.

CORONARY ARTERY DISEASE: STENT THERAPY USE OF TRIPLE ANTICOAGULATION TREATMENT—AMERICAN COLLEGE OF CARDIOLOGY/AMERICAN HEART ASSOCIATION/EUROPEAN SOCIETY OF CARDIOLOGY (*Continued*)

- However, the addition of DAPT to warfarin increases the bleeding risk by 3.7-fold.
- Therefore, awaiting a definitive clinical trial (WOEST trial), risk stratification of patients to evaluate the *thromboembolic potential of AF* vs. the *bleeding potential* should be performed.
- The HAS-BLED (see table page 210) bleeding risk score is the best measure of bleeding risk. A high risk of bleeding is defined by a score >3.

Source: January CT, Wann LS, Alpert JS, et al. 2014 AHA/ACC/HRS Guideline for the Management of Patients With Atrial Fibrillation. *Circulation.* 2014. (http://circ.ahajournals.org/content/early/2014/04/10/CIR.0000000000000041).

Hypertension (≥160 mm Hg), **a**bnormal kidney function (creatinine ≥2, chronic dialysis, transplant), **a**bnormal liver function (cirrhosis, bilirubin >2×, AST >3×), **s**troke, **b**leeding history or anemia, labile INR (<60% within range), elderly (age ≥65 y), **d**rugs/alcohol (use of ASA or clopidogrel) or alcohol (≥8 alcoholic drinks/wk). *Each risk factor is assigned 1 point for a total of 9 points.*

- If DAPT or TAT is required, *prophylactic GI therapy* with an H_2 blocker (except cimetidine) or PPI agent should be maintained. If omeprazole (Prilosec) is considered, the risk-to-benefit ratio needs to be considered because of its possible interference with clopidogrel function.
- In patients with a high risk of bleeding, TAT should be reserved for AF patients with a high thromboembolic risk. If the bleeding risk is high but the AF thromboembolic risk is low, DAPT therapy is suggested.

AF, atrial fibrillation; ASA, aspirin; AST, aspartate transaminase; DAPT, dual antiplatelet therapy; INR, international normalized ratio; GI, gastrointestinal; PPI, proton pump inhibitor; TAT, triple anticoagulation therapy.
Sources: Adopted from European Heart Rhythm Association; European Association for Cardio-Thoracic Surgery, Camm AJ, Kirchhof P, Lip GY, et al. Guidelines for the management of atrial fibrillation: the Task Force for the Management of Atrial Fibrillation of the European Society of Cardiology (ESC). *Eur Heart J.* 2010;31:2369-2429. Lip GY. Managing the anticoagulated patient with atrial fibrillation at high risk of stroke who needs coronary intervention. *BMJ.* 2008;337:a840. Rubboli A, Kovacic JC, Mehran R, Lip GY. Coronary stent implantation in patients committed to long-term oral anticoagulation: successfully navigating the treatment options. *Chest.* 2011;139:981-987. King SB III, Smith SC Jr, Hirshfeld JW Jr, et al. 2007 focused update of the ACC/AHA/SCAI 2005 guideline update for percutaneous coronary intervention: a report of the American College of Cardiology/American Heart Association Task Force on Practice guidelines. *J Am Coll Cardiol.* 2008;51:172-208. Wright RS, Anderson JL, Adams CD, et al. 2011 ACCF/AHA focused update of the Guidelines for the Management of Patients with Unstable Angina/Non-ST-Elevation Myocardial Infarction (updating the 2007 guideline): a report of the American College of Cardiology Foundation/American Heart Association Task Force on Practice Guidelines developed in collaboration with the American College of Emergency Physicians, Society for Cardiovascular Angiography and Interventions, and Society of Thoracic Surgeons. *J Am Coll Cardiol.* 2011;57:1920-1959. Abraham NS, Hlatky MA, Antman EM, et al. ACCF/ACG/AHA. ACCF/ACG/AHA 2010 expert consensus document on the concomitant use of proton pump inhibitors and thienopyridines: a focused update of the ACCF/ACG/AHA 2008 expert consensus document on reducing the gastrointestinal risks of antiplatelet therapy and NSAID use. A Report of the American College of Cardiology Foundation Task Force on Expert Consensus Documents. *J Am Coll Cardiol.* 2010;56:2051-2066. Holmes DR Jr, Kereiakes DJ, Kleiman NS, Moliterno DJ, Patti G, Grines CL. Combining antiplatelet and anticoagulation therapies. *J Am Coll Cardiol.* 2009;54:95-109. January CT, Wann LS, Alpert JS, et al. 2014 AHA/ACC/HRS Guideline for the Management of Patients with Atrial Fibrillation. *Circulation.* 2014. http://circ.ahajournals.org/content/early/2014/04/10/CIR.0000000000000041.

CORONARY ARTERY DISEASE: STENT THERAPY USE OF TRIPLE ANTICOAGULATION TREATMENT

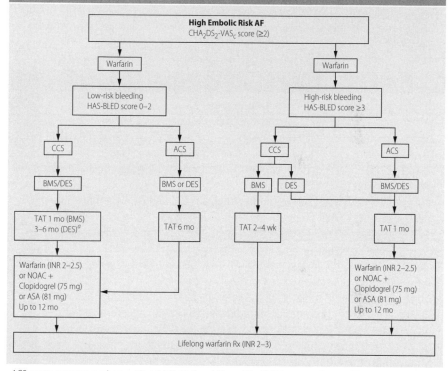

ACS, acute coronary syndrome; AF, atrial fibrillation; ASA, aspirin; BMS, bare-metal stent; CCS, patient with chronic coronary syndrome (stable coronary artery disease); DES, drug eluting stent; INR, international normalized ratio; Rx, therapy [warfarin (INR 2–2.5) + aspirin (81 mg daily) + clopidogrel (75 mg daily)]; TAT, triple anticoagulation therapy.

[a]DES stents if sirolimus, everolimus, or tacrolimus require 3-mo dual platelet therapy (ASA plus clopidogrel). If DES stent is paclitaxel, 6-mo dual therapy is required.

Sources: European Heart Rhythm Association; European Association for Cardio-Thoracic Surgery, Camm AJ, Kirchhof P, Lip GY, et al. Guidelines for the management of atrial fibrillation: the Task Force for the Management of Atrial Fibrillation of the European Society of Cardiology (ESC). *Eur Heart J.* 2010;31:2369-2429. Lip GY. Managing the anticoagulated patient with atrial fibrillation at high risk of stroke who needs coronary intervention. *BMJ.* 2008;337:a840. Rubboli A, Kovacic JC, Mehran R, Lip GY. Coronary stent implantation in patients committed to long-term oral anticoagulation: successfully navigating the treatment options. *Chest.* 2011;139:981-987. King SB III, Smith SC Jr, Hirshfeld JW Jr, et al. 2007 focused update of the ACC/AHA/SCAI 2005 guideline update for percutaneous coronary intervention: a report of the American College of Cardiology/ American Heart Association Task Force on Practice guidelines. *J Am Coll Cardiol.* 2008;51:172-208. 2014 AHA/ ACC/HRS Guideline for the Management of Patients With Atrial Fibrillation. CT January, LS Wann, JS Alpert, et al. *Circulation.* 2014. http://circ.ahajournals.org/content/early/2014/04/10/CIR.0000000000000041. Wright RS, Anderson JL, Adams CD, et al. 2011 ACCF/AHA focused update of the Guidelines for the Management of Patients with Unstable Angina/Non-ST-Elevation Myocardial Infarction (updating the 2007 guideline): a report of the American College of Cardiology Foundation/American Heart Association Task Force on Practice Guidelines developed in collaboration with the American College of Emergency Physicians, Society for Cardiovascular Angiography and Interventions, and Society of Thoracic Surgeons. *J Am Coll Cardiol.* 2011;57:1920-1959. Abraham NS, Hlatky MA, Antman EM, et al. ACCF/ACG/AHA. ACCF/ACG/AHA 2010 expert consensus document on the concomitant use of proton pump inhibitors and thienopyridines: a focused update of the ACCF/ACG/AHA 2008 expert consensus document on reducing the gastrointestinal risks of antiplatelet therapy and NSAID use. A Report of the American College of Cardiology Foundation Task Force on Expert Consensus Documents. *J Am Coll Cardiol.* 2010;56:2051-2066. Holmes DR Jr, Kereiakes DJ, Kleiman NS, Moliterno DJ, Patti G, Grines CL. Combining antiplatelet and anticoagulation therapies. *J Am Coll Cardiol.* 2009;54:95-109.

CAD IN WOMEN

- CVD is the leading cause of mortality in women.
- AHA recommends the risk assessment of CVD in women should begin at age 20 y, identifying women at higher risk.
- There are racial/ethnic differences in risk factors, with black and Hispanic women having a higher prevalence of hypertension and diabetes. The highest CVD morbidity and mortality occurs in black women.
- Autoimmune diseases (systemic lupus erythematosus, rheumatoid arthritis) and preeclampsia are significant risk factors for CVD in women.
- Psychological stress (anxiety, depression) and socioeconomic disadvantages are associated with a higher CVD risk in women.
- *Microvascular disease with endothelial dysfunction*, also known as *female pattern disease*, is the etiology of ischemia in more women than men.
- Women are more likely to have atypical cardiovascular symptoms such as sudden or extreme fatigue, dyspnea, sleep disturbances, anxiety, nausea, vomiting, and indigestion.
- *ACC/AHA guidelines recommend a routine exercise stress test* as the initial evaluation in symptomatic women who have a good exercise capacity and a normal baseline ECG. Exercise stress perfusion study (myocardial perfusion scintigraphy [MPS]) or exercise echo should be reserved for symptomatic women with higher pretest likelihood for CAD or indeterminate routine testing.
- Women often receive less medical therapy and lifestyle counseling than men.
- After PCI procedure, women experience higher rate of complications and mortality than men.
- Management of stable CAD should be the same as in men which include ASA, β-blocker, statin, ACE inhibitor (ejection fraction [EF] <40%), and nitrate/calcium channel blocker (CCB) for angina management.
- In microvascular disease, β-blockers have shown to be superior to CCB for angina management. Statins, ACE inhibitors, ranolazine, and exercise can improve angina scores and endothelial dysfunction in female pattern disease.

Sources: Moasca L, Benjamin EJ, Berra K, et al. Effectiveness-based guidelines for the prevention of cardiovascular disease in women—2011 update: a guideline from the American Heart Association. *Circulation.* 2011;123:1243-1262. Gulati M, Shaw LJ, Bairey Merz CN. Myocardial ischemia in women: lessons from the NHLBI WISE study. *Clin Cardiol.* 2012;35:141-148.

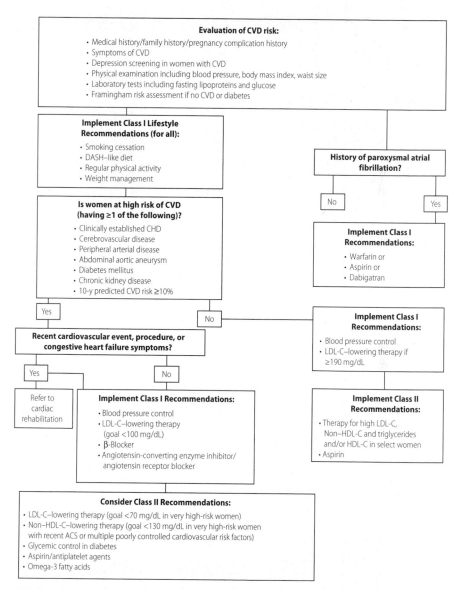

Evaluation of CVD risk:
- Medical history/family history/pregnancy complication history
- Symptoms of CVD
- Depression screening in women with CVD
- Physical examination including blood pressure, body mass index, waist size
- Laboratory tests including fasting lipoproteins and glucose
- Framingham risk assessment if no CVD or diabetes

Implement Class I Lifestyle Recommendations (for all):
- Smoking cessation
- DASH–like diet
- Regular physical activity
- Weight management

History of paroxysmal atrial fibrillation?

No   Yes

Is women at high risk of CVD (having ≥1 of the following)?
- Clinically established CHD
- Cerebrovascular disease
- Peripheral arterial disease
- Abdominal aortic aneurysm
- Diabetes mellitus
- Chronic kidney disease
- 10-y predicted CVD risk ≥10%

Implement Class I Recommendations:
- Warfarin or
- Aspirin or
- Dabigatran

Yes   No

Recent cardiovascular event, procedure, or congestive heart failure symptoms?

Implement Class I Recommendations:
- Blood pressure control
- LDL-C–lowering therapy if ≥190 mg/dL

Yes   No

Refer to cardiac rehabilitation

Implement Class I Recommendations:
- Blood pressure control
- LDL-C–lowering therapy (goal <100 mg/dL)
- β-Blocker
- Angiotensin-converting enzyme inhibitor/ angiotensin receptor blocker

Implement Class II Recommendations:
- Therapy for high LDL-C, Non–HDL-C and triglycerides and/or HDL-C in select women
- Aspirin

Consider Class II Recommendations:
- LDL-C–lowering therapy (goal <70 mg/dL in very high-risk women)
- Non–HDL-C–lowering therapy (goal <130 mg/dL in very high-risk women wirh recent ACS or multiple poorly controlled cardiovascular risk factors)
- Glycemic control in diabetes
- Aspirin/antiplatelet agents
- Omega-3 fatty acids

ACS, acute coronary syndrome; CHD, coronary heart disease; CVD, cardiovascular disease; DASH, dietary approaches to stop hypertension; HDL-C, high-density lipoprotein cholesterol; LDL-C, low-density lipoprotein cholesterol.
Source: Moasca L, Benjamin EJ, Berra K, et al. Effectiveness-based guidelines for the prevention of cardiovascular disease in women—2011 update: a guideline from the American Heart Association. *Circulation.* 2011;123:1243-1262.

CUSHING'S SYNDROME (CS)

Population

–Pediatric and adult patients with Cushing's syndrome.

Recommendations

▶ Endocrine Society 2015

–Treatment goals for Cushing's syndrome
  • Normalize cortisol levels to eliminate the signs and symptoms of CS.
–Recommend vaccinations against:
  • Influenza, herpes zoster, pneumococcus
–Recommend perioperative thromboprophylaxis for venous thromboembolism.
–Recommend surgical resection of primary adrenal or ectopic focus underlying CS.
–Assess postoperative serum cortisol levels.

Source

–https://guidelines.gov/summaries/summary/49658

DELIRIUM

Population

–Adults age ≥18 y in the hospital or in long-term care facilities.

Recommendations

▶ NICE 2010

1. Perform a short Confusion Assessment Method (CAM) screen to confirm the diagnosis of delirium.
2. Recommended approach to the management of delirium:
   a. Treat the underlying cause.
   b. Provide frequent reorientation and reassurance to patients and their families.
   c. Provide cognitively stimulating activities.
   d. Ensure adequate hydration.
   e. Prevent constipation.
   f. Early mobilization.
   g. Treat pain if present.
   h. Provide hearing aids or corrective lenses if sensory impairment is present.
   i. Promote good sleep hygiene.
   j. Consider short-term antipsychotic use (<1 wk) for patients who are distressed or considered at risk to themselves or others.

Source

–http://www.nice.org.uk/nicemedia/live/13060/49909/49909.pdf

▶ American Geriatrics Society 2015

–Do not use physical restraints for behavioral control in elderly patients with delirium.

Source

–http://www.choosingwisely.org/societies/american-geriatrics-society/

Comment

–Recommended antipsychotics are haloperidol or olanzapine given at the lowest effective dose.

DELIRIUM, POSTOPERATIVE

Population

–Older adults at risk for or who have postoperative delirium.

Recommendations

▶ AGS 2015

–Institutions should enact multi-component intervention programs to manage delirium.

–Consider regional anesthesia at the time of surgery to improve postoperative pain control.

–Avoid inappropriate medications postoperatively in older adults.

–Use antipsychotics at the lowest effective dose and for the shortest duration possible to treat severe agitated delirium.

–Avoid benzodiazepines for postoperative delirium.

–Avoid pharmacologic therapy for hypoactive delirium.

Source

–https://guidelines.gov/summaries/summary/49932

DEMENTIA

Population

–Adults with dementia.

Recommendations

▶ ACP 2008, AAFP 2008

1. Recommend a trial of therapy with a cholinesterase inhibitor or memantine based on individual assessment of relative risks vs. benefits.

2. The choice of medication is based on tolerability, side effect profile, ease of use, and medication cost.
3. The evidence is insufficient to compare the relative efficacy of different medications for dementia.
4. Evidence is insufficient to determine the optimal duration of therapy.

Source
–http://www.annals.org/content/148/5/370.full.pdf

Comments

1. A beneficial effect of cholinesterase inhibitors or memantine is generally observed within 3 mo.
2. Good-quality data in mild-to-moderate Alzheimer disease and vascular dementia show that cholinesterase inhibitors provide a modest improvement in global assessment, but no clinically important cognitive improvement. Subsets of patients may have significant cognitive improvement.
3. Five high-quality studies evaluated memantine use in moderate-to-severe Alzheimer disease and vascular dementia and show statistically significant improvement in global assessment, but no clinically important cognitive improvement.

DEMENTIA, ALZHEIMER DISEASE

Population
–Adults.

Recommendations

▶ NICE 2011

–Donepezil, galantamine, and rivastigmine are recommended as options for mild-to-moderate Alzheimer disease.
–Memantine is recommended as an option for managing moderate Alzheimer disease in patients who cannot tolerate acetylcholinesterase inhibitors.

Source
–http://www.nice.org.uk/nicemedia/live/13419/53619/53619.pdf

Comments

1. Common adverse effects of acetylcholinesterase inhibitors include diarrhea, nausea, vomiting, muscle cramps, and insomnia.
2. Common adverse effects of memantine are dizziness, headache, constipation, somnolence, and hypertension.

DEMENTIA, FEEDING TUBES

Population
–Patients with advanced dementia.

Recommendations
▶ American Geriatrics Society 2013
–Percutaneous feeding tubes are not recommended for older adults with advanced dementia.
–Careful hand-feeding should be offered.

Source
–http://americangeriatrics.org/health_care_professionals/clinical_practice/clinical_guidelines_recommendations/

Comment
–Careful hand-feedings and tube-feedings have identical outcomes of death, aspiration pneumonia, functional status, and patient comfort. In addition, tube-feeding is associated with agitation, increased use of physical and chemical restraints, and worsening pressure ulcers.

DEPRESSION

Population
–Children and adolescents.

Recommendations
▶ USPSTF 2009
–Adequate evidence showed that SSRIs, psychotherapy, and combined therapy will decrease symptoms of major depressive disorder in adolescents age 12–18 y.
–Insufficient evidence to support screening and treatment of depression in children age 7–11 y.

Source
–http://www.uspreventiveservicestaskforce.org/uspstf/uspschdepr.htm

Comments
1. Good evidence showed that SSRIs may increase absolute risk of suicidality in adolescents by 1%–2%. Therefore, SSRIs should be used only if close clinical monitoring is possible.
2. Fluoxetine and citalopram yielded statistically significant higher response rates than did other SSRIs

DIABETIC FOOT PROBLEMS, INPATIENT MANAGEMENT

Population
–Hospitalized adults older than 18 y with diabetic foot problems.

Recommendations
▶ NICE 2011

–Every hospital should have a multidisciplinary foot care team to assess and treat any diabetic patient with foot problems.
–Every patient with a diabetic foot problem should undergo an assessment for:
  • Need for debridement, pressure off-loading.
  • Vascular inflow.
  • Infection of the foot.
  • Glycemic control.
  • Neuropathy.
–If osteomyelitis is suspected, obtain an x-ray, and if x-ray is normal, obtain an MRI.
–Provide off-loading for diabetic foot ulcers.
–For mild diabetic foot infections, treat with empiric antibiotics that provide good gram-positive organisms coverage.
–For moderate-to-severe diabetic foot infections, treat with empiric antibiotics that provide coverage of gram-positive, gram-negative, and anaerobic bacteria.

Source
–http://www.nice.org.uk/nicemedia/live/13416/53556/53556.pdf

Comment
–The diabetic foot care team should include:
  • Diabetologist.
  • Surgeon with expertise managing DM foot problems.
  • DM nurse specialist.
  • Podiatrist.
  • Tissue viability nurse.

DIABETES MELLITUS, GESTATIONAL (GDM)

Population
–Pregnant women.

Recommendations
▶ ACOG 2013

–Women with gestational diabetes should be treated with nutrition therapy.

–For pharmacologic therapy of GDM, oral medications and insulin are equivalent in efficacy.

–Women with GDM and estimated fetal weight of 4500 g or more should be counseled regarding option of scheduled cesarean delivery vs. vaginal trial of labor.

–Women with GDM should follow fasting and 1 h postprandial glucose levels.

Source

–http://www.guideline.gov/content.aspx?id=47014

DIABETES MELLITUS (DM), TYPE 1

Population

–Adults and children

Recommendations

▶ ADA 2013

1. Recommends intensive insulin therapy with >3 injections daily using either basal and prandial insulin or an insulin pump.
2. Self-monitoring blood glucose >3 times daily in all patients using multiple insulin injections or an insulin pump.
3. Recommends assessment of psychological and social situation as part of diabetic evaluation.
4. Recommends glucose (15–20 g) for all conscious patients with hypoglycemia.
5. Advise all patients not to smoke.
6. Recommends beginning these screening tests after 5 y with type 1 DM
   a. Urine albumin-to-creatinine ratio and serum creatinine annually.
   b. Dilated funduscopic exam annually.
   c. Monofilament screening for diabetic neuropathy annually.
   d. Comprehensive foot examination at least annually.
7. Recommends screening at diagnosis for other autoimmune conditions
   a. Tissue transglutaminase IgA antibodies.
   b. Thyroperoxidase and thyroglobulin antibodies.
   c. TSH.
8. Fasting lipid panel at age 10 y or at puberty (consider as early as age 2 y for a strong family history of hyperlipidemia).
   a. Repeat annually if results abnormal or every 5 y if results acceptable.
9. Consider statin therapy if age ≥10 y and LDL >160 mg/dL despite good glycemic control and lifestyle modification.

10. Aspirin 75–162 mg/d if:

    b. Primary prevention of CVD if 10-y risk of coronary artery disease (CAD) >10%.

    c. Secondary prevention of CVD.

Source

–http://care.diabetesjournals.org/content/36/Supplement_1/S11.full

Comments

1. Glycemic control recommendations for **toddlers (age 0–6 y).**
   a. Before meals, capillary blood gas (CPG) 100–180 mg/dL.
   b. Bedtime, CPG 110–200 mg/dL.
   c. HgbA1c <8.5%.
2. Glycemic control recommendations for **school-age (age 6–12 y).**
   a. Before meals, CPG 90–180 mg/dL.
   b. Bedtime, CPG 100–180 mg/dL.
   c. HgbA1c <8%.
3. Glycemic control recommendations for **adolescents (age 13–19 y).**
   a. Before meals, CPG 90–130 mg/dL.
   b. Bedtime, CPG 90–150 mg/dL.
   c. HgbA1c <7.5%.

Population

–Adults with type 1 diabetes.

Recommendations

▶ NICE 2015

–Confirm diagnosis by checking C-peptide levels and auto-antibody testing.
–Provide all adults with DM 1 a structured education program.
–Offer carbohydrate counting education.
–Offer peer support groups.
–Measure glycohemoglobin every 3–6 mo.
  • Fructosamine level is an alternative test for anemic patients.
–Recommend self-glucose monitoring at least 4 times daily.
–Glucose targets are:
  • 90–126 mg/dL fasting.
  • 72–126 mg/dL before meals.
–Basal insulin
  • Daily insulin glargine.
  • Insulin detemir bid.
–Recommend rapid-acting prandial insulin before meals.

−Consider referral for islet cell transplantation in those with recurrent severe hypoglycemia.

−Screen adults with low BMI for celiac disease.

−Measure a TSH annually.

−Recommend therapy with ACEI or ARB for patients with hypertension or diabetic nephropathy.

−Offer digital retinopathy screening annually.

−Offer men with DM 1 and erectile dysfunction a phosphodiesterase-5 inhibitor.

Source

−https://guidelines.gov/summaries/summary/49529

DIABETES MELLITUS (DM), TYPE 2

Population

−Nonpregnant adults.

Recommendations

▶ AACE 2010

1. Endorses the use of HgbA1c ≥6.5% as a means of diagnosing type 2 DM.
2. HgbA1c is not recommended for diagnosing type 1 DM or gestational diabetes.

Source

−http://www.aace.com/pub/pdf/guidelines/AACEpositionA1cfeb2010.pdf

Population

−Adults.

Population

−Adults and children.

Recommendations

▶ ADA 2017

1. Self-monitoring blood glucose ≥3 times daily in all patients using multiple insulin injections or an insulin pump.
2. Recommends HgbA1c every 3 mo if therapy has changed or if blood glucose control is inadequate.
3. Provide diabetes self-management education, including education about hypoglycemia management and adjustments during illness.
4. Provide family planning for women of reproductive age.
5. Provide medical nutrition therapy.
6. Weight loss is recommended for all overweight or obese diabetic patients.

7. Keep saturated fat intake <7% of total calories.

8. Reduction of protein intake to 0.8–1.0 g/kg/d for early stages of CKD and 0.8 g/kg/d for later stages of CKD.

9. Recommends at least 150 min/wk of moderate physical activity.

10. The glucose range for critically ill patients is 100–180 mg/dL.

11. The glucose range for noncritically ill patients in the hospital is <140 mg/dL premeal (<7.8 mmol/L) and random blood glucose <180 mg/dL (<10 mmol/L).

12. Recommends the following:
    a. Immunizations
        i. Annual influenza vaccination if age ≥6 mo.
        ii. Pneumococcal polysaccharide vaccine if age >2 y.
        iii. 1× revaccination if age ≥65 y.
        iv. hepatitis B vaccination if unvaccinated and age 19–59 y.
    b. Target BP <130/80 mm Hg.
    c. Statin therapy if:
        i. Overt CVD present.
        ii. Age >40 y and ≥1 CV risk factor.[b]
        iii. LDL >100 mg/dL despite lifestyle modification.
        iv. LDL >70 mg/dL if DM2 and overt cardiovascular disease.
    d. ASA 75–162 mg/d if:
        i. Primary prevention of CVD if 10-y risk of CAD >10%.
        ii. Secondary prevention of CVD.
    e. Annual check of urine albumin-to-creatinine ratio and serum creatinine.
    f. Annual serum creatinine and fasting lipid profile.
    g. Annual dilated funduscopic exam.
    h. Annual monofilament screening for diabetic neuropathy.
    i. At minimum, annual comprehensive foot exam.

Source
–https://professional.diabetes.org/sites/professional.diabetes.org/files/media/dc_40_s1_final.pdf

Comments

1. Glycemic control recommendations:
    a. Preprandial CPG 70–130 mg/dL.
    b. Postprandial CPG <180 mg/dL (1–2 h postmeals).
    c. HgbA1c <7%.

2. Consider bariatric surgery if BMI >35 kg/m^2 and if diabetes is difficult to control with lifestyle modification and medications.

3. Angiotensin-converting enzyme inhibitors (ACEIs) or ARBs are first-line antihypertensives.

4. Second-line antihypertensives are a thiazide diuretic if GFR $\geq$30 mL/min/1.73 m^2 or a loop diuretic if GFR <30 mL/min/1.73 m^2.
5. Clopidogrel 75 mg/d is an alternative for persons ASA intolerant.
6. Nephrology referral indicated if GFR <60 mL/min/1.73 m^2, or if heavy proteinuria or structural kidney disease present.
7. Consider a serum TSH in women age >50 y.
8. Consider assessing patients for the following comorbidities that are increased with DM:
   a. Hearing impairment.
   b. Obstructive sleep apnea.
   c. Fatty liver disease.
   d. Low testosterone in men.
   e. Periodontal disease.
   f. Cognitive impairment.

Population
–Adults older than 18 y.

Recommendations
▶ ACP 2012
–Oral pharmacologic therapy should be added for treatment of type 2 DM when lifestyle modifications, including diet, exercise, and weight loss, have failed to adequately control hyperglycemia.
–Recommends metformin as the initial pharmacologic agent to treat most patients with type 2 DM.
–Recommends adding another oral agent to metformin if patients have persistent hyperglycemia despite metformin and lifestyle modifications.

Source
–http://www.annals.org/content/156/3/I-36.full.pdf+html

Comments
1. All dual-regimens were more effective than monotherapy and decreased the HbA1c levels by an average of 1% more.
2. Most monotherapy regimens had similar efficacy and reduced HbA1c levels by an average of 1%.
3. Studies suggest that metformin decreases all-cause mortality slightly more than sulfonylureas with a much lower rate of hypoglycemia.

Population
–Hospitalized adults older than 18 y.

Recommendations
▶ ACP 2011
–Avoid intensive insulin therapy in hospitalized patients (even if in SICU/MICU).

–Recommends a target blood glucose level of 140–200 mg/dL if insulin therapy is used in SICU/MICU patients.

Source

–http://www.annals.org/content/154/4/260.full.pdf+html

Comment

–Intensive insulin therapy (targeting blood glucose levels of 80–110 mg/dL) in SICU/MICU patients does not improve mortality, but has a 5-fold increased risk of hypoglycemia.

Population

–Children and adolescents with newly diagnosed DM2.

Recommendations

▶ AAP 2013

–Insulin therapy should be initiated for children with:
- Diabetic ketoacidosis.
- HbA1c >9%.
- Random glucose >250 mg/dL.

–Diet, exercise, and metformin are initial therapy for other situations.

–Recommend moderate-to-vigorous exercise for 60 min daily.

–Limit nonacademic screen time t <2 h/d.

–Monitor HbA1c every 3 mo.

–Desire HbA1c <7%.

Source

–pediatrics.aappublications.org/content/131/2/364.full.pdf

ORAL DIABETES MELLITUS TYPE 2 AGENTS—CPG 2015

Category	Metformin	DDP-4I	GLP-1 RA	TZD	AGI	Colesevelam	BCR-QR	SU/MGN	Insulin	SGLT-2	Pramlintide
Hypoglycemia	Neutral	Neutral	Neutral	Neutral	Neutral	Neutral	Neutral	Moderate/severe/mild	Moderate/severe	Neutral	Neutral
Weight	Slight loss	Neutral	Loss	Gain	Neutral	Neutral	Neutral	Gain	Gain	Loss	Loss
Renal/GU	Cl if Crt>1.4 (W) Crt>1.5 (M) CrCl <50 mL/min	Dose adjust if CrCl <30 mL/min	Cl if CrCl <30 mL/min	Fluid retention	Neutral	Neutral	Neutral	Renal impairment increases hypoglycemia	Renal impairment increases hypoglycemia	Infection; Cl if CrCl <45 mL/min	Neutral
Gastrointestinal[a]	Moderate	Neutral	Moderate	Cl in cirrhosis	Moderate	Mild	Moderate	Neutral	Neutral	Neutral	Moderate
CHF	Neutral	Neutral	Neutral	Moderate	Neutral	Neutral	Neutral	Neutral	Neutral	Neutral	Neutral
CVD	Benefit	Neutral	Neutral	Slight risk	Neutral	Neutral	Neutral	Unclear	Neutral	Orthostasis in elderly	Neutral
Bone loss	Neutral	Neutral	Neutral	Moderate	Neutral	Neutral	Neutral	Neutral	Neutral	Small	Neutral
Miscellaneous	B$_{12}$ deficiency	–	–	–	–	–	–	SIADH/headaches	–	–	Avoid with gastroparesis; headache

AGI, alphaglucosidase inhibitors; BCR-QR, bromocriptine quick release; Cl, contraindicated; CVD, cardiovascular disease; DPP-4I, dipeptidyl peptidase-4 inhibitor; GLP-1 RA, glucagon-like peptide-1 receptor antagonist; GU, genitourinary; MGN, meglitinides; SIADH, syndrome of inappropriate antidiuretic hormone; SGLT-2, salt glucose contransporter 2; SU, sulfonylurea; TZD, thiazolidindiones.

[a]GI symptoms can include nausea, vomiting, flatulence, diarrhea, anorexia, and pancreatitis (for GLP-1 RA).

Source: Garber A et al. *Endocr Pract.* 2013;19:327. Reprinted with permission from American Association of Clinical Endocrinologists © 2013 AACE.

INJECTABLE MEDICATIONS FOR DM 2

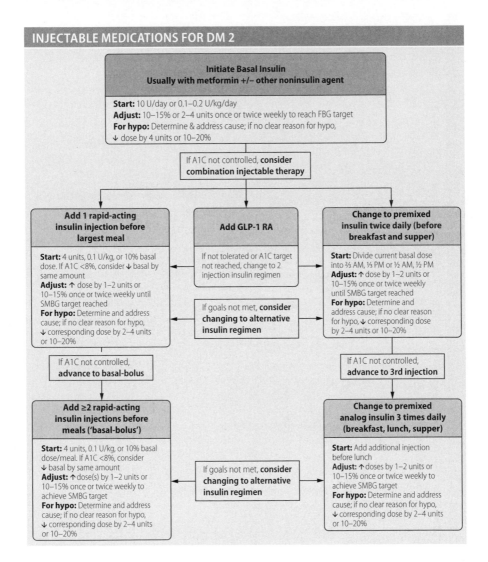

Initiate Basal Insulin
Usually with metformin +/– other noninsulin agent

Start: 10 U/day or 0.1–0.2 U/kg/day
Adjust: 10–15% or 2–4 units once or twice weekly to reach FBG target
For hypo: Determine & address cause; if no clear reason for hypo,
↓ dose by 4 units or 10–20%

If A1C not controlled, **consider combination injectable therapy**

Add 1 rapid-acting insulin injection before largest meal

Start: 4 units, 0.1 U/kg, or 10% basal dose. If A1C <8%, consider ↓ basal by same amount
Adjust: ↑ dose by 1–2 units or 10–15% once or twice weekly until SMBG target reached
For hypo: Determine and address cause; if no clear reason for hypo, ↓ corresponding dose by 2–4 units or 10–20%

Add GLP-1 RA

If not tolerated or A1C target not reached, change to 2 injection insulin regimen

If goals not met, **consider changing to alternative insulin regimen**

Change to premixed insulin twice daily (before breakfast and supper)

Start: Divide current basal dose into ⅔ AM, ⅓ PM or ½ AM, ½ PM
Adjust: ↑ dose by 1–2 units or 10–15% once or twice weekly until SMBG target reached
For hypo: Determine and address cause; if no clear reason for hypo, ↓ corresponding dose by 2–4 units or 10–20%

If A1C not controlled, **advance to basal-bolus**

If A1C not controlled, **advance to 3rd injection**

Add ≥2 rapid-acting insulin injections before meals ('basal-bolus')

Start: 4 units, 0.1 U/kg, or 10% basal dose/meal. If A1C <8%, consider ↓ basal by same amount
Adjust: ↑ dose(s) by 1–2 units or 10–15% once or twice weekly to achieve SMBG target
For hypo: Determine and address cause; if no clear reason for hypo, ↓ corresponding dose by 2–4 units or 10–20%

If goals not met, **consider changing to alternative insulin regimen**

Change to premixed analog insulin 3 times daily (breakfast, lunch, supper)

Start: Add additional injection before lunch
Adjust: ↑ doses by 1–2 units or 10–15% once or twice weekly to achieve SMBG target
For hypo: Determine and address cause; if no clear reason for hypo, ↓ corresponding dose by 2–4 units or 10–20%

DIABETES MELLITUS TYPE 2 MANAGEMENT

Start with Monotherapy unless:

A1C is greater than or equal to 9%, consider Dual Therapy.

A1C is greater than or equal to 10%, blood glucose is greater than or equal to 300 mg/dL, or patient is markedly symptomatic, consider Combination Injectable Therapy.

Monotherapy   Metformin   Lifestyle Management

EFFICACY*	high
HYPO RISK	low risk
WEIGHT	neutral/loss
SIDE EFFECTS	GI/lactic acidosis
COSTS*	low

If A1C target not achieved after approximately 3 months of monotherapy, proceed to 2-drug combination (order not meant to denote any specific preference–choice dependent on a variety of patient- & disease-specific factors):

Dual Therapy   Metformin +   Lifestyle Management

	Sulfonylurea	Thiazolidinedione	DPP-4 inhibitor	SGLT2 inhibitor	GLP-1 receptor agonist	Insulin (basal)
EFFICACY*	high	high	intermediate	intermediate	high	highest
HYPO RISK	moderate risk	low risk	low risk	low risk	low risk	high risk
WEIGHT	gain	gain	neutral	loss	loss	gain
SIDE EFFECTS	hypoglycemia	edema, HF, fxs	rare	GU, dehydration, fxs	GI	hypoglycemia
COSTS*	low	low	high	high	high	high

If A1C target not achieved after approximately 3 months of dual therapy, proceed to 3-drug combination (order not meant to denote any specific preference–choice dependent on a variety fo patient- & disease-specific factors):

Triple Therapy   Metformin +   Lifestyle Management

Sulfonylurea +		Thiazolidinedione +		DPP-4 inhibitor +		SGLT2 inhibitor +		GLP-1 receptor agonist +		Insulin (basal) +	
TZD		SU		SU		SU		SU		TZD	
DPP-4-i	or	DPP-4-i	or	TZD	or	TZD	or	TZD	or	DPP-4-i	or
SGLT2-i	or	SGLT2-i	or	SGLT2-i	or	DPP-4-i	or	SGLT2-i	or	SGLT2-i	or
GLP-1-RA	or	GLP-1-RA	or	Insulin§	or	GLP-1-RA	or	Insulin§	or	GLP-1-RA	or
Insulin§	or	Insulin§	or			Insulin§	or				

If A1C target not achieved after approximately 3 months of triple therapy and patient (1) on oral combination, move to basal insulin or GLP-1 RA, (2) on GLP-1 RA, add basal insulin, or (3) on optimally titrated basal insulin, add GLP-1 RA or mealtime insulin. Metformin therapy should be maintained, while other oral agents may be discontinued on an individual basis to avoid unnecessarily complex or costly regimens (i.e., adding a fourth antihyperglycemic agent).

Combination Injectable Therapy

–Prolonged metformin use can lead to vitamin B12 deficiency. SGLT-2 inhibitors are favored over sulfonylureas as an add-on to metformin in terms of cardiovascular mortality.

Sources
–https://professional.diabetes.org/sites/professional.diabetes.org/files/media/dc_40_s1_final.pdf
–Qaseem A, Barry MJ, Humphrey LL, Forciea MA; Clinical Guidelines Committee of the American College of Physicians. Oral pharmacologic treatment of type 2 diabetes mellitus: a clinical practice guideline update from the American College of Physicians. *Ann Intern Med.* 2017 Feb 21;166(4):279-290.

DIARRHEA, ACUTE

Population
– Adults with acute diarrheal illness.

Recommendations

APPROACH TO EMPIRIC THERAPY AND DIAGNOSTIC-DIRECTED MANAGEMENT OF THE ADULT PATIENT WITH ACUTE DIARRHEA (SUSPECT INFECTIOUS ETIOLOGY)

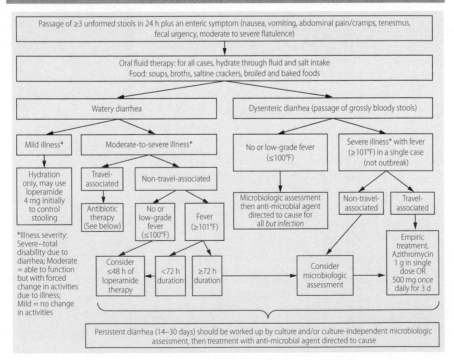

ACUTE DIARRHEA ANTIBIOTIC TREATMENT RECOMMENDATIONS

Antibiotic[a]	Dose	Treatment duration
Levofloxacin	500 mg by mouth	Single dose[b] or 3-d course
Ciprofloxacin	750 mg by mouth or	Single dose[b]
	500 mg by mouth	3-d course
Ofloxacin	400 mg by mouth	Single dose[b] or 3-d course
Azithromycin[c,d]	1,000 mg by mouth or	Single dose[b]
	500 mg by mouth	3-d course[d]
Rifaximin[e]	200 mg by mouth3 times daily	3-d

ETEC, Enterotoxigenic *Escherichia coli*.

[a]Antibiotic regimens may be combined with loperamide, 4 mg first dose, and then 2 mg dose after each loose stool, not to exceed 16 mg in a 24-h period.
[b]If symptoms are not resolved after 24 h, complete a 3-d course of antibiotics.
[c]Use empirically as first line in Southeast Asia and India to cover fluoroquinolone-resistant **Campylobacter** or in other geographical areas if **Campylobacter** or resistant ETEC are suspected.
[d]Preferred regimen for dysentery or febrile diarrhea.
[e]Do not use if clinical suspicion for **Campylobacter, Salmonella, Shigella,** or other causes of invasive diarrhea.

–The use of probiotics or prebiotics for the treatment of acute diarrhea in adults is not recommended.

–Bismuth subsalicylates can be administered to control rates of passage of stool and may help travelers function better during bouts of mild-to-moderate illness.

–In patients receiving antibiotics for traveler's diarrhea, adjunctive loperamide therapy should be administered to decrease duration of diarrhea and increase chance for a cure.

–Use of antibiotics for community-acquired diarrhea should be discouraged as epidemiological studies suggest that most community-acquired diarrhea is viral in origin (norovirus, rotavirus, and adenovirus) and is not shortened by the use of antibiotics.

Source

–ACG Clinical Guideline: Diagnosis, treatment, and prevention of acute diarrheal infections in adults. *Am J Gastroenterol.* 2016;111:602-622.

DIFFUSE LARGE ß CELL LYMPHOMA (DLBCL) STAGE I THROUGH IV

Population

–Complete remission of DLBCL following treatment with negative PET-CT scan.

Recommendations

▶ NCCN 2016

–**Clinical Follow-up Stages I and II**
- History and physical exam and labs (CBC, metabolic panel including LDH) every 3–6 mo for 5 y then yearly as clinically indicated.

–**Imaging**
- Repeat CT or PET scan only as clinically indicated (symptoms, palpable nodes, or abnormal labs—especially increased LDH).
- If recurrence is suspected, re-biopsy is mandatory to guide salvage therapy.

–**Clinical Decisions Stages III and IV**
- Observation or consider radiation therapy (RT) to initial area of bulky (>10 cm) disease or consider high-dose chemotherapy with autologous stem cell rescue in very high risk patients who have Stage IV disease and a significant chance of relapse.

–**Clinical Follow-up**
- History and physical with labs (CBC, metabolic panel including LDH every 2–4 mo for 5 y and then yearly or as clinically indicated).

–**Imaging**
- Controversial—either CT scans every 6 mo or only when signs or symptoms are suggestive of recurrence.

Sources

–*Mayo Clinic Proceedings.* 2015; 90:1574-1583 *J Clin Oncol.* 2014; 32:3039-30593067.

Comments

1. **Lymphoma Facts**
   - DLBCL most common non-Hodgkin's lymphoma (NHL)—30%.
   - Follicular lymphoma 2nd most common at 20%.
   - 71,000 cases of NHL with 19,000 deaths yearly. Total number of NHL diagnosis is increasing by 1% to 2% per year.

2. **Ann Arbor staging system**
   - Stage I—single nodal group either side of diaphragm.
   - Stage II—more than 1 nodal group involvement either side of diaphragm.
   - Stage III—nodal groups on both sides of the diaphragm.
   - Stage IV—disseminated disease to bone marrow and/or visceral organs.

- β symptoms include fever, night sweats, and weight loss.
- Bulk disease (>10 cm) increases risk of recurrence.
- There has been a reduction in frequency of surveillance CT scans due to concern about increased radiation exposure. (*JAMA*.2012;307:2400)
- Monitor for late events—secondary cancers, cardiovascular disease, hypothyroidism, and fertility issues.
- Bone marrow injury may evolve to myelodysplasia and acute myeloid leukemia.
- Always biopsy recurrent disease—10% to 15% will be follicular lymphoma with indolent biology.
- CNS prophylaxis in aggressive DLBCL (testis, sinus, bone marrow)—intrathecal vs. high-dose methotrexate with rescue.

DYSPEPSIA

▶ American College of Gastroenterology/Canadian Association of Gastroenterology 2017

Population

–Adults with dyspepsia.

WORK-UP OF UNDIAGNOSED DYSPEPSIA

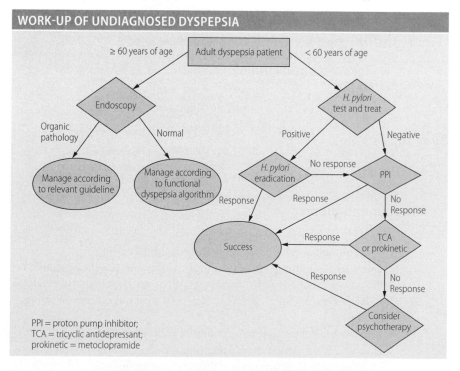

PPI = proton pump inhibitor;
TCA = tricyclic antidepressant;
prokinetic = metoclopramide

MANAGEMENT OF FUNCTIONAL DYSPEPSIA

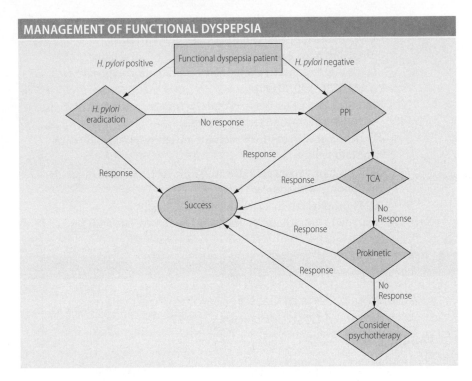

Recommendation

–Recommends against routine motility studies for patients with functional dyspepsia unless there is a strong suspicion for gastroparesis in which case a motility study is indicated.

Source

–ACG and CAG Clinical Guideline: Management of dyspepsia. *Am J Gastroenterol.* 2017 Jul;112(7):988-1013.

NICE 2014

Population

–Adults

Recommendations

▶ NICE 2014

1. Recommend smoking cessation and weight reduction.
2. Consider discontinuation of offending medications (calcium channel blockers, nitrates, theophylline, bisphosphonates, steroids, and NSAIDs).
3. Consider testing for *H. pylori* after a 2-wk washout off proton pump inhibitors.
4. Empiric trial of proton pump inhibitor therapy.
5. Consider laparoscopic fundoplication for patients who do not wish to continue with acid suppressive therapy long term.

6. Consider specialist referral for:
   a. Dyspepsia refractory to meds.
   b. Consideration of surgery.
   c. Refractory *H. pylori* infection.
   d. Barrett esophagus.

Source
   –http://www.guideline.gov/content.aspx?id=48563

DYSPHAGIA

Population
   –Adults.

Recommendations
▶ ASGE 2014

   –Recommend endoscopic dilation for benign esophageal strictures or eosinophilic esophagitis.
   –Recommend through-the-scope balloon dilation for complex esophageal strictures.
   –Concomitant antisecretory therapy with dilation for peptic strictures.
   –Reserve esophageal stents for refractory esophageal strictures.
   –Options for endoscopic management of achalasia include pneumatic dilation or botulinum toxin injections.

Source
   –http://www.guideline.gov/content.aspx?id=47786

EATING DISORDERS

Population
   –Adults and children with eating disorders.

Recommendations
▶ APA 2013

   –Psychiatric management begins with the establishment of a therapeutic alliance.
   –Recommend a multidisciplinary approach with a psychiatrist, dietician, social worker, and physician.
   –Components of the initial evaluation include:
      • A thorough history and physical examination.
      • Assessment of the social history.
      • An evaluation of the height and weight history.
      • Any family history of eating disorders or mental health disorders?

- Assess attitude of eating, exercising, and appearance.
- Assess for suicidality.
- Assess for substance abuse.
- Recommend nutritional rehab for seriously underweight patients.
  - Recommend nasogastric tube feeding over parenteral nutrition for patients not meeting caloric requirements with oral feeds alone.
- Psychosocial rehab for patients with both anorexia nervosa and bulimia nervosa.
- Prozac is preferred agent to prevent relapse during maintenance phase of bulimia nervosa.
- Labs
  - CBC.
  - Chemistry panel.
  - TSH.
- Additional testing
  - Bone mineral densitometry if amenorrhea for more than 6 mo.
  - Dental evaluation for history of purging.

Source
  –http://www.guideline.gov/content.aspx?id=9318

ECTOPIC PREGNANCY

Population
  –Pregnant women.

Recommendations
▶ NICE 2012
  –Recommended evaluation for stable women with an early pregnancy.
  - Transvaginal ultrasound (TVUS) with a crown-rump length ≥7 mm but no cardiac activity.
    - Repeat ultrasound in 7 d.
    - Quantitative β-hCG q48h × 2 levels.
  - TVUS with gestational sac ≥25 mm and no fetal pole.
    - Repeat ultrasound in 7 d.
    - Quantitative β-hCG q48h × 2 levels.
  –Management of ectopic pregnancies.
  - Methotrexate candidates.
    - No significant pain.
    - Adnexal mass <3.5 cm.
    - No cardiac activity on TVUS.
    - β-hCG <5000 IU/L.
    - Dose is 50 mg/m2 IM.

- Laparoscopy if:
  - Unstable patient.
  - Severe pain.
  - Adnexal mass >3.5 cm.
  - Cardiac activity seen.
  - β-hCG >5000 IU/L.
- Rhogam 250 IU to all Rh-negative women who undergo surgery for an ectopic.

Source
  -www.guidelines.gov/content.aspx?id=39274

Comments

1. Ectopic pregnancy can present with:
   - Abdominal or pelvic pain.
   - Vaginal bleeding.
   - Amenorrhea.
   - Breast tenderness.
   - GI symptoms.
   - Dizziness.
   - Urinary symptoms.
   - Rectal pressure.
   - Dyschezia.
2. Most normal intrauterine pregnancies will show an increase in β-hCG level by at least 63% in 48 h.
3. Intrauterine pregnancies are usually apparent by TVUS if β-hCG >1500 IU/L.

EPILEPSY

Population
  -Children and adults.

Recommendations

▶ NICE 2012
  -Educate adults about all aspects of epilepsy.
  -Diagnosis of epilepsy should be made by a specialist in epilepsy.
  -Evaluation of epilepsy
  - Electroencephalogram.
  - Sleep-deprived EEG if standard EEG is inconclusive.
  - Neuroimaging to evaluate for any structural brain abnormalities.
    - MRI is preferred for children <2 y, adults, refractory seizures, and focal seizures.

- Measurement of prolactin is not recommended.
- Chemistry panel.
- ECG in adults.
- Urine toxicology screen.

−Antiepileptic drugs (AED)
  - Start AED only after the diagnosis of epilepsy is made.
  - Focal seizures.
    ◦ Carbamazepine.
    ◦ Lamotrigine.
    ◦ Adjunctive AED: levetiracetam, oxcarbazepine, or sodium valproate.
  - Generalized tonic-clonic seizures.
    ◦ Sodium valproate.
    ◦ Lamotrigine.
    ◦ Carbamazepine.
    ◦ Oxcarbazepine.
    ◦ Adjunctive AED: levetiracetam or topiramate.
  - Absence seizures.
    ◦ Ethosuximide.
    ◦ Sodium valproate.
    ◦ Alternative: lamotrigine.
  - Myoclonic seizures.
    ◦ Sodium valproate.
    ◦ Alternatives: levetiracetam or topiramate.

Source
  −http://www.guidelines.gov/content.aspx?id=36082

Comment

  −AED can decrease the efficacy of combined oral contraceptive pills.

ERECTILE DYSFUNCTION (ED)

Population
  −Adult men.

Recommendations

▶ EAU 2009

  −Recommends a medical and psychosexual history on all patients.
  −Recommends a focused physical examination to assess CV status, neurologic status, prostate disease, penile abnormalities, and signs of hypogonadism.
  −Recommends checking a fasting glucose, lipid profile, and total testosterone levels.
  −Recommends psychosexual therapy for psychogenic ED.

–Recommends testosterone therapy for androgen deficiency if no contraindications present.[a]

–Selective phosphodiesterase 5 (PDE5) inhibitors are first-line therapy for idiopathic ED.

Source

–http://www.uroweb.org/gls/EU/2010%20Male%20Sex%20Dysfunction.pdf

Comments

1. Selective PDE5 inhibitors:
   a. Sildenafil.
   b. Tadalafil.
   c. Vardenafil.
2. Avoid nitrates and use α-blockers with caution when prescribing a selective PDE5 inhibitor.

GALLSTONES

Population

–Adults with or suspected of having gallstones.

Recommendations

▶ NICE 2014

1. Obtain liver function tests and ultrasound if suspected gallstone disease.
2. Consider magnetic resonance cholangiopancreatography (MRCP) if ultrasound has not detected common bile duct stones but the:
   a. Common bile duct is dilated.
   b. Liver function tests are abnormal.
3. Offer cholecystectomy for symptomatic gallstones or acute cholecystitis.
4. Offer percutaneous cholecystostomy for acute cholecystitis or gallbladder empyema if surgery is contraindicated.
5. Options for choledocholithiasis:
   a. Cholecystectomy and intraoperative clearance of CBD stones.
   b. ERCP prior to cholecystectomy.

Source

–http://www.guideline.gov/content.aspx?id=49014

GASTROINTESTINAL BLEEDING, LOWER

Population

– Adults with suspected lower GI bleeding.

Recommendations

▶ ACG 2016

[a]Prostate CA, breast CA, or signs of prostatism.

ALGORITHM FOR THE MANAGEMENT OF PATIENTS PRESENTING WITH ACUTE LGIB STRATIFIED BY BLEEDING SEVERITY

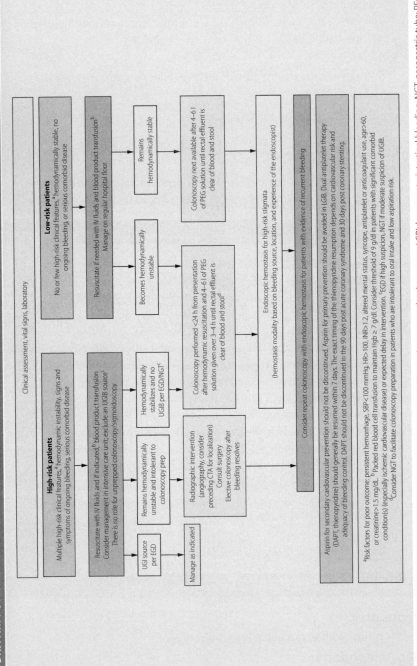

CTA, computed tomographic angiography; DAPT, dual antiplatelet therapy; EGD, esophagogastroduodenoscopy; LGIB, lower gastrointestinal bleeding; NGT, nasogastric tube; PEG, polyethylene glycol; UGIB, upper gastrointestinal bleeding.

Source: Strate LL, Gralnek IM. ACG Clinical Guideline: Management of Patients With Acute Lower Gastrointestinal Bleeding. Am J Gastroenterol. 2016; 111: 459–474, Fig 1.

-Platelet transfusion should be considered to maintain a platelet count of 50,000 in patients with severe bleeding and those requiring endoscopic hemostasis.

-Reversal of anticoagulation should be considered before endoscopy in patients with an INR >2.5

Source

-ACG Clinical Guideline: Management of patients with acute lower gastrointestinal bleeding. *Am J Gastroenterol.* 2016;111:459–474.

GASTROINTESTINAL BLEEDING, UPPER (UGIB)

Population

-Adults.

Recommendations

▶ NICE 2012

-Recommend a formal risk assessment for patients with an UGIB.
  • Blatchford score at first assessment.
  • Rockall score after endoscopy.
-Avoid platelet transfusions in patients who are not actively bleeding and are hemodynamically stable.
-For UGIB, give FFP if:
  • Fibrinogen <100 mg/dL.
  • Partial thromboplastin time >1.5× normal.
-Prothrombin complex concentrate (PCC) indicated for UGIB on warfarin.
-Timing of endoscopy.
  • Immediately for unstable patients.
  • Within 24 h for stable patients.
-Management of nonvariceal bleeding
  • Surgical clips.
  • Thermal coagulation.
  • Epinephrine injection.
  • Fibrin or thrombin glue.
  • Proton pump inhibitors.
  • Recurrent bleeding can be assessed by repeat endoscopy or by interventional radiology angioembolization.

–Management of variceal bleeding.
- Esophageal variceal band ligation.
- Terlipressin or octreotide infusions.
- Prophylactic third-generation cephalosporin.
- Transjugular intrahepatic portosystemic shunt for recurrent esophageal variceal bleeding or gastric variceal bleeding.

Source
–http://www.guidelines.gov/content.aspx?id=37563

Comments
1. Patients should stop NSAIDs.
2. Alcohol cessation if a factor.
3. Low-dose aspirin can be resumed if needed for secondary prevention of vascular events once hemostasis has been achieved.
4. Ongoing use of thienopyridine agents (eg, clopidogrel, ticagrelor, or prasugrel) should be only after discussion with appropriate specialist.

GERIATRICS

▲ Medication Use in Older Adults, Potentially Inappropriate

2012 AGS BEERS CRITERIA FOR POTENTIALLY INAPPROPRIATE MEDICATION USE IN OLDER ADULTS

Organ System/ Therapeutic Category/Drug(s)	Rationale	Recommendation	Quality of Evidence	Strength of Recommendation
Anticholinergics (exclude TCAs)				
First-generation antihistamines (as single agent or as part of combination products) • Brompheniramine • Carbinoxamine • Chlorpheniramine • Clemastine • Cyproheptadine • Dexbrompheniramine • Dexchlorpheniramine • Diphenhydramine (oral) • Doxylamine • Hydroxyzine • Promethazine • Triprolidine	Highly anticholinergic; clearance reduced with advanced age, and tolerance develops when used as hypnotic; increased risk of confusion, dry mouth, constipation, and other anticholinergic effects/toxicity. Use of diphenhydramine in special situations such as acute treatment of severe allergic reaction may be appropriate.	Avoid	Hydroxyzine and promethazine: high; all others: moderate	Strong
Antiparkinson agents • Benztropine (oral) • Trihexyphenidyl	Not recommended for prevention of extrapyramidal symptoms with antipsychotics; more effective agents available for treatment of Parkinson disease.	Avoid	Moderate	Strong

2012 AGS BEERS CRITERIA FOR POTENTIALLY INAPPROPRIATE MEDICATION USE IN OLDER ADULTS *(Continued)*

Organ System/Therapeutic Category/Drug(s)	Rationale	Recommendation	Quality of Evidence	Strength of Recommendation
Antispasmodics • Belladonna alkaloids • Clidinium-chlordiazepoxide • Dicyclomine • Hyoscyamine • Propantheline • Scopolamine	Highly anticholinergic, uncertain effectiveness.	Avoid except in short-term palliative care to decrease oral secretions.	Moderate	Strong
Antithrombotics				
Dipyridamole, oral short-acting*a* (does not apply to the extended-release combination with aspirin)	May cause orthostatic hypotension; more effective alternatives available; IV form acceptable for use in cardiac stress testing.	Avoid	Moderate	Strong
Ticlopidine*a*	Safer, effective alternatives available.	Avoid	Moderate	Strong
Anti-infective				
Nitrofurantoin	Potential for pulmonary toxicity; safer alternatives available; lack of efficacy in patients with CrCl <60 mL/min due to inadequate drug concentration in the urine.	Avoid for long-term suppression; avoid in patients with CrCl <60 mL/min.	Moderate	Strong

Cardiovascular

Drug	Recommendation	Rationale	Quality of Evidence	Strength of Recommendation
Alpha₁ blockers • Doxazosin • Prazosin • Terazosin	Avoid use as an antihypertensive.	High risk of orthostatic hypotension; not recommended as routine treatment for hypertension; alternative agents have superior risk/benefit profile.	Moderate	Strong
Alpha blockers, central • Clonidine • Guanabenz[a] • Guanfacine[a] • Methyldopa[a] • Reserpine (>0.1 mg/d)[a]	Avoid clonidine as a first-line antihypertensive. Avoid others as listed.	High risk of adverse CNS effects; may cause bradycardia and orthostatic hypotension; not recommended as routine treatment for hypertension.	Low	Strong
Antiarrhythmic drugs (Class Ia, Ic, III) • Amiodarone • Dofetilide • Dronedarone • Flecainide • Ibutilide • Procainamide • Propafenone • Quinidine • Sotalol	Avoid antiarrhythmic drugs as first-line treatment of atrial fibrillation.	Data suggest that rate control yields better balance of benefits and harms than rhythm control for most older adults. Amiodarone is associated with multiple toxicities, including thyroid disease, pulmonary disorders, and QT interval prolongation.	High	Strong
Disopyramide[a]	Avoid	Disopyramide is a potent negative inotrope and therefore may induce heart failure in older adults; strongly anticholinergic; other antiarrhythmic drugs preferred.	Low	Strong

	2012 AGS BEERS CRITERIA FOR POTENTIALLY INAPPROPRIATE MEDICATION USE IN OLDER ADULTS (Continued)			
Organ System/Therapeutic Category/Drug(s)	Rationale	Recommendation	Quality of Evidence	Strength of Recommendation
Dronedarone	Worse outcomes have been reported in patients taking dronedarone who have permanent atrial fibrillation or heart failure. In general, rate control is preferred over rhythm control for atrial fibrillation.	Avoid in patients with permanent atrial fibrillation or heart failure	Moderate	Strong
Digoxin >0.125 mg/d	In heart failure, higher dosages associated with no additional benefit and may increase risk of toxicity; decreased renal clearance may lead to increased risk of toxic effects.	Avoid	Moderate	Strong
Nifedipine, immediate release[a]	Potential for hypotension; risk of precipitating myocardial ischemia.	Avoid	High	Strong
Spironolactone >25 mg/d	In heart failure, the risk of hyperkalemia is higher in older adults if taking >25 mg/d.	Avoid in patients with heart failure or with a CrCl <30 mL/min.	Moderate	Strong

Central Nervous System

Tertiary TCAs, alone or in combination: • Amitriptyline • Chlordiazepoxide-amitriptyline • Clomipramine • Doxepin >6 mg/d • Imipramine • Perphenazine-amitriptyline • Trimipramine	Highly anticholinergic, sedating, and cause orthostatic hypotension; the safety profile of low-dose doxepin (≤6 mg/d) is comparable to that of placebo.	Avoid	High	Strong
Antipsychotics, first- (conventional) and second- (atypical) generation	Increased risk of cerebrovascular accident (stroke) and mortality in persons with dementia.	Avoid use for behavioral problems of dementia unless nonpharmacologic options have failed and patient is threat to self or others.	Moderate	Strong
Thioridazine Mesoridazine	Highly anticholinergic and greater risk of QT-interval prolongation.	Avoid	Moderate	Strong
Barbiturates • Amobarbital[a] • Butabarbital[a] • Butalbital • Mephobarbital[a] • Pentobarbital[a] • Phenobarbital • Secobarbital[a]	High rate of physical dependence; tolerance to sleep benefits; greater risk of overdose at low dosages.	Avoid	High	Strong

2012 AGS BEERS CRITERIA FOR POTENTIALLY INAPPROPRIATE MEDICATION USE IN OLDER ADULTS   *(Continued)*

Organ System/ Therapeutic Category/Drug(s)	Rationale	Recommendation	Quality of Evidence	Strength of Recommendation
Benzodiazepines *Short- and intermediate-acting:* • Alprazolam • Estazolam • Lorazepam • Oxazepam • Temazepam • Triazolam	Older adults have increased sensitivity to benzodiazepines and decreased metabolism of long-acting agents. In general, all benzodiazepines increase risk of cognitive impairment, delirium, falls, fractures, and motor vehicle accidents in older adults.	Avoid benzodiazepines (any type) for treatment of insomnia, agitation, or delirium.	High	Strong
Long-acting: • Chlorazepate • Chlordiazepoxide • Chlordiazepoxide-amitriptyline • Clidinium-chlordiazepoxide • Clonazepam • Diazepam • Flurazepam • Quazepam	May be appropriate for seizure disorders, rapid eye movement sleep disorders, benzodiazepine withdrawal, ethanol withdrawal, severe generalized anxiety disorder, periprocedural anesthesia, end-of-life care.			
Chloral hydrate[a]	Tolerance occurs within 10 d and risk outweighs the benefits in light of overdose with doses only 3 times the recommended dose.	Avoid	Low	Strong
Meprobamate	High rate of physical dependence; very sedating.	Avoid	Moderate	Strong

Nonbenzodiazepine hypnotics • Eszopiclone • Zolpidem • Zaleplon	Benzodiazepine-receptor agonists that have adverse events similar to those of benzodiazepines in older adults (e.g., delirium, falls, fractures); minimal improvement in sleep latency and duration.	Avoid chronic use (>90 d)	Moderate	Strong
Ergot mesylates[a] Isoxsuprine[a]	Lack of efficacy.	Avoid	High	Strong
Endocrine				
Androgens • Methyltestosterone[a] • Testosterone	Potential for cardiac problems and contraindicated in men with prostate cancer.	Avoid unless indicated for moderate-to-severe hypogonadism.	Moderate	Weak
Desiccated thyroid	Concerns about cardiac effects; safer alternatives available.	Avoid	Low	Strong
Estrogens with or without progestins	Evidence of carcinogenic potential (breast and endometrium); lack of cardioprotective effect and cognitive protection in older women. Evidence that vaginal estrogens for treatment of vaginal dryness is safe and effective in women with breast cancer, especially at dosages of estradiol <25 µg twice weekly.	Avoid oral and topical patch. Topical vaginal cream: Acceptable to use low-dose intravaginal estrogen for the management of dyspareunia, lower urinary tract infections, and other vaginal symptoms.	Oral and patch: high Topical: moderate	Oral and patch: strong Topical: weak

2012 AGS BEERS CRITERIA FOR POTENTIALLY INAPPROPRIATE MEDICATION USE IN OLDER ADULTS *(Continued)*

Organ System/ Therapeutic Category/Drug(s)	Rationale	Recommendation	Quality of Evidence	Strength of Recommendation
Growth hormone	Impact on body composition is small and associated with edema, arthralgia, carpal tunnel syndrome, gynecomastia, impaired fasting glucose.	Avoid, except as hormone replacement following pituitary gland removal.	High	Strong
Insulin, sliding scale	Higher risk of hypoglycemia without improvement in hyperglycemia management regardless of care setting.	Avoid	Moderate	Strong
Megestrol	Minimal effect on weight; increases risk of thrombotic events and possibly death in older adults.	Avoid	Moderate	Strong
Sulfonylureas, long-duration • Chlorpropamide • Glyburide	Chlorpropamide: prolonged half-life in older adults; can cause prolonged hypoglycemia; causes SIADH Glyburide: higher risk of severe prolonged hypoglycemia in older adults.	Avoid	High	Strong
Gastrointestinal				
Metoclopramide	Can cause extrapyramidal effects including tardive dyskinesia; risk may be further increased in frail older adults.	Avoid, unless for gastroparesis.	Moderate	Strong

Mineral oil, given orally	Potential for aspiration and adverse effects; safer alternatives available.	Avoid	Moderate	Strong
Trimethobenzamide	One of the least effective antiemetic drugs; can cause extrapyramidal adverse effects.	Avoid	Moderate	Strong
Pain Medications				
Meperidine	Not an effective oral analgesic in dosages commonly used; may cause neurotoxicity; safer alternatives available.	Avoid	High	Strong
Non-COX-selective NSAIDs, oral • Aspirin >325 mg/d • Diclofenac • Diflunisal • Etodolac • Fenoprofen • Ibuprofen • Ketoprofen • Meclofenamate • Mefenamic acid • Meloxicam • Nabumetone • Naproxen • Oxaprozin • Piroxicam • Sulindac • Tolmetin	Increases risk of GI bleeding/peptic ulcer disease in high-risk groups, including those >75 y old or taking oral or parenteral corticosteroids, anticoagulants, or antiplatelet agents. Use of proton pump inhibitor or misoprostol reduces but does not eliminate risk. Upper GI ulcers, gross bleeding, or perforation caused by NSAIDs occur in approximately 1% of patients treated for 3–6 mo, and in about 2%–4% of patients treated for 1 y. These trends continue with longer duration of use.	Avoid chronic use unless other alternatives are not effective and patient can take gastroprotective agent (proton-pump inhibitor or misoprostol).	All others: moderate	Strong

2012 AGS BEERS CRITERIA FOR POTENTIALLY INAPPROPRIATE MEDICATION USE IN OLDER ADULTS (Continued)

Organ System/Therapeutic Category/Drug(s)	Rationale	Recommendation	Quality of Evidence	Strength of Recommendation
Indomethacin Ketorolac, includes parenteral	Increases risk of GI bleeding/peptic ulcer disease in high-risk groups (see above Non-COX-selective NSAIDs) Of all the NSAIDs, indomethacin has most adverse effects.	Avoid	Indomethacin: moderate Ketorolac: high	Strong
Pentazocine[a]	Opioid analgesic that causes CNS adverse effects, including confusion and hallucinations, more commonly than other narcotic drugs; is also a mixed agonist and antagonist; safer alternatives available.	Avoid	Low	Strong
Skeletal muscle relaxants • Carisoprodol • Chlorzoxazone • Cyclobenzaprine • Metaxalone • Methocarbamol • Orphenadrine	Most muscle relaxants poorly tolerated by older adults, because of anticholinergic adverse effects, sedation, increased risk of fractures; effectiveness at dosages tolerated by older adults is questionable.	Avoid	Moderate	Strong

ACEI, angiotensin converting-enzyme inhibitors; ARB, angiotensin receptor blockers; CNS, central nervous system; COX, cyclooxygenase; CrCl, creatinine clearance; GI, gastrointestinal; NSAIDs, nonsteroidal anti-inflammatory drugs; SIADH, syndrome of inappropriate antidiuretic hormone secretion; TCAs, tricyclic antidepressants.

[a]Infrequently used drugs.

The primary target audience is the practicing clinician. The intentions of the criteria include (1) improving the selection of prescription drugs by clinicians and patients; (2) evaluating patterns of drug use within populations; (3) educating clinicians and patients on proper drug usage; and (4) evaluating health-outcome, quality of care, cost, and utilization data.

2012 AGS BEERS CRITERIA FOR POTENTIALLY INAPPROPRIATE MEDICATION USE IN OLDER ADULTS DUE TO DRUG-DISEASE OR DRUG-SYNDROME INTERACTIONS THAT MAY EXACERBATE THE DISEASE OR SYNDROME

Disease or Syndrome	Drug(s)	Rationale	Recommendation	Quality of Evidence	Strength of Recommendation
Cardiovascular					
Heart failure	NSAIDs and COX-2 inhibitors Nondihydropyridine CCBs (avoid only for systolic heart failure) • Diltiazem • Verapamil Pioglitazone, rosiglitazone Cilostazol Dronedarone	Potential to promote fluid retention and/or exacerbate heart failure.	Avoid	NSAIDs: moderate CCBs: moderate Thiazolidinediones (glitazones): high Cilostazol: low Dronedarone: moderate	Strong
Syncope	Acetylcholinesterase inhibitors (AChEIs) Peripheral alpha blockers • Doxazosin • Prazosin • Terazosin Tertiary TCAs Chlorpromazine, thioridazine, and olanzapine	Increases risk of orthostatic hypotension or bradycardia.	Avoid	AChEIs and alpha blockers: high TCAs and antipsychotics: Moderate	AChEIs and TCAs: strong Alpha blockers and antipsychotic: weak

2012 AGS BEERS CRITERIA FOR POTENTIALLY INAPPROPRIATE MEDICATION USE IN OLDER ADULTS DUE TO DRUG-DISEASE OR DRUG-SYNDROME INTERACTIONS THAT MAY EXACERBATE THE DISEASE OR SYNDROME (Continued)

Disease or Syndrome	Drug(s)	Rationale	Recommendation	Quality of Evidence	Strength of Recommendation
Central Nervous System					
Chronic seizures or epilepsy	Bupropion Chlorpromazine Clozapine Maprotiline Olanzapine Thioridazine Thiothixene Tramadol	Lowers seizure threshold; may be acceptable in patients with well-controlled seizures in whom alternative agents have not been effective.	Avoid	Moderate	Strong
Delirium	All TCAs Anticholinergics (see "Drugs with Strong Anticholinergic Properties" table for full list) Benzodiazepines Chlorpromazine Corticosteroids H₂-receptor antagonist Meperidine Sedative hypnotics Thioridazine	Avoid in older adults with or at high risk of delirium because of inducing or worsening delirium in older adults; if discontinuing drugs used chronically, taper to avoid withdrawal symptoms.	Avoid	Moderate	Strong

Disease or Syndrome	Drug(s)	Rationale	Recommendation	Quality of Evidence	Strength of Recommendation
Dementia and cognitive impairment	Anticholinergics (see "Drugs with Strong Anticholinergic Properties" table for full list) Benzodiazepines H$_2$-receptor antagonists Zolpidem Antipsychotics, chronic and as-needed use	Avoid due to adverse CNS effects. Avoid antipsychotics for behavioral problems of dementia unless non-pharmacologic options have failed and patient is a threat to themselves or others. Antipsychotics are associated increased risk of cerebrovascular accident (stroke) and mortality in persons with dementia.	Avoid	High	Strong
History of falls or fractures	Anticonvulsants Antipsychotics Benzodiazepines Nonbenzodiazepine hypnotics • Eszopiclone • Zaleplon • Zolpidem TCAs/SSRIs	Ability to produce ataxia, impaired psychomotor function, syncope, and additional falls; shorter-acting benzodiazepines are not safer than long-acting ones.	Avoid unless safer alternatives are not available; avoid anticonvulsants except for seizure.	High	Strong

2012 AGS BEERS CRITERIA FOR POTENTIALLY INAPPROPRIATE MEDICATION USE IN OLDER ADULTS DUE TO DRUG-DISEASE OR DRUG-SYNDROME INTERACTIONS THAT MAY EXACERBATE THE DISEASE OR SYNDROME *(Continued)*

Disease or Syndrome	Drug(s)	Rationale	Recommendation	Quality of Evidence	Strength of Recommendation
Insomnia	Oral decongestants • Pseudoephedrine • Phenylephrine • Stimulants • Amphetamine • Methylphenidate • Pemoline • Theobromines • Theophylline • Caffeine	CNS stimulant effects	Avoid	Moderate	Strong
Parkinson disease	All antipsychotics (except for quetiapine and clozapine) Antiemetics • Metoclopramide • Prochlorperazine • Promethazine	Dopamine receptor antagonists with potential to worsen parkinsonian symptoms. Quetiapine and clozapine appear to be less likely to precipitate worsening of Parkinson disease.	Avoid	Moderate	Strong

Gastrointestinal

Condition	Drug/Class	Rationale	Recommendation	Quality of evidence	Strength of recommendation
Chronic constipation	Oral antimuscarinics for urinary incontinence • Darifenacin • Fesoterodine • Oxybutynin (oral) • Solifenacin • Tolterodine • Trospium Nondihydropyridine CCB • Diltiazem • Verapamil First-generation antihistamines as single agent or part of combination products • Brompheniramine (various) • Carbinoxamine • Chlorpheniramine • Clemastine (various) • Cyproheptadine • Dexbrompheniramine • Dexchlorpheniramine (various) • Diphenhydramine • Doxylamine • Hydroxyzine • Promethazine • Triprolidine	Ability to worsen constipation; agents for urinary incontinence: antimuscarinics overall differ in incidence of constipation; response variable; consider alternative agent if constipation develops.	Avoid unless no other alternatives	For urinary incontinence: high All others: moderate/low	Weak

2012 AGS BEERS CRITERIA FOR POTENTIALLY INAPPROPRIATE MEDICATION USE IN OLDER ADULTS DUE TO DRUG-DISEASE OR DRUG-SYNDROME INTERACTIONS THAT MAY EXACERBATE THE DISEASE OR SYNDROME *(Continued)*

Disease or Syndrome	Drug(s)	Rationale	Recommendation	Quality of Evidence	Strength of Recommendation
	Anticholinergics/antispasmodics (see "Drugs with Strong Anticholinergic Properties" table for full list of drugs with strong anticholinergic properties) • Antipsychotics • Belladonna alkaloids • Clidinium-chlordiazepoxide • Dicyclomine • Hyoscyamine • Propantheline • Scopolamine • Tertiary TCAs (amitriptyline, clomipramine, doxepin, imipramine, and trimipramine)				
History of gastric or duodenal ulcers	Aspirin (>325 mg/d) Non-COX-2 selective NSAIDs	May exacerbate existing ulcers or cause new/additional ulcers.	Avoid unless other alternatives are not effective and patient can take gastroprotective agent (proton-pump inhibitor or misoprostol).	Moderate	Strong

Kidney/Urinary Tract

Chronic kidney disease stages IV and V	NSAIDs Triamterene (alone or in combination)	May increase risk of kidney injury. May increase risk of acute kidney injury.	Avoid Avoid	NSAIDs: moderate Triamterene: low	NSAIDs: strong Triamterene: weak
Urinary incontinence (all types) in women	Estrogen oral and transdermal (excludes intravaginal estrogen)	Aggravation of incontinence.	Avoid in women	High	Strong
Lower urinary tract symptoms, benign prostatic hyperplasia	Inhaled anticholinergic agents Strongly anticholinergic drugs, except antimuscarinics for urinary incontinence (see "Drugs with Strong Anticholinergic Properties" table for complete list)	May decrease urinary flow and cause urinary retention.	Avoid in men	Moderate	Inhaled agents: strong All others: weak
Stress or mixed urinary incontinence	Alpha-blockers • Doxazosin • Prazosin • Terazosin	Aggravation of incontinence.	Avoid in women	Moderate	Strong

AChEIs, acetylcholinesterase inhibitors; CCBs, calcium channel blockers; CNS, central nervous system; COX, cyclooxygenase; NSAIDs, nonsteroidal anti-inflammatory drugs; SSRIs, selective serotonin reuptake inhibitors; TCAs, tricyclic antidepressants.

The primary target audience is the practicing clinician. The intentions of the criteria include (1) improving the selection of prescription drugs by clinicians and patients; (2) evaluating patterns of drug use within populations; (3) educating clinicians and patients on proper drug usage; and (4) evaluating health-outcome, quality of care, cost, and utilization data.

2012 AGS BEERS CRITERIA FOR POTENTIALLY INAPPROPRIATE MEDICATIONS TO BE USED WITH CAUTION IN OLDER ADULTS

Drug(s)	Rationale	Recommendation	Quality of Evidence	Strength of Recommendation
Aspirin for primary prevention of cardiac events	Lack of evidence of benefit versus risk in individuals ≥80 y old.	Use with caution in adults ≥80 y old.	Low	Weak
Dabigatran	Increased risk of bleeding compared with warfarin in adults ≥75 y old; lack of evidence for efficacy and safety in patients with CrCl <30 mL/min	Use with caution in adults ≥75 y old or if CrCl <30 mL/min.	Moderate	Weak
Prasugrel	Increased risk of bleeding in older adults; risk may be offset by benefit in highest-risk older patients (eg, those with prior myocardial infarction or diabetes).	Use with caution in adults ≥75 y old.	Moderate	Weak
Antipsychotics Carbamazepine Carboplatin Cisplatin Mirtazapine SNRIs SSRIs TCAs Vincristine	May exacerbate or cause SIADH or hyponatremia; need to monitor sodium level closely when starting or changing dosages in older adults due to increased risk.	Use with caution.	Moderate	Strong
Vasodilators	May exacerbate episodes of syncope in individuals with history of syncope.	Use with caution.	Moderate	Weak

CrCl, creatinine clearance; SIADH, syndrome of inappropriate antidiuretic hormone secretion; SNRIs, serotonin–norepinephrine reuptake inhibitors; SSRIs, selective serotonin reuptake inhibitors; TCAs, tricyclic antidepressants.

The primary target audience is the practicing clinician. The intentions of the criteria include (1) improving the selection of prescription drugs by clinicians and patients; (2) evaluating patterns of drug use within populations; (3) educating clinicians and patients on proper drug usage; and (4) evaluating health-outcome, quality of care, cost, and utilization data.

DRUGS WITH STRONG ANTICHOLINERGIC PROPERTIES

Antihistamines	Antiparkinson agents	Skeletal muscle relaxants
• Brompheniramine • Carbinoxamine • Chlorpheniramine • Clemastine • Cyproheptadine • Dimenhydrinate • Diphenhydramine • Hydroxyzine • Loratadine • Meclizine	• Benztropine • Trihexyphenidyl	• Carisoprodol • Cyclobenzaprine • Orphenadrine • Tizanidine
Antidepressants	Antipsychotics	
• Amitriptyline • Amoxapine • Clomipramine • Desipramine • Doxepin • Imipramine • Nortriptyline • Paroxetine • Protriptyline • Trimipramine	• Chlorpromazine • Clozapine • Fluphenazine • Loxapine • Olanzapine • Perphenazine • Pimozide • Prochlorperazine • Promethazine • Thioridazine • Thiothixene • Trifluoperazine	
Antimuscarinics (urinary incontinence)	Antispasmodics	
• Darifenacin • Fesoterodine • Flavoxate • Oxybutynin • Solifenacin • Tolterodine • Trospium	• Atropine products • Belladonna alkaloids • Dicyclomine • Homatropine • Hyoscyamine products • Loperamide • Propantheline • Scopolamine	

GLAUCOMA, CHRONIC OPEN ANGLE

Population
–Adults.

Recommendations

▶ NICE 2009

1. All persons with known or suspected chronic open-angle glaucoma (COAG) or ocular hypertension (OHT) should undergo the following:
   a. Intraocular pressure monitoring using tonometry.
   b. Central corneal thickness measurement.
   c. Peripheral anterior chamber depth assessments using gonioscopy.
   d. Visual field testing.
   e. Optic nerve assessment using slit-lamp exam.
2. Recommends monitoring patients with OHT at least annually for COAG (every 6 mo for high-risk patients).
3. Recommends monitoring patients with COAG every 6–12 mo based on disease progression.
4. Recommends prostaglandin analogue therapy for early-to-moderate COAG patients at risk of visual loss.
5. Consider surgery with pharmacologic augmentation for advanced COAG.
6. Recommends β-blocker drops for mild OHT until age 60 y.
7. Recommends prostaglandin analogue drops for any degree of OHT.
8. Recommends additional medication therapy for uncontrolled OHT despite single-agent therapy.

Source
–http://www.guidelines.gov/content.aspx?id=14444

Comment

1. Alternative pharmacologic treatments for OHT or suspected COAG in patients whose intraocular pressures remain elevated on monotherapy include:
   a. Prostaglandin analogues.
   b. β-blockers.
   c. Carbonic anhydrase inhibitors.
   d. Sympathomimetics.

GOUT, ACUTE ATTACKS

Population
–Adults.

Recommendations
▶ ACR 2012
  –Therapy options for acute gout attacks.
  - Mild-to-moderate attacks involving 1–2 joints.
    ◦ NSAIDs: full-dose naproxen, sulindac, or indomethacin is preferred.
    ◦ Colchicine 1.2 mg PO × 1 then 0.6 mg 1 h later then 0.6 mg daily bid.
    ◦ Corticosteroids: prednisone or prednisolone 0.5 mg/kg PO daily for 5–10 d.
  - Severe attacks or polyarticular gout.
    ◦ Colchicine + NSAIDs.
    ◦ Colchicine + steroids.
  - Expert opinion to continue urate-lowering therapy (eg, allopurinol) during acute attacks
  - Ice applied to affected joints can help
  –Pharmacologic urate-lowering therapy.
  - Allopurinol.
    ◦ Starting dose should not exceed 100 mg/d.
    ◦ Uptitrate dose every 2–4 wk to max of 800 mg/d, unless renal impairment exists.
    ◦ Desire uric acid level of <6 mg/dL.
  - Consider adding a uricosuric agent (eg, probenecid) for refractory hyperuricemia despite urate-lowering therapy.
  - Initiate allopurinol after an acute gout attack has resolved and continue prophylactic anti-inflammatory agents for 3 mo beyond achieving urate level <6 mg/dL.
    ◦ Colchicine 0.6 mg daily bid.
    ◦ Naproxen 250 mg PO bid.

Sources
  –http://www.guideline.gov/content.aspx?id=38624
  –http://www.guideline.gov/content.aspx?id=38625

Comment
  –Consider HLAB*5801 testing prior to the initiation of allopurinol for patients at particularly high risk of allopurinol hypersensitivity reaction.
  - Highest risk group are those of Korean, Han Chinese, or Thai descent, especially if Stage 3 or higher CKD is present.

Population

–Adults with suspected gout.

Recommendation

▶ American College of Physicians 2017

–Clinicians should use synovial fluid analysis when diagnostic testing is necessary in patients with possible gout.

Sources

–http://guidelines.gov/summaries/summary/50607/diagnosis-of-acute-gout-a-clinical-practice-guideline-from-the-american-college-of-physicians?q=gout

–Qaseem A, McLean RM, Starkey M, Forciea MA; Clinical Guidelines Committee of the American College of Physicians. Diagnosis of acute gout: a clinical practice guideline from the American College of Physicians. *Ann Intern Med.* 2017 Jan 3;166(1):52-57.

Population

–Adults >18 y with acute or recurrent gout.

Recommendations

▶ American College of Physicians 2017

–Options for treatment of acute gout include corticosteroids, NSAIDs, or colchicine.

–Corticosteroids should be considered first-line therapy in patients without contraindications. Prednisolone 35 mg orally for 5 d.

–Recommends against using long-term urate-lowering therapy in most patients with infrequent attacks (<3 attacks per year).

–Febuxostat and allopurinol are equally effective at decreasing serum urate levels.

Sources

–http://guidelines.gov/summaries/summary/50608/management-of-acute-and-recurrent-gout-a-clinical-practice-guideline-from-the-american-college-of-physicians?q=gout

–Qaseem A, Harris RP, Forciea MA; Clinical Guidelines Committee of the American College of Physicians. Management of acute and recurrent gout: a clinical practice guideline from the American College of Physicians. *Ann Intern Med.* 2017 Jan 3;166(1):58-68.

HEADACHE

Population
–Adults

Recommendation
▶ ACR 2012
–Do not do imaging for uncomplicated headaches.

Source
–http://www.choosingwisely.org/societies/american-college-of-radiology/

HEADACHE, MIGRAINE PROPHYLAXIS

Population
–Adults.

Recommendations
▶ AAN 2012
–The following medications have **established efficacy** for migraine prophylaxis:
  • Divalproex sodium.
  • Sodium valproate.
  • Topiramate.
  • Metoprolol.
  • Propranolol.
  • Timolol.
–Frovatriptan is effective for menstrual migraine prophylaxis.
–The following medications are **probably effective** for migraine prophylaxis:
  • Amitriptyline.
  • Venlafaxine.
  • Atenolol.
  • Nadolol.

Source
–http://www.neurology.org/content/78/17/1337.full.pdf+html

Comment
–Lamotrigine and clomipramine are ineffective for migraine prevention.

HEADACHE DIAGNOSIS ALGORITHM—ICSI 2011

Patient presents with complaint of a headache **A**

Detailed History
- Characteristics of the headache
- Assess functional impairment
- Past medical history
- Family history of migraines
- Current medications and previous medications for headache (Rx and over-the-counter)
- Social history
- Review of systems-to rule out systemic illness

All algorithm boxes with an "A" and those that refer to other algorithm boxes link to annotaation content.

Causes for concern:
- Subacute and/or progressive headache over months
- New or different headache
- "Worst headache ever"
- Any headache of maximum severity at onset
- Onset after the age of 50 y old
- Symptoms of systemic illness
- Seizures
- Any neurological signs

Critical first steps:
- Detailed history
- Focused physical examination
- Focused neurological examination **A**

Causes for concern? **A** — Yes → Consider secondary headache disorder **A**

No

Headaches other than primary headache out of guideline

No ← Meets criteria for primary headache disorder **A**

Specialty consultation indicated? **A** — Yes → Refer to headache specialist

No

Perform diagnostic testing if indicated **A**

Diagnosis of primary headache confirmed? — Yes

No

Findings consistent with secondary headache? **A** — Yes → Determine secondary headache type out of guideline

No

Yes

Evaluate type of primary headache. Initiate patient education and lifestyle management **A**

Migraine (see Migraine algorithm)

Tension-type (see Tension-Type Headache algorithm)

Cluster (see Cluster Headache algorithm)

Chronic daily headache **A**

Other headache **A**

Sinus Headache

Migraine-associated symptoms are often misdiagnosed as "sinus headache" by patients and providers. Most headaches characterized as "sinus headaches" are migraines.

The International Classifications of Headache Disorders (ICHD-II) defines sinus headache by purulent nasal discharge, pathologic sinus finding by imaging, simultaneous onset of headache and sinusitis, and headache localized to specific facial and cranial areas of the sinuses.

A = Annotation

MIGRAINE TREATMENT ALGORITHM—ICSI 2011

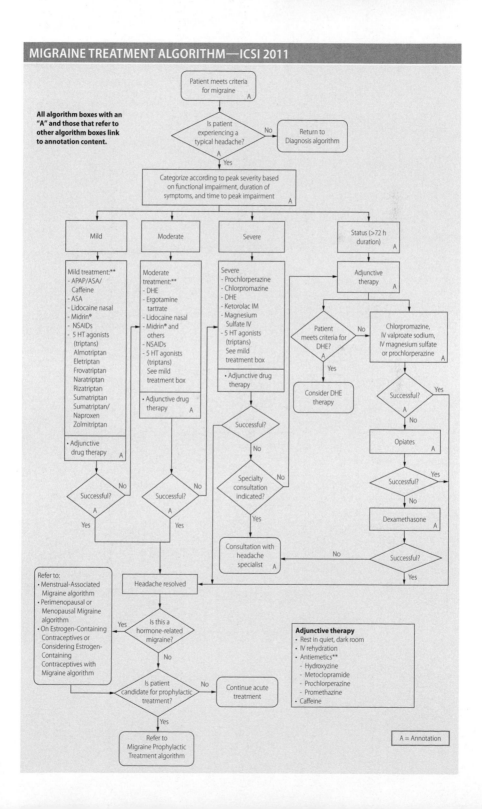

All algorithm boxes with an "A" and those that refer to other algorithm boxes link to annotation content.

Patient meets criteria for migraine — A

Is patient experiencing a typical headache? — A → No → Return to Diagnosis algorithm

Yes

Categorize according to peak severity based on functional impairment, duration of symptoms, and time to peak impairment — A

Mild

Mild treatment:**
- APAP/ASA/ Caffeine
- ASA
- Lidocaine nasal
- Midrin®
- NSAIDs
- 5 HT agonists (triptans)
  Almotriptan
  Eletriptan
  Frovatriptan
  Naratriptan
  Rizatriptan
  Sumatriptan
  Sumatriptan/ Naproxen
  Zolmitriptan

• Adjunctive drug therapy — A

Successful? — A → No

Yes

Moderate

Moderate treatment:**
- DHE
- Ergotamine tartrate
- Lidocaine nasal
- Midrin® and others
- NSAIDs
- 5 HT agonists (triptans)
  See mild treatment box

• Adjunctive drug therapy — A

Successful? — A → No

Yes

Severe

Severe
- Prochlorperazine
- Chlorpromazine
- DHE
- Ketorolac IM
- Magnesium Sulfate IV
- 5 HT agonists (triptans)
  See mild treatment box

• Adjunctive drug therapy

Successful? → No

Specialty consultation indicated? → No

Yes

Consultation with headache specialist — A

Status (>72 h duration) — A

Adjunctive therapy — A

Patient meets criteria for DHE? — A → No → Chlorpromazine, IV valproate sodium, IV magnesium sulfate or prochlorperazine — A

Yes

Consider DHE therapy

Successful? — A → Yes

No

Opiates — A

Successful? → Yes

No

Dexamethasone — A

Successful? → Yes

No

Headache resolved

Refer to:
• Menstrual-Associated Migraine algorithm
• Perimenopausal or Menopausal Migraine algorithm
• On Estrogen-Containing Contraceptives or Considering Estrogen-Containing Contraceptives with Migraine algorithm

Yes ← Is this a hormone-related migraine?

No

Is patient candidate for prophylactic treatment? → No → Continue acute treatment

Yes

Refer to Migraine Prophylactic Treatment algorithm

Adjunctive therapy
• Rest in quiet, dark room
• IV rehydration
• Antiemetics**
  - Hydroxyzine
  - Metoclopramide
  - Prochlorperazine
  - Promethazine
• Caffeine

A = Annotation

TENSION-TYPE HEADACHE ALGORITHM—ICSI 2011

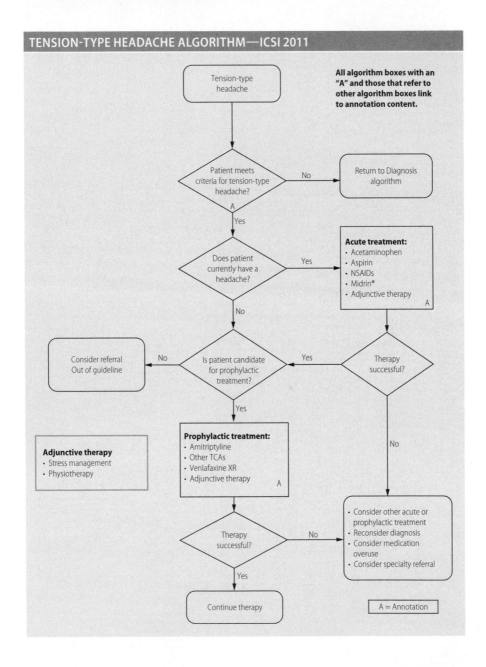

Tension-type headache

All algorithm boxes with an "A" and those that refer to other algorithm boxes link to annotation content.

Patient meets criteria for tension-type headache?

No → Return to Diagnosis algorithm

A

Yes

Does patient currently have a headache?

Yes → **Acute treatment:**
- Acetaminophen
- Aspirin
- NSAIDs
- Midrin®
- Adjunctive therapy

A

No

Is patient candidate for prophylactic treatment?

No → Consider referral Out of guideline

Yes ← Therapy successful?

Yes

Adjunctive therapy
- Stress management
- Physiotherapy

Prophylactic treatment:
- Amitriptyline
- Other TCAs
- Venlafaxine XR
- Adjunctive therapy

A

No

Therapy successful?

No →
- Consider other acute or prophylactic treatment
- Reconsider diagnosis
- Consider medication overuse
- Consider specialty referral

Yes

Continue therapy

A = Annotation

CLUSTER HEADACHE ALGORITHM—ICSI 2011

All algorithm boxes with an "A" and those that refer to other algorithm boxes link to annotation content.

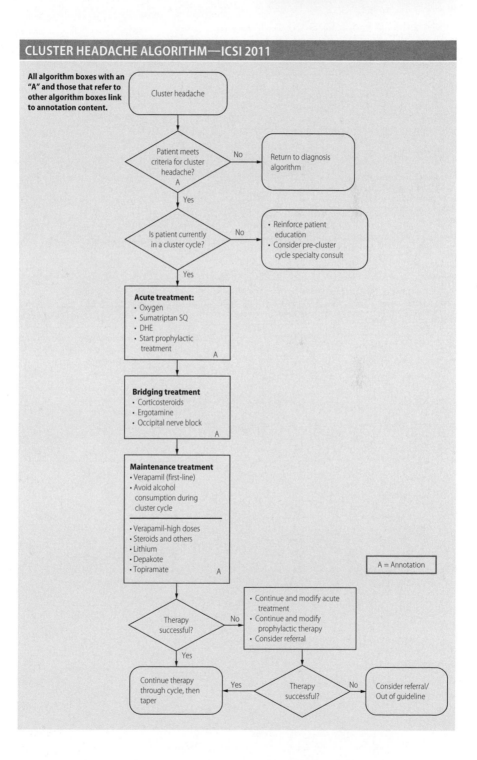

Cluster headache

Patient meets criteria for cluster headache? **A**

No → Return to diagnosis algorithm

Yes ↓

Is patient currently in a cluster cycle?

No → • Reinforce patient education
• Consider pre-cluster cycle specialty consult

Yes ↓

Acute treatment:
• Oxygen
• Sumatriptan SQ
• DHE
• Start prophylactic treatment **A**

Bridging treatment
• Corticosteroids
• Ergotamine
• Occipital nerve block **A**

Maintenance treatment
• Verapamil (first-line)
• Avoid alcohol consumption during cluster cycle

• Verapamil-high doses
• Steroids and others
• Lithium
• Depakote
• Topiramate **A**

A = Annotation

Therapy successful?

No → • Continue and modify acute treatment
• Continue and modify prophylactic therapy
• Consider referral

Yes ↓

Continue therapy through cycle, then taper

← Yes — Therapy successful? — No → Consider referral/ Out of guideline

MENSTRUAL-ASSOCIATED MIGRAINE ALGORITHM—ICSI 2011

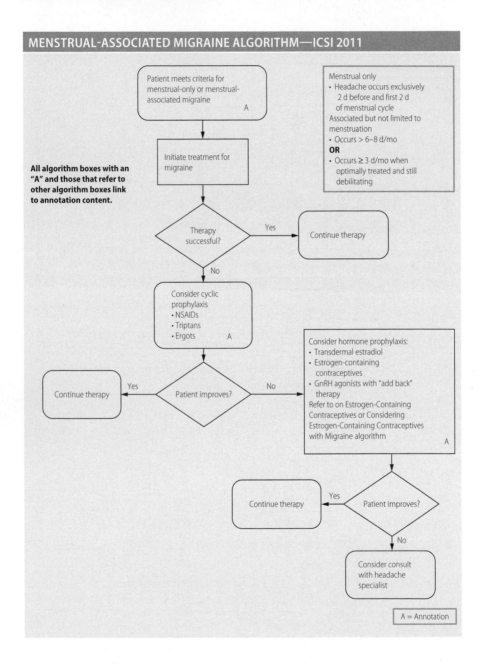

PERIMENOPAUSAL OR MENOPAUSAL MIGRAINE ALGORITHM—ICSI 2011

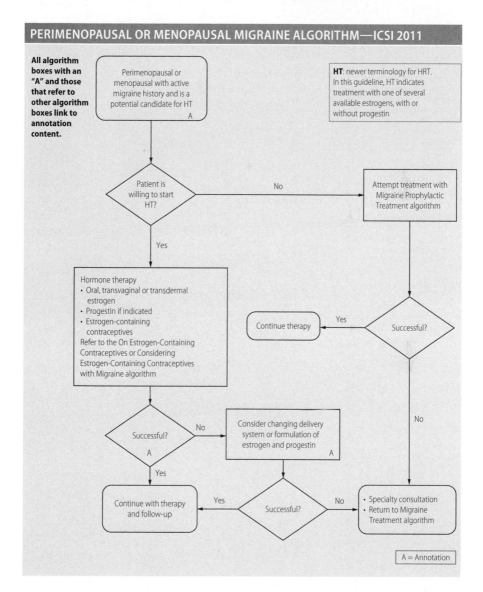

All algorithm boxes with an "A" and those that refer to other algorithm boxes link to annotation content.

Perimenopausal or menopausal with active migraine history and is a potential candidate for HT

A

HT: newer terminology for HRT. In this guideline, HT indicates treatment with one of several available estrogens, with or without progestin

Patient is willing to start HT?

No → Attempt treatment with Migraine Prophylactic Treatment algorithm

Yes

Hormone therapy
• Oral, transvaginal or transdermal estrogen
• Progestin if indicated
• Estrogen-containing contraceptives
Refer to the On Estrogen-Containing Contraceptives or Considering Estrogen-Containing Contraceptives with Migraine algorithm

Continue therapy ← Yes — Successful?

Successful?

A

No → Consider changing delivery system or formulation of estrogen and progestin

A

Yes

No

Continue with therapy and follow-up ← Yes — Successful?

No → • Specialty consultation
• Return to Migraine Treatment algorithm

A = Annotation

ON ESTROGEN-CONTAINING CONTRACEPTIVES OR CONSIDERING ESTROGEN-CONTAINING CONTRACEPTIVES WITH MIGRAINE ALGORITHM—ICSI 2011

All algorithm boxes with an "A" and those that refer to other algorithm boxes link to annotation content.

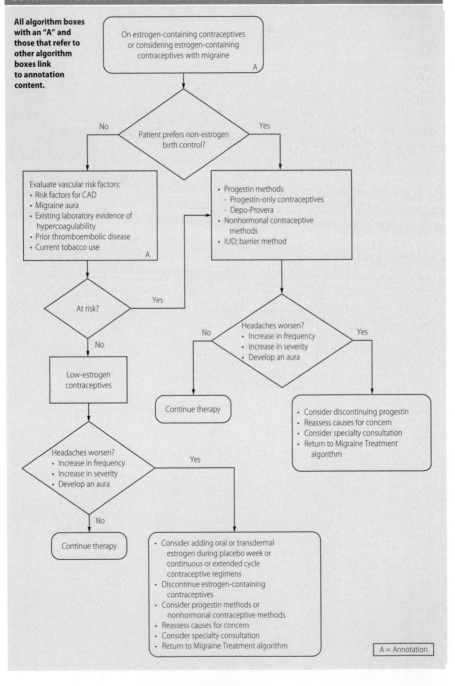

MIGRAINE PROPHYLACTIC TREATMENT ALGORITHM—ICSI 2011

All algorithm boxes with an "A" and those that refer to other algorithm boxes link to annotation content.

Patient meets criteria for migraine headache

↓

Prophylactic treatment
Assess factors that may trigger migraine
Treatment:
- Medication
  - β-blocker
  - Tricyclic antidepressants
  - Ca++ channel blockers
  - Antiepileptic drugs
    - Divalproex
    - Topiramate
    - Gabapentin
- Reinforce education and lifestyle management
- Consider other therapies (biofeedback, relaxation)
- Screen for depression and generalized anxiety

A

↓

Successful?* — Yes → Continue treatment for 6–12 mo, then reassess A

Successful?
Success as determined by:
- Headaches decrease by 50% or more
- An acceptable side effect profile

↓ No

Try different first-line medication or different drug of same class

A

↓

Successful? * — Yes → Continue treatment for 6–12 mo, then reassess

↓ No

Try combination of β-blockers and tricyclics

A

↓

Successful? * — Yes → Continue treatment for 6–12 mo, then reassess

↓ No

Third-line prophylaxis treatment or consultation with headache specialist

A

A = Annotation

HEARING LOSS, SUDDEN

Population
–Adults age 18 y and older.

Recommendations

▶ AAO-HNS 2012

–Distinguish –hearing loss into sensorineural or conductive hearing loss.
–Counsel patients with incomplete recovery of hearing about the benefits of hearing aids.
–Evaluate patients with idiopathic sudden sensorineural hearing loss (ISSNHL) for retrocochlear pathology by obtaining an MRI of the internal auditory canal, auditory brainstem responses, and an audiology exam.
–Consider treatment of ISSNHL with incomplete hearing recovery with systemic or intratympanic steroids or hyperbaric oxygen therapy.
–In patients with ISSNHL, recommend against antivirals, thrombolytics, vasodilators, or antioxidants for treatment and against CT scanning of the head or routine lab testing.

Source
–http://oto.sagepub.com/content/146/3_suppl/S1.full.pdf+html

HEART FAILURE

Population
–Patients with stable, symptomatic, chronic HF, in sinus rhythm, with LVEF ≤35%, who are in sinus rhythm with a resting HR ≥70 bpm, and either are on maximally tolerated doses of β-blocker or have a contraindication to β-blocker use.

Recommendations

▶ ACC/AHA HF Guidelines 2017

–Ivabradine (Corlanor*) was approved to reduce hospitalization from worsening HF. Ivabradine can be beneficial to reduce HF hospitalization for patients with symptomatic (NYHA Class II and III) stable chronic HFrEF(LVEF ≤35%) who are receiving goal-directed medical therapy, including a beta blocker at maximum tolerated dose, and who are in sinus rhythm with a heart rate of 70 bpm or greater at rest.
–*Starting dose*: 5 mg 1 tab bid. Maximum dose 7.5 mg bid (dose can be increased after 1 mo as needed based on resting HR and tolerability).

HEART FAILURE

Stage A: Patients with hypertension, atherosclerotic disease, diabetes mellitus, metabolic syndrome, *or* those using cardiotoxins or having a family history of cardiomyopathy.
Stage B: Patients with previous MI, LV remodeling including LVH and low EF, or asymptomatic valvular disease.
Stage C: Patients with known structural heart disease; shortness of breath and fatigue, reduced exercise tolerance.
Stage D: Patients who have marked symptoms at rest despite maximal medical therapy (eg, those who are recurrently hospitalized or cannot be safely discharged from the hospital without specialized interventions).

a. History of atherosclerotic vascular disease, diabetes mellitus, or hypertension and associated cardiovascular risk factors.
b. Recent or remote MI, regardless of ejection fraction; or reduced ejection fraction regardless of MI Hx.
c. Use ARB in patients post-MI who cannot tolerate ACE inhibitors.
d. Evidence suggests that isosorbide dinitrate plus hydralazine reduces mortality in blacks with advanced heart failure. (*NEJM*. 2004;351:2049)

Comments

Exercise training in patients with HF seems to be safe and beneficial overall in improving exercise capacity, quality of life, muscle structure, and physiologic responses to exercise.
*Source:*Adapted from the American College of Cardiology, American Heart Association, Inc. *Circulation*. 2017. doi: 10.1161/CIR.0000000000000509.

HEART FAILURE: ACCF/AHA 2013 CLASSIFICATION ON CLINICAL ASSESSMENT IN HEART FAILURE CLASS I RECOMMENDATIONS

1. Classification:
    i. Heart failure with reduced ejection fraction (HFrEF) referred to as *systolic heart failure* when LVEF ≤40%.
    ii. Heart failure with preserved ejection fraction (HFpEF) referred to as diastolic dysfunction:
    −HFpEF when LVEF >40%
2. Lifetime risk of developing HF for Americans ≥40 y old is 20%.
3. Overall mortality is 50% in 5 y; varies with HF stage with:
    −Stage B having a 5-y mortality of 4%.
    −Stage C having a 5-y mortality of 25%.
    −Stage D having a 5-y mortality of 80%.
4. Patients with idiopathic dilated cardiomyopathy should have a 3-generational family history obtained to exclude familial disease.
5. Risk score evaluation should be considered to help predict the ultimate outcome, chronic heart failure—Seattle Heart Failure Model. (http://depts.washington.edu/shfm/)
6. Identify prior cardiac or noncardiac disease that may lead to HF.
7. For patients at risk of developing HF (Stage A/B), natriuretic peptide biomarker–based screening (BNP or NT-pro-BNP) and optimizing GDMT can be useful to prevent the development of left ventricular dysfunction (systolic or diastolic) or new-onset HF

HEART FAILURE: ACCF/AHA 2013 CLASSIFICATION ON CLINICAL ASSESSMENT IN HEART FAILURE CLASS I RECOMMENDATIONS *(Continued)*

8. Obtain history to include diet or medicine nonadherence; current or past use of alcohol, illicit drugs, and chemotherapy; or recent viral illness.
9. Identify the patient's present activity level and desired post-treatment level.
10. Assess the patient's volume status, orthostatic BP changes, height and weight, and body mass index.
11. Hypertension and lipid disorders should be controlled in accordance with contemporary guideline to lower the risk of HF. Other risk factors should be controlled or avoided.
12. Initial blood work should measure N-terminal pro-brain natriuretic peptide (NT-proBNP) or BNP levels to support clinical judgment for diagnosis, especially in the setting of uncertainty for the diagnosis. Other labs to include CBC, chemistry panel, lipid profile, troponin I level, and TSH level.
13. 12-lead ECG should be obtained.
14. 2D echocardiogram is indicated to determine the systolic function, diastolic function, valvular function, and pulmonary artery pressure.
15. Coronary arteriography to be performed in patients with angina or significant ischemia with HF unless the patient is not eligible for surgery.
16. Initiate diuretic therapy and salt restriction if volume overloaded. Diuretics do not improve long-term survival, but improve symptoms and short-term survival. Once euvolemic and symptoms have resolved, carefully start to wean dosage as an outpatient to lowest dose possible to prevent electrolyte disorders and activation of the renin angiotensin system.
17. ACE inhibitor or ARB or ARNI (ARB plus a neprilysin inhibitor), which reduce morbidity and mortality, should be considered early in the initial course to decrease afterload unless contraindicated if decreased ejection fraction noted (systolic dysfunction). Both agents improve long-term survival. The only available ARNI is valsartan/sacubitril. Titrate dosage to that employed in clinical studies as BP allows.
18. In patients with chronic symptomatic HFrEF NYHA class II or III who tolerate an ACE inhibitor or ARB, replacement by an ARNI is recommended to further reduce morbidity and mortality.
19. Specific beta-blockers (carvedilol, sustained release metoprolol succinate, bisoprolol) should be added to reduce morbidity and mortality. These specific β-blockers improve survival the most in systolic heart failure. Titrate dosage to heart rate 65–70 beats/min.
20. Start aldosterone antagonist in patients with moderate or severe symptoms (NYHA Class II-IV) and reduced ejection fraction. Creatinine should be <2.5 mg/dL in men and <2 mg/dL in women, and the potassium should be <5 mEq/L.
21. The combination of hydralazine and nitrates should be employed to improve outcome in African Americans with moderate-to-severe HF with decreased ejection fraction in addition to optimal therapy. If ACE inhibitor or ARB agent is contraindicated, hydralazine and nitrates may be used as alternative therapy.
22. Statins are not beneficial as adjunctive therapy when prescribed solely for the diagnosis of HF. In all patients with a recent or remote hx of CAD, CVA, PAD, or hyperlipidemia, statins should be used according to guidelines.
23. Discontinue anti-inflammatory agents, diltiazem, and verapamil.

24. Nutritional supplements as treatment for HF are not recommended in patients with current or prior symptoms of systolic dysfunction (HFrEF).

25. Calcium channel blockers are not recommended as routine treatment for patients with HFrEF.

26. Remember that exercise training is beneficial in HF patients with decreased ejection fraction (systolic dysfunction) or preserved ejection fraction (diastolic dysfunction) once therapy is optimized.

27. Intracardiac cardiac defibrillator is indicated for secondary survival benefit in patients who survive cardiac arrest, ventricular fibrillation, or hemodynamically significant ventricular tachycardia.

28. Intracardiac cardiac defibrillator is indicated for primary survival benefit in patients with ischemic or nonischemic cardiomyopathy with EF ≤35% with New York Heart Association (NYHA) class II or III. The patient should be stable on GDMT (guideline-determined medical therapy) optimal chronic medical HF therapy and at least 40 d post-MI and a life-expectancy of at least 1 y.

29. Biventricular heart pacemaker (CRT) should be considered in refractory HF with ejection fraction equal to or less than 35% with NYHA class II and III or ambulatory class IV on GDMT. The rhythm should be sinus, with a QRS ≥150 ms, ± LBBB.

30. Long-term anticoagulation therapy is not recommended in patients with chronic systolic function while in sinus rhythm in the absence of AF, a prior thromboembolic event, or cardioembolic source.

31. In patient with nonvalvular AF and HFrEF anticoagulation with warfarin or a DOAC is recommended.

32. Aim for blood pressure less than 130/80 mm Hg.

33. In HF patients with preserved systolic function (diastolic dysfunction), randomized data on therapy are lacking. The goal is to control blood volume (diuretic), keep systolic blood pressure <130 mm Hg (β-blocker, ACE inhibitor, ARB agent, or diuretic), slow heart rate (β-blocker), and treat coronary artery ischemia. Whether β-blockers, ACE inhibitors, ARB agents, or aldosterone antagonists improve survival independently is yet to be proven.

34. Comprehensive written discharge instruction should be given to all patients. Diet, weight monitoring, medicine, and salt adherence should be emphasized. Activity should be discussed along with education of symptoms of worsening HF.

35. During a HF hospitalization, a predischarge natriuretic peptide level (BNP or NT-pro-BNP) can be useful to establish a post-discharge prognosis

36. Post-discharge appointment with physician and health care team with attention to information on discharge medications.

Sources: Adapted from: ACCF/AHA 2017 Guidelines. *Circulation. 2017.* doi: 10.1161/CIR.0000000000000509.; *N Engl J Med.* 2012; WARCET Trial; American Academy of Family Physicians; American Academy of Hospice and Palliative Medicine; American Nurses Association; American Society of Health-System Pharmacists; Heart Rhythm Society; Society of Hospital Medicine, Bonow RO, Ganiats TG, Beam CT, et al. ACCF/AHA/AMA-PCPI 2011 performance measures for adults with heart failure: a report of the American College of Cardiology Foundation/American Heart Association Task Force on Performance Measures and the American Medical Association-Physician Consortium for Performance Improvement. *J Am Coll Cardiol.* 2012;59(20):1812-1832. Yancy CW, Jessup M, Bozkurt B, et al. 2013 ACCF/AHA Guideline for the management of heart failure: a report of the American College of Cardiology Foundation/American Heart Association Task Force on practice guidelines. *Circulation.* 2013;128:e240-e327.

–*Contraindications*:

- Acute decompensated HF; BP <90/50 mm Hg, SSS, sinoatrial block, third-degree AV block (unless a functioning demand pacemaker is present), resting HR <60 bpm prior to treatment, severe hepatic impairment, pacemaker dependent, concomitant use of strong cytochrome P450 3A4(CYPRA4) inhibitors.

Sources

–*Circulation*. 2017. doi: 10.1161/CIR.0000000000000509

–http://www.fda.gov/NewsEvents/Newsroom/PressAnnouncements/ucm442978.htm

–http://pi.amgen.com/united_states/corlanor/corlanor_pi_hcp.pdf

Comment

–SHIFT study showed that ivabradine reduced the time to first occurrence of hospitalization for worsening heart failure compared to placebo.

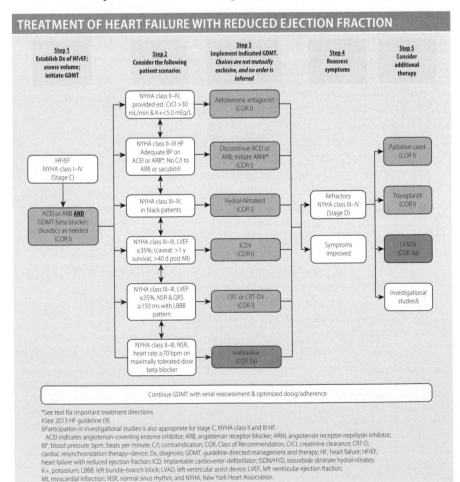

TREATMENT OF HEART FAILURE WITH REDUCED EJECTION FRACTION

*See text for important treatment directions.
‡See 2013 HF guideline (9).
§Participation in investigational studies is also appropriate for stage C, NYHA class II and III HF.
ACEI indicates angiotensin-coverting enzyme inhibitor; ARB, angiotensin receptor-blocker; ARNI, angiotensin receptor-neprilysin inhibitor; BP, blood pressure; bpm, beats per minute; C/I, contraindication; COR, Class of Recommendation; CrCl, creatinine clearance; CRT-D, cardiac resynchronization therapy–device; Dx, diagnosis; GDMT, guideline-directed management and therapy; HF, heart failure; HFrEF, heart failure with reduced ejection fraction; ICD, implantable cardioverter-defibrillator; ISDN/HYD, isosorbide dinitrate hydral-nitrates; K+, potassium; LBBB, left bundle-branch block; LVAD, left ventricular assist device; LVEF, left ventricular ejection fraction; MI, myocardial infarction; NSR, normal sinus rhythm; and NYHA, New York Heart Association.

BIOMARKERS IN CHF

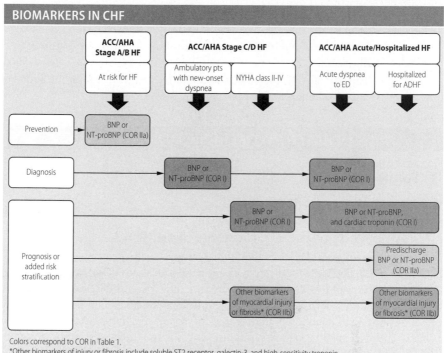

Colors correspond to COR in Table 1.
*Other biomarkers of injury or fibrosis include soluble ST2 receptor, galectin-3, and high-sensitivity troponin.
ACC indicates American College of Cardiology; AHA, American Heart Association; ADHF, acute decompensated heart failure; BNP, B-type natriuretic peptide; COR, Class of Recommendation; ED, emergency department; HF, heart failure; NT-proBNP, N-terminal pro-B-type natriuretic peptide; NYHA, New York Heart Association; and pts, patients.

Population

–Patients with chronic heart failure NYHA Class II-IV, with systolic dysfunction, in sinus rhythm, with resting HR ≥75 bpm, in combination with standard therapy including β-blocker therapy or when β-blocker therapy is contraindicated or not tolerated.

Recommendation

▶ EMA 2012

–Ivabradine was approved in treatment for HF.

Source

–http://www.ema.europa.eu/ema/index.jsp?curl=pages/ medicines/human/medicines/000598/human_med_000727. jsp&mid=WC0b01ac058001d124

Comments

1. 2014 EMA review based on SIGNIFY study showed:
   - –Ivabradine should not be used in combination with verapamil or diltiazem.
   - –The risk of AF is increased in patient treated with ivabradine and doctors should monitor patients for AF.

HELICOBACTER PYLORI INFECTION

Population

–Adults.

Recommendations

▶ American College of Gastroenterology 2017

- –The following patients should be screened for *Helicobacter pylori* (*H. pylori*) infection—active peptic ulcer disease (PUD), a past history of PUD (unless previous cure of *H. pylori* infection has been documented), low-grade gastric mucosa-associated lymphoid tissue (MALT) lymphoma, undiagnosed dyspepsia: patients who are under the age of 60 y, patients initiating chronic treatment with a nonsteroidal anti-inflammatory drug (NSAID), unexplained iron deficiency anemia, idiopathic thrombocytopenic purpura, or a history of endoscopic resection of early gastric cancer (EGC) should be tested for *H. pylori* infection.
- –Patients who test positive for *H. pylori* should be treated.
- –Choice of therapy depends on prior antibiotic exposure.
- –Clarithromycin triple therapy consisting of a PPI, clarithromycin, and amoxicillin or metronidazole for 14 d remains a recommended treatment in regions where *H. pylori* clarithromycin resistance is known to be <15% and in patients with no previous history of macrolide exposure for any reason.
- –Bismuth quadruple therapy consisting of a PPI, bismuth, tetracycline, and a nitroimidazole for 10–14 d is a recommended first-line treatment option. Bismuth quadruple therapy is particularly attractive in patients with any previous macrolide exposure or who are allergic to penicillin.
- –Levofloxacin triple therapy consisting of a PPI, levofloxacin, and amoxicillin for 10–14 d is a suggested first-line treatment option.

–Concomitant therapy consisting of a PPI, clarithromycin, amoxicillin, and a nitroimidazole for 10–14 d is a recommended first-line treatment option.

–Whenever *H. pylori* infection is identified and treated, testing to prove eradication should be performed using a urea breath test, fecal antigen test- or biopsy-based testing at least 4 wk after the completion of antibiotic therapy and after PPI therapy has been withheld for 1–2 wk.

–Bismuth quadruple therapy or levofloxacin salvage regimens are the preferred treatment options if a patient received a first-line treatment containing clarithromycin.

Source

–ACG Clinical Guideline: treatment of *Helicobacter pylori* infection. *Am J Gastroenterol.* 2017;112: 212–238

▶ Cochrane Database Systematic Reviews 2013

–Recommends using longer duration therapy for PPI-based *H. pylori* therapy.

Source

–http://www.cochrane.org/CD008337/UPPERGI_ideal-length-of-treatment-for-helicobacter-pylori-h.-pylori-eradication

HEMATURIA

Population

–Adults with microscopic hematuria.

Recommendations

▶ AUA 2012

–Work-up and Management of Microscopic Hematuria

Source

–Davis R, Jones JS, Barocas DA, et al. *Diagnosis, Evaluation and Follow-up of Asymptomatic Microhematuria (AMH) in Adults: AUA Guideline.* American Urological Association Education and Research, Inc., 2012: 1–30.

ALGORITHM FOR THE DIAGNOSIS AND MANAGEMENT OF INCIDENTALLY DISCOVERED MICROSCOPIC HEMATURIA

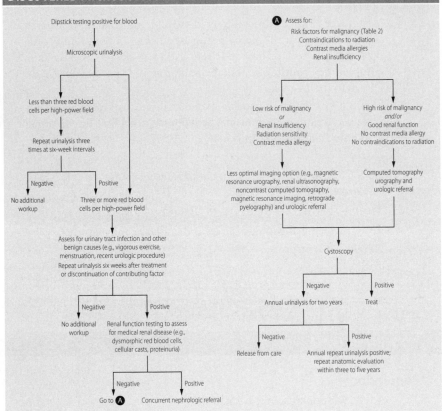

HEPATITIS B VIRUS (HBV)

Population
–Adults and children with HBV infection.

Recommendations
▶ NIH 2009, AASLD 2009

–Recommend HBV immunoglobulin and HBV vaccine to all infants born to HbsAg-positive women.
–Recommend antiviral therapy for adults and alanine transaminase (ALT) >2× normal, moderate-severe hepatitis on biopsy, compensated cirrhosis or advanced fibrosis and HBV DNA >20,000 IU/mL; or for reactivation of chronic HBV after chemotherapy or immunosuppression.

−Recommend antiviral therapy in children for ALT >2× normal and HBV DNA >20,000 IU/mL for at least 6 mo.

−Optimal monitoring practices have not been defined.

Sources

−http://www.guidelines.gov/content.aspx?id=14240

−http://www.guidelines.gov/content.aspx?id=15475

Comments

1. The most important predictors of cirrhosis or hepatocellular carcinoma (HCC) in chronic HBV infection are persistently elevated HBV DNA and serum ALT levels, HBV genotype C infection, male gender, older age, and coinfection with hepatitis C virus or human immunodeficiency virus (HIV).

   a. Persons at risk for HCC should be screened by ultrasound every 6–12 mo.

2. No randomized controlled trials have demonstrated a decrease in overall mortality, liver-specific mortality, or the rate of HCC with anti-HBV therapies.

3. Consider lamivudine or interferon-α for initial anti-HBV therapy.

HEPATITIS B VIRUS INFECTION

Population

−Adults.

Recommendations

▶ NICE 2013

−Offer antiviral therapy to adults if:

- Without a liver biopsy to adults with a transient elastography score ≥11 kPa.
- HBV DNA >2000 IU/mL and ALT >30 IU/mL (males) or >19 IU/mL (females).
- Cirrhosis and detectable HBV DNA.

−Initial antiviral options for HBV infection:

- Peginterferon α-2a.
- Entecavir.
- Tenofovir disoproxil.

−Coinfection with HBV and HCV:

- Peginterferon alfa-2a and ribavirin.

Population
  –Children and young adults.

Recommendations
▶ NICE 2013
  –Consider liver biopsy if HBV DNA >2000 IU/mL and ALT >30 IU/mL (males) or >19 IU/mL (females)
  –Initial antiviral options:
  • Peginterferon α-2a.

Source
  –http://www.guideline.gov/content.aspx?id=46933

Comments
  1. Consider a liver biopsy to confirm fibrosis for a transient elastography score 6–10 kPa.
  2. Monitor CBC, liver panel, and renal panel at 2, 4, 12, 24, 36, and 48 wk while on interferon therapy.
  3. Monitor CBC, liver panel, and renal panel at 4 wk and every 3 mo while on tenofovir therapy.

Population
  –Pregnant women.

Recommendation
▶ NICE 2013
  –Consider tenofovir disoproxil if HBV DNA >10^7 IU/mL in third trimester.

Source
  –http://www.guideline.gov/content.aspx?id=46933

Comment
  –Reduces risk of HBV transmission to baby.

HEPATITIS B VIRUS TREATMENT

Population
  –Adults and children with chronic hepatitis B virus infection.

Recommendations
▶ AASLD 2016
  –Recommends antiviral treatment for immune-active chronic hepatitis B to decrease the risk of liver-related complications:
  • Pegylated-interferon.
  • Entecavir.
  • Tenofovir.

–Recommends antiviral treatment for immune-active chronic hepatitis B with compensated cirrhosis and low-level viremia.

–Recommends against antiviral treatment for immune-tolerant chronic hepatitis B.

–Test alanine aminotransferase (ALT) levels every 6 mo for immune-tolerant chronic hepatitis B.

Source

–https://guidelines.gov/summaries/summary/50013

HEPATITIS C VIRUS (HCV)

Population

–Adults with HCV infection.

Recommendations

▶ AASLD 2009

1. Recommends education on methods to avoid transmission to others.
2. Recommends antiviral treatment for:
    a. Bridging fibrosis or compensated cirrhosis.
    b. Consideration of acute HCV infection.
3. Test quantitative HCV RNA before treatment and at 12 wk of therapy.
4. Patients who lack antibodies for hepatitis A and B viruses should receive vaccination.
5. Recommends abstaining from alcohol consumption.
6. Insufficient evidence to recommend herbal therapy.

Source

–http://www.guidelines.gov/content.aspx?id=14708

▶ WHO 2014

–Recommends pegylated interferon with ribavirin for adults and children with chronic HCV infection.

–Recommends telaprevir or boceprevier in combination with pegylated interferon with ribavirin for genotype 1 chronic HCV infection.

–Sofosbuvir in combination with ribavirin +/– pegylated interferon for genotypes 1, 2, 3, or 4 HCV infection.

Source

–http://www.guideline.gov/content.aspx?id=48895

Comment

1. Optimal therapy is the combination of peginterferon-α and ribavirin.
    a. Duration of therapy is 48 wk for HCV genotypes 1 and 4.
    b. Duration of therapy is 24 wk for HCV genotypes 2 and 3.

HEREDITARY HEMOCHROMATOSIS (HH)

Recommendations

▶ American Association for the Study of Liver Disease (AASLD) 2011

–**Clinical Features**

- Asymptomatic patients with abnormal iron studies (increased ferritin and iron saturation) should be evaluated for hemochromatosis.
- All patients with liver disease should be evaluated for hemochromatosis. (*Ann Intern Med.* 2006;145:209)

–**Diagnosis**

- Combination of transferrin saturation (TS) and ferritin should be done—if either abnormal (TS > 45% or ferritin > upper limit of normal) the HFE mutation analysis is indicated.
- Screening (iron studies and HFE mutation studies) is recommended for first-degree relatives. (*Ann Intern Med.* 2009;143:522)
- Liver biopsy is recommended for diagnosis and prognosis in patients with phenotypic markers of iron overload who are not C282Y homozygotes or compound heterozygotes (C282Y, H63D).
- Liver biopsy to stage the degree of liver disease in C282Y homozygote or compound heterozygotes if liver enzymes elevated or ferritin >1000 µg/L.

–**Treatment of Hemochromatosis**

- Therapeutic phlebotomy weekly until ferritin level 50 to 100 µg/L.
- C282Y homozygotes who have an elevated ferritin (but <1000 µg/L) should proceed to phlebotomy without liver biopsy.
- Patients with end-organ damage due to iron overload should undergo regular phlebotomy to keep ferritin between 50 to 100 µg/L.
- Vitamin C and iron supplements should be avoided but other dietary adjustments not necessary.
- Patients should be monitored on a regular basis for reaccumulation of iron and undergo maintenance with targeted ferritin levels of 50 to l00 µg/L.
- Use of iron chelation with deferoxamine or deferasirox is not recommended in hemochromatosis. (*Blood.* 2010;116:317-325. *Blood.* 2008;111:3373-3376; *Hepatology.* 2011; 54:328-343)

Source

–Practice guidelines. *Hepatology.* 2011;54:328-343

Comment

–**Problems in Hemochromatosis**

- Symptoms besides liver function abnormalities include skin pigmentation, pancreatic dysfunction with diabetes, arthralgias, impotence, and cardiac involvement with ECG changes and heart failure.
- Other rare mutations causing phenotypic hemochromatosis include transferrin receptor 2 mutation, ferroportin mutation, and H ferritin mutation.
- The most devastating complication of hemochromatosis is a 20-fold increase in the risk of hepatocellular carcinoma (HCC). Less than 1% of patients whose ferritin has never been >1000 µg/L develop HCC, while the risk rises considerably in patients with cirrhosis and ferritin level >1000 µg/L. These patients should be screened with hepatic ultrasound every 6 mo. Alfa fetoprotein (AFP) is elevated in only 60% of patients with HCC and should not be used as a single screening test. (*Liver Cancer.* 2014;3:31)
- Patients with hemochromatosis are at increased risk for certain bacterial infections whose virulence is increased in the presence of iron overload. These include *Listeria monocytogenes* (most common in renal dialysis patients), *Yersinia enterocolitica,* and *Vibrio vulniticus* (uncooked seafood is a common source). Infections are made more virulent by iron overload of macrophages impairing their anti-bacterial activity.
- Secondary iron overload (most commonly secondary to a transfusion requirement due to blood or bone marrow disease) is best managed by iron chelation beginning when the ferritin rises above 1000 µg/L. In contrast to HH excess iron is deposited primarily in the reticuloendothelial system, although visceral iron overload does occur over time. (*Blood.* 2014;124:1212)

HIP FRACTURES

Population

–Elderly patients with hip fractures.

Recommendations

▶ AAOS 2014

- Recommends preop pain control in patients with hip fractures.
- Insufficient evidence to support preop traction in hip fractures.
- Recommends hip fracture surgery within 48 h of admissions.
- Do not delay hip fracture surgery for patients on aspirin +/– clopidogrel.

- Recommends operative fixation for nondisplaced femoral neck fractures.
- Recommends unipolar or bipolar hemiarthroplasty for displaced femoral neck fractures.
- Recommends prolonged thromboprophylaxis to prevent venous thromboembolism after hip fracture surgery.
- Recommends intensive physical therapy post-discharge to improve functional outcomes.
- Recommends evaluation for osteoporosis in all patients who have sustained a hip fracture

Source
  –http://www.guideline.gov/content.aspx?id=48518

HOARSENESS

Population
  –Persons with hoarseness.

Recommendations
▶ AAO-HNS 2009
  –Recommends against the routine use of antibiotics to treat hoarseness.
  –Recommends voice therapy for all patients with hoarseness and a decreased voice quality of life.
  –All patients with chronic hoarseness >3 mo should undergo laryngoscopy.
  –Recommends against routine use of antireflux medications unless the patient exhibits signs or symptoms of gastroesophageal reflux disease.
  –Recommends against the routine use of corticosteroids to treat hoarseness.
  –Recommends against screening neck imaging (CT or MRI scanning) for chronic hoarseness prior to laryngoscopy.
  –Consider surgery for possible laryngeal CA, benign laryngeal soft-tissue lesions, or glottis insufficiency.
  –Consider botulinum toxin injections for spasmodic dysphonia.

Source
  –http://www.guidelines.gov/content.aspx?id=15203

Comment
  –Nearly one-third of Americans will have hoarseness at some point in their lives.

HUMAN IMMUNODEFICIENCY VIRUS (HIV)

Population
–HIV-infected adults and children.

Recommendations

▶ IDSA 2009

1. Recommends education to avoid high-risk behaviors to minimize risk of HIV transmission.
2. Assess for the presence of depression, substance abuse, or domestic violence.
3. Baseline labs: CD4 count; quantitative HIV RNA by PCR (viral load); HIV genotyping; CBCD, chemistry panel, G6PD testing; fasting lipid profile; HLA B5701 test (if abacavir is used); urinalysis; PPD; *Toxoplasma* antibodies; HBsAg, HBsAb, and HCV antibodies; VDRL; urine NAAT for gonorrhea; and urine NAAT for chlamydia (except in men age <25 y); Pap smear in women.[a]
4. Monitoring labs:
   a. CD4 counts and HIV viral load every 3–4 mo.
   b. Frequency of repeat sexually transmitted disease (STD) screening is undefined.
   c. Annual PPD test.
   d. Persons starting antiretroviral medications should have a repeat fasting glucose and lipid panel 4–6 wk after initiation of therapy.
5. Vaccination for pneumococcal infection, influenza, varicella, hepatitis A, and HBV according to standard immunization charts.
6. All HIV-infected women of childbearing age should be counseled regarding contraception.
7. Pap smear in women every 6 mo.
8. Consider annual mammography in all women age ≥40 y.
9. Hormone replacement therapy is not recommended.
10. All women age ≥65 y should have a dual-energy x-ray absorptiometry (DXA) test of spine/hips.

Source
–http://www.guidelines.gov/content.aspx?id=15440

---

[a]CBCD, complete blood count with differential; G6PD, glucose-6-phosphate dehydrogenase; HBsAb, hepatitis B surface antibody; HBsAg, hepatitis B surface antigen; HLA, human leukocyte antigen; NAAT, nucleic acid amplification test; PCR, polymerase chain reaction; PPD, purified protein derivative; RNA, ribonucleic acid; VDRL, Venereal Disease Research Laboratory.

Comments

1. Homosexual men and women with abnormal cervical Pap smear results and persons with a history of genital warts should undergo anogenital human papilloma virus (HPV) screening and anal Pap testing.
2. Serum testosterone level should be considered in men complaining of fatigue, ED, or decreased libido.
3. Chest x-ray should be obtained in persons with pulmonary symptoms or who have a positive PPD test result.

HUMAN IMMUNODEFICIENCY VIRUS (HIV), ANTIRETROVIRAL THERAPY (ART)

Population

–HIV-infected children.

Recommendations

▶ HHS 2010

1. ART is recommended for all children with symptomatic HIV disease.
2. Recommends ART for:
   a. Infants age <12 mo.
   b. Asymptomatic children with HIV RNA ≥100,000 copies/mL.
   c. Children age 1–5 y with CD4 <25%.
   d. Children age ≥5 y with CD4 <350 cells/mm^3.
   e. Children age ≥1 y with acquired immunodeficiency syndrome (AIDS) or symptomatic HIV infection.
3. HIV genotype testing is recommended:
   a. Prior to initiation of therapy in all treatment-naive children.
   b. Prior to changing therapy for treatment failure.
4. Recommends evaluating all children 4–8 wk after initiation of ART for possible side effects and to evaluate response to therapy.
   a. Reevaluate children every 3–4 mo thereafter.

Source

–http://www.guideline.gov/content.aspx?id=38702

Comment

–Specific ART recommendations are beyond the scope of this book.

HUMAN IMMUNODEFICIENCY VIRUS-1 (HIV-1), ANTIRETROVIRAL USE

Population
–Adults and adolescents.

Recommendations
▶ HHS 2013

–Antiretroviral-naive patients should start:
- Efavirenz/tenofovir/emtricitabine.
- Ritonavir-boosted atazanavir/ tenofovir/emtricitabine.
- Ritonavir-boosted darunavir/ tenofovir/emtricitabine.
- Raltegravir/tenofovir/ emtricitabine.
- Rilpivirine-based regimens are an alternative.
- Selection of a regimen should be individualized.
  - Efavirenz is teratogenic.
  - Tenofovir should be used cautiously with renal insufficiency.
  - Ritonavir-boosted atazanavir and rilpivirine should not be used with high-dose proton pump inhibitors.

–Coreceptor tropism assay is recommended whenever a CCR5 coreceptor antagonist is considered.

–HLA-B*5701 screening before starting abacavir.

–Interruption of HAART is recommended for drug toxicity, intercurrent illness, or operations that precludes oral intake.

–Management of a treatment—experienced patient is complex and should be managed by an HIV specialist.

Source
–http://aidsinfo.nih.gov/guidelines/html/1/adult-and-adolescent-arv-guidelines/0

Comments
1. This guideline focuses on antiretroviral management in HIV-1-infected individuals.
2. Baseline evaluation should include:
   - CD4 T-cell count.
   - HIV-1 antibody testing.
   - HIV RNA viral load.
   - CBC, chemistry panel, liver panel, urinalysis.
   - Serologies for HAV, HBV, and HCV.
   - Fasting glucose and lipid panel.
   - HIV-1 genotypic resistance testing.
   - STD screening.
   - Psychosocial assessment.

- Substance abuse screening.
- HIV risk behavior screening.
- CD_4 <350 cells/mm^3
- Consider for CD_4 350–500 cells/mm^3
- Pregnant women as soon as possible to prevent perinatal transmission.
- Consider for preventing heterosexual transmission.
- Patients must commit to strict adherence to HAART therapy.

HUMAN IMMUNODEFICIENCY VIRUS (HIV), PREGNANCY

Population

–HIV-infected pregnant women.

Recommendations

▶ CDC 2010

1. Recommends combination ART regimens during the antepartum period.
2. Women who were taking ART prior to conception should have their regimen reviewed (ie, teratogenic potential of drugs), but continue combination ART throughout the pregnancy.
3. Initial prenatal labs should include a CD4 count, HIV viral load, and HCV antibody.
   a. If HIV RNA is detectable (>500–1000 copies/mL), perform HIV genotypic resistance testing to help guide antepartum therapy.
4. Women who do not require ART for their own health should initiate combination ART between 14 and 28 gestational weeks and continue until delivery.
   a. Zidovudine should be a component of the regimen when feasible.
   b. Recommend against single-dose intrapartum/newborn nevirapine in addition to antepartum ART.
5. Antepartum monitoring:
   a. Monitor CD4 count every 3 mo.
   b. HIV viral load should be assessed 2–4 wk after initiating or changing ART, monthly until undetectable, and then at 34–36 wk.
   c. Recommend a first-trimester ultrasound to confirm dating.
   d. Screen for gestational diabetes at 24–28 wk.
6. Scheduled cesarean delivery is recommended for HIV-infected women who have HIV RNA levels >1000 copies/mL and intact membranes near term.
7. Intrapartum IV zidovudine is recommended for all HIV-infected pregnant women.
8. Avoid artificial rupture of membranes.
9. Avoid routine use of fetal scalp electrodes.
10. Breast-feeding is not recommended.

Source
–http://www.guideline.gov/content.aspx?id=38253

Comments

1. Avoid Methergine for postpartum hemorrhage in women receiving a protease inhibitor or efavirenz.
2. If women do not receive antepartum/intrapartum ART prophylaxis, infants should receive zidovudine for 6 wk.
3. Infants born to HIV-infected women should have an HIV viral load checked at 14 d, at 1–2 mo, and at 4–6 mo.

HYPERLIPIDEMIA

2013 ACC/AHA GUIDELINES ON THE TREATMENT OF CHOLESTEROL TO REDUCE ATHEROSCLEROTIC CV RISK IN ADULTS MAJOR STATIN BENEFIT GROUPS ALL SHOULD RECEIVE RX UNLESS CONTRAINDICATED

1. *Clinical ASCVD*
   Rx: High-intensity statin unless contraindicated or if age >70 y (moderate Rx).
2. *Primary elevation of LDL-C ≥190 mg/dL*
   Rx: High-intensity statin unless contraindicated, then moderate Rx.
3. *Diabetes (type 1 or 2) age 40–75 y with LDL-C 70–189 mg/dL and without clinical ASCVD*
   Rx: Moderate-intensity statin; high-intensity statin Rx if 10-y ASCVD risk ≥7.5%.
4. *Without clinical ASCVD or diabetes with LDL-C 70–189 mg/dL and estimated 10-y ASCVD ≥7.5%*[a]
   Rx: Moderate- to high-intensity statin.

[a]The pooled cohort equation.
Sources
–http://tools.cardiosource.org/ASCVD-Risk-Estimator/
–Also available as "ASCVD Risk" app from iTunes and Google Play.
–https://itunes.apple.com/us/app/ascvd-risk-estimator/id808875968?mt=8
– https://play.google.com/store/apps/details?id=org.acc.cvrisk&hl=en

INTENSITY STATIN DRUG LEVELS

High-Intensity Rx (lowers LDL-C >50%)	Atorvastatin 80 mg Rosuvastatin 40 mg
Moderate-Intensity Rx (lowers LDL-C 30%–50%)	Atorvastatin 10–20 mg Rosuvastatin 5–10 mg Simvastatin[a] 20–40 mg Pravastatin 40–80 mg Lovastatin 40 mg Fluvastatin *XL* 80 mg Fluvastatin 40 mg bid Pitavastatin 2–4 mg *[a]Simvastatin 80 mg should be avoided due to high risk of drug interactions*

INTENSITY STATIN DRUG LEVELS *(Continued)*	
Low-Intensity Rx	Simvastatin 10 mg
	Pravastatin 10–20 mg
	Lovastatin 20 mg
	Fluvastatin 20–40 mg
	Pitavastatin 1 mg

- If unable to tolerate moderate- to high-intensity statin therapy, consider the use of low-intensity dosages to reduce ASCVD risk.
- No RCTs have been identified that demonstrate that **titration of the drug dose** to specific LDL-C level improved ASCVD outcomes in primary or secondary prevention.

PRIMARY PREVENTION—GLOBAL RISK ASSESSMENT

1. Identify higher risk patients with a 10-y ASCVD risk as these are the patients mostly likely to benefit from Rx. The absolute benefit in ASCVD risk reduction is proportional to the baseline risk of the individual.
2. However, not all high-risk patients benefit; therefore, a **"patient-centered"** approach is required. The potential of ASCVD risk reduction, adverse effects, drug-drug interaction, and patient's preference all must be considered. Age ≥70 y should not restrict the use of moderated-intensity statin therapy if otherwise indicated.
3. Adults ≥21 y with primary LDL-C >190 mg/dL should receive high-intensity statin Rx (10-y risk estimate not required).
4. Diabetes (type 1 or 2) age 40–75 y with LDL-C 70–189 mg/dL and without clinical ASCVD. Rx: moderate-intensity statin; high-intensity statin Rx if 10-y ASCVD risk ≥7.5%.
5. Without clinical ASCVD or diabetes with LDL-C 70–189 mg/dL and estimated 10-y ASCVD ≥7.5%. Rx: moderate- to high-intensity statin.
6. Nontraditional risk factors to consider: LDL-C ≥160 mg/dL, genetic hyperlipidemia, premature family history of ASCVD with onset <55 y in first-degree male relative or <65 y in first-degree female relative; high-sensitivity CRP ≥2 mg/L, coronary artery calcium score score >300 Agatston units or >75% for age, sex, and ethnicity, ankle brachial index <0.9, or elevated lifetime risk of ASCVD. These should be considered when:
   a. Patients who are not in the 1 of the 4 statin benefit groups.
   b. Patients in whom the decision to start statin Rx remains unclear.
7. The panel emphasizes that the benefit of statin therapy outweighs the risk of newly diagnosed diabetes.
8. No RCTs have been identified that demonstrate that **titration of the drug dose** to specific LDL-C level improved ASCVD outcomes in primary or secondary prevention.

Sources: Stone NJ, Robinson J, Lichtenstein AH, et al. 2013 ACC/AHA Guideline on the Treatment of Blood Cholesterol to Reduce Atherosclerotic Cardiovascular Disease Risk in Adults: a report of the American College of Cardiology/American Heart Association Task Force on Practice Guidelines. Circulation published online November 12, 2013.
http://circ.ahajournals.org/content/early/2013/11/11/01.cir.0000437738.63853.7a.full.pdf
http://circ.ahajournals.org/content/early/2013/11/11/01.cir.0000437738.63853.7a.full.pdf+html

LIPID AND STATIN MONITORING

Initial

- Prior to initiating statin, consider fasting lipid panel, ALT, HbA1C (to R/O DM).
- Baseline CK levels if the patient is at increased risk of adverse muscle events based on personal or family history of statin intolerance, muscle disease, or concomitant drugs which may have interactions with statins.

Chronic

- Routine CK is not indicated unless symptoms appear.
- Follow-up hepatic function if symptoms suggesting hepatic toxicity arise.
- If confusion or memory impairment occurs while on statin, evaluate for nonstatin causes or drug interactions with statin.
- Repeat second lipid panel 4–12 wk after initiating therapy to determine patient's adherence. Then repeat lipid panel every 3–12 mo as clinically indicated.
- Statin use was associated with an increased likelihood of new diagnoses of DM, diabetic complications, and overweight/obesity in healthy people taking statin for primary prevention. *Source:* Mansi I, Frei CR, Wang CP, et al. Statins and new-onset diabetes mellitus and diabetic complications: a retrospective cohort study of US healthy adults. (*J Gen Intern Med*. 2015. doi:10.007/s11606-015-3335-1)
- In METSMIN (Metabolic Syndrome in Men) cohort, statin therapy (simvastatin, atorvastatin) was associated with a 46% increased risk of type 2 diabetes (after adjustment for confounding factors, worsening of hyperglycemia, a 24% reduction in insulin sensitivity, and a 12% reduction in insulin secretion). The risk of diabetes was increased in a dose-dependent and time-dependent manner by both simvastatin and atorvastatin.

Source: Diabetologia. 2015;58:1109-1117. doi:10.1007/s00125-015-3528-5.

NON-STATIN CHOLESTEROL LOWERING AGENTS

- No data have demonstrated that adding a **nonstatin lipid drug** to statin therapy further reduces ASCVD events.
- In high-risk patients (clinical ASCVD, age <75 y; LDL-C ≥190 mg/dL; 40–75 y old with DM) who are intolerant to statins, may consider the use of nonstatin cholesterol lowering drugs.
- *Niacin:* indicated for LDL-C elevation or fasting triglyceride ≥500 mg/dL; should be avoided with liver disease, persistent hyperglycemia, acute gout, or new onset AF.
- *BAS:* indicated for LDL-C elevation; should be avoided with triglycerides ≥300 mg/dL.
- *Ezetimibe:* indicated for LDL-C elevation when combine with statin monitor transaminase levels.
- *Fibrates:* indicated for fasting triglycerides ≥500 mg/dL; should avoid the addition of Gemfibrozil to statin agent due to increased risk of muscle symptoms. Fenofibrate should be avoided if moderate/severe renal impairment. If needed, fenofibrate should only be added to a low- or moderate-intensity statin.
- *Omega-3 fatty acids:* indicated in severe fasting triglycerides ≥500 mg/dL.
- *New class of LDL lowering agent:* PCSK9 (proprotein convertase subtilisin kexin 9).

NON-STATIN CHOLESTEROL LOWERING AGENTS (Continued)

- FDA Advisory Panel (June 2015) recommended approval of:
  1. Alirocumab (Praluent®) for lowering LDL cholesterol in patients with hypercholesterolemia, citing likely benefit especially for patients with heterozygous familial hypercholesterolemia (HeFH). Other groups predicted to get special benefit include those at high CV risk or who don't tolerate statin.
  2. Evolocumab (Repatha®) for lowering LDL-cholesterol. Studies have shown decrease in LDL cholesterol most notably in patients with heterozygous familial hypercholesterolemia.
- FOURIER trial is an ongoing study which is testing the use of evolocumab in combination with statin therapy against placebo plus statin therapy in patients with elevated cholesterol levels and existing cardiovascular disease.

Sources: http://www.medscape.com/viewarticle/846143 and http://www.medscape.com/viewarticle/846236.

2014 NLA (NATIONAL LIPID ASSOCIATION) GUIDELINES

- Population: adults >20 y old.
- **Targets of therapy: non-HDL-C is more predictive than LDL-C, both are primary targets. Apolipoprotein B (apo B) is considered a secondary, optional target for therapy.**
- If low/moderate ASCVD risk: Trial of lifestyle management prior to initiate drug therapy. Reduction of saturated fat and cholesterol intake, moderate physical activity, and weight loss, consider adding plant stanols/sterols, and increase viscous fiber intake. Evaluate every 6 wk for atherogenic cholesterol response. If after 12 wk, goal is not achieved, consider adding drug therapy/referral to dietician. Once goal achieved, follow every 4–6 mo to monitor adherence to lifestyle therapies.
- High/very high ASCVD risk: Lifestyle management concomitant with drug therapy. A moderate or high-intensity statin should be first-line drug therapy for treatment, unless contraindicated. In patients with very high TG, may consider TG-lowering drug (fibrates, high-dose omega 3 fatty acids, nicotinic acid) for first-line use to prevent pancreatitis. Follow every 6 wk, increasing the dosage/intensity if not at goal. If not at goal after 12 wk, refer to lipid specialist. Once at goal, follow every 4–6 mo for treatment adherence. Involve patient when making the decision to start statin.
- If TG ≥500, may consider TG-lowering drug as first-line therapy.
- If TG 500–1000 mg/dL, may start with statin if no history of pancreatitis.
- Nonstatin therapies (BAS, CAI, fibrate, nicotinic acid) may be considered (alone or in combination) in those with contraindications to statin therapy.
- For patients with statin intolerance, reducing the dose of statin, switching to a different statin or every other day statin may be considered.
- Goals: Attain levels below the goal cut points, non-HDL-C.
- For patients with ASCVD or DM, consideration should be given to use of moderate- or high-intensity statin therapy irrespective of baseline atherogenic cholesterol levels.

- Women with FH of childbearing age should receive prepregnancy counseling and instructions to stop statins, ezetimibe, and niacin at least 4 wk before discontinuing contraception and should not use these medications during pregnancy and lactation.
- During pregnancy in women with FH: Consider LDL apheresis if there is significant atherosclerotic disease or if the patient has homozygous FH.

Risk Category	Treatment Goal, Non-HDL-C (LDL-C)	Consider Drug Therapy, Non-HDL-C (LDL-C)
Low	<130 (<100)	≥190 (≥160)
Moderate	<130 (<100)	≥160 (≥130)
High	<130 (<100)	≥130 (≥100)
Very High	<100 (<70)	≥100 (≥70)

Source: NLA recommendations for patient-centered management of dyslipidemia. *J Clin Lipidol.* 2011;5:S1-S8. doi:10.1016/j.jacl.2011.04.003.(https://www.lipid.org/).

2014 AMERICAN DIABETES ASSOCIATION HYPERLIPIDEMIA GUIDELINES

- In all patients with hyperlipidemia and DM recommend lifestyle modifications including:
  - Diet: focusing on the reduction of saturated fat, trans fat, and cholesterol intake; increase of n-3 fatty acids, viscous fiber, and plant stanols/sterols.
  - Weight loss: if indicated.
  - Physical activity.
  - Smoke cessation.
- Regardless of baseline lipid levels, statin therapy should be added to lifestyle therapy in all patients with hyperlipidemia and DM who have overt CVD or who are without CVD, but are age >40, ≥1 CVD risk factors (family history of CVD, hypertension, smoking, dyslipidemia, or albuminuria).
- For low-risk patients, without overt CVD, age <40, consider statin in addition to lifestyle therapy if LDL-C remains >100 mg/dL or if >1 CVD risk factors.
- LDL-C targeted statin therapy remains the preferred strategy.
- LDL-C therapy goals:
  - Individuals without overt CVD: <100 mg/dL (2.6 mmol/L).
  - Individuals with overt CVD: <70 mg/dL (1.8 mmol/L) with high dose of statin is an option.
  - If drug-treated patients do not reach the above targets on maximum tolerated statin therapy, a reduction in LDL-C of 30%–40% from baseline is an alternative therapeutic goal.
- If severe hypertriglyceridemia with TG>1,000, focus on reducing the LDL-C.
- Triglyceride levels <150 mg/dL (1.7 mmol/L) and HDL-C >40 mg/dL (1 mmol/L) in men and >50 mg/dL (1.3 mmol/L) in women are desirable.

2014 AMERICAN DIABETES ASSOCIATION HYPERLIPIDEMIA GUIDELINES   (Continued)

- Combination therapy has been shown not to provide additional CV benefit above statin therapy alone and is not generally recommended.
- Statin therapy is contraindicated in pregnancy.
- Although there is an increased risk of incident diabetes with statin use, the CV rate reduction with statins outweighed the risk of incident diabetes even for patient with a highest risk for diabetes.

Source: Standards of medical care in diabetes 2014. Diabetes Care. 2014;37(1):S14-S80.

CHOLESTEROL GUIDELINES DIFFERENCES 2014

Guidelines	ACC/AHA 2013	ESC/EAS 2011
Risk stratification tools	ASCVD	SCORE
Scope of evidence	Randomized control trials	All data covering dyslipidemia
Therapy	Statin Rx only	Statin + additional cholesterol agents
F/U LDL-C levels	Only for evaluation of adherence	To evaluate adherence, allow risk stratification and consider additional cholesterol-lowering therapies
Quality risk scores	Not evaluated in Asia-Pacific population	European country specific
Present usage	USA	Europe

Source: Adapted from Ray KK, et al. The ACC/AHA 2013 guideline on the treatment of blood cholesterol to reduce atherosclerotic cardiovascular disease risk in adults: the good the bad and the uncertain: a comparison with ESC/EAS guidelines for the management of dyslipidemias 2011. Eur Heart J. 2014;35(15):960-8.

2011 EUROPEAN SOCIETY OF CARDIOLOGY/EUROPEAN ATHEROSCLEROSIS SOCIETY GUIDELINES FOR THE MANAGEMENT OF DYSLIPIDEMIA

ESC/EAS Guidelines
1. Screen with lipid profile:
   Men ≥40 y.
   Women ≥50 y or postmenopausal with additional risk factors.
   Evidence of atherosclerosis in any vascular bed.
   Diabetes type 2.
   Family history of premature cardiovascular disease (CVD).
2. Estimate total CV 10-y risk by SCORE (Systemic Coronary Risk Estimation), which has a large European cohort database, or the Framingham Risk Score.
   If the 10-y risk is ≥5% at increased risk, recommend heart score modified to include HDL-C.

VERY HIGH RISK—LDL-C goal <70 mg/dL

Documented CVD by invasive or noninvasive testing, previous MI, percutaneous coronary intervention (PCI), coronary artery bypass graft (CABG), other arterial revascularization procedures, ischemic cardiovascular accident (CVA), or peripheral arterial disease (PAD). Type 2 diabetes; type 1 with end-organ disease (microalbinuria).
Moderate-to-severe chronic kidney disease (CKD) GRF <60 mL/min/1.73 m²
Calculated 10-y risk SCORE ≥10%; FRS ≥20%.

HIGH RISK—LDL-C goal <100 mg/dL

Markedly elevated lipids or BP.
SCORE ≥5% and <10% for the 10-y risk of fatal cardiovascular disease (CVD); Framingham Risk Score (FRS) ≥20%.

MODERATE RISK—LDL-C goal <115 mg/dL

SCORE ≥1% and <5% at 10 y; FRS 10%–20%.
Family history (FH) of premature CAD.
Obesity.
Physical inactivity.
Low HDL-C, high TGs.

LOW RISK SCORE <1%; FRS ≤5%

3. Lipid analysis.

LDL-C is the primary marker.

TGs, HDL-C, non-HDL-C, apolipoprotein B (apoB) (with diabetes and MetS), lipoprotein A (LpA) in selected high-risk patients with FH of premature disease. Total cholesterol (TC) adds little to assessment.

4. Lifestyle management—same as ATP recommendations with additional use of phytosterols, soy protein, red yeast rice, and polycosanol supplements.

5. Secondary causes for hypercholesterolemia: hypothyroidism, nephrotic syndrome, pregnancy, Cushing syndrome, anorexia nervosa, immunosuppressant agents, corticosteroids.

6. Drug therapy, LDL-C.

Statins—initial agent in moderate-, high-, or very-high-risk patients.

Statin therapy in primary prevention should be limited to patients with moderate or high risk.
Combined therapy: bile acid sequestrant (BAS) + nicotinic acid, cholesterol absorption inhibitor + BAS + nicotinic acid.

7. TG >880 mg/dL—pancreatitis.

Fibrates, nicotinic acid, n-3 fatty acids.

HDL-C.

Nicotinic acid, statin, nicotinic acid + statin.

CKD stages 1–2.

Statin well tolerated; stage >3; more adverse events—use atorvastatin, fluvastatin, gemfibrozil.

Source: European Association for Cardiovascular Prevention & Rehabilitation, Reiner Z, Catapano AL, De Backer G, et al; ESC Committee for Practice Guidelines (CPG) 2008–2010 and 2010–2012 Committees. ESC/EAS Guidelines. *Eur Heart J.* 2011;32:1769-1818.

MANAGEMENT OF DYSLIPIDEMIA FOR CARDIOVASCULAR DISEASE RISK REDUCTION—VETERAN AFFAIRS AND U.S. DEPARTMENT OF DEFENSE CLINICAL PRACTICE GUIDELINE 2014

- Screen all men >35, women >45, and all patients with atherosclerotic CVD (ASCVD) or equivalents.
- Equivalents of ASCVD: ACS or MI, CABG or PCI, sable obstructive CAD, CVA/TIA, atherosclerotic PVD (claudication or AAA).
- If the patient has a history of CVD or ACS, calculate 10-y CVD risk, and measure lipid levels and BP.

10-y Risk	Statin Dose
ASCVD (second prevention)	Moderate to high
>12 %	Moderate
6%–12% (with shared decision making)	Moderate
<6%	None

- **Statin dose**

Statin	Moderate (mg)	High (mg)
Atorvastatin	10–20	40–80
Rosuvastatin	5–10	20–40
Simvastatin	20–40	
Pravastatin	40	
Lovastatin	40–80	
Fluvastatin	80 (80 daily or 40 bid)	

- If risk between 6% and 12%, the 10-y CVD risk should be repeated every 2 y. If risk <6%, the 10-y CVD risk should be repeated every 5 y.
- All patients should be encouraged to make positive lifestyle changes—to follow Mediterranean diet and to optimize comorbid conditions.

EXPERT PANEL ON INTEGRATED GUIDELINES FOR CARDIOVASCULAR HEALTH AND RISK REDUCTION IN CHILDREN AND ADOLESCENTS: SUMMARY REPORT 2013

SUMMARY:
- All children should have cholesterol screening once between age 9 and 11 y and once between age 17 and 21 y.
- Nonfasting total cholesterol and HDL cholesterol should be used as the screening tests.
- Clinicians may recommend low-fat or nonfat dairy at age 1 y for high-risk patients.
- If lifestyle changes are not effective, a lipid-lowering agent should be considered at age 10 y.

EVIDENCE-BASED RECOMMENDATIONS FOR DIETARY MANAGEMENT OF ELEVATED LDL-C, NON–HDL-C, AND TGs

Grades reflect the findings of the evidence review.

Recommendation levels reflect the consensus opinion of the Expert Panel.

Supportive actions represent expert consensus suggestions from the Expert Panel provided to support implementation of the recommendations; they are not graded.

NOTE: Values given are in mg/dL. To convert to SI units, divide the results for TC, LDL-C, HDL-C, and non–HDL-C by 38.6; for TGs, divide by 88.6.

ELEVATED LDL-C: CHILD 2—LDL		
2–21 y	Refer to a registered dietitian for family medical nutrition therapy:	Grade B Strongly recommend
	• 25%–30% of calories from fat, ≤7% from saturated fat, approximately 10% from monounsaturated fat; <200 mg/d of cholesterol; avoid trans fats as much as possible *Supportive actions:* • Plant sterol esters and/or plant stanol esters[a] up to 2 g/d as replacement for usual fat sources can be used after age 2 y in children with familial hypercholesterolemia. • Plant stanol esters as part of a regular diet are marketed directly to the public. Short-term studies show no harmful effects in healthy children. • The water-soluble fiber psyllium can be added to a low-fat, low-saturated-fat diet as cereal enriched with psyllium at a dose of 6 g/d for children 2–12 y, and 12 g/d for those ≥12 y. • As in all children, 1 h/d of moderate-to-vigorous physical activity and <2 h/d of sedentary screen time are recommended.	Grade A Recommend

[a]Can be found added to some foods, such as some margarines.

ELEVATED TGS OR NON–HDL-C: CHILD 2—TGs

2–21 y	Refer to a registered dietitian for family medical nutrition therapy:[a]	Grade B Strongly recommend
	• 25%–30% of calories from fat, ≤7% from saturated fat, ~10% from monounsaturated fat; <200 mg/d of cholesterol; avoid trans fats as much as possible	Grade A Recommend

	• Decrease sugar intake:
	  ◦ Replace simple with complex carbohydrates
	  ◦ No sugar sweetened beverages
		Grade B
		Recommend

	• Increase dietary fish to increase omega-3 fatty acids[b]	Grade D Recommend

[a]If child is obese, nutrition therapy should include calorie restriction, and increased activity (beyond that recommended for all children).

[b]The Food and Drug Administration (FDA) and the Environmental Protection Agency are advising women of childbearing age who may become pregnant, pregnant women, nursing mothers, and young children to avoid some types of fish and shellfish and eat fish and shellfish that are low in mercury. For more information, call the FDA's food information line toll free at 1-888-SAFEFOOD or visit http://www.fda.gov/downloads/Food/FoodborneIllnessContaminants/UCM312787.pdf-page=21.

Source: Expert Panel on Integrated Guidelines for Cardiovascular Health and Risk Reduction in Children and Adolescents: summary report. *Pediatrics.* 2011;128(5):S213-S258.

EVIDENCE-BASED RECOMMENDATIONS FOR PHARMACOLOGIC TREATMENT OF DYSLIPIDEMIA

Grades reflect the findings of the evidence review.
Recommendation levels reflect the consensus opinion of the Expert Panel.
When medication is recommended, this should always be in the context of the complete cardiovascular risk profile of the patient and in consultation with the patient and the family.

NOTE: Values given are in mg/dL. To convert to SI units, divide the results for TC, LDL-C, HDL-C, and non–HDL-C by 38.6; for TGs, divide by 88.6.

Birth–10 y	Pharmacologic treatment is limited to children with severe primary hyperlipidemia (homozygous familial hypercholesterolemia, primary hypertriglyceridemia with TG ≥500 mg/dL) or a high-risk condition or evident cardiovascular disease; all under the care of a lipid specialist.	Grade C Recommend
≥10–21 y	Detailed FH and risk factor (RF) assessment required before initiation of drug therapy.[a] High- to moderate-level RFs and risk conditions (RCs).	Grade C Strongly recommend

LDL-C:

If average LDL-C ≥250 mg/dL[a], consult lipid specialist.	Grade B Strongly recommend
If average LDL-C ≥130–250 mg/dL, or non-HDL ≥145 mg/dL: • Refer to dietitian for medical nutrition therapy with Cardiovascular Health Integrated Lifestyle Diet (CHILD 1) CHILD 2-LDL × 6 mo repeat fasting lipid panel (FLP).	Grade A Strongly recommend

Repeat FLP:

• →LDL-C <130 mg/dL, continue CHILD 2-LDL, reevaluate in 12 mo.	Grade A Strongly recommend
• →LDL-C ≥190[b] mg/dL, consider initiation of statin therapy.	Grade A Strongly recommend
• LDL-C ≥130–189 mg/dL, FH (–), no other RF or RC, continue CHILD 2-LDL, reevaluate q 6 mo.	Grade B Recommend
• →LDL-C = 160–189 mg/dL + FH positive or ≥1 high-level RF/RC or ≥2 moderate-level RFs/RCs, consider statin therapy.	Grade B Recommend
• →LDL-C ≥130–159 mg/dL + ≥2 high-level RFs/RCs or 1 high-level + 2 moderate-level RFs/RCs, consider statin therapy.	Grade B Recommend
Children on statin therapy should be counseled and carefully monitored.	Grade A Strongly recommend
Detailed FH and RF/RC assessment required before initiation of drug therapy.[c] High- and moderate-level RFs/RCs.[d]	Grade C Strongly recommend

TG:

If average TG ≥500 mg/dL, consult lipid specialist.	Grade B Recommend
If average TG ≥100 mg/dL in a child <10 y, ≥130 mg/dL in a child age 10–19 y, TG <500 mg/dL:	
• Refer to dietitian for medical nutrition therapy with CHILD 1 CHILD 2-TG × 6 mo.	Grade B Strongly recommend

EVIDENCE-BASED RECOMMENDATIONS FOR PHARMACOLOGIC TREATMENT OF DYSLIPIDEMIA *(Continued)*

Repeat FLP:	
• →TG <100 mg/dL, continue CHILD 2-TG, monitor 6–12 mo.	Grade B Strongly recommend
• →TG >100 mg/dL, reconsult dietitian for intensified CHILD 2 TG diet counseling.	Grade C Recommend
• →TG ≥200–499 mg/dL, non-HDL ≥145 mg/dL, consider fish oil ± consult lipid specialist.	Grade D Recommend
Non–HDL-C:	
Children ≥10 y with non–HDL-C ≥145 mg/dL after LDL-C goal achieved may be considered for additional treatment with statins, fibrates, or niacin in conjunction with a lipid specialist.	Grade D Optional

[a]Consideration of drug therapy based on the average of ≥2 FLPs, obtained at least 2 wk but no >3 mo apart.
[b]If average LDL-C ≥190 mg/dL after CHILD 2-LDL and child is age 8–9 y with + FH *or* ≥1 high-level RF/RC *or* ≥2 moderate-level RFs/RCs, statin therapy may be considered.
[c]Consideration of drug therapy based on the average of ≥2 fasting lipid profiles obtained at least 2 wk but no more than 3 mo apart.
[d]If child is obese, nutrition therapy should include calorie restriction and increased activity beyond that recommended for all children.
Source: Expert Panel on Integrated Guidelines for Cardiovascular Health and Risk Reduction in Children and Adolescents: summary report. *Pediatrics.* 2011;128(5):S213-S258.

MEDICATIONS FOR MANAGING HYPERLIPIDEMIA					
Type of Medication	Mechanism of Action	Major Effects	Examples	Adverse Reactions	FDA Approval in Youths as of This Writing
HMG CoA Reductase Inhibitors (Statins)	Inhibit cholesterol synthesis in hepatic cells, decreases cholesterol pool, resulting in upregulation of LDL receptors	Mainly lower LDL-C; some decrease in TG and modest increase in HDL-C	Atorvastatin Fluvastatin Lovastatin Pravastatin Rosuvastatin Simvastatin	Raised hepatic enzymes, raised creatine kinase, myopathy possibly progressing to rhabdomyolysis	All statins listed approved as an adjunct to diet to lower LDL-C in adolescent boys and postmenarchal girls age 10–18 y (8+ y for pravastatin) with heterozygous familial hypercholesterolemia (HeFH) and LDL-C ≥190 mg/dL, or ≥160 mg/dL with FH of premature CVD and 2+ CVD risk factors in the pediatric patient.
Bile Acid Sequestrants	Bind intestinal bile acids interrupting enterohepatic recirculation, more cholesterol converted into bile acids, decrease hepatic cholesterol pool, upregulate LDL receptors	Lower LDL-C; small increase in HDL; raises TG	Cholestyramine Colestipol Colesevelam	Limited to gastrointestinal tract: gas, bloating, constipation, cramps	No pediatric indication listed for cholestyramine or colestipol; colesevelam indicated as monotherapy or with statin for LDL-C reduction in boys and postmenarchal girls age 10–17 y with FH after diet trial if LDL-C ≥190 mg/dL or if LDL-C ≥160 mg/dL with family history of premature CVD or 2+ more CVD risk factors in the pediatric patient.

MEDICATIONS FOR MANAGING HYPERLIPIDEMIA (Continued)					
Type of Medication	Mechanism of Action	Major Effects	Examples	Adverse Reactions	FDA Approval in Youths as of This Writing
Cholesterol Absorption Inhibitors	Inhibit intestinal absorption of cholesterol and plant sterols, decrease hepatic cholesterol pool, upregulate LDL receptors	Mainly lower LDL-C; some decrease in TG and small increase in HDL-C	Ezetimibe	Myopathy, gastrointestinal upset, headache	No
Fibric Acid Derivatives	Agonist for peroxisome proliferator-activated receptor (PPAR) alfa nuclear receptors that upregulate lipoprotein lipase (LPL) and downregulate apolipoprotein C (apoC)-III, both increasing degradation of very-low-density lipoprotein C (VLDL-C) and TG. Hepatic synthesis of VLDL-C may also be decreased.	Mainly lower TG and raises HDL-C, with little effect on LDL-C	Fenofibrate Gemfibrozil	Dyspepsia, constipation, myositis, anemia	No

	Mechanism	Lipid Effects		Side Effects	Comments
Nicotinic Acid (Extended Release)	Inhibits release of free fatty acid (FFA) from adipose tissue; decreases VLDL-C and LDL-C production and HDL-C degradation	Lowers TG and LDL-C and raises HDL-C; can decrease Lp(a)	Niacin, extended release	Flushing, hepatic toxicity, can increase fasting blood glucose, uric acid; hyperacidity	Use not recommended in children <2 y of age.
Omega-3 Fish Oil	Decreases hepatic fatty acid (FA) and TG synthesis while enhancing FA degradation/oxidation, with subsequent reduced VLDL-C release	Lowers TG, raises HDL-C, increases LDL-C and LDL-C particle size	Omega-3 acid ethyl esters	Occasional gastrointestinal side effects, but no adverse effect on glucose levels or muscle or liver enzymes or bleeding	Only 1 FDA-approved fish oil preparation for adults, but many generic fish oil capsules commercially available.

Source: Expert Panel on Integrated Guidelines for Cardiovascular Health and Risk Reduction in Children and Adolescents: Summary Report 2013 Stephen R. Daniels, MD, PhD, Irwin Benuck, MD, PhD, Dimitri A. Christakis, MD, MPH et al. *Pediatrics.* 2011;128(6):S1–S44. (http://www.nhlbi.nih.gov/guidelines/cvd_ped/summary.htm#chap9).

HYPERTENSION

HYPERTENSION TREATMENT—JNC 8 2014

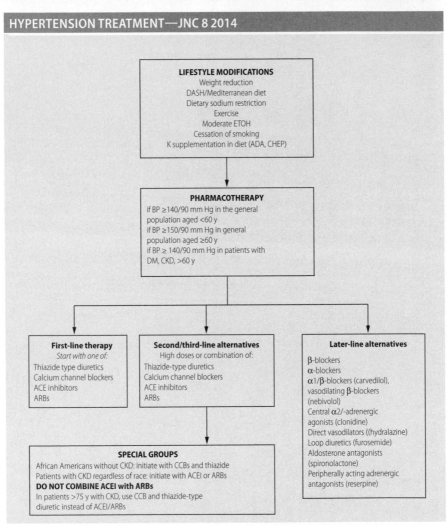

LIFESTYLE MODIFICATIONS
Weight reduction
DASH/Mediterranean diet
Dietary sodium restriction
Exercise
Moderate ETOH
Cessation of smoking
K supplementation in diet (ADA, CHEP)

PHARMACOTHERAPY
if BP ≥140/90 mm Hg in the general
population aged <60 y
if BP ≥150/90 mm Hg in general
population aged ≥60 y
if BP ≥ 140/90 mm Hg in patients with
DM, CKD, >60 y

First-line therapy
Start with one of:
Thiazide type diuretics
Calcium channel blockers
ACE inhibitors
ARBs

Second/third-line alternatives
High doses or combination of:
Thiazide-type diuretics
Calcium channel blockers
ACE inhibitors
ARBs

Later-line alternatives

β-blockers
α-blockers
α1/β-blockers (carvedilol),
vasodilating β-blockers
(nebivolol)
Central α2/-adrenergic
agonists (clonidine)
Direct vasodilators ((hydralazine)
Loop diuretics (furosemide)
Aldosterone antagonists
(spironolactone)
Peripherally acting adrenergic
antagonists (reserpine)

SPECIAL GROUPS
African Americans without CKD: initiate with CCBs and thiazide
Patients with CKD regardless of race: initiate with ACEI or ARBs
DO NOT COMBINE ACEI with ARBs
In patients >75 y with CKD, use CCB and thiazide-type
diuretic instead of ACEI/ARBs

Source: James PA, Oparil S, Carter BL. 2014 Evidence-based guideline for the management of high blood pressure in adults. Report from the panel members appointed to the Eighth Joint National Committee (JNC8). *JAMA.* 2014;311(5):507-520. doi:10.1001/jama.2013.284427.

JNC 8 2014 ANTIHYPERTENSIVE THERAPY

Initiate therapy
- BP ≥140/90 mm Hg in the general population age <60 y old.
- BP ≥150/90 mm Hg in general population age ≥60 y old.

Goal therapy
- BP <140/90 mm Hg in patients <60 y old.
- BP <150/90 mm Hg in patients ≥60 y old.
- BP <140/90 mm Hg in patients with DM, CKD who are <60 y old.

Antihypertensive therapy
- In the general non-black population, including those with DM, initial treatment should include a thiazide-type diuretic, CCB, ACEI, or ARB.
- In the general black population, including those with DM, initial treatment should include a thiazide-type diuretic or CCB.
- In all population age ≥18 y old with CKD (+/-DM), treatment should include an ACEI/ARB to improve kidney outcomes.
- Patients with CKD regardless of race: initiate with ACEI or ARBs.
- In patients >75 y old with CKD, use CCB and thiazide-type diuretic instead of ACEI/ARBs.
- If BP cannot be reached within 1 mo increase the dose of the initial drug or add a second and then third drug from the recommended classes.

Do not use an ACEI and ARB together!
- β-blockers, α-blockers, central α-2-adrenergic agonists (eg, clonidine), direct vasodilators (eg, hydralazine), aldosterone receptor antagonists (eg, spironolactone), peripherally acting adrenergic antagonists (eg, reserpine), and loop diuretics (eg, furosemide) are not recommended as a first-line therapy.

Source: James PA, Oparil S, Carter BL. 2014 Evidence-based guideline for the management of high blood pressure in adults. Report from the panel members appointed to the Eighth Joint National Committee (JNC8). *JAMA.* 2014;311(5):507-520. doi:10.1001/jama.2013.284427.

ACC/AHA/ASH 2015 ANTIHYPERTENSIVE THERAPY FOR PATIENTS WITH CAD

1. *Patients with HTN and chronic stable angina*
   - Goal therapy: <140/90 mm Hg for secondary prevention of CV events on patients with HTN and CAD.
   - <130/80 mm Hg may be appropriate for patients with CAD, previous MI, stroke or TIA, or CAD equivalents (CAD, PAD, AAA).
   - Treatment should include:
     1. β-blocker in patients with a history of prior MI.
     2. ACEI/ARB if prior MI, LV systolic dysfunction, DM, or CKD.
     3. A thiazide or thiazide-like diuretic.
   - If β-blocker is contraindicated or produce intolerable side effects, a nondihydropyridine CCB may be substituted but NOT if there is LV dysfunction.

ACC/AHA/ASH 2015 ANTIHYPERTENSIVE THERAPY FOR PATIENTS WITH CAD *(Continued)*

- If either angina or HTN remains uncontrolled, a long-acting dihydropyridine CCB can be added to the basic regimen of β-blocker, ACEI/ARB, and thiazide/thiazide-like diuretic. Combination of β-blocker and either of the nondihydropyridine CCB should be used with caution in patients with symptomatic CAD and HTN because of the increased risk of significant bradyarrhythmias and HF.
- There are no special contraindications in HTN patients for the use of antiplatelet or anticoagulant drugs, except that in patients with uncontrolled severe HTN who are taking antiplatelet or anticoagulant drugs, the BP should be lowered without delay to reduce the risk of hemorrhagic stroke.

2. *Patients with HTN and ACS*
- BP target <140/90 mm Hg in patients with HTN and ACS that are hemodynamically stable. BP target <130/80 mm Hg at the time of hospital discharge is reasonable. BP should be lowered slowly and caution is advised to avoid decreases in DBP to <60 mm Hg because this may reduce coronary artery perfusion and worsen ischemia.
- If no contraindication to β-blockers, the initial therapy of HTN should include a short-acting $β_1$-selective β-blocker without intrinsic sympathomimetic activity (metoprolol tartrate or bisoprolol). β-Blocker therapy should typically be initiated orally within 24 h of presentation. For patients with severe HTN or ongoing ischemia, an intravenous β-blocker (esmolol) can be considered. For hemodynamically unstable patients or when decompensated HF exists, the initiation of β-blocker therapy should be delayed until stabilization has been achieved.
- Nitrates should be considered to lower BP or relieve ongoing ischemia or pulmonary congestion. Nitrates should be avoided in patients with suspected RV infarction and in those with hemodynamic instability. Sublingual or IV nitroglycerin therapy is preferred for initial treatment and can be transitioned later to a longer-acting form if needed.
- If contraindication/intolerance/side effects to β-blocker and no presence of LV dysfunction or HF, okay to substitute with nondihydropyridine CCB (verapamil, diltiazem). If the angina or HTN is not controlled on β-blocker alone, a longer-acting dihydropyridine CCB may be added after optimal use of ACEI.
- ACEI/ARB should be added if anterior MI, persistent HTN, LV dysfunction, HF, or DM. For lower-risk ACS patients with preserved LV function and no DM, ACEI can be considered a first-line agent for BP control.
- Aldosterone antagonists are indicated for patients who are already receiving a β-blocker and ACEI after MI and have LV dysfunction and either HF or DM. Serum K levels must be monitored. These agents should be avoided in patients with elevated serum creatinine levels (≥2.5mg/dL in men, ≥2.0 mg/dL in women) or elevated K levels (≥5.0 mEq/L).
- Loop diuretics are preferred over thiazide/thiazide-type diuretics for patients with ACS who have HF (NYHA III or IV) or for patients with CKD and estimated glomerular filtration rate <39 mL/min. If HTN remains uncontrolled despite a β-blocker, an ACEI, and an aldosterone antagonist, a thiazide/thiazide-type diuretic may be added in selected patients for BP control.

3. *Patients with HTN and HF of ischemic origin*
- BP target is <130/80 mm Hg, but consideration can be given to lowering the BP even further, to <130/80 mm Hg. In patients with an elevated DBP who have CAD and HF with evidence of myocardial ischemia, the BP should be lowered slowly. In older hypertensive individuals with wide pulse pressures, lowering SBP may cause very low DBP values (<60 mm Hg). This should alert the clinician to assess carefully any untoward signs or symptoms, especially those caused by myocardial ischemia and worsening HF. Octogenarians should be checked for orthostatic changes with standing, and an SBP <130 mm Hg and a DBP <65 mm Hg should be avoided.
- Treatment should include management of risk factors (dyslipidemia, obesity, DM, smoking, dietary sodium, and closely monitored exercise program).
- The patient should be treated with ACEI/ARB, β-blocker (carvedilol, metoprolol succinate, bisoprolol, or nebivolol), and aldosterone receptor antagonists. These drugs have shown to improve outcomes for patients with HF and reduced EF.
- Thiazide/thiazide-type diuretic should be used for BP control and to reverse volume overload and associated symptoms. In patients with severe HF (NYHA III or IV), or those with severe renal impairment (eGFR <30 mL/min), loop diuretics should be used for volume control, but they are less effective than thiazide/thiazide-type diuretics in lowering BP. Diuretics should be used together with an ACE/ARB and a β-blocker.
- Studies have shown equivalence of benefit of ACEI and ARB (candesartan or valsartan) in HF with reduced EF. Either class of agents is effective in lowering BP.
- The aldosterone receptor antagonists spironolactone and eplerenone have been shown to be beneficial in HF and should be included in the regimen if there is HF (NYHA III or IV) with reduced EF <40%. One or the other may be substituted for a thiazide diuretic in patients requiring a K-sparing agent. If an aldosterone receptor antagonist is administered with an ACEI/ARB in the presence of renal insufficiency, serum K level should be monitored frequently. Should not be used if creatinine level ≥2.5 mg/dL in men or ≥2.0 mg/dL in women, or if serum K level ≥5mEq/L. Spironolactone or eplerenone may be used with a thiazide/thiazide-type diuretic in resistant HTN.
- Hydralazine plus isosorbide dinitrate should be added to the regimen of diuretic, ACE inhibitor, or ARB, and β-blocker in African American patients with NYHA class III or IV HF with reduced ejection fraction. Others may benefit similarly, but this has not yet been tested.
- In patients who have hypertension and HF with preserved ejection fraction, the recommendations are to control systolic and diastolic hypertension, ventricular rate in the presence of atrial fibrillation, and pulmonary congestion and peripheral edema.
- Use of β-adrenergic blocking agents, ACEI/ARBs, or CCB in patients with HF with preserved ejection fraction and hypertension may be effective to minimize symptoms of HF.
- In IHD, the principles of therapy for acute hypertension with pulmonary edema are similar to those for STEMI and NSTEMI, as described above. If the patient is hemodynamically unstable, the initiation of these therapies should be delayed until stabilization of HF has been achieved.

ACC/AHA/ASH 2015 ANTIHYPERTENSIVE THERAPY FOR PATIENTS WITH CAD   (Continued)

- Drugs to avoid in patients with hypertension and HF with reduced ejection fraction are nondihydropyridine CCBs (such as verapamil and diltiazem), clonidine, moxonidine, and hydralazine without a nitrate. α-Adrenergic blockers such as doxazosin should be used only if other drugs for the management of hypertension and HF are inadequate to achieve BP control at maximum tolerated doses. Nonsteroidal anti-inflammatory drugs should also be used with caution in this group, given their effects on BP, volume status, and renal function.

Sources: Rosendorff C, Lackland DT, Allison M, et al. Treatment of hypertension in patients with coronary artery disease: a scientific statement from the American Heart Association, American College of Cardiology, and American Society of Hypertension. *JACC.* 2015;65(18):1998-2038. *Circulation.* 2017. doi: 10.1161/CIR.0000000000000509.

AMERICAN SOCIETY OF HYPERTENSION (ASH) 2013 ANTIHYPERTENSIVE THERAPY

Goal therapy
- BP <150/90 mm Hg in patients ≥80 y old.
- BP <140/90 mm Hg in patients 60–79 y old.
- BP <140/90 mm Hg or <130/80 mm Hg (if tolerated), in patients <50 y old.
In patients with CKD or diabetes:
- BP <140/90 mm Hg (without proteinuria).
- BP <130/80 mm Hg (with proteinuria) or if they are at "high risk of cardiovascular disease"—no consensus.

Antihypertensive therapy
- Start lifestyle changes.
- In stage I (140–159/90–99) in patients without CV risks, some months of regularly monitored lifestyle management without drugs can be considered.
- In black patients initiate with CCB or thiazide. If unable to control BP, add ACEI/ARB. If needed add spironolactone, centrally acting agents, and β-blockers.
- In nonblack patients <60 y old initiate with ACEI/ARB. If uncontrolled, add CCB or thiazide. If needed add spironolactone, centrally acting agents, and β-blockers. In nonblack patients ≥60 y old initiate with CCB or thiazide. If needed add spironolactone, centrally acting agents, and β-blockers.

Source: Clinical practice guidelines for the management of hypertension in the community: a statement by the American Society of Hypertension and the International Society of Hypertension. *J Clin Hypertens.* 2014. doi: 10.1111/jch.12237. *Diabetes Care.* 2017;40(Suppl 1):S1–S142.

AMERICAN DIABETES ASSOCIATION (ADA) 2017 ANTIHYPERTENSIVE THERAPY

Goal therapy
- BP <140/80 mm Hg in patients with diabetes and HTN.
- BP <130/80 mm Hg in young patients and those at "high risk of cardiovascular disease."
- BP 110–129/65–79 in pregnant patients with diabetes and chronic HTN (lower than this may be associated with impaired fetal growth).

Antihypertensive therapy
- Start lifestyle changes.
- Initiate with ACEI or ARB.
- Administer one or more antihypertensive medications at bedtime. Closely monitor eGFR, serum K levels if any ACEI/ARB/ diuretic is used.
- Safe in pregnancy: methyldopa, labetalol, diltiazem, clonidine, and prazosin.

Source: Standards of medical care in diabetes. *Diabetes Care.* 2017;40(Suppl 1):S1–S142. (www.care. diabetesjournals.org).

CANADIAN HYPERTENSION EDUCATION PROGRAM (CHEP) 2014/2015 ANTIHYPERTENSIVE THERAPY

- The diagnosis of HTN should be based on out-of-office measurements (home or ambulatory). Electronic (oscillometric) measurement methods are preferred to manual measurements. HBPM and ABPM identify white-coat hypertension (as well as diagnose masked hypertension). (10% may have marked hypertension).
- Risk factors cluster; therefore, the management of HTN is combining global cardiovascular risk management and vascular protection including advice and treatment for smoking cessation.
- Structured exercise prescription as lifestyle modification.
- Resistance or weight training does not adversely affect BP in normotensive or mildly hypertensive individuals.
- Stress management should be considered as an intervention in hypertensive patients in whom stress may be contributing to BP elevation.

Initiate therapy
- BP ≥160/100 mm Hg in patients without macrovascular target organ damage or other CV risk factors.
- BP ≥140/90 mm Hg in patients with macrovascular target organ damage or high cardiovascular risk.
- BP >130/80 mm Hg in patients with diabetes.
- SBP >160 mm Hg in elderly (≥60 y).

Goal therapy
- BP <140/90 mm Hg in the general population, including those with CKD.
- BP <130/80 mm Hg in patients with DM.
- SBP <150 mm Hg in the elderly (≥60 y).
- SBP<140 mmHg in the elderly with cerebrovascular disease (history of CVA/TIA).
- Caution in elderly patients who are frail and in patients with CAD and have low DBP <60 mm Hg.

Antihypertensive agents
- Combination of both lifestyle modifications and antihypertensive medicines are generally necessary to achieve target blood pressures. Adopting health behaviors is integral to the management of hypertension.
- Optimum management of the hypertensive patient requires assessment and communication of overall cardiovascular risk.

CANADIAN HYPERTENSION EDUCATION PROGRAM (CHEP) 2014/2015 ANTIHYPERTENSIVE THERAPY (*Continued*)

- Initial therapy should be monotherapy with a thiazide diuretic, a beta-blocker, an ACEI in non-black patients, a long-acting CCB or an ARB in patients <60 y.
- First-line combinations: thiazide diuretic or CCB with an ACEI, ARB, or β-blocker. **Combination of ACEI and ARB is not recommended!** Caution in combination of nondihydropyridine and a β-blocker.
- In patients with diabetes, the combination preferred: ACEI with dihydropyridine rather than ACEI with HCTZ.
- Single pill combination therapies improve achieving optimal BP control.
- **ISH:** initial monotherapy with a thiazide diuretic, a long-acting dihydropyridine CCB, or an ARB. Combination of 2 or more first-line agents or other classes like α-blockers, ACEI, centrally acting agents, or nondihydropyridine CCBs.
- β-blockers are not recommended as first-line therapy for uncomplicated hypertension/ uncomplicated ISH in patients ≥60 y. ACEIs are not recommended as first-line therapy for uncomplicated hypertension in black patients. α-blockers are not recommended as first-line agents for uncomplicated hypertension/uncomplicated ISH.
- The patient with hypertension attributable to atherosclerotic renal artery stenosis should be primarily medically managed, because renal angioplasty and stenting offer no benefits over optimal medical therapy alone. Renal artery angioplasty and stenting for atherosclerotic hemodynamically significant renal artery stenosis *could be considered* for patients with uncontrolled HTN resistant to maximally tolerated pharmacotherapy, progressive renal function loss, and acute PE.
- Global cardiovascular risk should be assessed in all hypertensive patients. Informing patients of their global risk improves the effectiveness of risk factor modification.
- Statin therapy is recommended in high-risk hypertensive patients based on having established atherosclerotic disease or at least 3 of the following: male, ≥55 y, smoking, type 2 diabetes, total-C/HDL-C ratio ≥6, premature family history of CV disease, previous stroke or TIA, LVH, ECG abnormalities, microalbuminuria or proteinuria, and peripheral vascular disease.
- Low-dose ASA should be started in hypertensive patients ≥50 y for vascular protection. Caution should be exercised if BP is not controlled.
- Advice in combination with pharmacotherapy (eg, varenicline, bupropion, nicotine replacement therapy) should be offered to all smokers with a goal of smoking cessation.

ABPM, ambulatory BP measurement; HBPM, home BP measurement.
Sources: https://www.hypertension.ca/en/chep. Padwal R, Poirier L, Quinn R, et al. The 2013 Canadian Hypertension Education Program Recommendations.
http://guidelines.gov/summaries/summary/50733/pharmacologic-treatment-of-hypertension-in-adults-aged-60-years-or-older-to-higher-versus-lower-blood-pressure-targets-a-clinical-practice-guideline-from-the-american-college-of-physicians-and-the-american-academy-of-family-physicians?q=hypertension·
Qaseem A, Wilt TJ, Rich R, Humphrey LL, Frost J, Forciea MA. Pharmacologic treatment of hypertension in adults age 60 y or older to higher versus lower blood pressure targets: a clinical practice guideline from the American College of Physicians and the American Academy of Family Physicians. *Ann Intern Med.* 2017 Mar 21;166(6):430-437.

IMPACT OF HEALTH BEHAVIOR MANAGEMENT ON BLOOD PRESSURE

Intervention	Systolic BP (mm Hg)	Diastolic BP (mm Hg)
Diet and weight control	−6.0	−4.8
Reduced salt/sodium intake <2000 mg sodium (Na)[a]	−5.4	−2.8
Reduced alcohol intake (<2 drinks/d)	−3.4	−3.4
DASH diet	−11.4	−5.5
Physical activity (30–40 min 5–7× week)	−3.1	−1.8
Relaxation therapies	−5.5	−3.5

[a]2000 mg sodium (Na) = 87 mmol sodium (Na) = 5 g of salt (NaCl) ~1 teaspoon of table salt.

Source: Adapted from Canadian Hypertension Education Program (CHEP) Recommendations. 2015. (www.hypertension.ca/en/chep).

LIFESTYLE MODIFICATIONS FOR TREATMENT OF HYPERTENSION[a,b]

Modification	Recommendation	Approximate SBP Reduction (Range)
Weight reduction	Maintain normal body weight (BMI 18.5–24.9 kg/m²).	5–20 mm Hg per 10-kg weight loss
Adopt DASH eating plan	Consume diet rich in fruits, vegetables, and low-fat dairy products with a reduced content of saturated and total fat.	8–14 mm Hg
Dietary sodium reduction	Reduce dietary sodium intake to less than 100 mmol/d (2.4 g sodium or 6 g sodium chloride).	2–8 mm Hg
Physical activity	Engage in regular aerobic physical activity such as brisk walking (at least 30 min/d, most days of the week).	4–9 mm Hg
Moderation of alcohol consumption	Limit consumption to no more than 2 drinks (1 oz or 30 mL ethanol; eg, 24 oz beer, 10 oz wine, or 3 oz 80-proof whiskey) per day in most men and to no more than 1 drink per day in women and lighter-weight persons.	2–4 mm Hg

DASH, dietary approaches to stop hypertension.
[a]For overall cardiovascular risk reduction, stop smoking.
[b]The effects of implementing these modifications are dose- and time-dependent and could be greater for some individuals.
DASH diet found to be effective in lowering SBP in adolescents.

Sources: Couch SC, Saelens BE, Levin L, Dart K, Falciglia G, Daniels SR. The efficacy of a clinic-based behavioral nutrition intervention emphasizing a DASH-type diet for adolescents with elevated blood pressure. *J Pediatr.* 2008;152:494-501. Aronow WS, Fleg JL, Pepine CJ, et al. ACCF/AHA 2011 expert consensus document on hypertension in the elderly: a report of the American College of Cardiology Foundation Task Force on Clinical Expert Consensus documents developed in collaboration with the American Academy of Neurology, American Geriatrics Society, American Society for Preventive Cardiology, American Society of Hypertension, American Society of Nephrology, Association of Black Cardiologists, and European Society of Hypertension. *J Am Coll Cardiol.* 2011:57:2037-2110.

RECOMMENDED MEDICATIONS FOR COMPELLING INDICATIONS

Compelling Indication[a]	Diuretic	BB	ACEI	ARB	CCB	AldoANT
Heart failure	X	X	X	X		X
Post-MI		X	X			X
High coronary disease risk	X	X	X		X	
Diabetes	X	X	X	X	X	
Chronic kidney disease[b]			X	X		
Recurrent stroke prevention	X		X			

ACEI, ACE inhibitor; AldoANT, aldosterone antagonist; ARB, angiotensin receptor blocker; BB, beta-blocker; CCB, calcium channel blocker.

[a]Compelling indications for antihypertensive drugs are based on benefits from outcome studies or existing clinical guidelines; the compelling indication is managed in parallel with the BP.

[b]ALLHAT: Patients with hypertension and reduced GFR: no difference in renal outcomes (development of end-stage renal disease [ESRD] and/or decrement in GFR of ≥50% from baseline) comparing amlodipine, lisinopril, and chlorthalidone. (*Arch Intern Med.* 2005;165:936-946) Data do *not* support preference for CCB, alfa-blockers, or ACEI compared with thiazide diuretics in patients with metabolic syndrome. (*Arch Intern Med.* 2008;168:207-217; *J Am Coll Cardiol.* 2011;57:2037-2110; 2012 CHEP Recommendations (http://www.hypertension.ca).

COMPLICATED HYPERTENSION CHEP 2014

- **HTN and documented CAD**
  - ACEI is recommended for patients with HTN and documented CAD.
  - For patients with stable angina, β-blockers are preferred as initial therapy.
  - Combination of ACEI with ARB is not recommended in HTN patients with CAD but absence of LV systolic dysfunction.
  - In high-risk patients, combination of ACEI and a dihydropyridine CCB is preferable to an ACEI and a thiazide/thiazide-like diuretic in selected patients.
  - Myocardial ischemia may be exacerbated when DBP ≤60 mm Hg—caution in lowering DBP too much. (grade D)
- **HTN and recent STEMI/NSTEMI**
  - Initial therapy should include β-blocker and an ACEI or ARB. CCB may be used if β-blockers are contraindicated. Should not use nondihydropyridine CCBs with heart failure.
- **HTN with heart failure**
  - When LVEF <40% ACEI/ARBs and β-blockers are recommended as initial therapy.
  - Aldosterone antagonists may be added for patients with a recent CV hospitalization, acute MI, elevated BNP/NT-proBNP levels, or symptomatic cardiomyopathy NYHA class II-IV. Diuretics can be used if needed: thiazide/thiazide-like diuretic for BP control, loop diuretics for volume control.

- If ACEI/ARB contraindicated or not tolerated, a combination of hydralazine and isosorbide dinitrate is recommended.
- For HTN patients whose BP is not controlled, and ARB may be added to an ACEI and other antihypertensive drug treatment. (grade A) (Watch for hypotension, hyperkalemia, and worsening renal function.)

- **HTN with stroke/TIA**
  Acute stroke (72 h)
  - For patients eligible for thrombolytic therapy very high BP >185/110 mm Hg should be treated concurrently in patient receiving thrombolytic therapy for acute ischemic stroke to reduce the risk of intracranial hemorrhage.
  - For patients not eligible for thrombolytic therapy, extreme SBP elevation >220 or DBP> 120 mm Hg may be treated to reduce BP by 15% and not more than 25% over the first 24 h.

  After acute stroke
  - Strong consideration should be given to the initiation of antihypertensive therapy after the acute phase of a stroke or TIA.

- **HTN with LVH**
  - Initial therapy with ACEI/ARB, long-acting CCB, or thiazide/thiazide-like diuretics. Hydralazine and minoxidil should not be used.

- **HTN with nondiabetic CKD**
  - Goal BP <140/90 mm Hg.
  - If proteinuric CKD initiate with ACEI or ARB.
  - ACEI in combination with ARB is not recommended for patients with nonproteinuric CKD.

- **HTN with diabetes**
  - Goal BP 130/80 mm Hg.
  - Initiate with ACEI, dihydropyridine CCBS, thiazide/thiazide-like diuretic, or ARB.
  - If additional CVD, CKD, microalbuminuria, or CV risk factors, initiate with an ACEI or ARB.
  - Combination preferred: ACEI with dihydropyridine rather than ACEI with HCTZ.

Source: http://www.hypertension.ca/en/chep.

REFRACTORY HYPERTENSION

Definition:
Failure to reach BP goal (<140/90 mm Hg, or 130/80 mm Hg in patients with diabetes, heart disease, or chronic kidney disease) using three different antihypertensive drug classes.
Incidence: 20%–30% of HTN patients.
Common Causes:
1. Nonadherence to drugs/diet.
2. Suboptimal therapy/BP measurement (fluid retention, inadequate dosage).
3. Diet/drug interactions (caffeine, cocaine, alcohol, nicotine, NSAIDs, steroids, BCP, erythropoietin, natural licorice, herbs).
4. Common secondary causes:
   Obstructive sleep apnea.
   Diabetes.
   Chronic kidney disease.

REFRACTORY HYPERTENSION   *(Continued)*

Renal artery stenosis.

Obesity.

Endocrine disorders (primary hyperaldosteronism, hyperthyroidism, hyperparathyroidism, Cushing syndrome), pheochromocytoma.

Therapy:

- Exclude nonadherence and incorrect BP measurement.
- Review drug and diet history.
- Screen for secondary causes:

 History of sleep disorders/daytime sleepiness/tachycardias/BPs in both arms; routine labs: sodium, potassium, creatinine, CBC, ECG, urinalysis, blood glucose, cholesterol; additional evaluation: aldosterone: renin ratio, renal ultrasound with Doppler flow study, serum or urine catecholamine levels, morning cortisol level.

- Lifestyle therapy:

 Weight loss (10-kg weight loss results in a 5–20 mm Hg decrease in SBP); diet consult for low sodium (2.3 g daily), high fiber, and high potassium (DASH diet results in an 8–14 mm Hg decrease in SBP); exercise aerobic training results in a 4–9 mm Hg decrease in SBP; and restriction of excess alcohol (1 oz in men and 0.5 oz in women) results in a 2– 4 mm Hg decrease in SBP.

- Pharmacologic therapy:

 Consider volume overload.

- Switch from HCTZ to chlorthalidone (especially if GFR <40 mL/min).
- Switch to loop diuretic if GFR <30 mL/min (eg, furosemide 40 mg bid).
- Use CCB (amlodipine or nifedipine) + ACE inhibitor or ARB:

 Consider catecholamine excess.

- Switch to vasodilating β-blocker (carvedilol, labetalol, nebivolol):

 Consider aldosterone excess (even with normal serum K+ level).

- Spironolactone or eplerenone

 Finally, consider hydralazine or minoxidil.

- If already on β-blocker, clonidine adds little BP benefit.
- Nonpharmacologic therapy: Still under investigation.
- Carotid baroreceptor stimulation (*Hypertension.* 2010;55:1-8):

 May lower BP 33/22 mm Hg.

- Renal artery nerve denervation (SYMPLICITY HTN-3) did not show a significant reduction of SBP in patients with resistant hypertension, 6 mo after the procedure.

ACE, angiotensin-converting enzyme; ARB, angiotensin receptor blocker; BCP, birth control pill; bid, twice a day; BP, blood pressure; CBC, complete blood count; CCB, calcium channel blocker; DASH diet, Dietary Approaches to Stop Hypertension diet; ECG, electrocardiogram; GFR, glomerular filtration rate; HCTZ, hydrochlorothiazide; HTN, hypertension; NSAIDs, nonsteroidal anti-inflammatory drugs; SBP, systolic blood pressure.

Sources: Bhatt DL, Kandzari DE, O'Neill WW, et al. A controlled trial of renal denervation for resistant hypertension. N Engl J Med. 2014;370:1393-1401. Calhoun DA, Jones D, Textor S, et al; American Heart Association Professional Education Committee. Resistant hypertension: diagnosis, evaluation, and treatment: a scientific statement from the American Heart Association Professional Education Committee of the Council for High Blood Pressure Research. *Circulation.* 2008;117:e510–e526. JNC VII. *Arch Intern Med.* 2003;289:2560-2572; *European* 2007 Guidelines. 2007;28:1462-1536.
American College of Cardiology/American Heart Association/European Society of Cardiology.

HYPERTENSION: CHILDREN AND ADOLESCENTS

Indications for antihypertensive drug therapy in children and adolescents:

- Symptomatic hypertension.
- Secondary hypertension.
- Hypertensive target organ damage.
- Diabetes (types 1 and 2).
- Persistent hypertension despite nonpharmacologic measures (weight management counseling if overweight; physical activity; diet management).

Sources: Pediatrics. 2011;128(5):S213-S258. Kavey RE, Allada V, Daniels SR, et al; American Heart Association Expert Panel on Population and Prevention Science; American Heart Association Council on Cardiovascular Disease in the Young; American Heart Association Council on Epidemiology and Prevention, et al. Cardiovascular risk reduction in high-risk pediatric patients: a scientific statement from the American Heart Association Expert Panel on Population and Prevention Science; the Councils on Cardiovascular Disease in the Young, Epidemiology and Prevention, Nutrition, Physical Activity and Metabolism, High Blood Pressure Research, Cardiovascular Nursing, and the Kidney in Heart Disease; and the Interdisciplinary Working Group on Quality of Care and Outcomes Research: endorsed by the American Academy of Pediatrics. Circulation. 2006;114:2710-2738.

HYPERTENSION: TREATMENT IN SPECIAL POPULATIONS ESH/ESC GUIDELINES 2013

- *White-coat HTN* is defined as elevated BP in doctor's office with normal home BPs.
  - White-coat hypertension at low risk (unassociated with additional risk factors) should receive lifestyle intervention and close follow-up.
  - White-coat hypertension at higher risk (associated with additional risk factors, metabolic disorders, or organ damage) should receive lifestyle intervention and drug therapy.
- *Masked HTN* is defined as normal BP in the doctor's office with elevated BPs at home.
  - Masked hypertension at low risk (with or without additional risk factors) should receive lifestyle intervention and drug therapy due to the higher CV risk.
- *Elderly HTN occurs in patients ≥65 y old.*
  - In all elderly hypertensive patients SBP >160 mm Hg should be reduced to SBP between 140 and 150 mm Hg based upon good evidence.
  - In *fit* elderly hypertensive patients <80 y old, SBP >160 mm Hg may be reduced to <140 mm Hg, if therapy is well tolerated.
  - Diuretics and calcium antagonist may be preferred in isolated systolic hypertension, although all medications have been used with success.
- *Very elderly HTN* occurs in patients ≥80 y old.
  - In *fit* very elderly patients >80 y old, SBP should be reduced to 140–150 mm Hg.
  - In *frail* very elderly patients >80 y old, SBP goal needs to be individualized.
- Hypertensive therapy during *pregnancy*.
  - Drug therapy should be started with persistent BP ≥150/95 mm Hg and BP ≥140/90 mm Hg if associated with gestational hypertension, subclinical organ damage, or if associated with symptoms.
  - Women with hypertension with childbearing potential should not receive renin-angiotensin system (RAS) blockers.

HYPERTENSION: TREATMENT IN SPECIAL POPULATIONS ESH/ESC GUIDELINES 2013 (*Continued*)

- ○ Methyldopa and nifedipine should be initial therapy for hypertension. Labetalol and nitroprusside are the intravenous drugs of choice.
- Hypertension goal with CAD, diabetes, and nephropathy.
  - ○ SBP goal <140 mm Hg should be considered.

Source: Adapted from Mancia G, Fagard R, Narkiewicz K, et al. 2013 ESH/ESC guidelines for the management of arterial hypertension: the Task Force for the management of arterial hypertension of the European Society of Hypertension (ESH) and the European Society of Cardiology (ESC). *Eur Heart J.* 2013;34:2159-2219.

HYPERTENSIVE TREATMENT IN PREGNANCY— AHA/ASA 2014 GUIDELINES

- Risk factors of pregnancy-induced hypertension: obesity, age >40 y old, chronic HTN, personal or family history of preeclampsia, gestational HTN, nulliparity, multiple pregnancy, preexisting vascular disease, collagen vascular disease, diabetes, renal disease.
- Severe hypertension per JNC VII: BP ≥160/110 mm Hg (high risk of stroke and eclampsia).
- BP goal during pregnancy: 130–155/80–105 mm Hg.
- **Prevention of eclampsia recommendations**
  - ○ Women with chronic primary or secondary hypertension, or previous pregnancy-related hypertension, should take low-dose aspirin from the 12th week of gestation until delivery.
  - ○ Calcium supplementation (of at least 1 g/d, orally) should be considered for women with low dietary intake of calcium (<600 mg/d) to prevent preeclampsia.
- **Treatment of hypertension in pregnancy and postpartum recommendations**
  - ○ Severe hypertension in pregnancy should be treated with safe and effective antihypertensive medications such as methyldopa, labetalol, and nifedipine, with consideration of maternal and fetal side effects.
  - ○ Atenolol, ARBs, and direct renin inhibitors are contraindicated in pregnancy and should not be used.
  - ○ Because of the increased risk of future hypertension and stroke 1 to 30 y after delivery in women with a history of preeclampsia it is reasonable to:
    - –Consider evaluating all women starting 6 mo to the 1 y postpartum, as well as those who are past childbearing age, for a history of preeclampsia/eclampsia, and document their history of preeclampsia/eclampsia as a risk factor.
    - –Evaluate and treat for cardiovascular risk factors including hypertension, obesity, smoking, and dyslipidemia.
  - ○ After giving birth, women with chronic hypertension should be continued on their antihypertensive regime, with dosage adjustments to reflect the decrease in volume of distribution and glomerular filtration rate that occurs following delivery. They should also be monitored carefully for the development of postpartum preeclampsia.

Source: Bushnell C, McCullough LD, Awad IA, et al. Guidelines for the prevention of stroke in women: a statement for healthcare professionals from the American Heart Association/American Stroke Association. *Stroke.* 2014;45. doi: 10.1161/01.str.0000442009.06663.48.

HYPOGONADISM, MALE

Population
–Adults.

Recommendations
▶ EAU 2012
–Testosterone testing should be done in:
- Pituitary masses.
- ESRD.
- Moderate-to-severe COPD.
- Infertility.
- Osteoporosis.
- HIV infection.
- DM type 2.
- Signs and symptoms of hypogonadism.

–Indications for testosterone treatment are patients with low testosterone and:
- Hypogonadism.
- Delayed puberty.
- Klinefelter syndrome.
- Sexual dysfunction.
- Low bone mass.
- Hypopituitarism.

–Contraindications to testosterone use:
- Prostate CA.
- PSA >4 ng/mL.
- Male breast CA.
- Severe sleep apnea.
- Male infertility.
- Hematocrit >50%.
- Symptomatic BPH.

–Monitor response to therapy, PSA, and hematocrit 3, 6, and 12 mo after starting therapy.

Source
–http://www.uroweb.org/gls/pdf/16_Male_Hypogonadism_LR%20II.pdf

Comments
1. Caused by androgen deficiency.
2. Primary hypogonadism:
   - Klinefelter syndrome.

- Cryptorchidism.
- Congenital anorchia.
- Testicular CA.
- Orchitis.
- Chemotherapy.
3. Secondary hypogonadism:
    - Kallmann syndrome.
    - Pituitary tumor.
    - Renal failure.
    - Hemochromatosis.
    - Hypothyroidism.
    - Anabolic steroid abuse.
    - Morbid obesity.
    - Radiotherapy.
    - Idiopathic hypogonadotrophic hypogonadism.
    - Androgen insensitivity syndrome.

IDENTIFYING RISK OF SERIOUS ILLNESS IN CHILDREN UNDER 5 Y

TRAFFIC LIGHT SYSTEM FOR DENTIFYING RISK OF SERIOUS ILLNESS IN CHILDREN UNDER 5 Y

Category	Green—Low Risk	Yellow—Intermediate Risk	Red—High Risk
Color of skin, lips, or tongue	Normal color	Pallor	Mottled, ashen, or blue
Activity	• Responds normally to social cues • Smiles • Awakens easily • Strong cry	• Abnormal response to social cues • No smile • Wakes only with prolonged stimulation • Decreased activity	• No response to social cues • Appears toxic • Stuporous • Weak, high-pitched cry
Respiratory	• Normal breathing	• Nasal flaring • Tachypnea ∘ >50 breaths/min (6–12 mo) ∘ >40 breaths/min (>1 y) • SpO$_2$ ≤95% • Pulmonary rales	• Grunting • Marked tachypnea ∘ >60 breaths/min • Moderate to severe chest retractions

| Circulation | • Normal skin and eyes
• Moist mucous membranes | • Tachycardia
  ∘ >160 beats/min (<12 mo)
  ∘ >150 beats/min (12–24 mo)
  ∘ >140 beats/min (2–5 y)
• Capillary refill ≥3 s
• Dry mucous membranes
• Poor feeding
• Decreased urine output | • Findings in yellow zone PLUS
• Reduced skin turgor |
| Other | • Nontoxic appearance | • Temperature ≥39°C (age 3–6 mo)
• Fever ≥5 d
• Rigors
• Swelling of a limb or joint
• Nonweight bearing on one extremity | • Temperature ≥38°C (<3 mo)
• Nonblanching rash
• Bulging fontanelle
• Neck stiffness
• Status epilepticus
• Focal neurological signs
• Focal seizures |

Source: Adapted from National Institute for Health and Care Excellence (NICE) Guideline on Feverish Illness in children: assessment and initial management in children younger than 5 years; 2013 May (Clinical Guideline no. 160).

INDWELLING URINARY CATHETERS OR INTERMITTENT CATHETERIZATION

Recommendation

▶ AUA 2015

–Recommends against empiric antibiotics unless the patient has symptoms of a urinary tract infection.

Source

–http://www.choosingwisely.org/clinician-lists/american-urological-association-antimicrobials-indwelling-or-intermittent-bladder-catheterization/

INFERTILITY, MALE

Population
–Adults.

Recommendations
▶ EAU 2012
–Assessment of male infertility includes:
- Semen analysis.
- Checking FSH, LH, and testosterone levels.
- Screening for gonorrhea and *Chlamydia*.
- *Substance abuse screening.*

–Refer patients with abnormal screens to a specialist in male infertility for potential treatments that may include clomiphene citrate, tamoxifen, human chorionic gonadotropin (hCG), dopamine agonists, or surgical treatments depending on the underlying etiology.

Source
–http://www.uroweb.org/gls/pdf/15_Male_Infertility_LR%20II.pdf

Comment
–Infertility is defined as the inability of a sexually active couple not using contraception to conceive in 1 y.

INFLAMMATORY BOWEL DISEASE, CROHN'S DISEASE

Population
–Children, young adults, and adults with Crohn's disease.

Recommendations
▶ NICE 2012
–Inducing remission in Crohn's disease.
- Glucocorticoids are recommended for a single exacerbation in a 12-mo period.
  ◦ Prednisolone, methylprednisolone, or IV hydrocortisone.
- Add azathioprine or mercaptopurine to steroids if steroids cannot be tapered or ≥2 exacerbations in last 12 mo.
- Infliximab or adalimumab are indicated with active fistulizing refractory to conventional therapy.

–Maintaining remission.
- Azathioprine.
- Mercaptopurine.

−Managing strictures.
  • Balloon dilation is an option for single stricture that is short, straight, and accessible by colonoscopy.
−Recommend routine surveillance for osteopenia or osteoporosis.

Source
−www.guideline.gov/content.aspx?id=38574

▼ INFLAMMATORY BOWEL DISEASE, ULCERATIVE COLITIS

Population
−Children, young adults, and adults.

Recommendations
▶ NICE 2013
−Mild-to-moderate proctitis and proctosigmoiditis to achieve and maintain remission.
  • Aminosalicylate suppository or enemas.
  • Oral aminosalicylate.
  • Topical corticosteroid.
−Mild-to-moderate extensive left-sided colitis.
  • Induction dose oral aminosalicylate.
  • Consider adding oral tacrolimus to oral prednisolone if remission not achieved after 4 wk of prednisolone therapy.
  • Maintain remission with low-dose aminosalicylate.
−Severe acute ulcerative colitis
  • IV methylprednisolone.
  • Consider IV cyclosporine for those in whom steroids cannot be used or have not improved after 72 h of steroid therapy.
  • Consider a colectomy for:
    ◦ Persistent diarrhea >8 bowel movements/d.
    ◦ Fevers.
    ◦ Hemodynamic instability.
    ◦ Toxic megacolon.
    ◦ CRP >4.5 mg/dL.

Source
−http://www.guideline.gov/content.aspx?id=46936

Comments

1. Oral prednisolone is an adjunct to aminosalicylates for proctitis or colitis if remission is not attained within 4 wk.
2. Consider adding oral azathioprine or oral mercaptopurine to maintain remission if not maintained by aminosalicylates alone.
3. Monitor bone health in children and young adults with chronic active disease or who require frequent steroid therapy.

Population

–Patients with ulcerative colitis (UC).

Recommendations

▶ ASCRS 2014

–Indications for colectomy:
  • Actual or impending colonic perforation.
  • Chronic UC refractory to medical therapy.
  • Development of a colonic stricture, high-grade dysplasia, or carcinoma.
–Options for patients with a UC flare that is worsening despite 96 h of primary medical therapy:
  • Add a second-line agent.
  • Surgery.

Source

–https://guidelines.gov/summaries/summary/47756

Comments

1. Procedure of choice for emergency surgery is a total or subtotal colectomy with end ileostomy.
2. Procedure of choice for elective surgery is a total proctocolectomy with ileostomy or ileal pouch-anal anastomosis.

INFLAMMATORY BOWEL DISEASE, ULCERATIVE COLITIS, SURGICAL TREATMENT

Population

–Patients with UC.

Recommendation

▶ American Society of Colon and Rectal Surgeons 2014

–Indications for surgery in UC:
  • Patients with acute colitis and actual or impending perforation.
  • Chronic UC refractory to medical therapy.
  • Presence of carcinoma or high-grade dysplasia in colon.

- Development of a colonic stricture.
- Consider a second-line agent or surgery for acute colitis that is worsening after 96 h of first-line medical therapy.

Source
–https://guidelines.gov/summaries/summary/47756

Comment
–Patient with severe diarrhea (>8 stools/d) in absence of *C. difficile* colitis and a c-reactive protein >4.5 mg/dL despite medical therapy for 72 h has an 85% chance of requiring a colectomy.

INFLUENZA

Population
–Adults and children.

Recommendations
▶ IDSA 2009

1. Antiviral treatment is recommended for:
   a. Lab-confirmed cases of influenza within 48 h of symptom onset.
   b. Strongly suspected influenza within 48 h of symptom onset.
   c. Hospitalized patients with severe, complicated, or progressive lab-confirmed influenza or influenza-like illness with high likelihood of complications even if >48 h from symptom onset.
2. Antiviral options include oseltamivir and zanamivir.
   a. Oseltamivir for influenza A or B: 75 mg by mouth (PO) twice daily (bid) (adults); 30 mg PO bid (≤15 kg); 45 mg PO bid (16–23 kg); 60 mg PO bid (24–40 kg); 75 mg PO bid (>40 kg or age ≥13 y) × 5 d. Avoid in children age <1 y.
   b. Zanamivir for influenza A or B: 2 puffs bid × 5 d (children age ≥7 y and adults); avoid in asthmatic patients.

Source
–http://www.guidelines.gov/content.aspx?id=14173

Population
–Children age 6 mo and older.

Recommendations

▶ AAP 2013

–Oseltamivir remains the antiviral drug of choice for the management of influenza infections.

–Treatment indicated if symptom onset within 48 h and:

- Any child hospitalized with presumed influenza or with severe, complicated, or progressive illness attributable to influenza, regardless of influenza immunization status.
- Influenza infection of any severity in children at high risk of complications of influenza infection.

Source

–http://www.guideline.gov/content.aspx?id=47372

Comments

1. Consider an influenza nasal swab for diagnosis during influenza season in:
   a. Persons with acute onset of fever and respiratory illness.
   b. Persons with fever and acute exacerbation of chronic lung disease.
   c. Infants and children with fever of unclear etiology.
   d. Severely ill persons with fever or hypothermia.
2. Rapid influenza antigen tests have a 70%–90% sensitivity in children and a 40%–60% sensitivity in adults.
3. Direct or indirect fluorescent antibody staining is useful in screening tests.
4. Influenza PCR may be used as a confirmatory test.

IRON DEFICIENCY ANEMIA

Population

–Adults.

Recommendations

▶ British Society of Gastroenterology

Scope of Problem

–Iron deficiency anemia (IDA) is the most common cause of anemia and occurs in 2%–5% of adult men and postmenopausal women in the developed world.

–More than 25% of the world's population is anemic with one-half attributed to iron deficiency. (*N Engl J Med.* 2015;372:1832)

Diagnosis

–Serum ferritin <30, iron transferrin saturation <10%, and hypochromic, microcytic RBCs on peripheral smear. MCV Usually

>80 until hemoglobin drops to <10 g/dL, random distribution of width (RDW) is elevated. (*N Eng J Med.* 2005;352:1741-1744. *N Eng J Med.* 1999. 341:1986-1995)

Clinical Evaluation

–Upper and lower gastrointestinal investigations (esophagogastroduodenoscopy and colonoscopy preferred) should be done in all postmenopausal females and all male patients unless there is a history of recent non-Gl significant blood loss. (*Am J Med.* 2001;111:439-445)

–Gastrointestinal evaluation should proceed whether or not fecal occult blood testing is positive. Iron deficiency without significant anemia should also be worked up with Gl evaluation in postmenopausal women and men >40 y old. (*N Engl J Med.* 1993.329:1691-1695)

–If the patient is postgastrectomy upper and lower Gl investigation is indicated in those >40y old. If upper and lower Gl tracts are normal, small bowel visualization is indicated if the patient has symptoms of small bowel disease and/or continued fecal occult blood positive stools. (*Best Pract Res Clin Haematol.* 2005;18:319-322)

Iron Replacement Therapy

–Ferrous sulfate (65-mg elemental iron) should be administered 2 to 3 times a day depending on tolerance. Taking iron 15-30 min before a meal with orange juice or 500 mg of vitamin C will enhance absorption. Treatment should be continued for 4–8 mo to fully replete iron stores.

–20%-25% of patients on iron therapy will have Gl side effects (abdominal bloating, pain, nausea, vomiting, diarrhea/constipation). Reducing the elemental iron concentration of each dose may avoid side effects.

–In patients who continue to be intolerant of iron, noncompliant, or have diminished iron absorption intravenous iron (iron sucrose-Venofer preferred) should be given to replete iron stores and correct the anemia.

Refractory Iron Deficiency

–In patients who have been compliant but do not correct their iron deficiency with oral iron must have further evaluation. Many gastric bypass patients have reduced iron absorption due to bypass of the duodenum where the majority of iron absorption takes place.

–Occasionally patients have significant continued blood loss for which oral iron is insufficient to maintain iron stores. Other possible causes such as celiac sprue, *H. pylori* infection, and autoimmune gastritis must be evaluated and treated. (*Haematologica.* 2005; 90:585-595)

–Antacids and protein pump inhibitors will also reduce iron absorption. Hereditary iron-refractory iron deficiency syndrome is an autosomal recessive disorder caused by mutations affecting iron transport.

–Patients with refractory iron deficiency anemia due to poor absorption are treated successfully with intravenous iron preparations.

Sources

–http://www.guideline.gov/search/search.aspx?term=iron + deficiency+ management. *N Engl J Med.* 2015;372:1832

–*Gut.* 2011;60:1309-1316

Comments

Clinical Correlates

–Symptoms of IDA include weakness, headache, irritability, fatigue, exercise intolerance, and restless leg syndrome. Symptoms may occur without anemia in patients with iron depletion (ferritin <30 ng/mL). As many as 40% of patients with IDA will experience pica (appetite for clay, starch, and paper products) and/or pagophagia (craving for ice) which resolves rapidly with iron repletion.

–Rarely, in severe iron deficiency, dysphagia and esophageal webs (Plummer-Vinson syndrome) occur as well as koilonychia (spoon nails), glossitis with decreased salivary flow, and alopecia also occur with severe prolonged IDA.

–Besides Gl and genitourinary blood loss, other infrequent causes of iron deficiency include intravascular hemolysis (especially paroxysmal nocturnal hemoglobinuria and microangiopathic hemolytic anemia), pulmonary hemosiderosis, and congenital IDA (germline mutation in the TMPRSS6 gene which leads to a reduction in iron absorption and mobilization).

–Optimal absorption of oral iron occurs when iron is taken 15–30 min before a meal with 500 mg of vitamin C or a glass of orange juice. 20%–25% of patients will have Gl side effects including abdominal pain, nausea, constipation, and diarrhea. Side effects are related to the amount of elemental iron delivered with each dose. The most commonly used iron preparation is ferrous sulfate that contains 65 mg of elemental iron. If patients have intolerable Gl problems, lowering the elemental iron intake by giving ferrous gluconate (28–36 mg of elemental iron) or titrating liquid ferrous sulfate (44 mg iron per 5 mL) can be successful although duration of therapy will be extended. Patients who continue to be intolerant of oral iron can be successfully treated with IV iron preparations (iron sucrose preferred). (*Blood.* 2014; 123:326-333. *Transfusion.* 2008;48:988-995)

–A simple iron absorption test can determine whether or not a patient has iron malabsorption. Check a baseline iron level and then a second iron level 2–4 h after ingesting a single 325 mg ferrous sulfate tablet with water. An increase in the iron level of at least l00 µg/dL indicates adequate absorption.

–Other hypochromic, microcytic anemias should be ruled out (see Table I). Diagnosing iron deficiency in patients who also have anemia of chronic disease (ACD) is difficult. Circulating transferrin receptor (sTFR) is elevated when iron deficiency is present and a high sTFR/ferritin index is consistent with concurrent IDA and ACD. A bone marrow examination with absent stainable iron stores, although invasive, will also confirm a diagnosis of IDA in the presence of ACD. Recombinant erythropoietin is not effective in treating anemia in patients who are iron deficient. (*N Engl J Med.* 2014;371:324)

–Indications for IV iron therapy includes refractory noncompliance or side effects, gastric bypass, iron malabsorption, and continued blood loss with IDA and inadequate iron repletion with oral therapy. IV iron causes a modest early increase in reticulocytes compared to oral iron but it still takes 8–10 wk for hemoglobin levels to normalize. Iron dextran was the first IV preparation of iron used but problems with anaphylaxis were significant. Iron sucrose (Venofer®) is effective and has a 15-fold reduction in the risk of anaphylaxis compared to iron dextran. This can be dosed at 150–200 mg once or twice a week until the calculated iron deficit is administered. Ferric gluconate complex (Ferrlecit®) is similar to iron sucrose. Ferumoxytol (Feraheme®) is composed of iron oxide nanoparticle and is approved for use only in patients with renal failure. Ferric carboxymaltose (Ferinject®) is the newest IV iron option with 1,000 mg elemental iron weekly with more rapid infusion times. Low phosphate levels have been reported with this drug. It has also been shown to be helpful in patients with iron deficiency and heart failure. (*Ann Int Med.* 2010;152:4-5)

–In patients who malabsorb iron, further diagnostic studies should be done to look for celiac disease (IgA anti-tissue transglutamine antibody, duodenal biopsy), *Helicobacter pylori* infection of the stomach (dx by stool antigen, urea breath test, gastric biopsy), and autoimmune gastritis (gastrin level, intrinsic factor, and parietal cell antibodies, gastric biopsy) and congenital iron deficiency (recessive germ line mutation in TMPRSS6). (*N Engl J Med.* 2012;366:376-377. *Arch Int Med.* 2000;160:1229-1230. *Blood.* 2014;123:326-333. *Am Fam Physician.* 2013;87:98)

TABLE I

THE COMMON CAUSES OF MICROCYTIC HYPOCHROMIC ANEMIA

Microcytic, Hypochromic Anemia	Ferritin Level	RDW	Hgb Electrophoresis	Iron/TIBC	Mentzer Index[a]
Iron deficiency	<30	High	Normal	<10%	>13
Beta thalassemia	Normal	Normal	↑A$_2$, F hemoglobin	~20%	<13
Alfa thalassemia	Normal	Normal	Normal	~20%	<13
Anemia of chronic disease	High	High	Normal	10%–15% Low transferrin	>13
Hemoglobin E (mutation in beta-globin gene—common in Asia)	Normal	Normal	↑HgbE (30% if trait 90% if homozygote)	~20%	<13

[a]Mentzer index, MCV-red cell number in millions. Iron deficiency >13. Thalassemia minor <13. RDW, random distribution of width ↑ in iron deficiency.

IRRITABLE BOWEL SYNDROME (IBS)

Population
–Adults with symptoms of IBS.

Recommendations
▶ NICE 2015
–Consider IBS for any adult with any of these symptoms for at least 6 mo.
  • Abdominal pain.
  • Bloating.
  • Change in bowel habit.
–Assess all patients with possible IBS for red flag indicators that argue against IBS.
  • Unintentional weight loss.
  • Rectal bleeding.
  • Anemia.
  • Abdominal mass.
  • Change in bowel habit to looser and more frequent stools if over 60 y.
–Recommend for all patients with suspected IBS.
  • Complete blood count.
  • ESR.
  • C-reactive protein.
  • Anti-endomysial antibody and anti-tissue transglutaminase antibody to rule out celiac disease.
–Lifestyle recommendations for IBS.
  • Eat regular meals.
  • Drink at least 8 cups of non-caffeinated beverage daily.
  • Limit intake of tea, coffee, and alcohol.
  • Reduce intake of "resistant starch."
  • Avoid sorbitol, an artificial sweeteners, for diarrhea-predominant IBS.
–Pharmacologic therapy for IBS.
  • Consider laxatives as needed (except lactulose) for constipation.
  • Consider linaclotide for refractory constipation for longer than 12 mo.
  • Consider antispasmodic agents as needed for pain.
  • Loperamide is the antimotility agent of choice for diarrhea.
  • Consider low-dose tricyclics (TCAs) as second-line treatment if antispasmodics or antimotility agents have not helped.
  • Consider SSRI therapy if TCAs are ineffective.
  • Consider cognitive behavioral therapy or hypnotherapy for IBS refractory to above therapies.

Source
–https://guidelines.gov/summaries/summary/49049

KIDNEY DISEASE, CHRONIC

Population
–Adults.

Recommendations

▶ NICE 2008

1. Recommends the modification of diet in renal disease (MDRD) equation to estimate GFR.
   a. Advise patients not to eat any meat in the 12 h before a blood test for GFR estimation.
   b. Frequency of GFR testing by CKD stage:
      i. Stages 1–2: annually.
      ii. Stage 3: every 6 mo.
      iii. Stage 4: every 3 mo.
      iv. Stage 5: every 6 wk.
2. Recommends urine albumin-to-creatinine ratio (ACR) to detect low levels of proteinuria.
   a. Levels ≥30 mg/mmol are significant.
3. Recommends checking for urinary tract malignancy for persistent hematuria.
4. Recommend renal ultrasound for:
   a. A GFR decline >5 mL/min/1.73 m^2 in 1 y or >10 mL/min/1.73 m^2 in 5 y.
   b. Persistent hematuria.
   c. Symptoms of urinary tract obstruction.
   d. Age >20 y and has a family history of polycystic kidney disease.
   e. Stages 4–5 CKD.
   f. Being considered for a renal biopsy.
5. Recommends nephrology referral for:
   a. Stages 4–5 CKD.
   b. ACR ≥70 mg/mmol.
   c. Proteinuria ≥1 g/24 h.
   d. Poorly controlled HTN.
   e. Suspected renal artery stenosis.
   f. Rapidly progressive renal impairment.
   g. Metabolic complications of CKD (anemia or hyperparathyroidism).
   h. Nephrolithiasis.

6. Recommends a check of serum calcium, phosphate, intact parathyroid hormone (iPTH), 25-OH vitamin D, and hemoglobin levels for all Stages 4–5 CKD.

Source
   –http://www.nice.org.uk/nicemedia/live/12069/42117/42117.pdf

▶ Va/DoD 2014

   –Recommends dietary sodium restriction to reduce hypertension and proteinuria.
   –Protein restriction 0.6–0.8 g/kg/d for patients with Stage 3–4 CKD.
   –Recommends administration of vaccinations against influenza, Tdap, 13-valent pneumococcal conjugate vaccine, hepatitis B virus, Zoster, and MMR vaccines.
   –Recommends ACEI or ARB therapy for patients with diabetes, hypertension, or albuminuria.
   –Recommends bicarbonate supplementation in CKD with metabolic acidosis.
   –Recommends oral iron therapy for Stage 3 or worse CKD.
   –Recommends erythropoietic-stimulating agents if hemoglobin <10 g/dL.

Source
   –http://www.guideline.gov/content.aspx?id=48951

KIDNEY DISEASE, CHRONIC–MINERAL AND BONE DISORDERS (CKD-MBDS)

Population
   –Adults and children.

Recommendations

▶ NKF 2009

1. Recommends monitoring serum calcium, phosphorus, immunoreactive parathyroid hormone (iPTH), and alkaline phosphatase levels for:
   a. Stage 3 CKD (adults).
   b. Stage 2 CKD (children).
2. Measure 25-OH vitamin D levels beginning in stage 3 CKD.
3. Recommends treating all vitamin D deficiency with vitamin D supplementation.
4. In Stages 3–5 CKD, consider a bone biopsy before bisphosphonate therapy if a dynamic bone disease is a possibility.

5. In Stages 3–5 CKD, aim to normalize calcium and phosphorus levels.
6. In Stage 5 CKD, maintain a parathyroid hormone (PTH) level of 130–600 pg/mL.

Source
–http://kdigo.org/home/mineral-bone-disorder/

Comment
1. Options for oral phosphate binders:
   a. Calcium acetate.
   b. Calcium carbonate.
   c. Calcium citrate.
   d. Sevelamer carbonate.
   e. Lanthanum carbonate.

KIDNEY INJURY, ACUTE

Population
–Children and adults.

Recommendations
▶ NICE 2013
–Perform a urinalysis in all patients with AKI.
–Do not routinely obtain a renal ultrasound when the cause of the AKI has been identified.
–Detect AKI with any of the following criteria:
   • Rise in serum creatinine ≥0.3 mg/dL in 48 h.
   • 50% or more rise in creatinine in last 7 d.
   • Urine output <0.5 mL/kg/h.
–Refer for renal replacement therapy patients with any of the following refractory to medical management:
   • Hyperkalemia.
   • Metabolic acidosis.
   • Uremia.
   • Fluid overload.

Source
–http://www.guideline.gov/content.aspx?id=47080

KIDNEY STONES

Population
–Adults and children with kidney stone disease.

Recommendations

▶ EAU 2010, AUA 2014

1. Recommended imaging study for patients with acute flank pain is a noncontrast CT urogram.
2. Recommended evaluation for renal colic:
   a. Urinalysis
   b. Serum CBC, creatinine, uric acid, calcium, and albumin +/– intact parathyroid hormone.
   c. Stone analysis by x-ray crystallography or infrared spectroscopy.
3. Recommends 24-h urine analysis for complicated calcium stone disease: calcium; oxalate; citrate; creatinine; urate; magnesium; phosphate; sodium; and potassium.
4. Recommends a thiazide diuretic for patients with hypercalciuria.
5. Recommends treatment with an alkaline citrate for hypocitraturia, type 1 renal tubular acidosis (RTA), hypercalciuria, and hyperoxaluria.
6. Recommends that adults with a history of urinary stones drink sufficient water to maintain a urine output >2.5 L/d.
7. Consider use of an α-receptor blocker to facilitate spontaneous passage of ureteral stones <10 mm.
8. Consider active ureteral stone removal for persistent obstruction, failure of spontaneous passage, or the presence of severe, unremitting colic.
   a. Options include shockwave lithotripsy or ureteroscopy.
9. For calcium stones and hypercalciuria
   a. Limit sodium intake and consume 1–2 g/d of dietary calcium.
   b. Thiazide diuretic.
10. For calcium oxalate stones
    a. If high urinary oxalate, limit intake of oxalate-rich foods and maintain normal calcium consumption.
    b. If hyperuricosuria, treat with allopurinol.
11. For uric acid stones and high urinary uric acid, limit intake of non-dairy animal protein.
12. For struvite stones refractory to surgical management, consider acetohydroxamic acid therapy.
13. For uric acid or cystine stones, consider potassium citrate therapy to raise urinary pH to optimal level.

Sources
   –http://www.uroweb.org/gls/pdf/18_Urolithiasis.pdf
   –http://www.guideline.gov/content.aspx?id=48229

Comment

1. Patients at high risk for recurrent stone formation:
   a. ≥3 stones in 3 y.
   b. Infection stones.
   c. Urate stones.
   d. Children and adolescents with stones.
   e. Cystinuria.
   f. Primary hyperoxaluria.
   g. Type 1 RTA.
   h. Cystic fibrosis.
   i. Hyperparathyroidism.
   j. Crohn's disease.
   k. Malabsorption syndromes.
   l. Nephrocalcinosis.
   m. Family history of kidney stone disease.

Population

   –Adults with kidney stone disease.

Recommendations

▶ EAU 2013

   –Recommended evaluation for renal colic:
   • Sodium, potassium.
   • CRP.
   • PT, PTT (if intervention is likely).
   –Contrast-enhanced CT scan recommended if stone removal is planned and the renal anatomy needs to be assessed.
   –Hyperoxaluria.
   • Oxalate restriction.
   • Pyridoxine.
   –Renal colic analgesia.
   • NSAIDs.
   • Opiates.
   • Alpha-blockers.
   –Management of sepsis with obstructed kidney.
   • Requires urgent decompression with a ureteral stent or percutaneous nephrostomy tubes.
   • Start antibiotics immediately.

–Indications for active kidney stone treatment:
- Stone growth.
- Acute or chronic pain.
- Kidney infection.
- Kidney obstruction.

▶ EAU 2013

–Stop antiplatelets and anticoagulation before stone removal.
–Goal is to drink water to maintain a urine output >2.5 L/d.
–Struvite and infection stones:
- Surgical removal of stones.
- Antibiotics.
- Urinary acidification.
- Urease inhibition.

–Cystine stones.
- Potassium citrate.

–Tiopronin.

Source
–http://www.guideline.gov/content.aspx?id=45324

Population
–Children with kidney stone disease.

Recommendations

▶ EAU 2013

–Recommends a complete metabolic work-up based on stone analysis.
–Ultrasound is the preferred imaging method in children.
–Percutaneous nephrolithotripsy is recommended for treatment of renal pelvic or calyceal stones with a diameter >20 mm.

Source
–http://www.guideline.gov/content.aspx?id=45324

LARYNGITIS, ACUTE

Population
–Adults.

Recommendation

▶ Cochrane Database Systematic Reviews 2015

–Insufficient evidence to support the use of antibiotics for acute laryngitis.

Source
–http://www.cochrane.org/CD004783/ARI_antibiotics-to-treat-adults-with-acute-laryngitis

Comment

–Many methodological flaws in studies evaluated.

MALIGNANT SPINAL CORD COMPRESSION (MSCC)

Population

–Adults with MSCC.

Recommendation

▶ Scottish Palliative Care Guidelines 2014, National Collaborating Centre for Cancer—Metastatic Spinal Cord Compression (MSCC) 2012

–**Stratify Patient for Therapy**

- Patients presenting with >48 h for paraplegia—radiation for pain control, surgery only if spine is unstable.
- The chance for neurological recovery is zero. (*Lancet Oncol.* 2005;6:15)
- Patients presenting with significant or progressing weakness of lower extremities—if no previous history of cancer biopsy non-neural cancer if accessible. If biopsy not possible and lymphoma or myeloma unlikely give decadron 40 to 100 mg daily and take to surgery to make tissue diagnosis and relieve compression of spinal cord. (*Neurology.* 1989;39:1255. *Lancet Neurol.* 2008;7:459) If unstable, the spine should be stabilized. Taper steroids (decrease by ½ every 3 d) and begin radiation in 2–3 w. If tumor is lymphoma or myeloma, consider initiating chemotherapy and high-dose decadron. Recovery of lower extremity strength dependent on degree of paraparesis initially.
- Patients presenting with back pain but mild neurologic symptoms—if no previous cancer find site to biopsy, check PSA, serum protein electrophoresis, beta-2 microglobulin, and alfa-fetoprotein. Begin moderate-dose decadron (16 mg/d) with radiation therapy initially. Surgery reserved for progression of symptoms after starting radiation especially in radioinsensitive cancers (renal cell, sarcoma, melanoma). Recovery of neurologic function in 80%–90% range.
- Patients presenting with back pain but no neurologic symptoms—if no previous diagnosis of cancer search for site to biopsy (physical exam, PET CT scan, tumor markers) and consult radiation therapy. If myeloma or lymphoma, treat with systemic chemotherapy. Radiation is primary treatment with surgery only on progression. Low dose or no steroids is acceptable. Chance of continued lower extremity strength approaches 100%.

Sources
  –*Int J Radiat Oncol Biol/Phys.* 2012;84:312
  –*Quart J Med.* 2014;107:277–282
  –N Engl J Med. 2017;376:1358

Comment

  –**Clinical Considerations**
   • MRI with and without gadolinium of the entire spine is mandatory. 30% of patients will have cord compression in more than 1 area.
   • 20% of patients presenting with MSCC have not had a previous diagnosis of cancer.
   • 5%–8% of patients with known cancer will develop MSCC during their course of disease.
   • Most common tumors associated with MSCC are lung, breast, prostate, myeloma, and lymphoma.
   • Most common site of MSCC is the thoracic spine (70%) and least common is cervical spine (10%).
   • Back pain presents in 95% of patients with average time to MSCC being 6–7 wk. Once motor, sensory, or autonomic dysfunction occur—time to total paraplegia is rapid (hours to days).
   • Indications for surgery in MSCC include lack of diagnosis, progression on radiation, unstable fracture or bone in spinal canal, and previous radiation to site of MSCC. (*Int J Oncol.* 2011;38:5. *J Clin Onc.* 2011;29:3072)
   • Posterior decompression laminectomy was standard surgery for MSCC, but now resection of tumor with bone reconstruction and stabilization is done most commonly at centers of excellence.
   • Stereotactic body radiation therapy is being used more commonly with improved results especially in radiation-resistant cancers. (*Cancer.* 2010;116:2258)

MANAGEMENT OF VENOUS THROMBOSIS IN PATIENTS WITH CANCER

Population

  –Adult men and women with cancer.

Recommendation

▶ ASCO Clinical Practice Guidelines

  –Most hospitalized patients with active cancer require thromboprophylaxis throughout hospitalization. Data are inadequate to support routine thromboprophylaxis in patients for minor procedures or short chemotherapy infusions.

–Routine thrombophylaxis is not recommended for ambulatory patients with cancer. It may be considered for selected high-risk patients.

–Patients with multiple myeloma receiving antiangiogenesis agents with chemotherapy and/or dexamethasone should receive prophylaxis with either low-molecular-weight heparin (LMWH) or low-dose aspirin to prevent venous thromboembolism (VTE).

–Patients undergoing major cancer surgery should receive prophylaxis starting before surgery and continuing for at least 7 to 10 d after discharge (30-mg enoxaparin bid).

–Extending postoperative prophylaxis up to 4 wk should be considered in those undergoing major abdominal or pelvic surgery with high-risk features.

–LMWH is recommended for the initial 5 to 10 d of treament of established deep vein thrombosis and pulmonary embolism as well as for long-term secondary prophylaxis for at least 6 mo. If the cancer remains active, LMWH should be given indefinitely.

–Use of novel oral anticoagulants is not currently recommended for patients with malignancy and VTE but trials are ongoing to prove benefit.

–Anticoagulation should not be used to extend survival of patients with end-stage cancer in the absence of other indications.

–Patients with cancer should be periodically assessed for VTE risk.

–Oncology professionals should educate patients about signs and symptoms of VTE.

Source

–*J Clin Oncol.* 2015;33:654-656
–*J Clin Oncol.* 2013;31:2189-2204

Comments

1. VTE is the second leading cause of death among cancer patients. The highest risk cancers related to VTE are stomach and pancreas (15%). Significant risk is also associated with lung cancer, lymphoma, gynecological cancer, bladder, and testis cancer (6%).

2. Prostate and breast cancer have a significantly lower risk of VTE (0.8%-2%). Other risk factors include platelet count greater than 350,000, use of red cell growth factors, white blood cell count greater than 12,000, and BMI 35 kg/m^2 or higher. Inferior vena cava (IVC) filters should only be used when there is documented DVT but a contraindication to anticoagulation active bleed, melanoma, renal cell cancer or choriocarcinoma with untreated brain metastasis, platelets below 30,000 or severe platelet dysfunction. The IVC filter must be removed as soon as anticoagulation is begun. The new direct oral anticogulants are in trials but thus far have not been approved for patients with cancer and VTE.

3. It has been shown that in patients who present with unprovoked VTE, routine evaluation will discover 3%-5% of patients who have an underlying malignancy. A more extended work-up will find additional cancers, but this has not been shown to decrease the risk of dying from the underlying cancer. Therefore, extensive evaluation is not indicated.

4. Chemotherapy (1.8-fold risk) and tamoxifen (5.5-fold risk) also predispose to VTE and these patients should be followed closely. In patients who develop clot in a vein with an indwelling venous catheter are initially managed with anticoagulation with the catheter in place. If there is pain, edema, or progression of the clot, the catheter must be removed.

Sources
–*Ann Oncol.* 2011;22(Suppl 6):v85-v92.

–*Blood.* 2013;122:2310-2317.

–*J Thromb Thrombolysis.* 2016;41:81-91

–*NCCN guidelines on cancer associated venous thromboembolic disease.* 2014.

MENINGITIS, BACTERIAL

Population
–Children and adults.

Recommendation

▶ Cochrane Database of Systematic Reviews 2013
–Recommends corticosteroids prior to or when antibiotics are administered for presumed bacterial meningitis in high-income countries.

Source
–http://onlinelibrary.wiley.com/doi/10.1002/14651858.CD004405.pub4/pdf/abstract

Comments
1. Corticosteroids significantly reduced the incidence of hearing loss and neurological sequelae in bacterial meningitis.

2. Corticosteroids reduced mortality in meningitis from *Streptococcus pneumoniae*, but not with *Haemophilus influenzae* or *Neisseria meningitidis* infections.

3. No beneficial effect of corticosteroids in low-income countries.

MENOPAUSE

Population
–Menopausal women.

Recommendations

▶ AACE 2011

–Indications for menopausal hormone therapy:
- Severe menopausal symptoms.
- Severe vulvovaginal atrophy.
- Consider transdermal or topical estrogens which may reduce the risk of VTE.
- Treatment of osteoporosis.

–Cautions with menopausal hormone therapy:
- Avoid unopposed estrogen use in women with an intact uterus.
- Use hormonal therapy in the lowest effective dose for the shortest duration possible.
- Custom-compounded bioidentical hormone therapy is *not* recommended.
- Not appropriate for prevention or treatment of dementia.
- Avoid if at high risk for VTE.
- Not recommended for prevention or treatment of cardiovascular disease.

–Contraindications of menopausal hormone therapy:
- History of breast CA.
- Suspected estrogen-sensitive malignancy.
- Undiagnosed vaginal bleeding.
- Endometrial hyperplasia.
- History of VTE.
- Untreated hypertension.
- Active liver disease.
- Porphyria cutanea tarda.

Source
–https://www.aace.com/files/menopause.pdf

Comment
–Use of hormone therapy should always occur after a thorough discussion of the risks, benefits, and alternatives of this treatment with the patient.

Recommendations

▶ NICE 2015

  –Consider short-term hormone replacement therapy (HRT) for:
  - Severe vasomotor symptoms.
  - Menopause-related depression.
  - Poor libido.
  - Urogenital atrophy.

  –Consider adjuvant testosterone therapy for decreased libido despite HRT.

  –Offer vaginal estrogen cream for urogenital atrophy.

Source

  –https://guidelines.gov/summaries/summary/49904

Comment

  –Review risks of HRT before initiating:
  - Venous thromboembolism (VTE).
  - May slightly increase risk of breast CA.

Recommendations

▶ Endocrine Society 2015

  –Recommends HRT for severe vasomotor symptoms in women less than 60 y who do not have excess cardiovascular or breast cancer risk.

  –Recommends nonhormonal remedies for women at high risk of cardiovascular disease or breast cancer.
  - Options include a SSRI, SNRI, gabapentin, or pregabalin.

  –For women at increased risk of VTE, recommend transdermal estrogen and progesterone for severe vasomotor symptoms.

  –Recommends vaginal estrogen cream for urogenital atrophy unless history of a hormone-dependent cancer.

  –Consider ospemifene trial for moderate-to-severe dyspareunia.

Source

  –https://guidelines.gov/summaries/summary/49985

METABOLIC SYNDROME

METABOLIC SYNDROME: IDENTIFICATION AND MANAGEMENT

Clinical Identification

Risk Factor	Defining Level[a]
Abdominal obesity (waist circumference)[b]	
Men	>102 cm (>40 in.)
Women	>88 cm (>35 in.)

METABOLIC SYNDROME: IDENTIFICATION AND MANAGEMENT   *(Continued)*

Clinical Identification

Risk Factor	Defining Level[a]
Triglycerides	≥150 mg/dL
HDL cholesterol	
Men	<40 mg/dL
Women	<50 mg/dL
Blood pressure	≥135/≥85 mm Hg
Fasting glucose	≥100 mg/dL

Management

- First-line therapy: Lifestyle modification leading to weight reduction and increased physical activity.
- Goal: ↓ Body weight by approximately 7%–10% over 6–12 mo.
- At least 30 min of daily moderate-intensity physical activity.
- Low intake of saturated fats, trans fats, and cholesterol.
- Reduced consumption of simple sugars.
- Increased intake of fruits, vegetables, and whole grains.
- Avoid extremes in intake of either carbohydrates or fats.
- Smoking cessation.
- Drug therapy for HTN, elevated LDL cholesterol, and diabetes.
- Consider combination therapy with fibrates or nicotinic acid plus a statin.
- Low-dose ASA for patients at intermediate and high risk.
- Bariatric surgery for BMI >35 mg/kg^2.
- If one component is identified, a systematic search for the others is indicated, together with an active approach to managing all risk factors. (*Eur Heart J.* 2007;28:2375-2414)
- Metabolic syndrome is associated with the presence of subclinical ischemic brain lesions independent of other risk factors. (*Stroke.* 2008;39:1607-1609)
- In patients with atherosclerosis, the presence of metabolic syndrome is associated with an increased risk of cardiovascular event and all-cause mortality, independent of the presence of diabetes. (*Eur Heart J.* 2008;29:213-223)

ASA, aspirin; BMI, body mass index; HDL, high-density lipoprotein; HTN, hypertension; LDL, low-density lipoprotein.
[a]NCEP ATP III definition (*Circulation.* 2005;112:2735-2752)—requires any three of the listed components.
[b]Waist circumference can identify persons at greater cardiometabolic risk than are identified by BMI alone. However, further studies are needed to establish waist circumference cutpoints that assess risk not adequately captured by BMI (*Am J Clin Nutr.* 2007;85:1197-1202).

Note: The WHO and International Diabetes Federation (IDF, http://www.idf.org) define metabolic syndrome slightly differently. One study found a 5-fold difference in the prevalence of metabolic syndrome depending on which of seven diagnostic criteria were used. (*Metabolism.* 2008;57:355-361) There is no official definition of metabolic syndrome in children, but a constellation of conditions confers significant increased risk of coronary heart disease. (*Circulation.* 2007;115:1948-1967)
Source: NCEP 2005, ATP III 2005.

METHICILLIN-RESISTANT *STAPHYLOCOCCUS AUREUS* INFECTIONS

TREATMENT OF METHICILLIN-RESISTANT *STAPHYLOCOCCUS AUREUS* INFECTIONS (MRSA) IN ADULTS AND CHILDREN

Infection	Primary Therapy	Alternative Therapy	Comments

Abscess associated with extensive involvement; cellulitis; systemic illness; immuno-suppression; extremes of age; involvement of face, hands, or genitalia; septic phlebitis; trauma; infected ulcer or burn; or poor response to incision and drainage	1. Incision and drainage
	2. Antibiotics
	  a. Outpatient
	    i. Clindamycin
	    ii. Trimethoprim-sulfamethoxazole (TMP-SMX)
	  b. Inpatient
	    i. Vancomycin
	    ii. Linezolid
	    iii. Daptomycin
		1. Outpatient antibiotics
		  a. Tetracycline
		  b. Linezolid
		2. Inpatient antibiotics
		  a. Telavancin
		  b. Clindamycin
			1. Tetracyclines should not be used in children age <8 y.
			2. Vancomycin is recommended for hospitalized children.
			3. Clindamycin and linezolid are alternative choices for children.

Recurrent skin and soft-tissue infections (SSTIs)	1. Cover draining wounds.
	2. Maintain good hygiene.
	3. Avoid reusing or sharing personal toiletries.
	4. Use oral antibiotics only for active infections.
		1. Decolonization only if recurrent SSTI despite good hygiene
		  a. Mupirocin per nares bid × 5–10 d
		  b. Chlorhexidine or dilute bleach baths twice weekly (BIW) × 1–2 wk
			Screening cultures prior to decolonization or surveillance cultures after decolonization is not recommended.

Uncomplicated MRSA bacteremia[a]	Vancomycin × 2 wk	Daptomycin × 2 wk	Echocardiography is recommended for all MRSA bacteremia.

TREATMENT OF METHICILLIN-RESISTANT *STAPHYLOCOCCUS AUREUS* INFECTIONS (MRSA) IN ADULTS AND CHILDREN *(Continued)*

Infection	Primary Therapy	Alternative Therapy	Comments
MRSA native valve endocarditis	Vancomycin × 6 wk	Daptomycin × 6 wk	1. Synergistic gentamicin or rifampin is not indicated for native valve endocarditis. 2. Vancomycin is the drug of choice for children.
MRSA prosthetic valve endocarditis	1. Vancomycin plus rifampin × 6 wk 2. Gentamicin 1 mg/kg IV q8h × 2 wk		Recommend early evaluation for valve replacement surgery.
MRSA pneumonia	1. Vancomycin 2. Linezolid	Clindamycin	1. Duration of therapy is 7–21 d. 2. Vancomycin for children.
MRSA osteomyelitis	1. Surgical débridement 2. Vancomycin 3. Daptomycin 4. Duration of therapy is at least 8 wk	1. Linezolid 2. TMP-SMX plus rifampin 3. Clindamycin	
MRSA septic arthritis	1. Drain or débride the joint space 2. Vancomycin	Daptomycin	Duration of therapy is 3–4 wk.
MRSA meningitis	1. Vancomycin × 2 wk	1. Linezolid 2. TMP-SMX	Consider adding rifampin.

aNo endocarditis, no implanted prostheses, defervescence within 72 h, sterile blood cultures within 72 h, and no evidence of metastatic sites of infection.

Source: IDSA 2011 Clinical Practice Guideline. *Clin Infect Dis.* 2011;52:1-38.

MULTIPLE SCLEROSIS (MS)

Population
–Adults.

Recommendations

▶ AAN 2014

1. Consider oral cannabis extract or Sativex oromucosal cannabinoid spray to patients with MS with spasticity and pain (central neuropathic pain).
2. May consider a trial of Gingko biloba or magnetic therapy for reducing fatigue.
3. Recommend against a low-fat diet with ω-3 fatty acid or lofepramine use or bee venom therapy to reduce relapses, depression, or fatigue.
4. Reflexology may benefit paresthesias.

Source
–http://www.guideline.gov/content.aspx?id=47909

MUSCLE CRAMPS

Population
–Patients with idiopathic muscle cramps.

Recommendations

▶ AAN 2010

–Data are insufficient on the efficacy of calf stretching in reducing the frequency of muscle cramps.
–AAN recommends that although quinine is likely effective, it should not be used for routine treatment of cramps. Quinine derivatives should be reserved for disabling muscle cramps.
–Quinine derivatives are effective in reducing the frequency of muscle cramps, although the magnitude of benefit is small and than the serious side effects.

Source
–Katzberg HD, Khan AH, So YT. Assessment: symptomatic treatment for muscle cramps (an evidence-based review): report of the Therapeutics and Technology Assessment Subcommittee of the American Academy of Neurology. *Neurology.* 2010 Feb 23;74(8):691-696.

NEUROCYSTICERCOSIS

Population
–Adults and children with intraparenchymal neurocysticercosis.

Recommendations

▶ AAN 2013

–For symptomatic intraparenchymal neurocysticercosis, use albendazole plus either dexamethasone or prednisolone to decrease the number of active lesions and reduce the long-term seizure frequency.

–No evidence to support steroids alone in patients with intraparenchymal neurocysticercosis.

–It is reasonable to treat these patients with anti-epileptic drugs until the active lesions have subsided (expert opinion).

Source

–Baird RA, Wiebe S, Zunt JR, Halperin JJ, Gronseth G, Roos KL. Evidence-based guideline: treatment of parenchymal neurocysticercosis: Report of the Guideline Development Subcommittee of the American Academy of Neurology. *Neurology.* 2013 Apr 9;80(15):1424-1429.

NEUTROPENIA, FEBRILE

Population
–Patients with single temperature >100.9°F (38.3°C) or ≥100.4°F (38.0°C) for >1 h in the setting of neutropenia (absolute neutrophil count including granulocytes and bands <500/mm^3).

Recommendation

▶ Infectious Disease Society of America 2011

–**Evaluation and Therapy**

• Two sets of blood cultures/urine C+S/chemistries. CXR/ancillary studies based on clinical evaluation. Begin antibiotics as rapidly as possible within 60 min.

- Stratify into **LOW RISK**[a] (absence of comorbidity, no cardiovascular compromise, expected duration of neutropenia <7 d, compliant) vs. **HIGH RISK**[a] (absolute neutrophil count [ANC] <100 comorbidity, cardiovascular compromise, unreliable, expected duration of neutropenia >7 d).
- High-risk patients must be admitted to hospital with rapid initiation of single-agent antibiotic (cefepime, imipenem, ceftazidime) or combination therapy (extended spectrum beta-lactam plus either aminoglycoside or fluoroquinolone) depending on clinical features. Add antifungal agent if continued fever and negative cultures after 4–7 d.
- Selected low-risk patients can be treated as an outpatient with oral ciprofloxacin 500 mg bid and Augmentin 875 mg bid with <5% requiring hospitalization for worsening symptoms. Close communication with patient is essential.
- Continue broad-spectrum antibiotics in both low- and high-risk groups until ANC >500. Adjust antibiotics based on positive cultures and switch to oral to complete a 10–14 d course of antibiotics.

Sources
–*Clin Infect Dis.* 2011;52:e56-e93
–*J Clin Oncol.* 2013;31:794-810
–*J Oncol Pract.* 2015;11:450.

Comment
–**Clinical Concerns**
- Prophylactic granulocyte colony-stimulating factor (GCSF) should be used in patients on chemotherapy with an expected rate of FN of ≥20%. Secondary use of GCSF after FN shortens hospital stay by 1 d but has no impact on survival.
- Vancomycin should not be given empirically unless history of MRSA, catheter tunnel infection, presence of pneumonia, or soft-tissue infection.

---

[a]Multinational Association for Supportive Care in Cancer (MASCC)
- Symptoms no or mild = 5, moderate = 3, severe = 0
- No hypotension–5
- No COPD–4
- No previous fungal infection–4
- No dehydration requiring parenteral fluids–3
- Outpatient status–3
- Age <60–2
- High risk ≤ 21; Low risk ≥ 21

- Three other unique organisms requiring antibiotic adjustment:
  - Vancomycin-resistant enterococci (VRE)—use linezolid or daptomycin or ceftarolin.
  - Extended-spectrum beta-lactamase (ESBL) producing gram-negative bacteria—use imipenem, meropenem, or ertapenum.
  - Carbapenemase-producing organism (*Klebsiella*)—use polymyxin-colistin or tigecycline; meropenem can be added.
- If central venous catheter (CVC) line infection suspected, draw blood cultures from CVC and peripheral vein. If CVC culture grows out >120 min before peripheral blood cultures, then CVC is the source of infection.
- CVC must be removed if infected with *Staphylococcus aureus*, *Pseudomonas*, and other gram-negative bacteria, fungi, or mycobacteria, as well as tunnel or port pocket infection. If the organism is coagulation-negative *Staphylococcus*, retain CVC and treat with an antibiotic for 4 to 6 wk with 85% cure rate.
- In afebrile patients with ANC <100 give oral fluoroquinolone to lower risk of severe infection.
- With ANC <100 risk of serious infection is 10% per day.

NON-SMALL CELL LUNG CANCER (NSCLC) FOLLOW-UP CARE

Population
–Non-small cell lung cancer patients treated with curative intent.

Recommendation
▶ American College of Chest Physicians (ACCP) 2013
–Follow-up Program
- Chest CT scan should be performed every 6 mo for first 2 y after resection then once a year thereafter out to 10 y (second primary in 10% who survive 1st lung cancer).
- Routine imaging with PET scanning is not recommended.
- Patients should be seen every 3–4 mo for 2 y then less frequently. Health-related quality of life should be assessed with each visit.
- Surveillance biomarker testing should not be done outside of clinical trials.
- Smoking cessation interventions recommended. Annual influenza vaccine and every 5 y pneumococcal vaccinations encouraged.

Source
–*JAMA*. 2010;303:1070

Comment

–Lung Cancer Facts

- Only 30%–35% of patients diagnosed with NSCLC are candidates for surgery with curative intent. Lung CA is responsible for 165,000 deaths/y.
- Cure rates are reflective of stage:
  - ◦ Stage I— 65%–70%
  - ◦ Stage II—40%
  - ◦ Stage IIIA—25%
  - ◦ Stage IIIB—18%
- Platinum-based chemotherapy is standard of care for NSCLC resected for cure. This adjuvant therapy reduces recurrence risk by 5%–10%.
- Symptoms of local recurrence include increase or change in cough, dyspnea, and chest pain.
- Lung cancer is the most common malignancy to metastasize to brain—headache or neurologic symptoms should be an indication for brain MRI with gadolinium.
- In older, compromised patients with a Stage I lung cancer, less than 3 cm in size, treatment with radiosteriotactic body radiation has a 70%–75% chance of prolonged disease-free survival.

NORMAL PRESSURE HYDROCEPHALUS (NPH)

Population

–Patients with normal pressure hydrocephalus.

Recommendations

▶ AAN 2015

–Shunting is a treatment option for NPH with gait abnormalities.

–A positive response to a therapeutic lumbar puncture increases the chance of success with shunting.

–Patients with an impaired cerebral blood flow reactivity to acetazolamide, measured by SPECT, are more likely to respond to shunting.

Source

–https://guidelines.gov/summaries/summary/49957

OBESITY

MANAGEMENT OF OBESITY IN MATURE ADOLESCENTS AND ADULTS

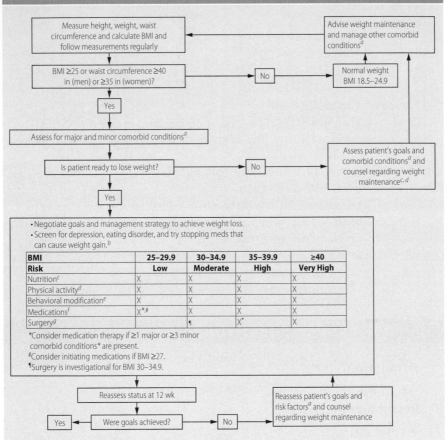

^a**Minor comorbid conditions:** cigarette smoking; hypertension; LDL cholesterol >130 mg/dL; HDL cholesterol <40 mg/dL (men) or <50 mg/dL (women); glucose intolerance; family history of premature CAD; age ≥65 y (men) or 55 y (women).

Major comorbid conditions: waist circumference ≥40 in. (men) or ≥35 in. (women); CAD; peripheral vascular disease; abdominal aortic aneurysm; symptomatic carotid artery disease; type 2 diabetes; and obstructive sleep apnea.

^bSulfonylureas; thiazolidinediones; olanzapine, clozapine; risperidone, quetiapine; lithium; paroxetine, citalopram, sertraline; carbamazepine; pregabalin; corticosteroids; megestrol acetate; cyproheptadine; tricyclic antidepressants; monoamine oxidase inhibitors; mirtazapine; valproic acid; and gabapentin.

^cEncourage a healthy, balanced diet including daily intake of ≥5 servings of fruits/vegetables; 35 g fiber; <30% calories from fat; eliminate takeout, fast foods, soda, and desserts; dietician consultation for a calorie reduction between 500 and 1000 kcal/kg/d to achieve a 1–2 lb weight reduction per week.

^dRecommend 30–60 min of moderate activity at least 5 d a week.

^eIdentify behaviors that may contribute to weight gain (stress, emotional eating, boredom) and use cognitive behavioral counseling, stimulus control, relapse prevention, and goal setting to decrease caloric intake and increase physical activity.

ᶠMedications that are FDA approved for weight loss: phentermine; orlistat; lorcaserin phendimetrazine; diethylpropion; and benzphetamine can be used for up to 3 mo as an adjunct for weight loss.
ᵍBariatric surgery is indicated for patients at high risk for complications. They should be motivated, psychologically stable, have no surgical contraindications, and must accept the operative risk involved.

Source: Adapted from the ICSI Guideline on the Prevention and Management of Obesity available at http://www.icsi.org/obesity/obesity_3398.html and from pharmacologic management of obesity: an Endocrine Society CPG available at https://academic.oup.com/jcem/article/100/2/342/2813109/Pharmacological-Management-of-Obesity-An-Endocrine.

Population
–Adults with DM 2.

Recommendations

▶ NICE 2015

–Desire BP <140/90 mm Hg.

–Desire BP <130/80 mm Hg if patient has nephropathy, retinopathy, or history of CVA.

–Recommend against antiplatelet therapy for primary prophylaxis of cardiovascular disease.

–Monitor glycohemoglobin every 3–6 mo.

–First-line therapy is metformin.

Source
–https://guidelines.gov/summaries/summary/49931

OSTEOARTHRITIS (OA)

Population
–Adults.

Recommendations

▶ ACR 2012

–Nonpharmacologic recommendations for the management of hand OA
- Evaluate ability to perform activities of daily living (ADLs).
- Instruct in joint-protection techniques.
- Provide assistive devices to help perform ADLs.
- Instruct in use of thermal modalities.
- Provide splints for trapeziometacarpal joint OA.

–Nonpharmacologic recommendations for the management of knee or hip OA
- Participate in aquatic exercise.
- Lose weight.
- Start aerobic exercise program.

- Instruct in use of thermal modalities.
- Consider for knee OA:
  - Medially directed patellar taping.
  - Wedged insoles for either medial or lateral compartment OA.
- –Pharmacologic options for OA
  - Topical capsaicin.
  - Topical or PO NSAIDs.
  - Acetaminophen.
  - Tramadol.
  - Intraarticular steroids is an option for refractory knee or hip OA.

Source
  –http://www.rheumatology.org/practice/clinical/guidelines/PDFs/ACR_
  OA_Guidelines_FINAL.pdf

Comment
1. The following should *not* be used for OA:
   - Chondroitin sulfate.
   - Glucosamine.
   - Opiates (if possible).

Population
  –Adults with osteoarthritis.

Recommendations
▶ NICE 2014
  –Recommends exercise as a core treatment to include muscle
  strengthening and general aerobic fitness.
  –Recommends weight loss for people who are obese.
  –Recommends against acupuncture, glucosamine, chondroitin, or intra-
  articular hyaluronan for OA.
  –Recommends against arthroscopic lavage and debridement unless knee
  OA with mechanical locking.
  –Recommends oral analgesics include acetaminophen and/or topical
  NSAIDs first line.
  - Oral NSAIDs or COX-2 inhibitors at the lowest effective dose for
    breakthrough pain.
  - Topical capsaicin can be used as an adjunct for knee or hand OA.
  –Consider referral for joint surgery for people with OA and severe joint
  symptoms refractory to nonsurgical treatments.

Source
  –https://guidelines.gov/summaries/summary/47862

Comment

–For chronic NSAID use, consider concomitant therapy with a proton pump inhibitor to prevent NSAID-induced ulcers.

OSTEOPOROSIS

Population

–Adults at risk for osteoporosis or who have confirmed osteoporosis.

Recommendations

▶ ICSI 2011

–Evaluate all patients with a low-impact fracture for osteoporosis.

–Advise smoking cessation and alcohol moderation (≤2 drinks/d).

–Advise 1500-mg elemental calcium daily for established osteoporosis, glucocorticoid therapy, or age >65 y.

–Assess for vitamin D deficiency with a 25-hydroxy vitamin D level.

   • Treat vitamin D deficiency if present.

–Treatment of osteoporosis.

   • Bisphosphonate therapy.

   • Consider estrogen therapy in menopausal women <50 y of age.

   • Consider parathyroid hormone in women with very high risk for fracture.

–Fall prevention program.

   • Home safety evaluation.

   • Avoid medications that can cause sedation and orthostatic hypotension, or affect balance.

   • Assistive walking devices as necessary.

Source

–https://www.icsi.org/_asset/vnw0c3/Osteo.pdf

Comments

1. All patients should have serial heights and observed for kyphosis.

2. Obtain a lateral vertebral assessment with DXA scan or x-ray if height loss exceeds 4 cm.

3. DXA bone mineral densitometry should be repeated no more than every 12–24 mo.

Population
–Postmenopausal women.

Recommendations
▶ NAMS 2010, AACE 2010, ACOG 2012

1. Recommend maintaining a healthy weight, eating a balanced diet, avoiding excessive alcohol intake, avoiding cigarette smoking, and utilizing measures to avoid falls.
2. Recommend supplemental calcium 1200 mg/d and vitamin D_3 800–1000 international units (IU)/d.
3. Recommend an annual check of height and weight, and assess for chronic back pain.
4. DXA of the hip, femoral neck, and lumbar spine should be measured in women age ≥65 y or postmenopausal women with a risk factor for osteoporosis.[a]
5. Recommend repeat DXA testing every 1–2 y for women taking therapy for osteoporosis and every 2–5 y for untreated postmenopausal women.
6. Recommend against measurement of biochemical markers of bone turnover.
7. Recommend drug therapy for osteoporosis for:
   a. Osteoporotic vertebral or hip fracture.
   b. DXA with T score ≤ –2.5.
   c. DXA with T score ≤ –1 to –2.4 and a 10-y risk of major osteoporotic fracture of ≥20% or hip fracture ≥3% based on FRAX calculator, available at http://www.shef.ac.uk/FRAX/
8. Consider the use of hip protectors in women at high risk of falling.

Sources
–http://www.guidelines.gov/content.aspx?id=15500
–https://www.aace.com/files/osteo-guidelines-2010.pdf
–http://www.guidelines.gov/content.aspx?id=38413

---

[a]Previous fracture after menopause, weight <127 lb, BMI <21 kg/m², parent with a history of hip fracture, current smoker, rheumatoid arthritis, or excessive alcohol intake.

Comments

1. Options for osteoporosis drug therapy:
   a. Bisphosphonates
      i. First-line therapy.
      ii. Options include alendronate, ibandronate, risedronate, or zoledronic acid.
      iii. Potential risk for jaw osteonecrosis.
   b. Denosumab.
      i. Consider for women at high fracture risk.
   c. Raloxifene.
      i. Second-line agent in younger women with osteoporosis.
   d. Teriparatide is an option for high fracture risk when bisphosphonates have failed.
      i. Therapy should not exceed 24 mo.
   e. Calcitonin.
      i. Third-line therapy for osteoporosis.
      ii. May be used for bone pain from acute vertebral compression fractures.
2. Vitamin D therapy should maintain a 25-OH vitamin D level between 30 and 60 ng/mL.

OSTEOPOROSIS, GLUCOCORTICOID-INDUCED

Population

–Glucocorticoid-induced osteoporosis.

Recommendations

▶ ACR 2010

1. All patients receiving glucocorticoid therapy should receive education and assess risk factors for osteoporosis.
2. FRAX calculator should be used to place patients at low risk, medium risk, or high risk for major osteoporotic fracture.
3. If glucocorticoid treatment is expected to last >3 mo, recommend:
   a. Weight-bearing activities.
   b. Smoking cessation.
   c. Avoid >2 alcoholic drinks/d.
   d. Calcium 1200–1500 mg/d.
   e. Vitamin D 800–1000 IU/d.
   f. Fall risk assessment.
   g. Baseline DXA test and then every 2 y.
   h. Annual 25-OH vitamin D.
   i. Baseline and annual height measurement.

      j. Assessment of prevalent fragility fractures.

      k. X-rays of spine.

      l. Assessment of degree of osteoporosis medication compliance, if applicable.

4. For postmenopausal women or men age >50 y:

    a. Low-risk group.

      i. Bisphosphonate if equivalent of prednisone ≥7.5 mg/d.

    b. Medium-risk group.

      i. Bisphosphonate if equivalent of prednisolone ≥5 mg/d.

    c. High-risk group.

      i. Bisphosphonate for any dose of glucocorticoid.

5. For premenopausal women or men age <50 y with a prevalent fragility (osteoporotic) fracture and glucocorticoid use ≥3 mo:

    a. For prednisone ≥5 mg/d, use alendronate or risedronate.

    b. For prednisone ≥7.5 mg/d, use zoledronic acid.

    c. Consider teriparatide for bisphosphonate failures.

Source

    –http://www.rheumatology.org/practice/clinical/guidelines/ACR_2010_GIOP_Recomm_Clinicians_Guide.pdf

Comments

1. Clinical factors that may increase the risk of osteoporotic fracture estimated by FRAX calculator:

    a. BMI <21 kg/m^2

    b. Parental history of hip fracture.

    c. Current smoking.

    d. ≥3 alcoholic drinks/d.

    e. Higher glucocorticoid doses or cumulative dose.

    f. IV pulse glucocorticoid use

    g. Declining central bone mineral density measurement

2. Bisphosphonates recommended:

    a. Low- to medium-risk patients.

      i. Alendronate.

      ii. Risedronate.

      iii. Zoledronic acid.

    b. High-risk patients.

      i. Same + teriparatide.

OTITIS EXTERNA, ACUTE (AOE)

Population
–Children age 2 y or older and adults.

Recommendations
▶ AAO-HNS 2014

–Recommends against systemic antimicrobials as initial therapy for diffuse, uncomplicated acute otitis externa (AOE).

–Recommends topical antibiotics for initial therapy of AOE.

–In the presence of a perforated tympanic membrane or tympanostomy tubes, prescribe a non-ototoxic topical antibiotic.

Source
–https://guidelines.gov/summaries/summary/47795

Comment
–Recommends reassessment of the diagnosis if the patient fails to respond within 72 h of topical antibiotics.

OTITIS MEDIA, ACUTE

Population
–Children age 3 mo to 18 y.

Recommendations
▶ AAP 2013

1. Diagnosis should be made with pneumatic otoscopy.
2. Children at low risk[a] should use a wait-and-see approach for 48–72 h with oral analgesics.
3. Recommends symptomatic relief with acetaminophen or ibuprofen and warm compresses to the ear.
4. Educate caregivers about prevention of otitis media: encourage breast-feeding, feed child upright if bottle fed, avoid passive smoke exposure, limit exposure to groups of children, careful handwashing prior to handling child, avoid pacifier use >10 mo, ensure immunizations are up to date.
5. Amoxicillin is the first-line antibiotic for low-risk children.
6. Alternative medication if failure to respond to initial treatment within 72 h; penicillin allergy; presence of a resistant organism found on culture.

[a]Children older than age 2 y without severe disease (temperature >102°F [39°C] and moderate-to-severe otalgia), otherwise healthy, do not attend daycare, and have had no prior ear infections within the last month.

7. Recommends referral to an ear, nose, and throat (ENT) specialist for a complication of otitis media: mastoiditis, facial nerve palsy, lateral sinus thrombosis, meningitis, brain abscess, or labyrinthitis.
8. Recommends against routine recheck at 10–14 d in children feeling well.
9. Management of otitis media with effusion:
   a. Educate that effusion will resolve on its own.
   b. Recommends against antihistamines or decongestants.
   c. Recommends a trial of antibiotics for 10–14 d prior to referral for tympanostomy tubes.

Source
  –*Pediatrics.* 2013;131: e964-e999.

▶ AAFP 2013
  –Do not prescribe antibiotics to children age 2–12 y with non-severe AOM when observation is an option.

Source
  –http://www.choosingwisely.org/societies/american-academy-of-family-physicians/

Comments
1. Amoxicillin is first-line therapy for low-risk children:
   a. 40 mg/kg/d if no antibiotics used in last 3 mo.
   b. 80 mg/kg/d if child is not low risk.
2. Alternative antibiotics:
   a. Amoxicillin-clavulanate.
   b. Cefuroxime axetil.
   c. Ceftriaxone.
   d. Cefprozil.
   e. Loracarbef.
   f. Cefdinir.
   g. Cefixime.
   h. Cefpodoxime.
   i. Clarithromycin.
   j. Azithromycin.
   k. Erythromycin.

Population
  –Children 6 mo to 12 y.

Recommendations
▶ AAP 2013
  –**Diagnosis of AOM**
    • Moderate-severe bulging of the tympanic membrane.
    • New-onset otorrhea not due to otitis externa.

- Mild bulging of an intensely red tympanic membrane and new otalgia <48 h duration.
  - –Treatment of AOM
    - Analgesics and antipyretics.
    - Indications for antibiotics.
      - ◦ Children <24 mo old with bilateral AOM.
      - ◦ Symptoms that are not improving or worsening during a 48-h to 72-h observation period.
      - ◦ AOM associated with severe symptoms (extreme fussiness or severe otalgia).
    - Observation for 48–72 h is recommended in the absence of severe symptoms and fever <102.2°F.
  - –Consider tympanostomy tubes for recurrent AOM (3 episodes in 6 mo or 4 episode in 1 y).

Source
- –http://www.guidelines.gov/content.aspx?id=43892

Comments

1. AOM is **not** present in the absence of a middle ear effusion based on pneumatic otoscopy or tympanometry.
2. Amoxicillin is the preferred antibiotics if the child has not received amoxicillin in the last 30 d.
3. Augmentin is the preferred antibiotic if the child has received amoxicillin in the last 30 d.

OVARIAN CANCER FOLLOW-UP CARE

Population
- –Women treated for ovarian cancer with complete response (Stage I–IV).

Recommendation
▶ NCCN 2015
- –Follow-up Plan
  - Office visits every 2–4 mo for 2 y, then 3–6 mo for 3 y, then annually after 5 y.
  - Physical exam including pelvic exam and measurement of CA-125 with each visit.
  - Refer for genetic risk evaluation if not previously done.
  - Chest/abdominal/pelvic CT, MRI, PET-CT, or PET as clinically indicated due to symptoms or rising CA-125.

Source
- –https://www/nccn.org/professionals/physician_gls/pdf/ovarian/pdf

Comment

–Clinical Points

- All patients with ovarian cancer should be screened for *BRCA 1* and *2* mutations. 10% of patients with Lynch syndrome will develop ovarian cancer.
- 23,000 new cases of ovarian cancer in the United States with 14,000 deaths. 5-y survival is related to stage:
  - Stage I—86% alive at 5 y.
  - Stage II—68%.
  - Stage III—38%.
  - Stage IV—19%.
- Relapsed ovarian cancer is rarely curable, but sequential treatments and intraperitoneal chemotherapy have extended survival to 50–60 mo.

PAIN, CHRONIC

Population

–Adults with chronic noncancer pain outside of palliative and end-of-life care.

Recommendations

▶ CDC 2016

–This guideline is focused on opioid use for chronic pain management.

When to initiate or continue opioids for chronic pain

1. Nonpharmacologic therapy and nonopioid medications are preferred for chronic pain.
2. Opioid therapy should be used for both pain and function only if the anticipated benefits outweigh the risks.
3. Treatment goals, including goals for pain and function, should be established before starting opioid therapy for chronic pain. This plan should also address how opioid therapy will be discontinued if benefits do not outweigh the risks.
4. Clinicians must discuss with patients the risks and benefits of opioid therapy before starting opioids and periodically during therapy.

Opioid selection, follow-up and discontinuation

1. When starting opioid therapy, use immediate-release opioids, and prescribe the lowest effective dose.
2. Carefully reassess benefits and risks when increasing daily dosage to >50 morphine milligram equivalents.
3. Avoid increasing daily dosage to >90 morphine milligram equivalents or carefully justify such large doses.

4. Reassess efficacy within 4 wk
5. of starting opioid therapy for chronic pain and consider discontinuing opioids if benefits do not outweigh risks.

Assessing risk of opioid use

1. Clinicians should evaluate risks of opioid-related harms.
2. Consider offering naloxone when patients have an increased risk of opioid overdose.
3. Frequent review of prescription drug monitoring program data.
4. Recommend periodic urine drug testing.
5. Avoid concurrent opioid and benzodiazepine therapy concurrently whenever possible.
6. Offer or arrange for medication-assisted treatment for patients with opioid use disorders (e.g., buprenorphine or methadone).

Source

–Dowell D, Haegerich TM, Chou R. CDC guideline for prescribing opioids for chronic pain—United States, 2016. *MMWR Recomm Rep.* 2016 Mar 18;65(1):1-49.

▶ ICSI 2016

1. Use validated tools to assess patient's functional status, pain, and quality of life.
2. Assess for current or prior exposure to opioids and consider checking prescription drug monitoring program data before prescribing opioids.
3. Prescribe NSAIDS and acetaminophen for dental pain.
4. Assess for mental health comorbidities in patients with chronic pain.
5. Screen all patients with chronic pain for substance use disorders.
6. Recommend a multidisciplinary approach to patients with chronic pain.
7. Recommend incorporating cognitive behavioral therapy or mindfulness-based stress reduction and exercise/physical therapy to pharmacologic therapy in chronic pain patients.
8. Minimize benzodiazepine or carisoprodol use for chronic pain. If used, limit duration of therapy to 1 wk.
9. Before initiating opioids for chronic pain, providers should seeks a diagnostic cause of the pain and document objective findings on physical exam.
10. Opioid risk assessment tools and knowledge of patient's risk of opioid-related harm should guide decision about initiation or continuation of opioids.
11. Geriatric patients should be assessed for their fall risk, cognitive impairment, respiratory function and renal/hepatic impairment prior to initiation of opioids.

12. Patients who are initiating opioids or who have their opioid dose increased should be advised not to operate heavy machinery, drive a car, or participate in any activity that may be affected by the sedating effect of opioids.
13. Long-acting opioids should be reserved for patients with opioid tolerance and in whom prescriber is confident of medication adherence.
14. Avoid daily opioid doses of >100 morphine milligram equivalents.
15. Avoid opioid use for patients with substance use disorders.
16. Urine drug screening should be done at least annually.
17. If an opioid use disorder is suspected, refer patient to an addiction specialist.

Source
–Hooten M, Thorson D, Bianco J, et al. Pain: assessment, non-opioid treatment approaches and opioid management. Bloomington (MN): Institute for Clinical Systems Improvement (ICSI); 2016 Sep. 160 pp.

PAIN, CHRONIC, CANCER RELATED

Management of Chronic Pain in Survivors of Adult Cancers: ASCO Clinical Practice Guideline

Population
–Women treated for ovarian cancer with complete response (Stage I–IV).

Recommendations

▶ A. SCREENING AND COMPREHENSIVE ASSESSMENT
–Screen for paint at each encounter, document using quantitative or semi-quantitative tool (strength of recommendation (SOR): strong).
–Conduct comprehensive pain assessment.
–Explore multidimensional nature of pain (pain descriptors, distress, impact on function and related physical, psychological, social, and spiritual factors)—explore information about cancer treatment history, comorbid conditions, and psychiatric history, including substance abuse as well as prior treatment for pain.
–The assessment should characterize the pain, and clarify probable cause. A physical exam and diagnostic testing (if appropriate) should be done (SOR: moderate).
–Clinicians should be aware of chronic pain syndromes resulting from cancer treatment, the prevalence of the syndrome, risk factors for an individual patient, and appropriate treatment options.
–Common cancer pain syndromes.
–Evaluate and monitor for recurrent disease, second cancer or late-onset treatment effects in patients with new-onset pain (SOR: moderate).

▶ B. TREATMENT AND CARE OPTIONS

–Clinicians should aim to enhance, comfort, improve function, limit adverse events, and ensure safety in the management of pain in cancer survivors. (SOR: moderate).

–Clinicians should engage patient and family/caregivers in all aspects of pain assessment and management (SOR: moderate)

–Clinicians should decide if other health professionals can provide further care for patients with complex needs. If necessary a referral should be made (SOR: moderate).

–Clinicians should directly refer selected patients to other professionals with expertise in physical medicine and rehabilitation, integrative therapies, interventional therapies, psychological approaches, and neurostimulation therapies (SOR: moderate).

▶ C. PHARMACOLOGICAL INTERVENTIONS

Miscellaneous analgesics

–Clinicians may prescribe nonopiod analgesics to relieve chronic pain or improve function in cancer survivors. This includes nonsteroidal anti-inflammatory drugs, acetaminophen, and adjuvant analgesics including antidepressants and selected anticonvulsants with evidence of analgesic efficacy (antidepressant duloxetine and anticonvulsants gabapentin and pregabalin) for neuropathic pain (SOR: moderate).

–Clinicians may prescribe topical analgesics (nonsteroidal anti-inflammatory drugs, local anesthetics or compounded creams/gels containing baclofen, amitriptyline and ketamine) (SOR: moderate).

–Long-term corticosteroids are not recommended solely to relieve chronic pain (SOR: moderate).

–Clinicians may follow specific state regulations that allow access to medical canabis for patients with chronic pain after consideration of benefits and risk (SOR: moderate).

▶ D. OPIOIDS

–Clinicians may prescribe a trial of opioids in carefully selected cancer survivors with chronic pain who do not respond to more conservative management and who continue to experience pain-related distress or functional impairment. Non-opioid analgesics and/or adjuvants can be added as clinically necessary (SOR: moderate).

–Clinicians should assess risks of adverse effects of opioids used for pain management.

▶ **E. RISK ASSESSMENT, MITIGATION, AND UNIVERSAL PRECAUTIONS WITH OPIOID USE**

–Clinicians should assess the potential risks and benefits when initiating treatment that will incorporate long-term use of opioids (SOR: moderate).

–Clinicians should clearly understand terminology such as tolerance, dependence, abuse, and addiction as it relates to the use of opioids for pain control (SOR: moderate).

–Clinicians should incorporate a universal precautions approach to minimize abuse, addiction, and adverse consequences of opioid use such as opioid-related deaths. Clinicians should be cautious in co-prescribing other centrally acting drugs especially benzodiazepines (SOR: moderate).

–Clinicians should educate patients and their family regarding risk and benefits of long-term opioid therapy and the safe storage use and disposal of controlled substances.

–If opioids are no longer warranted clinicians should taper the dose to avoid withdrawal symptoms (SOR: moderate).

▶ **F. ADVERSE EFFECTS ASSOCIATED WITH LONG-TERM OPIOID USE**

1. Persistent common adverse effects.
   a. Constipation mental clouding, upper GI symptoms.
2. Endocrinopathy (hypogonadism, hyperprolactinemia).
   a. Fatigue, infertility, reduced libido.
   b. Osteoporosis/osteopenia, reduced or absence of menses.
3. Neurotoxicity.
   a. Myoclonus, changes in mental status.
   b. Risk of opioid induced hyperalgesia.
   c. New onset or worsening of sleep apnea syndrome.

Sources
–*J Clin Oncol.* 2016;34:3325-3345
–*J Pain Symptom Manage.* 2016;51:1070-1090
–*J Clim Oncol.* 2014;32:1739-1747
–*JAMA.* 2016;315:1624-1645

PAIN, NEUROPATHIC

Population
–Adults with neuropathic pain.

Recommendations
▶ NICE 2013

–Offer a choice of amitriptyline, duloxetine, gabapentin, or pregabalin as initial treatment for neuropathic pain (except trigeminal neuralgia).
–Consider tramadol only if acute rescue therapy.
–Consider capsaicin cream for localized neuropathic pain.
–Recommend against the following agents:
- Cannabis sativa extract.
- Capsaicin patch.
- Lacosamide.
- Lamotrigine.
- Levetiracetam.
- Morphine.
- Oxcarbazepine.
- Topiramate.
- Tramadol (for long-term use).
- Venlafaxine.

–Recommend carbamazepine as initial therapy for trigeminal neuralgia.

Source
–http://www.guideline.gov/content.aspx?id=47701

PALLIATIVE CARE OF DYING ADULTS

Population
–Dying adults.

Recommendations
▶ NICE 2015

–Care of the dying patient should be aligned with the patient's goals and wishes and cultural values.
–Symptom management should address physical, emotional, social, and spiritual needs.
–Determine who should be the surrogate decision maker if they cannot make their own decisions.
–Establish if the patient has a preferred care setting.

–Medical management of symptoms:
- Pain is typically managed with opioids.
- Breathlessness can be managed with opioids or benzodiazepines +/– oxygen.
- Nausea can be managed with sublingual ondansetron or promethazine suppositories.
- Anxiety can be managed with benzodiazepines.
- Delirium or agitation can be managed with antipsychotics.
- Secretions can be managed with a scopolamine patch.

Source
–https://guidelines.gov/summaries/summary/49956

PALLIATIVE AND END-OF-LIFE CARE: PAIN MANAGEMENT

Principles of Analgesic Use

By the mouth	The oral route is the preferred route for analgesics, including morphine.
By the clock	Persistent pain requires round-the-clock treatment to prevent further pain. As-needed (PRN) dosing is irrational and inhumane; it requires patients to experience pain before becoming eligible for relief. Relief is accomplished with long-acting delayed-release preparations (fentanyl patch, slow-release morphine, or oxycodone).
By the WHO ladder	If a maximum dose of medication fails to adequately relieve pain, move up the ladder, not laterally to a different drug in the same efficiency group. Severe pain requires immediate use of an opioid recommended for controlling severe pain, without progressing sequentially through Steps 1 and 2. When using a long-acting opioid, the dose for breakthrough pain should be 10% of the 24-h opioid dose (ie, if a patient is on 100 mg/d of an extended-release morphine preparation, their breakthrough dose is 10 mg of morphine or equivalent every 1–2 h until pain relief is achieved).
Individualize treatment	The right dose of an analgesic is the dose that relieves pain with acceptable side effects for a specific patient.
Monitor	Monitoring is required to ensure the benefits of treatment are maximized while adverse effects are minimized.

Use adjuvant drugs	For example, a nonsteroidal anti-inflammatory drug (NSAID) is often helpful in controlling bone pain. Nonopioid analgesics, such as NSAIDs or acetaminophen, can be used at any step of the ladder. Adjuvant medications also can be used at any step to enhance pain relief or counteract the adverse effects of medications. Neuropathic pain should be treated with gabapentin, duloxetine, nortriptyline, or pregabalin. Moderate- to high-dose dexamethasone is effective as an adjunct to opioids in a pain crisis situation.

Source: Reprinted with permission from the American Academy of Hospice and Palliative Medicine. *Pocket Guide to Hospice/Palliative Medicine.*

▼ PANCREATITIS, ACUTE (AP)

Population
–Individuals with acute pancreatitis.

Recommendations

▶ ACG 2013

–**The diagnosis of acute pancreatitis** usually includes the presence of 2 of the 3 following criteria: (i) abdominal pain consistent with the disease, (ii) serum amylase and/or lipase greater than 3 times the upper limit of normal, and/or (iii) characteristic findings from abdominal imaging.
  • Recommend a contrast-enhanced CT scan or MRI of the pancreas if the diagnosis is unclear or if symptoms are not improving within 72 h.
  • A gallbladder ultrasound should be performed in all patients with AP.
  • All patients without a history of alcohol abuse or gallstones should have a serum triglyceride level checked.
  • Consider ICU or intermediate-level monitoring for any organ dysfunction.

–**Initial management**
  • Aggressive isotonic fluids at 250–500 mL/h.
  • ERCP indicated for AP associated with choledocholithiasis.
  • In the absence of cholangitis or jaundice, recommend MRCP or endoscopic ultrasound to screen for choledocholithiasis.
  • Prophylactic antibiotics for severe necrotizing AP is not recommended.
  • In patients with infected necrosis, antibiotics known to penetrate pancreatic necrosis, such as carbapenems, quinolones, and

metronidazole, may be useful in delaying or sometimes totally avoiding intervention, thus decreasing morbidity and mortality.

- In mild AP, oral feedings with clear liquids or low-fat diet can be started immediately if there is no nausea and vomiting, and the abdominal pain has resolved.
- In severe AP, enteral nutrition is recommended to prevent infectious complications. Parenteral nutrition should be avoided, unless the enteral route is not available, not tolerated, or not meeting caloric requirements.
- Nasogastric delivery and nasojejunal delivery of enteral feeding appear comparable in efficacy and safety.
- In patients with mild AP, found to have gallstones in the gallbladder, a cholecystectomy should be performed before discharge to prevent a recurrence of AP.

–In a patient with necrotizing biliary AP, in order to prevent infection, cholecystectomy is to be deferred until active inflammation subsides and fluid collections resolve or stabilize.

–In stable patients with infected necrosis, surgical, radiologic, and/or endoscopic drainage should be delayed preferably for more than 4 wk to allow liquefaction of the contents and the development of a fibrous wall around the necrosis (walled-off necrosis).

Source
–http://www.guideline.gov/content.aspx?id=47155

PAP SMEAR, ABNORMAL

ABNORMAL PAP SMEAR ALGORITHM

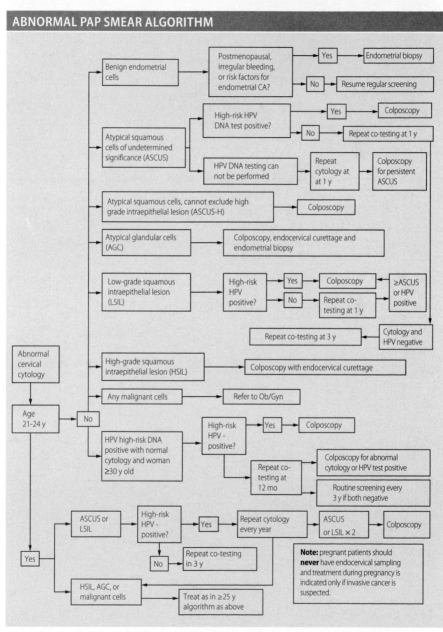

Source: Modified from the ASCCP 2013 Updated Consensus Guidelines for Managing Abnormal Cervical Cancer Screening Tests and Cancer Precursors at http://www.asccp.org/ConsensusGuidelines/tabid/7436/Default.aspx.

PREOPERATIVE CARDIAC CLEARANCE FOR NONCARDIAC SURGERY

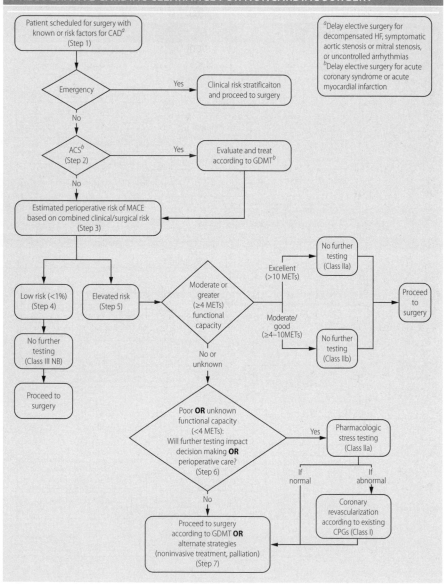

PERIOPERATIVE CARDIOVASCULAR EVALUATION AND MANAGEMENT OF PATIENTS UNDERGOING NONCARDIAC ACC/AHA/ESC 2014 GUIDELINES

Risk of surgical procedures:

–**Low risk:** when the combined surgical and patient characteristic predicts a risk of a major adverse cardiac event (MACE) of death or MI of <1% (eg, cataract and plastic surgery).

–**Elevated risk:** when risk of MACE ≥1%.

Calculation of risk to predict perioperative cardiac morbidity

• **RCRI** (Revised Cardiac Risk Index for perioperative risk) calculator (Lee index) assesses perioperative risk of major cardiac complications (MI, pulmonary edema, ventricular fibrillation or primary cardiac arrest, and complete heart block).
  ◦ It can be found at http://www.mdcalc.com/revised-cardiac-risk-index-for-pre-operative-risk/
  ◦ **For patients with a low risk of perioperative MACE, further testing is not recommended before the planned operation.**
• The NSQIP MICA model (American College of Surgeons National Surgical Quality Improvement Program), also known as myocardial infarction or cardiac arrest "GUPTA" risk calculator: http://www.surgicalriskcalculator.com/miorcardiacarrest
• ACS NSQIP Surgical Risk Calculator (American College of Surgeons) to calculate vascular surgery risk: http://riskcalculator.facs.org/PatientInfo/PatientInfo
• Revised Cardiac Risk Index for Pre-Operative Risk "LEE" calculator estimates risk of cardiac complications after surgery: http://www.mdcalc.com/revised-cardiac-risk-index-for-pre-operative-risk/

Perioperative β-blocker therapy ACC/AHA	Perioperative β-blocker therapy ESC
–β-blockers should be continued in patients undergoing surgery who have been on β-blockers chronically. –It is reasonable for the management of β-blockers after surgery to be guided by clinical circumstances (eg, hypotension, bradycardia, bleeding), independent of when the agent was started. –In patients with intermediate- or high-risk myocardial ischemia noted in preoperative risk stratification tests, it may be reasonable to begin perioperative β-blockers. Per ESC, for patients testing positive for preoperative stress, long-term β-blocker therapy should be used.	–Perioperative continuation of β-blockers is recommended in patients currently receiving this medication. –Preoperative initiation of β-blockers may be considered in patients scheduled for high-risk surgery and who have 2 clinical risk factors or ASA (American Society of Anesthesiologists) class III (patient has severe systemic disease that is not incapacitating). –Preoperative initiation of β-blockers may be considered in patients who have known IHD or myocardial ischemia. –When oral β-blockade is initiated in patients who undergo noncardiac surgery, the use of atenolol or bisoprolol as a first choice may be considered.

PERIOPERATIVE CARDIOVASCULAR EVALUATION AND MANAGEMENT OF PATIENTS UNDERGOING NONCARDIAC ACC/AHA/ESC 2014 GUIDELINES   *(Continued)*

–In patients with 3 or more RCRI risk factors (eg, diabetes mellitus, HF, CAD, renal insufficiency, cerebrovascular accident), it may be reasonable to begin β-blockers before surgery.

–In patients with a compelling long-term indication for β-blocker therapy but no other RCRI risk factors, initiating β-blockers in the perioperative setting as an approach to reduce perioperative risk is of uncertain benefit.

–In patients in whom β-blocker therapy is initiated, it may be reasonable to begin perioperative β-blockers long enough in advance to assess safety and tolerability, preferably more than 1 d before surgery.

–**β-blocker therapy should not be started on the day of surgery!!!**

–Abrupt withdrawal of long-term β-blockers is harmful.

–β-blocker therapy should be initiated ideally >1 d (when possible at least 1 wk and up to 30 d) before surgery, starting with a low dose (atenolol or bisoprolol as first choice).

–Initiation of perioperative high-dose β-blockers without titration **is not recommended.**

–Preoperative initiation of β-blockers is not recommended in patients scheduled for low-risk surgery.

Perioperative statin therapy ACC/AHA

–Statins should be continued in patients currently taking statins and scheduled for noncardiac surgery.

–Perioperative initiation of statin use is reasonable in patients undergoing vascular surgery.

–Perioperative initiation of statins may be considered in patients with clinical indications according to GDMT who are undergoing elevated-risk procedures.

Perioperative statin therapy ESC

–Perioperative continuation of statins is recommended, favoring statins with a long half-life or extended-release formulation (atorvastatin, lovastatin).

–Preoperative initiation of statin therapy should be considered in patients undergoing vascular surgery, ideally at least 2 wk before surgery.

Perioperative antiplatelet therapy ACC/AHA

–In patients undergoing urgent noncardiac surgery during the first 4 to 6 wk after BMS or DES implantation, dual antiplatelet therapy (DAPT) should be continued unless the relative risk of bleeding outweighs the benefit of the prevention of stent thrombosis.

Perioperative antiplatelet therapy ESC

–It is recommended that aspirin be continued for 4 wk after BMS implantation and for 3–12 mo after DES implantation, unless the risk of life-threatening surgical bleeding on aspirin is unacceptably high.

–In patients who have received coronary stents and must undergo surgical procedures that mandate the discontinuation of P2Y$_{12}$ platelet receptor–inhibitor therapy, it is recommended that aspirin be continued if possible and the P2Y$_{12}$ platelet receptor–inhibitor be restarted as soon as possible after surgery.

–Management of the perioperative antiplatelet therapy should be determined by a consensus of the surgeon, anesthesiologist, cardiologist, and patient, who should weigh the relative risk of bleeding versus prevention of stent thrombosis.

–Continuation of aspirin, in patients previously thus treated, may be considered in the perioperative period, and should be based on an individual decision that depends on the perioperative bleeding risk, weighed against the risk of thrombotic complications.

–Discontinuation of aspirin therapy, in patients previously treated with it, should be considered in those in whom hemostasis is anticipated to be difficult to control during surgery.

–In patients undergoing nonemergency/nonurgent noncardiac surgery who have not had previous coronary stenting, it may be reasonable to continue aspirin when the risk of potential increased cardiac events outweighs the risk of increased bleeding.

–Initiation or continuation of aspirin is not beneficial in patients undergoing elective noncardiac noncarotid surgery who have not had previous coronary stenting unless the risk of ischemic events outweighs the risk of surgical bleeding.

–Continuation of P2Y$_{12}$ inhibitor treatment should be considered for 4 wk after BMS implantation and for 3–12 mo after DES implantation, unless the risk of life-threatening surgical bleeding on this agent is unacceptably high.

–In patients treated with P2Y$_{12}$ inhibitors, who need to undergo surgery, postponing surgery for at least 5 d after cessation of ticagrelor and clopidogrel—and for 7 d in the case of prasugrel—if clinically feasible, should be considered unless the patient is at high risk of an ischemic event.

Perioperative anticoagulation therapy ACC/AHA

–The role of anticoagulants (warfarin, NOAC agents) other than platelet inhibitors in the secondary prevention of myocardial ischemia or MI has not been elucidated.

–The risk of bleeding for any surgical procedure must be weighed against the benefit of remaining on anticoagulants on a case-by-case basis.

Perioperative anticoagulation therapy ESC

–Patients at high risk of thromboembolism treated with vitamin K antagonists (VKAs) such as AF with CHA$_2$DS$_2$-VASc score ≥4, or mechanical prosthetic heart valves, newly inserted biological prosthetic valves, mitral valvular repair (within the last 3 mo) or recent venous thromboembolism (within 3 mo), or thrombophilia.

PERIOPERATIVE CARDIOVASCULAR EVALUATION AND MANAGEMENT OF PATIENTS UNDERGOING NONCARDIAC ACC/AHA/ESC 2014 GUIDELINES   *(Continued)*

	WILL NEED BRIDGING with unfractionated heparin (UFH) or therapeutic-dose LMWH. There is better evidence for the efficacy and safety of LMWH in comparison with UFH in bridging to surgery.
–In minor procedures (cataract, minor dermatologic procedures) it may be reasonable to continue anticoagulation preoperatively. –NOAC agents do not appear to be acutely reversible, no reversible agent available at this time. –Patients with prosthetic valves taking vitamin K antagonists may require bridging therapy. –For patients with AF and normal renal function undergoing elective procedures during which hemostatic control is essential, such as major surgery, spine surgery, and epidural catheterization, discontinuation of anticoagulants for ≥48 h is suggested. Monitoring activated partial thromboplastin time for dabigatran and prothrombin time for apixaban and rivaroxaban may be helpful; a level consistent with control levels suggests a low serum concentration of the anticoagulant.	–The overall recommendation is to stop NOACs for 2–3 times their respective biological half-lives prior to surgery in surgical interventions with "normal" bleeding risk, and 4–5 times the biological half-lives before surgery in surgical interventions with high bleeding risk. –Because of the fast "on" effect of NOACs (in comparison with VKAs), resumption of treatment after surgery should be delayed for 1–2 (in some cases 3–5) d, until postsurgical bleeding tendency is diminished.
Timing of elective noncardiac surgery in patients with previous PCI ACC/AHA –Elective noncardiac surgery should be delayed 14 d after balloon angioplasty and at least 30 d (ideally 3 mo) after BMS implantation. –Elective noncardiac surgery should optimally be delayed 365 d after drug-eluting stent (DES) implantation. –In patients in whom noncardiac surgery is required, a consensus decision among treating clinicians as to the relative risks of surgery and discontinuation or continuation of antiplatelet therapy can be useful.	**Timing of elective noncardiac surgery in patients with previous PCI ESC** –It is recommended that, except for high-risk patients, asymptomatic patients who have undergone CABG in the past 6 y be sent for nonurgent, noncardiac surgery without angiographic evaluation. –Consideration should be given to performing nonurgent, noncardiac surgery in patients with recent BMS implantation after a minimum of 4 wk and ideally 3 mo following the intervention.

–Elective noncardiac surgery after DES implantation may be considered after 180 d if the risk of further delay is greater than the expected risks of ischemia and stent.

–Elective noncardiac surgery should not be performed within 30 d after BMS implantation or within 12 mo after DES implantation in patients in whom dual antiplatelet therapy (DAPT) will need to be discontinued perioperatively.

–Elective noncardiac surgery should not be performed within 14 d of balloon angioplasty in patients in whom aspirin will need to be discontinued perioperatively.

–Consideration should be given to performing nonurgent, noncardiac surgery in patients who have had recent DES implantation no sooner than 12 mo following the intervention. This delay may be reduced to 6 mo for the new generation DES.

–In patients who have had recent balloon angioplasty, surgeons should consider postponing noncardiac surgery until at least 2 wk after the intervention.

Sources: Fleisher LA, Fleischmann KE, Auerbach AD, et al. 2014 ACC/AHA Guideline on perioperative cardiovascular evaluation and management of patients undergoing noncardiac surgery: executive summary. *J Am Coll Cardiol.* 2014. doi:10.1016/j.jacc.2014.07.945. 2014 ESC/ESA Guidelines on non-cardiac surgery: cardiovascular assessment and management. Kristensen SD, Knuuti J, Saraste A, et al. The Joint Task Force on non-cardiac surgery: cardiovascular assessment and management of the European Society of Cardiology (ESC) and the European Society of Anaesthesiology (ESA). *Eur Heart J.* 2014;35:2383-2431. doi:10.1093/eurheartj/ehu282.

PARACENTESIS

Population
–Adults with ascites

Recommendation
▶ AASLD 2014
–Do not routinely administer fresh frozen plasma prior to a paracentesis.

Source
–http://www.choosingwisely.org/societies/american-association-for-the-study-of-liver-diseases/

PERIPHERAL ARTERIAL DISEASE

Population
–Adults with lower extremity peripheral arterial disease (PAD).

Recommendations
▶ ACC/AHA 2016, NICE 2012
–In patients with history or physical examination findings suggestive of PAD, the resting ankle-brachial index (ABI), with or without segmental pressures and waveforms, is recommended to establish the diagnosis

–Resting ABI results should be reported as abnormal (ABI ≤0.90), borderline (ABI 0.91–0.99), normal (1.00–1.40), or noncompressible (ABI >1.40).

–Toe-brachial index (TBI) should be measured to diagnose patients with suspected PAD when the ABI >1.40 (noncompressible)

–Duplex ultrasound, CTA, or MRA of the lower extremities is useful to diagnose anatomic location and severity of stenosis for patients with symptomatic PAD in whom revascularization is considered.

–Antiplatelet therapy with aspirin alone (range 75–325 mg/d) or clopidogrel alone (75 mg/d), smoking cessation, a statin, and good glycemic control are recommended to reduce MI, stroke, and vascular death in patients with symptomatic PAD.

–Cilostazol is an effective therapy to improve symptoms and increase walking distance in patients with claudication.

–Patients with PAD should have an annual influenza vaccination.

–In patients with claudication, a supervised exercise program is recommended to improve functional status and QoL and to reduce leg symptoms.

–Patients with PAD and diabetes mellitus should be counseled about self–foot examination and healthy foot behaviors

–Endovascular procedures are effective as a revascularization option for patients with lifestyle-limiting claudication and hemodynamically significant aortoiliac occlusive disease.

–Endovascular procedures are recommended to establish in-line blood flow to the foot in patients with nonhealing wounds or gangrene

–When surgical revascularization is performed, bypass to the popliteal artery with autogenous vein is recommended in preference to prosthetic graft material

–In patients with critical limb ischemia, revascularization should be performed when possible and bypass to the popliteal or infrapopliteal arteries (ie, tibial, pedal) should be constructed with suitable autogenous vein.

–In patients with acute limb ischemia (ALI), systemic anticoagulation with heparin should be administered immediately unless contraindicated.

–Patients with ALI should be monitored and treated (e.g., fasciotomy) for compartment syndrome after revascularization

–Amputation should be performed as the first procedure in patients with a nonsalvageable limb

Source
–2016 AHA/ACC Guideline on the Management of Patients with Lower Extremity Peripheral Artery Disease: executive summary. *Circulation.* 2017;135:e686–e725.

Source
–https://guidelines.gov/summaries/summary/38409

Comments

1. Recommend bare metal stents when stenting people with intermittent claudication.
2. An autologous vein bypass is preferred when possible for infrainguinal bypass surgery.
3. Bypass surgery is recommended over stenting for aortoiliac or femoropopliteal stenosis causing intermittent claudication or critical limb ischemia.
4. Stenting is an option for **complete** aortoiliac occlusion.

PHARYNGITIS, ACUTE

APPROACH TO ACUTE PHARYNGITIS

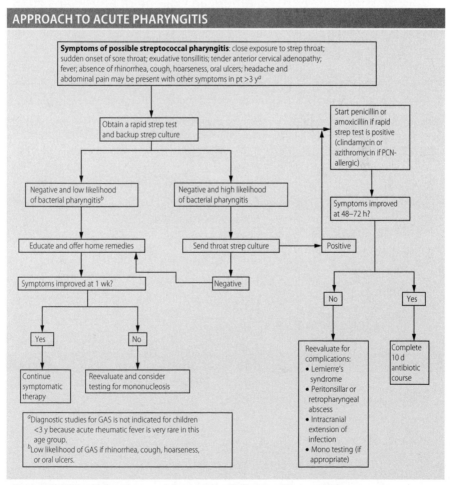

Source: IDSA 2012 guidelines on group A Streptococcus (GAS) pharyngitis.

▶ Choosing Wisely 2013, Society of Thoracic Surgeons 2013
  –Recommends against preoperative stress testing prior to noncardiac thoracic surgery in patients who have no cardiac history and good functional status.
  –Recommends against routine evaluation of carotid artery disease prior to cardiac surgery in the absence of symptoms or other high-risk criteria.

Source
  –http://www.choosingwisely.org/wp-content/uploads/2015/02/STS-Choosing-Wisely-List.pdf

▶ Choosing Wisely 2013, American College of Physicians 2013
  –Recommends against preoperative chest radiography in the absence of a clinical suspicion for intrathoracic pathology.

Source
  –http://www.choosingwisely.org/societies/american-college-of-physicians/

DELAY TIMES FOR NON-EMERGENT SURGERY

Event	Wait Times
PTCA	14 d
Bare metal stent	30 d
Drug-eluting stent	At least 6 mo
CABG	6–8 wk
After ischemic stroke	3–6 mo
After acute MI	2–3 mo

Sources
  –*Ann Surgery*. 2011;253:857-867
  –*JAMA*. 2014;312:269-277

WHEN TO BRIDGE ANTICOAGULATION FOR NONEMERGENT OPERATION

- AF with MS
- AF with prosthetic valve
- AF with ischemic stroke <3 mo
- NVAF and CHA_2DS_2-VASc score ≥6
- Mechanical MV
- Caged or tilted mechanical AV
- VT <3 mo or severe thrombophilia

▶ Choosing Wisely 2013, American Society of Echocardiography 2013

–Recommends avoiding echocardiograms for preoperative/perioperative assessment of patients with no history of symptoms of heart disease.

Sources
–*JACC.* 2017;69:871
–*NEJM.* 2015;373:823
–*JAMA Intern Med.* 2015;175:1163
–http://www.choosingwisely.org/societies/american-society-of-echocardiography/

PLATELET TRANSFUSION

Population
–Adults and children.

Recommendation
▶ American Association of Blood Banks (AABB) 2014
–**Practical Considerations**
  • Transfusion with a single apheresis unit or a pool of 4 to 6 whole-blood-derived platelet concentrates is indicated for patients with therapy-induced platelet counts of <10,000 (<20,000 if infection).
  • Prophylactic platelet transfusions are indicated for patients having elective central venous catheter (CVC) placement with platelet count <20,000 and for those having elective diagnostic lumbar puncture or major nonneurological surgery with <50,000 platelets.
  • Platelet transfusions are not recommended for nonthrombocytopenic patients having cardiopulmonary bypass surgery unless they have perioperative bleeding with thrombocytopenia or evidence of platelet dysfunction.

Sources
–*Ann Intern Med.* 2015;162:205-213
–*Blood.* 2014;123:1146-1151

Comment
–**Clinical Correlation**
  • These guidelines do not pertain to ITP, TTP, or heparin-induced thrombocytopenia. Platelet transfusion may worsen these immune-mediated diseases and should not be given unless there is major life-threatening bleeding. (*Blood.* 2015; 125:1470)
  • No strong evidence was found for platelet transfusion with intracranial bleed in patients taking antiplatelet drugs or in patients

undergoing neurosurgery with platelets <100,000 although platelets >100,000 is current clinical practice.

- Guidelines emphasize that clinical judgment and not a specific platelet count should be paramount in decision making.
- Beware that the risk of bacterial infection with platelet transfusion is 1 in 3000 (5 times more common than RBC transfusions). (*Transfusion.* 2013; 55:1603)

PLEURAL EFFUSION, MALIGNANT

Symptomatic Patients

1. Patients with symptoms should have initial therapeutic thoracentesis to relieve symptoms. The recommended amount of fluid removed per session is 1000-1500 mL. The rate of reaccumulation of the pleural effusion, and the patient's clinical and symptomatic response and prognosis will help to guide the subsequent choice of therapy.
2. Outpatient therapeutic thoracentesis alone may be indicated for patients with survival expected to be less than 1 mo and/or poor performance status (PS) and/or slow reaccumulation of the pleural effusion (ie, more than 1 mo).
3. Patients should be considered for more definitive intervention after the first or second thoracentesis.
4. Treatment options:
   (A) Indwelling (tunneled) pleural catheter (considered for patients with trapped lung who obtain some relief following thoracentesis) or patients who want to avoid hospitalization or discomfort of pleurodesis. (*Chest.* 2012; 142:394).
   (B) Talc pleurodisis (Talc poudrage) via thoracoscopy consider for patients with longer projected survival and those who don't want an indwelling catheter. This approach is contraindicated for patients with trapped lung.
   (C) Talc pleurodesis (slurry) via chest tube - Indicated for patients with longer anticipated survival or contraindication to thoracoscopy. Contraindicated for patients with trapped lung.
   (D) Chemotherapy may be considered as an adjunct treatment option. In particular, patients undergoing first line systemic therapy for tumors with high response rates (small cell lung cancer and lymphoma), may avoid the previously discussed definitive treatments.

Population

–Adult men and women with lung cancer or metastatic malignancy to the lung with a malignant pleural effusion.

Recommendations

▶ British Thoracic Society 2014, American College of Chest Physicians 2014

- –All treatment decisions should be guided by patient preferences.
- –Selection of a treatment approach is largely dependent on projected duration of survival and availability of adequate resources.
- –The management of a malignant pleural effusion (MPE) should be individualized and these patients should be commonly presented to a multidisciplinary Tumor Board for advice. (*JAMA*. 2012;307:2432).
- –Management of MPE is palliative and treatment decisions should focus on type of malignancy, patient's symptoms, life expectancy, functional status, quality of life, and goals of therapy. Palliative therapy goals should improve patient's quality of life through (1) relief of dyspnea and (2) less need for reintervention and reduced hospitalizations and length of stay.

Diagnostic and Baseline Investigations

1. A chest x-ray (CXR) should be used to detect the presence of a pleural effusion. A lateral decubitus CXR may be used to differentiate pleural liquid from pleural thickening.
2. CT scans can detect very small effusions (less than 10 mL of fluid). A thoracic ultrasound can also document the presence of pleural effusions.
3. Undiagnosed effusions of more than 1 cm from the chest wall on lateral decubitus CXR should be diagnostically evaluated by ultrasound-assisted thoracentesis. In patients with advanced cancer thoracentesis for small effusions is unnecessary.
4. All effusions should be sent for cytology if a patient does not have a diagnosis of a MPE. A minimum of 50-60 mL. of pleural fluid should be withdrawn for analysis. Other studies including cell count and differential, gram stain and culture, pH, glucose, protein, and lactate dehydrogenase (LDH) will help separate transudate from exudate. Increased amounts of fluid (100 to 200 cc) can be sent for a cell block and molecular testing (eg, epidermal growth factor receptor mutation, Alk gene rearrangement and ROS 1 rearrangement).
5. All patients with a diagnosis of significant MPE should be referred to pulmonologist and/or thoracic surgery for treatment options.
6. Chest ultrasound is recommended at point of care for any thoracentesis or percutaneous chest drain placement (including indwelling pleural catheter (IPC)).
7. Treatment is not required in asymptomatic patients but follow-up should be frequent especially if large MPE present.

Comment

–Indwelling pleural catheter (IPC-pleurex catheter) requires a regular outpatient drainage schedule that may be a burden for the patient or caregiver. This issue needs to be addressed. Complications from IPCs are uncommon. The infection rate is 5% with more than half the patients responding to antibiotics without removing the catheter. (*Chest*. 2013; 144:1597). Other problems with IPCs includ–e pneumothorax (5.9%), cellulitis (3.4%), obstruction/clogging (3.7%), and unspecified catheter malfunction (9.1%). The most common adverse events with talc pleurodesis include fever, pain, and GI symptoms. Less common are cardiac arrhythmia, dyspnea, systemic inflammatory response, empyema, and talc dissemination.

Sources

–https://www.guideline.gov/summaries/summary/49355/management-of-malignant-pleural-effusion.

–*Chest*. 2013;143(5)(Suppl):e4555-e4975

–*J Natl Compr Canc Nefw*. 2012;10:975

–*Thoracic Society Pleural Disease Guideline*. 2010; *Thorax*. 2010; 65(Suppl 2):132

POLYCYSTIC OVARY SYNDROME

Population

–Adolescent and adult women.

Recommendations

▶ Endocrine Society 2013

1. Diagnosis if 2 of 3 criteria are met:
   a. Androgen excess.
   b. Ovulatory dysfunction.
   c. Polycystic ovaries.
2. Treatment
   a. Hormonal contraceptives for menstrual irregularities, acne, and hirsutism.
   b. Exercise and diet for weight management.
   c. Clomiphene citrate recommended for infertility.
   d. Recommends against the use of metformin, inositols, or thiazolidinediones.

Source

–http://www.guideline.gov/content.aspx?id=47899

AAP AND AFP PERINATAL AND POSTNATAL GUIDELINES

Breast-feeding	Strongly recommends education and counseling to promote breast-feeding.
Hemoglobinopathies	Strongly recommends ordering screening tests for hemoglobinopathies in neonates.
Hyperbilirubinemia	Perform ongoing systematic assessments during the neonatal period for the risk of an infant developing severe hyperbilirubinemia.
Phenylketonuria	Strongly recommends ordering screening tests for phenylketonuria in neonates.
Thyroid function abnormalities	Strongly recommends ordering screening tests for thyroid function abnormalities in neonates.

Sources: Pediatrics. 2004;114:297-316. *Pediatrics.* 2005;115:496-506.

▼ PNEUMONIA

PNEUMONIA, COMMUNITY-ACQUIRED: EVALUATION

Diagnostic Testing
- CXR or other chest imaging required for diagnosis
- Sputum Gram stain and culture
  ° Outpatients: optional
  ° Inpatients: if unusual or antibiotic resistance suspected

Admission Decision
- Severity of illness (eg, CURB-65) and prognostic indices (eg, PSI) support decision
- One must still recognize social and individual factors

CURB-65
(*Thorax.* 2003;58:337-382)

Clinical Factor	Points
Confusion	1
BUN >19 mg/dL	1
Respiratory rate ≥30 breaths/min	1
Systolic BP <90 mm Hg **OR** Diastolic BP ≤60 mm Hg	1
Age >65 y	1
Total points	
• CURB-65 ≥2 suggests need for hospitalization	

Pneumonia Severity Index
(*N Engl J Med.* 1997;336:243-250)

Demographic Factor	Points
Men age	Age in years
Women age	Age in years −10
Nursing home resident	+10
Coexisting illnesses	
Neoplastic disease	+30
Liver disease	+20
Congestive heart failure	+10

PNEUMONIA, COMMUNITY-ACQUIRED: EVALUATION (*Continued*)

Score	In-hospital mortality
0	0.7%
1	3.2%
2	3.0%
3	17%
4	42%
5	57%

Cerebrovascular disease	+10
Renal disease	+10
Physical exam findings	
Altered mental status	+20
Respiratory rate 30 breaths/min	+20
Systolic BP <90 mm Hg	+20
Temperature <95°F (35°C)	+15
Temperature >104°F (40°C)	+15
Pulse >125 beats/min	+10
Laboratory and radiographic findings	
Arterial blood pH <7.35	+30
BUN >30 mg/dL	+20
Sodium level <130 mmol/L	+20
Glucose level >250 mg/dL	+10
Hematocrit <30%	+10
PaO_2 <60 mm Hg or O_2 saturation <90%	+10
Pleural effusion	+10

Add up total points to estimate mortality risk

Class	Points	Overall Mortality
I	<51	0.1%
II	51–70	0.6%
III	71–90	0.9%
IV	91–130	9.5%
V	>130	26.7%

BP, blood pressure; BUN, blood urea nitrogen; CURB-65, confusion, urea nitrogen, respiratory rate, blood pressure, 65 of age and older; CXR, chest x-ray; PSI, pneumonia severity index.
Sources: Mandell LA, Wunderink RG, Anzueto A, et al; Infectious Diseases Society of America; American Thoracic Society. Infectious Diseases Society of America/American Thoracic Society consensus guidelines on the management of community-acquired pneumonia in adults. *Clin Infect Dis.* 2007;44 Suppl 2:S27-S72. Fine MJ, Auble TE, Yealy DM, et al. A prediction rule to identify low-risk patients with community-acquired pneumonia. *N Engl J Med.* 1997;336:243-250.

PNEUMONIA, COMMUNITY-ACQUIRED: SUSPECTED PATHOGENS
Source: IDSA, ATS, 2007

Condition and Risk Factors	Commonly Encountered Pathogens
Alcoholism	*Streptococcus pneumoniae,* oral anaerobes, *Klebsiella pneumoniae, Acinetobacter* species, *Mycobacterium tuberculosis*
COPD and/or smoking	*Haemophilus influenzae, Pseudomonas aeruginosa, Legionella* species, *S. pneumoniae, Moraxella catarrhalis, Chlamydia pneumoniae*
Aspiration	Gram-negative enteric pathogens, oral anaerobes
Lung abscess	CA-MRSA, oral anaerobes, endemic fungal pneumonia, *M. tuberculosis,* and atypical mycobacteria
Exposure to bat or bird droppings	Histoplasma capsulatum
Exposure to birds	*Chlamydophila psittaci* (if poultry: avian influenza)
Exposure to rabbits	*Francisella tularensis*
Exposure to farm animals or parturient cats	*Coxiella burnetii* (Q fever)
HIV infection (early)	*S. pneumoniae, H. influenzae,* and *M. tuberculosis*
HIV infection (late)	The pathogens listed for early infection plus *Pneumocystis jirovecii, Cryptococcus, Histoplasma, Aspergillus,* atypical mycobacteria (especially *Mycobacterium kansasii), P. aeruginosa, H. influenzae*
Hotel or cruise ship stay in previous 2 wk	*Legionella* species
Travel to or residence in southwestern United States	*Coccidioides* species, *hantavirus*
Travel to or residence in Southeast and East Asia	*Burkholderia pseudomallei,* avian influenza, SARS
Influenza active in community	Influenza, *S. pneumoniae, Staphylococcus aureus, H. influenzae*
Cough ≥2 wk with whoop or posttussive vomiting	*Bordetella pertussis*
Structural lung disease (eg, bronchiectasis)	*P. aeruginosa, Burkholderia cepacia,* and *S. aureus*
Injection drug use	*S. aureus,* anaerobes, *M. tuberculosis,* and *S. pneumoniae*
Endobronchial obstruction	Anaerobes, *S. pneumoniae, H. influenzae, S. aureus*
In context of bioterrorism	*Bacillus anthracis* (anthrax), *Yersinia pestis* (plague), *F. tularensis* (tularemia)

CA-MRSA, community-acquired methicillin-resistant *S. aureus;* COPD, chronic obstructive pulmonary disease; SARS, severe acute respiratory syndrome.
Sources: IDSA 2007, ATS 2007.

PREGNANCY, POSTPARTUM HEMORRHAGE (PPH)

Population
–Pregnant women.

Recommendations
▶ WHO 2012
–Uterotonics for the treatment of PPH.
- Intravenous oxytocin is the recommended agent.
- Alternative uterotonics:
  ◦ Misoprostol 800 μg sublingual.
  ◦ Methylergonovine 0.2 mg IM.
  ◦ Carboprost 0.25 mg IM.
–Additional interventions for PPH.
- Isotonic crystalloid resuscitation.
- Bimanual uterine massage.
–Therapeutic options for persistent PPH.
- Tranexamic acid is recommended for persistent PPH refractory to oxytocin.
- Uterine artery embolization.
- Balloon tamponade.
–Therapeutic options for a retained placenta.
- Controlled cord traction with oxytocin 10 IU IM/IV.
- Manual removal of placenta.
  ◦ Give single dose of first-generation antibiotic for prophylaxis against endometritis.
- Recommend against methylergonovine, misoprostol, or carboprost (Hemabate) for retained placenta.

Source
–http://www.guidelines.gov/content.aspx?id=39383

Comment
–Misoprostol 800–1000 μg can also be administered as a rectal suppository for PPH related to uterine atony.

PREGNANCY, PREMATURE RUPTURE OF MEMBRANES

Population
–Pregnant women.

Recommendations

▶ ACOG 2013

–Women with preterm premature rupture of membranes before 32 gestational weeks at risk for imminent delivery should be considered for intravenous magnesium sulfate treatment for its fetal neuroprotective effect.

–For women with premature rupture of membranes at 37 gestational weeks or more, labor should be induced if spontaneous labor does not occur near the time of presentation.

–At 34 gestational weeks or greater, delivery is recommended for all women with ruptured membranes.

–In the setting of ruptured membranes, therapeutic tocolysis is not recommended.

–Outpatient management of preterm premature rupture of membranes is not recommended.

Source
–http://www.guideline.gov/content.aspx?id=47106

▶ Cochrane Database of Systematic Reviews 2013

–Routine antibiotics should be prescribed for women with preterm rupture of membranes prior to 37 gestational weeks.

Source
–http://www.cochrane.org/CD001058/PREG_antibiotics-for-preterm-rupture-of-membranes

Comment

–22 studies involving over 6800 pregnant women with PROM prior to 37 gestational weeks were analyzed. Routine antibiotics decreased the incidence of chorioamnionitis (RR 0.66), prolonged pregnancy by at least 7 d (RR 0.79), and decreased neonatal infection (RR 0.67), but had no effect on perinatal mortality compared with placebo.

PREGNANCY, PRETERM LABOR

Population
–Pregnant women.

Recommendations

▶ ACOG 2012, Cochrane Database of Systematic Reviews 2013

–Single dose of corticosteroids for pregnant women between 24 and 34 gestational weeks who may deliver within 7 d.

–Magnesium sulfate for possible preterm delivery prior to 32 wk for neuroprotection.

–Tocolytic options for up to 48 h.

- β-agonists.
- Nifedipine.
- Indomethacin.

–No role for antibiotics in preterm labor and intact membranes.

–Bedrest and hydration have not been shown to prevent preterm birth and should not be routinely recommended.

Sources

–http://www.guidelines.gov/content.aspx?id=38621

–http://www.cochrane.org/CD003096/PREG_hydration-for-treatment-of-preterm-labour

Comments

1. Magnesium sulfate administered prior to 32 wk reduces the severity and risk of cerebral palsy.
2. Cochrane analysis found no difference in the incidence of preterm delivery comparing hydration and bedrest with bedrest alone.

PREGNANCY, PRETERM LABOR, TOCOLYSIS

Population

–Pregnant women in preterm labor.

Recommendations

▶ RCOG 2011

–There is no clear evidence that tocolysis improves perinatal outcomes and therefore it is reasonable not to use them.

–Nifedipine and atosiban have comparable effectiveness in delaying birth up to 7 d.

–Avoid the use of multiple tocolytic drugs simultaneously.

–Maintenance tocolytic therapy following threatened preterm labor is not recommended.

Source

–http://www.rcog.org.uk/files/rcog-corp/GTG1b26072011.pdf

Comment

–Tocolysis may be considered for women with suspected preterm labor who require in utero transfer or to complete a course of corticosteroids.

PREGNANCY, ROUTINE PRENATAL CARE

ROUTINE PRENATAL CARE

Preconception Visit
1. Measure height, weight, blood pressure, and total and HDL cholesterol.
2. Determine rubella, rubeola, and varicella immunity status.
3. Assess all patients for pregnancy risk: substance abuse, domestic violence, sexual abuse, psychiatric disorders, risk factors for reterm labor, exposure to chemicals or infectious agents, hereditary disorders, gestational diabetes, or chronic medical problems.
4. Educate patients about proper nutrition; offer weight reduction strategies for obese patients.
5. Immunize if not current on the following: Tdap (combined tetanus, diphtheria, and pertussis vaccine), MMR (measles, mumps, rubella), varicella, or hepatitis B vaccine.
6. Initiate folic acid 400–800 µg/d; 4 mg/d for a history of a child affected by a neural tube defect.

Initial Prenatal Visit
1. Medical, surgical, social, family, and obstetrical history, and do complete examination.
2. Pap smear, urine NAAT for gonorrhea and Chlamydia, and assess for history of genital herpes.
3. Consider a varicella antibody test if the patient unsure about prior varicella infection.
4. Urinalysis for proteinuria and glucosuria, and urine culture for asymptomatic bacteriuria.
5. Order prenatal labs to include a complete blood count, blood type, antibody screen, rubella titer, VDRL, hepatitis B surface antigen, and an HIV test.
6. Order an obstetrical ultrasound for dating if any of the following: beyond 16-wk gestational age, unsure of last menstrual period, size/date discrepancy on examination, or for inability to hear fetal heart tones by 12 gestational weeks.
7. Discuss fetal aneuploidy screening and counseling regardless of maternal age.
8. Prenatal testing offered for sickle cell anemia (African descent), thalassemia (African, Mediterranean, Middle Eastern, Southeast Asians), Canavan disease and Tay-Sachs (Jewish patients), cystic fibrosis (whites and Ashkenazi Jews), and fragile X syndrome (family history of nonspecified mental retardation).
9. Place a tuberculosis skin test for all medium- to high-risk patients.[a]
10. Consider a 1-h 50-g glucose tolerance test for certain high-risk groups.[b]
11. Obtain an operative report in all women who have had a prior cesarean section.
12. Psychosocial risk assessment for mood disorders, substance abuse, or domestic violence.

Frequency of Visits for Uncomplicated Pregnancies
1. Every 4 wk until 28 gestational weeks; q 2 wk from 28 to 36 wk; weekly >36 wk.

Routine Checks at Follow-up Prenatal Visits
1. Assess weight, blood pressure, and urine for glucose and protein.
2. Exam: edema, fundal height, and fetal heart tones at all visits; fetal presentation starting at 36 wk.
3. Ask about regular uterine contractions, leakage of fluid, vaginal bleeding, or decreased fetal movement.
4. Discuss labor precautions.

Antepartum Lab Testing

1. All women should be offered first trimester, second trimester, or combined testing to screen for fetal aneuploidy; invasive diagnostic testing for fetal aneuploidy should be available to all women regardless of maternal age.
   a. First trimester.
   b. Second trimester screening options: amniocentesis at 14 wk; a Quad Marker Screen at 16–18 wk; and/or a screening ultrasound with nuchal translucency assessment.
2. Consider serial transvaginal sonography of the cervix every 2–3 wk to assess cervical length for patients at high risk for preterm delivery starting at 16 wk.
3. No role for routine bacterial vaginosis screening.
4. 1-h 50-g glucose tolerance test in all women between 24 and 28 wk.
5. Rectovaginal swab for group B streptococcal (GBS) testing between 35 and 37 wk.
6. Recommend weekly amniotic fluid assessments and twice weekly nonstress testing starting at 41 wk.

Prenatal Counseling

1. Cessation of smoking, drinking alcohol, or use of any illicit drugs.
2. Avoid cat litter boxes, hot tubs, certain foods (ie, raw fish or unpasteurized cheese)
3. Proper nutrition and expected weight gain: National Academy of Sciences advises weight gain 28–40 lb (prepregnancy BMI <20), 25–35 lb (BMI 20–26), 15–25 lb (BMI 26–29), and 15–20 lb (BMI ≥30).
4. Inquire about domestic violence and depression at initial visit, at 28 wk, and at post-partum visit.
5. Recommend regular mild-to-moderate exercise 3 or more times a week.
6. Avoid high-altitude activities, scuba diving, and contact sports during pregnancy.
7. Benefits of breast-feeding vs. bottle-feeding.
8. Discuss postpartum contraceptive options (including tubal sterilization) during third trimester.
9. Discuss analgesia and anesthesia options and offer prenatal classes at 24 wk.
10. Discuss repeat C-section vs. vaginal birth after cesarean (if applicable).
11. Discuss the option of circumcision if a boy is delivered.
12. Avoid air travel and long train or car trips beyond 36 wk.

Prenatal Interventions

1. Suppressive antiviral medications starting at 36 wk for women with a history of genital herpes.
2. Cesarean delivery is indicated for women who are HIV positive or have active genital herpes and are in labor.
3. For patients who report a history of abuse, offer interventions and resources to increase their safety during and after pregnancy.
4. For patients with severe depression, consider treatment with an SSRI (avoid parox-etine if possible).

5. Rh immune globulin 300 μg IM for all Rh-negative women with negative antibody screens between 26 and 28 wk.
6. Refer for nutrition counseling at 10–12 wk for BMI <20 kg/m² or at any time during pregnancy for inadequate weight gain.
7. Start prenatal vitamins with iron and folic acid 400–800 μg/d and 1200 mg elemental calcium/d starting at 4 wk preconception (or as early as possible during pregnancy) and continued until 6 wk postpartum.
8. Give inactivated influenza vaccine IM to all pregnant women during influenza season.
9. Consider progesterone therapy IM weekly or intravaginally daily to women at high risk for preterm birth.
10. Recommend an external cephalic version at 37 wk for all noncephalic presentations.
11. Offer labor induction to women at 41 wk by good dates.
12. Treat all women with confirmed syphilis with penicillin G during pregnancy.
13. Treat all women with gonorrhea with ceftriaxone; follow treatment with a test of cure.
14. Treat all women with *Chlamydia* with azithromycin; follow treatment with a test of cure.
15. Treat all GBS-positive women with penicillin G when in labor or with spontaneous rupture of membranes.

Postpartum Interventions
1. Treat all infants born to HBV-positive women with hepatitis B immunoglobulin (HBIG) and initiate HBV vaccine series within 12 h of life.
2. All women with a positive tuberculosis skin test and no evidence of active disease should receive a postpartum chest x-ray; treat with isoniazid 300 mg PO daily for 9 mo if chest x-ray is negative.
3. Administer a Tdap booster if tetanus status is unknown or the last Td (tetanus-diphtheria) vaccine was >10 y ago.
4. Administer an MMR vaccine to all rubella nonimmune women.
5. Offer HPV vaccine to all women ≤26 wk who have not been immunized.
6. Initiate contraception.
7. Repeat Pap smear at 6-wk postpartum check.

aPostgastrectomy, gastric bypass, immunosuppressed (HIV-positive, diabetes, renal failure, chronic steroid/immunosuppressive therapy, head/neck or hematologic malignancies), silicosis, organ transplant recipients, malabsorptive syndromes, alcoholics, intravenous drug users, close contacts of persons with active pulmonary tuberculosis, medically underserved, low socioeconomic class, residents/employees of long-term care facilities and jails, health care workers, and immigrants from endemic areas.
bOverweight (BMI ≥25 kg/m² and an additional risk factor: physical inactivity; first-degree relative with DM; high-risk ethnicity (eg, African American, Latino, Native American, Asian American, Pacific Islander); history of gestational diabetes mellitus (GDM); prior baby with birthweight >9 lb; unexplained stillbirth or malformed infant; HTN on therapy or with BP ≥140/90 mm Hg; HDL cholesterol level <35 mg/dL (0.90 mmol/L) and/or a triglyceride level >250 mg/dL (2.82 mmol/L); polycystic ovary syndrome; history of impaired glucose tolerance or HgbA1c ≥5.7%; acanthosis nigricans; cardiovascular disease; or ≥2+ glucosuria.

Source: Adapted from ACOG ICSI Guideline on Routine Prenatal Care, July 2010. (http://www.icsi.org/prenatal_care_4/prenatal_care_routine_full_version_2.html).

PREGNANCY, SUBSTANCE ABUSE

Population
–Pregnant or postpartum patients using alcohol or illicit drugs.

Recommendations
▶ WHO 2014

–Health care providers should ask all pregnant women about their use of alcohol and other illicit drugs at every prenatal visit.
–Health care providers should offer a brief intervention and individualized care to all pregnant women using alcohol or drugs.
–Health care providers should refer pregnant women with alcohol or cocaine or methamphetamine abuse to a detoxification center.
  • Women with opioid addiction should continue a structured opioid maintenance program with either methadone or buprenorphine.
  • Women with a benzodiazepine addiction should gradually wean the dose.
–Mothers with a substance abuse history should be encouraged to breast-feed unless the risks outweigh the benefits.
–Carefully monitor and treat infants of substance abusing mothers.

Source
–https://guidelines.gov/summaries/summary/48894

PREOPERATIVE CLEARANCE

Population
–Asymptomatic population without cardiac history.

Recommendations
▶ Choosing Wisely 2014, ACC 2014

–Recommends against stress cardiac imaging or advanced noninvasive imaging as a preoperative assessment in patients scheduled to undergo low-risk noncardiac surgery.

Source
–http://www.choosingwisely.org/societies/american-college-of-cardiology/

PRESSURE ULCERS

Population
–Adults at risk for pressure ulcers.

Recommendations

▶ NICE 2014

1. Regular documentation of ulcer size.
2. Debride any necrotic tissue if present with sharp debridement or autolytic debridement.
3. Nutritional supplementation for patients who are malnourished.
4. Recommend a pressure-redistributing foam mattresses.
5. Negative pressure wound therapy, electrotherapy, or hyperbaric oxygen therapy is not routinely recommended.
6. Antibiotics are only indicated for superimposed cellulitis or underlying osteomyelitis.

Source

–http://www.guideline.gov/content.aspx?id=48026

Population

–Patients with pressure ulcers.

Recommendations

▶ ACP 2015

–Recommends nutritional supplementation with protein and amino acids to reduce wound size.
–Use hydrocolloid or foam dressings to reduce wound size.
–Use electrical stimulation as adjunctive therapy to accelerate wound healing.

Source

–https://guidelines.gov/summaries/summary/49050

Comment

–Moderate-quality evidence supports the addition of electrical stimulation to standard therapy to accelerate healing of Stage II–IV ulcers.

PROCEDURAL SEDATION

▶ ACEP 2014

Population

–Adults or children.

Recommendations

1. No preprocedural fasting needed prior to procedural sedation.
2. Recommends continuous capnometry and oximetry to detect hypoventilation.

3. During procedural sedation, a nurse or other qualified individual must be present for continuous monitoring in addition to the procedural operator.

4. Safe options for procedural sedation in children and adults include ketamine, propofol, and etomidate.

Source
  –http://www.guideline.gov/content.aspx?id=47772

Comments
1. The combination of ketamine and propofol is also deemed to be safe for procedural sedation in children and adults.
2. Alfentanil can be safely administered to adults for procedural sedation.

PROSTATE CANCER FOLLOW-UP CARE

Population
  –Prostate cancer survivors.

Recommendations
▶ ASCO 2015

  –**Surveillance for Prostate Cancer Patient Recurrence**
  • Measure serum PSA (prostate-specific antigen) every 4–12 mo (depending on recurrence risk) for the first 5 y then recheck annually thereafter.
  • Survivors with elevated or rising PSA levels should be evaluated as soon as possible by their primary treating specialist.
  • Perform an annual direct rectal examination.
  • Adhere to ASCO screening and early detection guidelines for 2nd cancers (increased risk of bladder and colon cancer after pelvic radiation).

  –**Assessment and Management of Physical and Psychosocial Effects of PC and Treatment**
  • Anemia related to androgen deprivation therapy (ADT).
  • Bowel dysfunction and symptoms especially rectal bleeding.
  • Cardiovascular and metabolic effects for men receiving ADT— follow USPSTF guidelines for evaluation and screening for cardiovascular risk factors.
  • Assess for distress and depression and refer to appropriate specialist.
  • Osteoporosis and fracture risk in men on ADT—do baseline DEXA (dual energy x-ray absorptiometry) scan and support with calcium, vitamin D, and bisphosphonates as indicated.
  • Sexual dysfunction—phosphodiesterase type 5 inhibitors may help—refer to appropriate specialist.

- Urinary dysfunction (incontinence and leakage)—refer to urology specialist.
- Vasomotor symptoms (hot flushes) in men receiving ADT—selective serotonin or noradrenergic reuptake inhibitors or gabapentin may be helpful. Low-dose progesterone may be helpful in refractory patients.

Source
  –Prostate cancer survivorship care guidelines. *J Clin Oncol.* 2015;33:1078-1085

Comments
  –**General health promotion can be helpful**
  - Counsel survivors to achieve and maintain a healthy weight by limiting consumption of high-caloric food and beverages.
  - Counsel survivors to engage in at least 150 min/wk of physical activity.
  - Improve dietary pattern with more fruits and vegetables and whole grains.
  - Encourage intake of at least 600 IU of vitamin D per day as well as sources of calcium not to exceed 1200 mg/d.
  - Counsel survivors to avoid or limit alcohol consumption to no more than 2 drinks/d.
  - Counsel survivors to avoid tobacco products.

  –**Rising PSA in patients with nonmetastatic PC**
  - A PSA $\geq$ 0.2 ng/mL on 2 consecutive tests is reflective of recurrent prostate cancer. These patients are treated with pelvic radiation with improvement in 10-y survival and freedom from recurrence. The earlier radiation is started after a PSA rise, the better the outcome. Patients who have had previous radiation to the prostate occasionally undergo surgery but most are treated with ADT or cryoablation. (*JCO.* 2009;27:4300-4305) A recent trial adding ADT to radiation in this setting increased disease-free progression. (*Eur Urol.* 2016; 69:802)
  - Routine CT or bone scanning is not indicated but evaluate new symptoms even if PSA not rising (transformation to small cell carcinoma in 5% of patients).
  - In newly relapsed patients with visceral metastasis and/or more than 4 separate bone lesions a combination of concurrent androgen deprivation and taxotere chemotherapy is associated with a 15%–20% increased survival at 5 y vs. sequential therapy. (*N Engl J Med.* 2015;373:737. *Lancet.* 2016;387:1163)

PSORIASIS AND PSORIATIC ARTHRITIS

Population
  –Adults.

Recommendations

▶ AAD 2010
  –Treatment options for patients with limited plaque-type psoriasis.
  • First-line therapy:
    ◦ Topical corticosteroids.
    ◦ Topical calcipotriene/calcitriol.
    ◦ Topical calcipotriene/steroid.
    ◦ Topical tazarotene.
    ◦ Topical calcineurin inhibitors (flexural surfaces and face).
    ◦ Targeted phototherapy.
  • Second-line therapy:
    ◦ Systemic agents.
  –Treatment of extensive plaque-type psoriasis.
  • First-line therapy:
    ◦ UVB phototherapy ± acitretin.
    ◦ Topical PUVA.
  • Second-line therapy:
    ◦ Acitretin + biologic.
    ◦ Cyclosporine + biologic.
    ◦ Cyclosporine + methotrexate.
    ◦ Methotrexate + biologic.
    ◦ UVB + biologic.
  –Treatment of palmoplantar psoriasis.
  • First-line therapy:
    ◦ Topical corticosteroids.
    ◦ Topical calcipotriene/calcitriol.
    ◦ Topical calcipotriene/steroid.
    ◦ Topical tazarotene.
  • Second-line therapy:
    ◦ Acitretin.
    ◦ Targeted UVB.
    ◦ Topical PUVA.
  • Third-line therapy:
    ◦ Adalimumab.
    ◦ Alefacept.
    ◦ Cyclosporine.

     ◦ Etanercept.
     ◦ Infliximab.
     ◦ Methotrexate.
     ◦ Ustekinumab.
  −Treatment of erythrodermic psoriasis.
    • Acitretin.
    • Adalimumab.
    • Cyclosporine.
    • Infliximab.
    • Methotrexate.
    • Ustekinumab.
  −Treatment of psoriatic arthritis.
    • First-line therapy:
     ◦ Adalimumab.
     ◦ Etanercept.
     ◦ Golimumab.
     ◦ Infliximab.
     ◦ Methotrexate.
     ◦ Tumor necrosis factor (TNF) blocker + methotrexate.
    • Second-line therapy:
     ◦ Ustekinumab and methotrexate.

Sources
  −http://www.guideline.gov/content.aspx?id=15650
  −http://www.aad.org/File%20Library/Global%20navigation/
    Education%20and%20quality%20care/Guidelines-psoriasis-sec-2.pdf

Comment
  −Use of potent topical corticosteroids should be limited to 4 wk duration.

PSORIASIS, PLAQUE-TYPE

Population
  −Adults.

Recommendations
▶ AAD 2009

Topical Therapies
1. Topical therapies are most effective for mild-to-moderate disease.
2. Topical corticosteroids daily—bid:
    a. Cornerstone of therapy.
    b. Limit Class I topical steroids to 4 wk maximum.

3. Topical agents that have proven efficacy when combined with topical corticosteroids:

   a. Topical vitamin D analogues.

   b. Topical tazarotene.

   c. Topical salicylic acid.

4. Emollients applied 1–3 times daily are a helpful adjunct.

Source

–http://www.aad.org/File%20Library/Global%20navigation/
   Education%20and%20quality%20care/Guidelines-psoriasis-sec-3.pdf

Comments

1. Approximately 2% of population has psoriasis.

2. 80% of patients with psoriasis have mild-to-moderate disease.

3. Topical steroid toxicity:

   a. Local: skin atrophy, telangiectasia, striae, purpura, or contact dermatitis.

   b. Hypothalamic-pituitary—adrenal axis may be suppressed with prolonged use of medium- to high-potency steroids.

Recommendations

▶ AAD 2009

–Systemic Therapies

1. Indicated for severe, recalcitrant, or disabling psoriasis.

2. Methotrexate (MTX):

   a. Dose: 7.5–30 mg PO weekly.

   b. Monitor CBC and liver panel monthly.

3. Cyclosporine:

   a. Initial dose: 2.5–3 mg/kg divided bid.

   b. Monitor for nephrotoxicity, HTN, and hypertrichosis.

4. Acitretin:

   a. Dose: 10–50 mg PO daily.

   b. Monitor: liver panel.

Source

–http://www.aad.org/File%20Library/Global%20navigation/
   Education%20and%20quality%20care/Guidelines-psoriasis-sec-4.pdf

Comments

1. MTX contraindications: pregnancy; breast-feeding; alcoholism; chronic liver disease; immunodeficiency syndromes; cytopenias; hypersensitivity reaction.

2. Cyclosporine contraindications: CA; renal impairment; uncontrolled HTN.

3. Acitretin contraindications: pregnancy, chronic liver, or renal disease.

PSYCHIATRIC PATIENTS IN THE EMERGENCY DEPARTMENT

Population

–Adult patients presenting to ED with psychiatric symptoms

Recommendations

- No role for routine laboratory testing. Medical history, examination, and previous psychiatric diagnoses should guide testing.
- No role for routine neuroimaging studies in the absence of focal neurological deficits.
- Risk assessment tools should not be used in isolation to identify low-risk adults who are safe for ED discharge if they presented with suicidal ideations.
- Ketamine is one option for immediate sedation in severely agitated adults who may be violent or aggressive.

Source

–Nazarian DJ, Broder JS, Thiessen ME, Wilson MP, Zun LS, Brown MD, American College of Emergency Physicians. Clinical policy: critical issues in the diagnosis and management of the adult psychiatric patient in the emergency department. Ann Emerg Med. 2017 Apr; 69(4):480-98.

PULMONARY NODULES

Population

–Adults with pulmonary nodules.

Recommendations

▶ BTS 2015

–Do not recommend nodule follow-up or further work-up for nodules with:
- Size <5 mm.
- Diffuse, central, or laminated pattern of calcification or fat.
- Perifissural or subpleural nodules that are <1 cm and homogenous, smooth or solid with a lentiform or triangular shape.

–Recommend thin-slice CT surveillance for nodules 5–8 mm after 3 mo and 1 y.
- No further surveillance needed for stable nodules after 1 y.

–Recommend using the Brock model for initial risk assessment of pulmonary nodules 8 mm or larger in patients who have ever smoked.

–Consider a PET-CT scan for patients with a pulmonary nodule and an initial risk of malignancy >10%.

–Suggestions for pulmonary nodules management:
- Serial CT scans when the malignancy risk is <10%.
- CT-guided biopsy when the risk of malignancy is 10%–70%.
- Video-assisted thoracoscopic surgery when the chance of malignancy exceeds 70%.
- Consider bronchoscopy when a bronchus sign is present on CT scan.

Source
–https://guidelines.gov/summaries/summary/49569

RED BLOOD CELL (RBC) TRANSFUSION

Population
–General population, male and female.

Recommendation

▶ American Association of Blood Banks (AABB)

–**Hospitalized, hemodynamically stable patients—restrictive transfusion strategy preferred (see Table II).**
- For nonsurgical patients transfusion considered at hemoglobin of 7 g/dL or less.
- In post-op surgical patients transfusion considered at hemoglobin of 8 g/dL or less.
- Patients with heart disease should be treated with restrictive transfusion strategy (trigger hemoglobin 7-8 g/dL). Erythrocyte-stimulating agents should not be used because of increased thrombotic risk.
- In symptomatic patients (chest pain, tachycardia, hypotension, or heart failure) or with continued hemorrhage, clinical judgment should supervene.
- In patients meeting criteria for transfusion, give only as much as necessary to raise hemoglobin to recommended levels (1 unit of red blood cells will raise hemoglobin by 1 g/dL).
- Leukocyte reduction (either at the time of collection or filtration at the time of transfusion) is necessary to decrease febrile, nonhemolytic transfusion reactions, decrease risk of cytomegalovirus (CMV) transmission, and decrease risk of HLA-allo immunization but does not prevent transfusion associated graft vs. host disease (TA-GVHD).

TABLE II

RED BLOOD CELL—TRANSFUSION GUIDELINES FOR HEMODYNAMICALLY STABLE PATIENTS		
Patient Situation	**Transfusion Threshold**	**Strength of Evidence**
ICU[a]	Hgb ≤7 g/dL	High
Post-op	Hgb ≤8 g or symptoms[b]	High
Cardiovascular disease	Hgb ≤8 or symptoms[b]	Moderate

[a]Guidelines for non-ICU hospitalized patients have not been determined.
[b]Includes chest pain, hypoxia, hypotension and tachycardia, CHF, and ischemic bowel.

Comment

–**Important Information**
  - 15 million units of red blood cells are transfused annually in the US and 85 million transfused annually worldwide.
  - Transfusion carries significant risk of infection, immunosupression, hemolytic transfusion reaction, transfusion related acute lung injury (TRALI) (see Table III).
  - Nineteen trials were evaluated by AABB assessing noninferiority of restrictive vs liberal transfusion policy. There was no statistically significant difference although a trend for lower mortality in the patients treated by the restrictive transfusion policy was noted.
  - Patients with pharmacologically treatable anemia such as iron deficiency or B_{12} or folate deficiency should not be transfused unless they are significantly symptomatic.
  - Transfusion of red cells should be given slowly over first 15 min and completed within 4 h.

TABLE III

NONINFECTIOUS COMPLICATIONS OF BLOOD TRANSFUSION			
Complication	**Incidence**	**Diagnosis**	**Rx and Outcome**
Acute hemolytic transfusion reaction (AHTR)	1:40,000	Serum-free hemoglobin, Coombs	Fluids to keep urine output >1 mL/kg/h, pressors, treat DIC, fatal in 1:1.8 × 10⁶ RBC exposures
Delayed transfusion reaction (HTR)	1:3000–5000	Timing (10–14 d after tx)–(+) Coombs, ↑ LDH, indirect bilirubin, reticulocyte count— Ab often to Kidd or Rh	Identify responsible antigen, transfuse compatible blood if necessary

NONINFECTIOUS COMPLICATIONS OF BLOOD TRANSFUSION *(Continued)*			
Complication	**Incidence**	**Diagnosis**	**Rx and Outcome**
Febrile non-HTR	0.1%–1%	Exclude AHTR —↓ risk with leucocyte depletion—starts within 2 h of transfusion	Acetaminophen PO, support and reassurance
Allergic (urticarial)	1%–3%	Urticaria, pruritus but no fever—caused by antibody to donor-plasma proteins	Hold tx—give antihistamines and complete tx. when symptoms resolve
Anaphylactic	1:20,000–50,000	Hypotension, bronchospasm, urticaria, anxiety, rule out hemolysis	Epinephrine 1:1000—0.2–0.5 mL. SQ, steroids, antihistamine
Transfusion-related acute lung injury (TRALI)	1:10,000	HLA or neutrophil antibodies in donor blood hypoxia, bilateral lung infiltrates, and fever within 6 h of transfusion	Supportive care—steroids ineffective mortality—10%–20% (most common cause of transfusion-related fatality)

Recommendation

▶ AABB

–Prevention of TA-GVHD[a]—High risk

- High-risk situations include product donated by family member or HLA-selected donor.
- Acute leukemia and Hodgkin and non-Hodgkin lymphoma patients on therapy.
- Allogenic or autologous hemopoietic progenitor cell transplant recipient.
- Aplastic anemia patients on antithymocyte globulin and/or cyclosporine.
- Purine analogues and other drugs affecting T-cell count and function—fludarabine, clofarabine, bendamustine, nelarabine, alemtuzumab, and temozolomide.
- Recommended preventive strategy is 2500 cGy of radiation to product to be transfused. This dose will destroy T cells. Shelf life of irradiated product is 28 d.
- Infection complications of transfusion are now very rare (see Table IV).

[a]A-GVHD, transfusion-associated graft-versus-host disease

TABLE IV

INFECTIOUS COMPLICATIONS OF TRANSFUSION	
Transfusion-Transmitted Organism	**Risk per Unit of Blood Transfused**
HIV	1 in 1,467,000
Hepatitis C	1 in 1,149,000
Hepatitis B	1 in 282,000
West Nile virus	Rare
Cytomegalovirus (CMV)	70%–80% of donors are carriers, leukodepletion ↓ risk but in situation of significant immunosuppression gives CMV-negative blood
Bacterial infection	1 in 3000—5-fold more common in platelet vs. RBC transfusion
Parasitic infection (Babesiosis, malaria, Chagas disease)	Rare

Sources
–*Ann Intern Med.* 2012;157:49-58
–*Blood.* 2012;119:1757-1767
–*N Engl J Med.* 2011;365:2433-2462
–*Crit Care Med.* 2008;36:2667-2674
–*JAMA* 2016;316:1984

Comment
–Caution in the immunosuppressed:
- Must be aware of circumstances that increase risk of TA-GVHD in order to initiate protective strategy. If TA-GVHD does occur mortality approaches 100%.
- In immunosuppressed patients and in donating family members with shared genes, targeting T cells from the donor may not be eliminated through immunologic attack. These surviving T cells then interact with host cellular antigens damaging skin, liver, GI tract, and lung with high mortality.
- With polymerase chain reaction (PCR) and antibody screening transfusion-related infection complications are rare. Bacterial infection and sepsis occurs 50-fold more commonly with platelet transfusion vs. red blood cell transfusion.
- Immune-compromised patients needing transfusion should have CMV serology checked and if antibodies not present CMV-negative blood should be given (70%-80% of recipients are antibody positive).

RENAL CANCER (RCC) FOLLOW-UP CARE

Recommendations

▶ NCCN 2016

- –Stage I—Follow-up after a partial or radical nephrectomy
  - History and physical (H&P) every 6 mo for 2 y then annually up to 5 y after surgery.
  - Comprehensive metabolic panel or other blood tests as indicated every 6 mo for 2 y then annually until 5 y.
- –Abdominal imaging after partial nephrectomy
  - Baseline abdominal CT, MRI, or US within 3–9 mo of surgery. If initial scan-negative abdominal imaging may be considered annually for 3 y based on overall risk factors.
- –After radical nephrectomy
  - Abdominal CT, MRI, or US within 3–12 mo of surgery.
  - If initial post-op imaging is negative, abdominal imaging beyond 12 mo may be done at the discretion of the physician.
  - Chest x-ray or CT annually for 3 y then as indicated clinically.
- –Stage II or III—follow-up after radical nephrectomy
  - H & P every 3–6 mo for 3 y then annually up to 5 y after radical nephrectomy, then as clinically indicated.
  - Comprehensive metabolic panel, LDH, and C-reactive protein every 6 mo for 2 y then annually up to 5 y.
- –Abdominal imaging after radical nephrectomy
  - Baseline abdominal CT or MRI within 3–6 mo then CT, MRI, or US every 3–6 mo for 3 y then annually up to 5 y.
  - Chest imaging—baseline chest CT within 3–6 mo.
  - Pelvic, brain, or spinal imaging as clinically indicated. Nuclear bone scan as clinically indicated.

Source
–*J Clin Onc.* 2014; j32:4059

Comments

- –RCC staging
  - Stage I—Tumor <7 cm N0M0
  - Stage II—Tumor >7cm limited to kidney N0M0
  - Stage III—Any tumor size with regional node metastasis
  - Stage IV—T4 (spread beyond Gerota's fascia—any T, any N, M (systemic metastases)

–**Features of high risk for relapse**
  • Stage III, size of tumor, high grade (Fuhrman 3 or 4), coagulative tumor necrosis (5x increase risk of death). (*British J Urol.* 2009; 103:165)
–**Paraneoplastic syndromes in RCC and clinical caveats**
  • Anemia, hepatic dysfunction, fever, hypercalcemia, cachexia, erythrocytosis, thrombocytosis, polymyalgia rheumatica. (*Lancet.* 1998; 352:1691)
  • Chemotherapy no longer used in treatment of RCC. Multi-targeted tyrosine kinase inhibitors and checkpoint immune blockade are treatments of choice. High-dose interleukin-2 is used occasionally in young, fit patients. (*NEJM.* 2015;373:1803. *NEJM.* 2013;369:722)
  • In patients with small-volume metastasis a nephrectomy to remove the primary has resulted in a prolongation of survival. (*N Engl J Med.* 2001;345:1655)
  • In selected patients with low-volume, limited, resectable metastatic disease, surgical removal of the metastasis increases overall survival with occasional long-term remission. (*Cancer.* 2011;117:2873)
  • The use of adjuvant therapy with multi-targeted tyrosine kinase inhibitors does not extend progression-free or overall survival in a placebo-controlled trial. (*Lancet.* 2016; published online March 14, 2016). A 2nd trial in higher risk patients did show a survival benefit with adjuvant TKI inhibitors. (*N Engl J Med.* 2016; 375:2246)

CANCER SURVIVORSHIP: LATE EFFECTS OF CANCER TREATMENTS

CA Treatment History	Late Effects	Periodic Evaluation
Any CA experience	Psychosocial disorders[b]	
Any chemotherapy	Oral and dental abnormalities	Dental examination and cleaning (every 6 mo)
Chemotherapy— alkylating agents (cyclophosphamide, melphelan, ifosfamide, chlorambucil, nitrosoureas)[a]	Gonadal dysfunction Hematologic disorders[c] Ocular toxicity[d] Pulmonary toxicity Renal toxicity[f] Urinary tract toxicity[g]	Pubertal assessment (yearly) in adults if symptoms of hypogonadism present History, examination for bleeding disorder; CBC/differential (yearly) Visual acuity, funduscopic examination, evaluation by ophthalmologist (yearly if ocular tumors, TBI, or ≥30 Gy; otherwise, every 3 y) CXR, PFTs (at entry into long-term follow-up, then as clinically indicated)

CANCER SURVIVORSHIP: LATE EFFECTS OF CANCER TREATMENTS *(Continued)*		
CA Treatment History	**Late Effects**	**Periodic Evaluation**
		Blood pressure (yearly); electrolytes, BUN, creatinine, Ca^{++}, Mg^{++}, PO_4^- urinalysis (at entry into long-term follow-up, then clinically as indicated) Bone marrow injury with myelodysplasia
Chemotherapy—antitumor antibiotics (anthracycline, epirubicin)[a]	Cardiac toxicity[h]	ECHO or MUGA; ECG at entry into long-term follow-up, periodic thereafter (↑ frequency if chest radiation); fasting glucose, lipid panel (every 3–5 y)
	Hematologic disorders[c]	See "Chemotherapy—Alkylating agents"—risk of acute myelocytic leukemia
Chemotherapy—antitumor antibiotics (mitomycin C[f], bleomycin[e])	Pulmonary toxicity[e] Renal injury[f]	Chest x-ray and pulmonary function tests at end of exposure to bleomycin, with re-evaluation as clinically indicated Monitor urinalysis and creatinine (mito C)
Chemotherapy—antimetabolites (cytarabine, MTX) (high-dose IV, intrathecal)[b]	Clinical leukoencephalopathy[i] Neurocognitive deficits	Full neurologic examination (yearly) Neuropsychological evaluation (at entry into long-term follow-up, then as clinically indicated)
Chemotherapy—epipodophyllotoxins (Ixabepilone)[a]	Hematologic disorders (causes AML with specific 11q 23 translocation[c])	See "Chemotherapy—alkylating agents" Hematologic disorders, AML gonadal dysfunction
Chemotherapy heavy metals (cis-platinum, carboplatin)	Dyslipidemia/hypertension and increased risk of cardiovascular disease Gonadal dysfunction Hematologic disorders[c] Ototoxicity[j] Peripheral sensory neuropathy Renal toxicity[f]	See "Chemotherapy—alkylating agents" Fasting lipid panel at entry. Complete pure tone audiogram or brainstem auditory-evoked response (yearly × 2 then as indicated by symptoms) Examination yearly for at least 5 y Increased risk of renal insufficiency, neuropathy and cardiac events – lab work and careful F/U at least yearly

Chemotherapy—microtubular inhibitors (taxanes, eribulin)	Peripheral neuropathy	Examination yearly for 2–3 y If neuropathy persistent – duloxetine or venlafaxine may help
Chemotherapy—nonclassical alkylators (dacarbazine and temazolomide)	Gonadal dysfunction Reduced CD4 count Hematologic disorders[c]	See "Chemotherapy—alkylating agents" Monitor for opportunistic infections (CD_4 count at 6 and 12 mo)
Chemotherapy—plant alkaloids (vincristine, vinorelbine, vinblastin)	Peripheral sensory neuropathy Raynaud phenomenon	Yearly history/examination. May have persistent neuropathy—duloxetine may help
Chemotherapy—purine agonists (fludarabine, pentostatin)	Hematologic disorders[c] Reduction in CD4 count	See "Chemotherapy—alkylating agents" Monitor for infection
Corticosteroids (dexamethasone, prednisone)	Ocular toxicity[d] Avascular osteonecrosis Osteopenia/ osteoporosis	Musculoskeletal examination (yearly)
Targeted biologic therapy • Monoclonal antibodies • Trastuzumab (anti–HER-2) • Rituximab (anti-CD20 antibody to B lymphocyte receptor) • Panitumumab, cetuximab (anti-EGFR)	Cardiac dysfunction is usually reversible Reduction in immunoglobulins and increased risk of infection	Monitor 2D echo for ejection fraction every 3 mo during therapy and as needed for symptoms Monitor quantitative immunoglobulins if increased frequency of infection
Multi-targeted tyrosine kinase inhibitors (TKIs) • Erlotinib • Carbozantinib • Regorafenib • Sunitinib • Sorafenib • Axitinib • Pazopanib • Imatinib • Lenvatinib • Dasatinib • Nilotinib • Lapatinib	Fatigue, diarrhea, hypertension, liver injury while on drug but little long-term toxicity. Hand and foot syndrome (palmar–plantar, erythrodysethesia) vascular injury, fluid retention, renal dysfunction	Routine monitoring for end-organ damage after completion of therapy not indicated

CANCER SURVIVORSHIP: LATE EFFECTS OF CANCER TREATMENTS   (Continued)

CA Treatment History	Late Effects	Periodic Evaluation
Immune-mediated therapy (checkpoint inhibitors) • Pembrolizumab • Ipilimumab • Nivolumab	Autoimmunity— colitis, hepatitis, dermatitis, thyroiditis, hypophysitis, rare myocardial injury Adrenal insufficiency, pneumonitis—often reversible but not always Gonadal dysfunction Growth hormone deficiency (children and adolescents) Hyperthyroidism Hyperprolactinemia Hypothyroidism	Check hormone levels every 4 to 6 mo Cortisol and ACTH stimulation testing based on clinical symptoms TSH, free thyroxine (T$_4$) yearly Prolactin level (as clinically indicated) Monitor for pituitary insufficiency based on clinical findings Major activity in Lung cancer, Hodgkin's lymphoma, and renal cell cancer
Chemotherapy drugs with minimal long-term toxicity effects • Topoisomerase I inhibitors (Camptosar, topotecan) • Antibiotics (actinomycin) • Antimetabolites (L-asparaginase, 5-fluorouracil (5-FU), capecitabine, gemcitabine, 6-mercaptopurine) **Drug-Antibody Conjugates** • Bretuximb vedotin (anti-CD30 antibody—in Hodgkin lymphoma and T-cell lymphoma) • TDM1 (Kadcyla®) Her2-directed Herceptin linked to chemo for Her2 positive breast cancer	Mild reduction in bone marrow and renal reserve Neuropathy Mild bone marrow suppression	Routine monitoring for end-organ dysfunction is not indicated Monitor neuropathy and platelet count. These problems largely reversed when treatment stops

| Radiation therapy (field- and dose-dependent) | Cardiac toxicity[h] (chest radiation)
Central adrenal insufficiency (pediatric brain tumors)
Cerebrovascular complications[i]
Pulmonary injury with symptoms[e]
Functional asplenia
Bowel injury and obstruction | 8 AM serum cortisol (yearly × 15 y, and as clinically indicated)
Neurologic examination (yearly)
Head/neck examination (yearly)—persistent dry mouth
Blood culture when temperature ≥101°F (38.3°C), rapid institution of empiric antibiotics—increased infection risk with poor spleen function
Increased risk of breast cancer with mediastinal radiation in women 15–35 y old—breast MRI yearly
Surveillance for 2nd cancers related to therapeutic radiation |

AML, acute myelocytic leukemia; BMI, body mass index; BUN, blood urea nitrogen; CBC, complete blood count; CXR, chest x-ray; ECG, electrocardiogram; ECHO, echocardiogram; IV, intravenous; MTX, methotrexate; MUGA, multiple-gated acquisition scan; PFTs, pulmonary function tests; TBI, total-body irradiation; TSH, thyroid-stimulating hormone.

[a]Chemotherapeutic agents, by mechanism of action:
- Alkylating agents: busulfan, carmustine (BCNU), chlorambucil, cyclophosphamide, ifosfamide, lomustine (CCNU), mechlorethamine, melphalan, procarbazine, thiotepa.
- Antimetabolites: MTX, cytosine arabinoside, gemcitabine.
- Heavy metals: carboplatin, cisplatin, oxaliplatin.
- Nonclassical alkylators: dacarbazine (DTIC), temozolomide.
- Anthracycline antibiotics: daunorubicin, doxorubicin, epirubicin, idarubicin, mitoxantrone.
- Antitumor antibiotics: bleomycin, mitomycin C.
- Plant alkaloids: vinblastine, vincristine, vinorelbine.
- Purine agonists: fludarabine, pentostatin, cladribine.
- Microtubular inhibitors: docetaxel, paclitaxel, cabazitaxel, ixabepilone.
- Epipodophyllotoxins: etoposide (VP16), teniposide (VM26).

[b]Psychosocial disorders: mental health disorders, risky behaviors, psychosocial disability because of pain, fatigue, limitations in health care/insurance access, "chemo brain" syndrome.

[c]Hematologic disorders: acute myeloid leukemia, myelodysplasia.

[d]Ocular toxicity: cataracts, orbital hypoplasia, lacrimal duct atrophy, xerophthalmia, keratitis, telangiectasias, retinopathy, optic chiasm neuropathy, endophthalmos, chronic painful eye, maculopathy, glaucoma.

[e]Pulmonary toxicity: pulmonary fibrosis, interstitial pneumonitis, restrictive lung disease, obstructive lung disease. Increased sensitivity to oxygen toxicity—keep FiO_2 ≤28% in patients with previous bleomycin exposure.

[f]Renal toxicity: glomerular and tubular renal insufficiency, hypertension, hemolytic uremic syndrome.

[g]Urinary tract toxicity: hemorrhagic cystitis, bladder fibrosis, dysfunctional voiding, vesicoureteral reflux, hydronephrosis, bladder malignancy.

[h]Cardiac toxicity: cardiomyopathy, arrhythmias, left ventricular dysfunction, congestive heart failure, pericarditis, pericardial fibrosis, valvular disease, myocardial infarction, atherosclerotic heart disease.

[i]Clinical leukoencephalopathy: spasticity, ataxia, dysarthria, dysphagia, hemiparesis, seizures.

[j]Ototoxicity: sensorineural hearing loss, tinnitus, vertigo, tympanosclerosis, otosclerosis, eustachian tube dysfunction, conductive hearing loss.

CANCER SURVIVORSHIP: LATE EFFECTS OF CANCER TREATMENTS   *(Continued)*

[k]Oncologic disorders: secondary benign or malignant neoplasm, especially breast CA after mantle radiation, gastrointestinal malignancy after paraaortic radiation for seminoma of the testis.
[l]Cerebrovascular complications: stroke and occlusive cerebral vasculopathy.

Note: Guidelines for surveillance and monitoring for late effects after treatment for adult CAs, available via the National Comprehensive Cancer Network, Inc. (NCCN). (http://www.nccn.org/professionals/physician_gls).

Source: Long-Term Follow-Up Guidelines for Survivors of Childhood, Adolescent, and Young Adult Cancers. Children's Oncology Group, Version 3.0, October 2008. (For full guidelines and references, see http://www.survivorshipguidelines.org).
See also: *N Engl J Med.* 2006;355:1722-1782; *J Clin Oncol.* 2007;25:3991-4008. *JAMA.* 2011;305:2311.

RENAL MASSES, SMALL

Population
  –Adults with small renal masses SRM (<4 cm).

Recommendations

▶ ASCO Guidelines (*J Clin Oncol.* 2017; 35:668-680)

  –Based on tumor-specific findings and competing risks of mortality all patients with an SRM (<4 cm in size) should be considered for renal tumor biopsy (RTB) when the results may alter management (strength of recommendation: strong).

  –Active surveillance should be an initial management option for patients who have significant comorbidities and limited life expectancy (end-stage renal disease, SRM <1 cm, life expectancy <5 y).

  –Partial nephrectomy (PN) for SRM is the standard treatment that should be offered to all patients for whom an intervention is indicated and who possess a tumor that is amenable to this approach (recommendation: strong).

  –Percutaneous thermal ablation should be considered an option for patients who possess tumors such that complete ablation will be achieved. A biopsy should be obtained before or at the time of ablation (recommendation: moderate).

  –Radical nephrectomy for SRM should be reserved only for patients who possess a tumor of significant complexity that is not amenable to PN or where PN may result in unacceptable morbidity even when performed at centers of excellence. Referral to experienced surgeon and a center with experience should be considered (recommendation: strong).

  –Referral to a nephrologist should be considered if CKD (GFR<45 mL/min) or progressive CKD develops after treatment, especially if associated with proteinuria (recommendation: moderate).

Comments

–SRM are commonly discovered incidentally during diagnostic evaluation for other medical conditions. A significant number of SRM are benign. As the size increases (especially >4 cm), the likelihood of malignancy increases. Imaging with MRI, CT scans, and ultrasound cannot make an absolute diagnosis of malignancy, necessitating a core biopsy if possible. About 10%-15% of patients will have a nondiagnostic biopsy and must be followed closely and rebiopsied if the mass is growing. Radiofrequency ablation (RFA) is commonly used to ablate small cancers but should have a biopsy done first to document malignancy.

–Decision regarding therapy in patients with significant comorbidities is difficult. The Charleston Comorbidity Index (CCI) is a tool that can predict 1-y mortality. In patients with a short life expectancy, surveillance and supportive care are the best approach for this population. Partial nephrectomy is the treatment of choice for SRM that are amenable to nephron-sparing surgery. Radical nephrectomy in the past has been the procedure of choice in managing small RCC. Today partial nephrectomy is preferred and radical nephrectomy now is the treatment of choice in <30% of patients with SRM.

Sources

–*N Engl J Med*. 2010;362:624.
–*Eur Urol*. 2016;69:116
–*JAMA*. 2015;150:664.
–*Eur Urol*. 2015;67

RESPIRATORY TRACT INFECTIONS, LOWER

Population

–Adults.

Recommendations

▶ ESCMID 2011

–For *Streptococcus* pneumonia:
  • Erythromycin MIC >0.5 mg/L predicts clinical failure.
  • Penicillin MIC ≤8 mg/L predicts IV penicillin susceptibility.
–The role of community-acquired MRSA in community-acquired pneumonia (CAP) is poorly defined in Europe.
–A C-reactive protein (CRP) <2 mg/dL at presentation with symptoms >24 h makes pneumonia highly unlikely; a CRP >10 mg/dL makes pneumonia likely.

–Indications for antibiotics in lower respiratory tract infections (LRTIs):
- Suspected pneumonia.
- Acute exacerbation of COPD with increased dyspnea, sputum volume, and sputum purulence.

–Evaluation of patients admitted for CAP.
- Two sets of blood cultures.
- Pleural fluid analysis is indicated when a significant parapneumonic effusion exists.
- Sputum Gram stain and culture should be obtained if a purulent sputum sample can be obtained.
- Consider testing for urine pneumococcal antigen.
- Antibiotic duration for CAP should not exceed 8 d.

Source
–http://www.escmid.org/fileadmin/src/media/PDFs/4ESCMID_ Library/2Medical_Guidelines/ESCMID_Guidelines/Woodhead_et_al_ CMI_Sep_2011_LRTI_GL_fulltext.pdf

Comments
1. Consider aspiration pneumonia in patients with a pneumonia and dysphagia.
2. Empiric antibiotics of choice for LRTI in outpatient setting are amoxicillin or tetracycline.

RESPIRATORY TRACT INFECTIONS, UPPER

Population
–Adults.

Recommendation
▶ IDSA 2015

–Do not prescribe antibiotics for upper respiratory tract infections.

Source
–http://www.choosingwisely.org/societies/infectious-diseases-society-of-america/

Comments
1. Consider aspiration pneumonia in patients with a pneumonia and dysphagia.
2. Empiric antibiotic of choice for LRTI in outpatient setting is amoxicillin or tetracycline.

RESTLESS LEGS SYNDROME AND PERIODIC LIMB MOVEMENT DISORDERS

Population
  –Adults.

Recommendation
▶ American Academy of Neurology 2016, American Academy of Sleep Medicine 2012
  –Recommends for moderate to severe restless legs syndrome (RLS).
  • Strong evidence for following meds:
    ◦ Pramipexole.
    ◦ Rotigotine.
    ◦ Cabergoline.
    ◦ Gabapentin.
  • Moderate evidence for:
    ◦ Ropinirole.
    ◦ Pregabalin.
    ◦ IV ferric carboxymaltose.
  –For primary RLS with periodic limb movements of sleep.
    ◦ Ropinirole .
  –For primary RLS with concomitant anxiety or depression.
    ◦ Ropinirole.
    ◦ Pramipexole.
    ◦ Gabapentin.
  –For RLS and ferritin <75 μg/L.
  • Ferrous sulfate with vitamin C.
  –For RLS with ESRD on hemodialysis.
    ◦ Vitamin C and E supplementation.
    ◦ Consider adding ropinirole, levodopa, or exercise.

Sources
  –Winkelman JW, Armstrong MJ, Allen RP, et al. Practice guideline summary: treatment of restless legs syndrome in adults: report of the Guideline Development, Dissemination, and Implementation Subcommittee of the American Academy of Neurology. *Neurology.* 2016 Dec 13;87(24): 2585-2593. (http://guidelines.gov/summaries/summary/50689/)
  –www.guidelines.gov/content.aspx?id=38320

Comments
  1. Potential for heart valve damage with pergolide and cabergoline.
  2. Insufficient evidence to support any pharmacological treatment for periodic limb movement disorder.

RHEUMATOID ARTHRITIS (RA), BIOLOGIC DISEASE-MODIFYING ANTIRHEUMATIC DRUGS (DMARDS)

Population
–Adults.

Recommendations
▶ ACR 2008
1. Anti–TNF-α agents
   a. A tuberculosis (TB) skin test or IGRA must be checked before initiating these medications.
   b. Any patient with latent TB needs at least 1 mo treatment prior to the initiation of a TNF-α or biologic agent.
   c. Recommended for all patients with high disease activity and presence of poor prognostic features of any duration of disease
2. Recommended for patients with disease ≥6 mo who have failed nonbiologic DMARD therapy and have moderate-to-high disease activity, especially if poor prognostic features are present.
3. Abatacept has same indications as anti–TNF-α agents.
4. Rituximab has same indications as anti–TNF-α agents.
5. Recommends withholding all biologic DMARDs 1 wk before or after surgery.

Comment
1. Anti–TNF-α agents, abatacept, and rituximab all contraindicated in:
   a. Serious bacterial, fungal, and viral infections, or with latent TB.
   b. Acute viral hepatitis or Child's B or Child's C cirrhosis.
   c. Instances of a lymphoproliferative disorder treated ≤5 y ago; decompensated congestive heart failure (CHF); or any demyelinating disorder.

Recommendations
▶ ACR 2012
1. Target low disease activity or remission.
2. MTX or leflunomide monotherapy may be used for patients with any disease severity or duration.
3. Hydroxychloroquine or minocycline monotherapy recommended if low disease activity and duration ≤24 mo.
4. Sulfasalazine recommended for all disease durations and without poor prognostic features.[a]

---

[a]Functional limitation, presence of rheumatoid nodules, secondary Sjögren syndrome, RA vasculitis, Felty syndrome, and RA lung disease.

5. MTX plus either hydroxychloroquine or leflunomide recommended for moderate-to-high disease activity regardless of disease duration.
6. MTX plus sulfasalazine recommended for high disease activity and poor prognostic features.

RHINITIS

MANAGEMENT OF NONINFECTIOUS RHINITIS

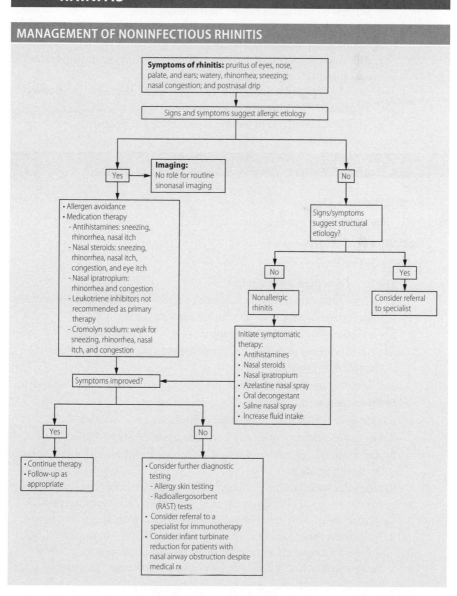

Sources
　　–ICSI, JAN 2011; AAO-HNSF, FEB 2015
　　–http://www.rheumatology.org/practice/clinical/guidelines/Singh_ACR_
　　　RA_GL_May_2012_AC-R.pdf

Comment

　　1. Contraindications to DMARD therapy:
　　　　a. Serious bacterial, fungal, or viral infections.
　　　　b. Only DMARDs safe with latent TB are hydroxychloroquine,
　　　　　 minocycline, and sulfasalazine.
　　　　c. Avoid MTX for interstitial pneumonitis and for creatinine clearance
　　　　　 <30 mL/min.
　　　　d. Avoid MTX and leflunomide for cytopenias, hepatitis, pregnancy,
　　　　　 and breast-feeding (also minocycline).
　　　　e. Avoid all DMARDs in Child's B or Child's C cirrhosis.

SCIATICA

Population

　　–People age ≥16 y with suspected sciatica.

Recommendations

▶ NICE 2016

For low-back pain with sciatica
　　1. Do not routinely offer imaging in a primary care setting to patient
　　　 with low-back pain with or without sciatica.
　　2. Continue aerobic exercise program.
　　3. Consider spinal manipulation or soft tissue massage as part of
　　　 treatment for sciatica.
　　4. Consider cognitive behavioral therapy as part of treatment for sciatica.
　　5. Promote return to work and normal activities.
　　6. Consider NSAIDs and low-dose opioids for acute sciatica.
　　7. For acute, severe sciatica can consider epidural steroid injection.
　　8. Recommend against opioids and anticonvulsants for chronic low-back
　　　 pain with sciatica.
　　9. Consider spinal decompression for people with disabling sciatica
　　　 for neurological deficits or chronic symptoms refractory to medical
　　　 management, and spine imaging is consistent with sciatica symptoms.
　　10. No proven benefit for belts, corsets, foot orthotics, rocker sole shoes,
　　　　 spine traction, acupuncture, ultrasound, transcutaneous electrical
　　　　 nerve stimulation (TENS), and interferential therapy for patients with
　　　　 sciatica.

Source
    –National Guideline Centre. *Low Back Pain and Sciatica in Over 16s:
    Assessment and Management*. London (UK): National Institute for
    Health and Care Excellence (NICE); 2016 Nov 30. 18 pp.

SEIZURES

Population
    –Adults.

Recommendations
▶ ACEP 2014

1. For first generalized convulsive seizure, ED physicians need not
   initiate chronic antiepileptic therapy.
   a. A precipitating medical condition should be sought.
   b. Need not admit patients who have returned to their clinical
      baseline.
2. If known seizure disorder, antiepileptic therapy in ED can be
   administered orally or by IV.
3. For status epilepticus:
   a. First-line therapy is benzodiazepines.
   b. Options for second-line therapy: phenytoin, fosphenytoin, valproic
      acid, levetiracetam.

Source
    –http://www.guideline.gov/content.aspx?id=47921

Comment
    –For refractory status epilepticus, consider intubation and use of a
    propofol infusion.

Population
    –Adults with first unprovoked seizure.

Recommendations
▶ AAN 2015

    –Patient education.
        • Recurrent seizures occur most frequently in the first 2 y.
        • Over the long term (>3 y), immediate antiepileptic drug (AED)
          therapy in unlikely to improve the prognosis for sustained seizure
          remission.
    –Indications for immediate antiepileptic therapy are based on clinical
    risk of a recurrent seizure.

–Risk factors for a recurrent seizure include:
- Brain injury.
- Prior stroke.
- Abnormal EEG with epileptiform activity.
- Structural abnormality on brain imaging.
- Nocturnal seizure.

Source
–https://guidelines.gov/summaries/summary/49218

SEIZURES, FEBRILE

Population
–Children 6 mo to 5 y old.

Recommendations
▶ AAP 2011

–A lumbar puncture should be performed in any child who presents with a fever and seizure and has meningeal signs or whose history is concerning for meningitis.

–Lumbar puncture is an option in children 6–12 mo of age who present with a fever and seizure and are not up to date with their *Haemophilus influenzae* or *Streptococcus pneumoniae* vaccinations.

–Lumbar puncture is an option in a child presenting with a fever and a seizure who has been pretreated with antibiotics.

–Studies that should not be performed for a simple febrile seizure:
- An EEG.
- Routine labs including a basic metabolic panel, calcium, phosphorus, magnesium, glucose, or CBC.
- Neuroimaging.

Source
–http://pediatrics.aappublications.org/content/127/2/389.full.pdf+html

Comment
–A febrile seizure is a seizure accompanied by fever (T ≥100.4°F [38°C]) without CNS infection in a child age 6 mo to 5 y.

SEXUALLY TRANSMITTED DISEASES

SEXUALLY TRANSMITTED DISEASES TREATMENT GUIDELINES

Infection	Recommended Treatment	Alternative Treatment
Chancroid	• Azithromycin 1 g PO × 1 • Ceftriaxone 250 mg IM × 1	• Ciprofloxacin 500 mg PO bid for 3 d • Erythromycin base 500 mg PO tid for 7 d
First episode of genital HSV	• Acyclovir 400 mg PO tid × 7–10 d[a] • Famciclovir 250 mg PO tid × 7–10 d[a] • Valacyclovir 1 g PO bid × 7–10 d[a-]	• Acyclovir 200 mg PO 5 times a day for 7–10 d[a]
Suppressive therapy for genital HSV	• Acyclovir 400 mg PO bid • Famciclovir 250 mg PO bid	• Valacyclovir 1 g PO daily
Episodic therapy for recurrent genital HSV	• Acyclovir 400 mg PO tid × 5 d • Famciclovir 125 mg PO bid × 5 d • Valacyclovir 500 mg PO bid × 3 d	• Acyclovir 800 mg PO bid × 5 d • Acyclovir 800 mg PO tid × 2 d • Famciclovir 1000 mg PO bid × 1 d • Famciclovir 500 mg PO × 1 then 250 mg bid × 2 d • Valacyclovir 1 g PO daily × 5 d
Suppressive therapy for HIV-positive patients	• Acyclovir 400–800 mg PO bid–tid • Famciclovir 500 mg PO bid • Valacyclovir 500 mg PO bid	
Episodic therapy for recurrent genital HSV in HIV-positive patients	• Acyclovir 400 mg PO tid × 5–10 d • Famciclovir 500 mg PO bid × 5–10 d • Valacyclovir 1 g PO bid × 5–10 d	
Granuloma inguinale (Donovanosis)	• Doxycycline 100 mg PO bid × ≥3 wk and until all lesions have completely healed	• Azithromycin 1 g PO weekly × ≥3 wk • Ciprofloxacin 750 mg PO bid × ≥3 wk • Erythromycin base 500 mg PO QID × ≥3 wk

SEXUALLY TRANSMITTED DISEASES TREATMENT GUIDELINES *(Continued)*

Infection	Recommended Treatment	Alternative Treatment
		• TMP-SMX 1 double-strength (160/800 mg) tablet PO bid × ≥3 wk • Continue all of these treatments until all lesions have completely healed
Lymphogranuloma venereum	• Doxycycline 100 mg PO bid for × 21 d	• Erythromycin base 500 mg PO qid × 21 d
Syphilis in adults	• Benzathine penicillin G 2.4 million units IM × 1	
Syphilis in infants and children	• Benzathine penicillin G 50,000 units/kg IM, up to the adult dose of 2.4 million units × 1	
Early latent syphilis in adults	• Benzathine penicillin G 2.4 million units IM × 1	
Early latent syphilis in children	• Benzathine penicillin G 50,000 units/kg IM, up to the adult dose of 2.4 million units × 1	
Late latent syphilis or latent syphilis of unknown duration in adults	• Benzathine penicillin G 2.4 million units IM weekly × 3 doses	
Late latent syphilis or latent syphilis of unknown duration in children	• Benzathine penicillin G 50,000 units/kg, up to the adult dose of 2.4 million units, IM weekly × 3 doses	
Tertiary syphilis	• Benzathine penicillin G 2.4 million units IM weekly × 3 doses	
Neurosyphilis	• Aqueous crystalline penicillin G 3–4 million units IV q4h × 10–14 d	• Procaine penicillin 2.4 million units IM daily × 10–14 d **PLUS** • Probenecid 500 mg PO qid × 10–14 d
Syphilis, pregnant women	• Pregnant women should be treated with the penicillin regimen appropriate for their stage of infection	

Congenital syphilis	• Aqueous crystalline penicillin G 50,000 units/kg/dose IV q12h × 7 d; then q8h × 3 more days	• Procaine penicillin G 50,000 units/kg/dose IM daily × 10 d • Benzathine penicillin G 50,000 units/kg/dose IM × 1
Older children with syphilis	• Aqueous crystalline penicillin G 50,000 units/kg IV q4–6h × 10 d	
Nongonococcal urethritis	• Azithromycin 1 g PO × 1 • Doxycycline 100 mg PO bid × 7 d	• Erythromycin base 500 mg PO qid × 7 d • Erythromycin ethylsuccinate 800 mg PO qid × 7 d • Levofloxacin 500 mg PO daily × 7 d • Ofloxacin 300 mg PO bid × 7 d
Recurrent or persistent urethritis	• Metronidazole 2 g PO × 1 • Tinidazole 2 g PO × 1 • Azithromycin 1 g PO × 1	
Cervicitis[b]	• Azithromycin 1 g PO × 1 • Doxycycline 100 mg PO bid × 7 d	
Chlamydia infections in adolescents, adults[b]	• Azithromycin 1 g PO × 1 • Doxycycline 100 mg PO bid × 7 d	• Erythromycin base 500 mg PO qid × 7 d • Erythromycin ethylsuccinate 800 mg PO qid × 7 d • Levofloxacin 500 mg PO daily × 7 d • Ofloxacin 300 mg PO bid × 7 d
Chlamydia infections in pregnancy[b]	• Azithromycin 1 g PO × 1 • Amoxicillin 500 mg PO tid × 7 d	• Erythromycin base 500 mg PO qid × 7 d • Erythromycin ethylsuccinate 800 mg PO qid × 7 d
Ophthalmia neonatorum from *Chlamydia*	• Erythromycin base or ethylsuccinate 50 mg/kg/d PO qid × 14 d	
Chlamydia trachomatis pneumonia in infants	• Erythromycin base or ethylsuccinate 50 mg/kg/d PO qid × 14 d	
Chlamydia infections in children <45 kg	• Erythromycin base or ethylsuccinate 50 mg/kg/d PO qid × 14 d	
Chlamydia infections in children ≥45 kg and age <8 y	• Azithromycin 1 g PO × 1	

SEXUALLY TRANSMITTED DISEASES TREATMENT GUIDELINES *(Continued)*

Infection	Recommended Treatment	Alternative Treatment
Chlamydia infections in children age ≥8 y	• Azithromycin 1 g PO × 1 • Doxycycline 100 mg PO bid × 7 d	
Uncomplicated gonococcal infections of the cervix, urethra, pharynx, or rectum in adults or children >45 kg	• Ceftriaxone 250 mg IM × 1 **PLUS** • Azithromycin 1 g PO × 1 **OR** • Doxycycline 100 mg daily × 7 d	
Gonococcal conjunctivitis in adults or children >45 kg	• Ceftriaxone 1 g IM × 1	
Gonococcal meningitis or endocarditis in adults or children >45 kg	• Ceftriaxone 1 g IV q12h	
Disseminated gonococcal infection in adults or children >45 kg	• Ceftriaxone 1 g IV/IM daily	• Cefotaxime 1 g IV q8h • Ceftizoxime 1 g IV q8h
Ophthalmia neonatorum caused by gonococcus	• Ceftriaxone 25–50 mg/kg, not to exceed 125 mg, IV/IM × 1	
Prophylactic treatment of infants born to mothers with gonococcal infection	• Ceftriaxone 25–50 mg/kg, not to exceed 125 mg, IV/IM × 1	
Uncomplicated gonococcal infections of the cervix, urethra, pharynx, or rectum in children ≤45 kg	• Ceftriaxone 125 mg IM × 1	
Gonococcal infections with bacteremia or arthritis in children or adults	• Ceftriaxone 50 mg/kg (maximum dose 1 g) IM/IV daily × 7 d	

Ophthalmia neonatorum prophylaxis	• Erythromycin (0.5%) ophthalmic ointment in each eye × 1	
Bacterial vaginosis	• Metronidazole 500 mg PO bid × 7 d[c] • Metronidazole gel 0.75%, 1 applicator (5 g) IVag daily × 5 d • Clindamycin cream 2%, 1 applicator (5 g) IVag qhs × 7 d[d]	• Tinidazole 2 g PO daily × 3 d • Clindamycin 300 mg PO bid × 7 d • Clindamycin ovules 100 mg IVag qhs × 3 d
Bacterial vaginosis in pregnancy	• Metronidazole 500 mg PO bid × 7 d • Metronidazole 250 mg PO tid × 7 d • Clindamycin 300 mg PO bid × 7 d	
Trichomoniasis	• Metronidazole 2 g PO × 1[c] • Tinidazole 2 g PO × 1	• Metronidazole 500 mg PO bid × 7 d[c]
Candidal vaginitis	• Butoconazole 2% cream 5 g IVag × 3 d • Clotrimazole 1% cream 5 g IVag × 7–14 d • Clotrimazole 2% cream 5 g IVag × 3 d • Nystatin 100,000-unit vaginal tablet, 1 tablet IVag × 14 d • Miconazole 2% cream 5 g IVag × 7 d • Miconazole 4% cream 5 g IVag × 3 d • Miconazole 100-mg vaginal suppository, one suppository IVag × 7 d • Miconazole 200-mg vaginal suppository, one suppository IVag × 3 d • Miconazole 1200-mg vaginal suppository, one suppository IVag × 1	• Fluconazole 150-mg oral tablet, 1 tablet in single dose

SEXUALLY TRANSMITTED DISEASES TREATMENT GUIDELINES   *(Continued)*

Infection	Recommended Treatment	Alternative Treatment
	• Tioconazole 6.5% ointment 5 g IVag × 1 • Terconazole 0.4% cream 5 g IVag × 7 d • Terconazole 0.8% cream 5 g IVag × 3 d • Terconazole 80-mg vaginal suppository, 1 suppository IVag × 3 d	
Severe pelvic inflammatory disease	• Cefotetan 2 g IV q12h **OR** • Cefoxitin 2 g IV q6h **PLUS** • Doxycycline 100 mg PO/IV bid	• Clindamycin 900 mg IV q8h **PLUS** • Gentamicin loading dose IV or IM (2 mg/kg of body weight), followed by a maintenance dose (1.5 mg/kg) q8h. Single daily dosing (3–5 mg/kg) can be substituted. **OR** • Ampicillin/sulbactam 3 g IV q6h **PLUS** • Doxycycline 100 mg PO/IV bid
Mild-to-moderate pelvic inflammatory disease	• Ceftriaxone 250 mg IM × 1 **OR** • Cefoxitin 2 g IM × 1 and probenecid 1 g PO × 1 **PLUS** • Doxycycline 100 mg PO bid × 14 d ± metronidazole 500 mg PO bid × 14 d[c]	
Epididymitis	• Ceftriaxone 250 mg IM × 1 **PLUS** • Doxycycline 100 mg PO bid × 10 d	• Levofloxacin 500 mg PO daily × 10 d • Ofloxacin 300 mg PO bid × 10 d
External genital warts	**Provider-Administered:** • Cryotherapy every 1–2 wk • Podophyllin resin 10%–25% in a compound tincture of benzoin	**Patient-Applied:** • Podofilox 0.5% solution or gel • Imiquimod 5% cream • Sinecatechins 15% ointment

	• TCA or BCA 80%–90% • Surgical removal by tangential scissor excision, tangential shave excision, curettage, or electrosurgery	
Cervical warts	• Biopsy to exclude high-grade SIL must be performed before treatment is initiated	
Vaginal warts	• TCA or BCA 80%–90% applied only to warts, repeated weekly	
Urethral meatal warts	• Cryotherapy every 1–2 wk • TCA or BCA 80%–90% applied only to warts, repeated weekly	
Anal warts	• Cryotherapy every 1–2 wk • TCA or BCA 80%–90% applied only to warts, repeated weekly	• Surgical removal by tangential scissor excision, tangential shave excision, curettage, or electrosurgery
Proctitis	• Ceftriaxone 250 mg IM × 1 **PLUS** • Doxycycline 100 mg PO bid × 7 d	
Pediculosis pubis	• Permethrin 1% cream rinse applied to affected areas and washed off after 10 min • Pyrethrins with piperonyl butoxide applied to the affected area and washed off after 10 min	• Malathion 0.5% lotion applied for 8–12 h and then washed off • Ivermectin 250 μg/kg PO, repeated in 2 wk
Scabies	• Permethrin cream (5%) applied to all areas of the body from the neck down and washed off after 8–14 h • Ivermectin 200 μg/kg PO, repeat in 2 wk	• Lindane (1%) 1 oz of lotion (or 30 g of cream) applied in a thin layer to all areas of the body from the neck down and thoroughly washed off after 8 h

BCA, bichloroacetic acid; bid, twice a day; h, hour(s); HIV, human immunodeficiency virus; HSV, herpes simplex virus; IM, intramuscular; IV, intravenous; IVag, intravaginally; PO, by mouth; q, every; qhs, at bedtime; qid, four 4 times a day; SIL, squamous intraepithelial lesion; TCA, trichloroacetic acid; tid, 3 times a day; TMP-SMX, trimethoprim-sulfamethoxazole.

[a]Treatment can be extended if healing is incomplete after 10 d of therapy.
[b]Consider concomitant treatment of gonorrhea.
[c]Avoid alcohol during treatment and for 24 h after treatment is completed.
[d]Clindamycin cream may weaken latex condoms and diaphragms during treatment and for 5 d thereafter.

Source: Adapted from CDC Guidelines. MMWR Recomm Rep. 2010;59(RR-12):1-116.

SINUSITIS

Population
–Children age 1–18 y.

Recommendation
▶ ACEP 2013

–Avoid prescribing antibiotics in the ER for patients presenting with uncomplicated acute sinusitis.

Source
–http://www.choosingwisely.org/societies/american-college-of-emergency-physicians/

Comment
–Improvement of symptoms should occur within 72 h of antibiotic initiation.

SINUSITIS, ACUTE BACTERIAL

Population
–Children age 1–18 y with acute bacterial sinusitis.

Recommendations
▶ AAP 2013

–Presumptive acute sinusitis if child with acute URI and one of the following:
  • Nasal discharge or persistent cough lasting more than 10 d.
  • Worsening course.
  • Severe onset with fever ≥102.2°F and purulent nasal discharge for at least 3 d.
–Recommend against imaging studies for uncomplicated sinusitis.
–Contrast-enhanced CT scan of sinuses for any suspicion of orbital or CNS involvement.
–Recommend antibiotics for any sinusitis with a severe onset or worsening course.
  • Amoxicillin +/– clavulanate is first-line therapy.
  • Persistent cough or rhinorrhea in the absence of severe symptoms may be managed with ongoing observation.

Source
–https://guidelines.gov/summaries/summary/46939

STROKE, ACUTE ISCHEMIC

Population
–Adults age 18 y and older presenting to the emergency department with an acute ischemic stroke.

Recommendations
▶ AHA/ASA 2016
–For otherwise medically eligible patients ≥18 y of age, intravenous alteplase administration within 3 h is equally recommended for patients <80 y of age **AND >80 y of age.**
–For severe stroke symptoms, intravenous alteplase is indicated within 3 h from symptom onset of ischemic stroke (even for NIHSS >22).
–Intravenous alteplase treatment in the 3- to 4.5-h time window is also recommended for those patients <80 y of age without a history of both diabetes mellitus and prior stroke, NIHSS score <25, not taking any anticoagulants, and without imaging evidence of ischemic injury involving more than one-third of the MCA territory
–In patients with end-stage renal disease on hemodialysis and normal aPTT, intravenous alteplase is recommended.

Stroke Rehabilitation
–It is recommended that stroke survivors receive rehabilitation at an intensity commensurate with anticipated benefit and tolerance.
–During hospitalization and inpatient rehabilitation, regular skin assessments are recommended with objective scales of risk such as the Braden scale.
–Regular turning, good skin hygiene, and use of specialized mattresses, wheelchair cushions, and seating are recommended until mobility returns.
–Resting ankle splints used at night and during assisted standing may be considered for prevention of ankle contracture in the hemiplegic limb.
–In ischemic stroke, prophylactic-dose subcutaneous heparin (UFH or LMWH) should be used for the duration of the acute and rehabilitation hospital stay or until the stroke survivor regains mobility.
–Remove a Foley catheter within 24 h of hospitalization if possible.
–Assessment of urinary retention through bladder scanning or intermittent catheterizations after voiding while recording volumes is recommended for patients with urinary incontinence or retention.
–It is recommended that individuals with stroke discharged to the community participate in exercise programs with balance training to reduce falls.

–It is recommended that individuals with stroke be provided a formal fall prevention program during hospitalization.

–Administration of a structured depression inventory such as the Patient Health Questionnaire-2 is recommended to routinely screen for poststroke depression. Antidepressants should be prescribed to all patients with depression.

–It is recommended that individuals with stroke residing in long-term care facilities be evaluated for calcium and vitamin D supplementation.

–It is recommended that all individuals with stroke be provided a formal assessment of their ADLs and IADLs, communication abilities, and functional mobility before discharge from acute care hospitalization and the findings be incorporated into the care transition and the discharge planning process.

–Assess speech, language, cognitive communication, pragmatics, reading, and writing; identify communicative strengths and weaknesses; and identify helpful compensatory strategies.

Sources

–Scientific rationale for the inclusion and exclusion criteria for intravenous alteplase in acute ischemic stroke: a statement for healthcare professionals from the American Heart Association/ American Stroke Association. *Stroke.* 2016;47:581-641.

–Guidelines for Adult Stroke Rehabilitation and Recovery: a guideline for healthcare professionals from the American Heart Association/ American Stroke Association. *Stroke.* 2016;47:e98-e169.

▶ ACEP 2015, AAN 2015

–IV tissue plasminogen activator (tPA) should be offered to patients presenting to the ED with an acute ischemic stroke if within 3 h of symptom onset and the hospital has systems in place to safely administer the medication.

–IV tPA may be offered to patients presenting to the ED with an acute ischemic stroke if between 3–4.5 h of symptom onset and the hospital has systems in place to safely administer the medication.

Source

–https://guidelines.gov/summaries/summary/49538

STROKE, RECURRENCE

Population
–Atrial fibrillation.

Recommendations

▶ AHA/ASA 2014

1. For most patients with a stroke or TIA in the setting of AF, it is reasonable to initiate oral anticoagulation within 14 d after the onset of neurological symptoms. In the presence of high risk for hemorrhagic conversion (ie, large infarct, hemorrhagic transformation on initial imaging, uncontrolled hypertension, or hemorrhage tendency), it is reasonable to delay initiation of oral anticoagulation beyond 14 d.

2. VKA therapy (Class I; Level of Evidence A), apixaban (Class I; Level of Evidence A), and dabigatran (Class I; Level of Evidence B) are all indicated for the prevention of recurrent stroke in patients with nonvalvular AF, whether paroxysmal or permanent. Rivaroxaban is reasonable for the prevention of recurrent stroke in patients with nonvalvular AF.

3. For patients with ischemic stroke or TIA and AF who are unable to take oral anticoagulants, aspirin alone is recommended. The addition of clopidogrel to aspirin therapy might be reasonable.

4. The usefulness of closure of the left atrial appendage with the WATCHMAN device in patients with ischemic stroke or TIA and AF is uncertain.

Population
–Hypertension.

Recommendation

▶ AHA/ASA 2014

–Initiation of BP therapy is indicated for previously untreated patients with ischemic stroke or TIA who after the first several days have an established SBP ≥140 mm Hg or DBP ≥90 mm Hg. In patients previously treated for HTN, resumption of BP therapy is indicated beyond the first several days for both prevention of recurrent stroke and other vascular events. Goals: <140/90 mm Hg; for recent lacunar stroke reasonable SBP target <130 mm Hg.

Population
–Dyslipidemia.

Recommendation

▶ AHA/ASA 2014

–Intensive lipid-lowering effects are recommended in patients with ischemic stroke or TIA presumed to be of atherosclerotic origin, an LDL-C ≥100 mg/dL and with/without evidence of other clinical ASCVD.

Population
–Glucose disorders.

Recommendation

▶ AHA/ASA 2014

–All patients should be screened for DM (HgbA1c).

Population
–Obesity

Recommendation

▶ AHA/ASA 2014

–Calculate BMI for all patients and start weight-loss management when necessary.

Population
–Sleep apnea.

Recommendation

▶ AHA/ASA 2014

–A sleep study might be considered for patients with history of CVA or TIA on the basis of very high prevalence in this population.

Population
–MI and thrombus.

Recommendation

▶ AHA/ASA 2014

–VKA therapy (INR: 2–3) for 3 mo may be considered in patients with ischemic stroke or TIA in the setting of acute anterior STEMI.

Population
–Cardiomyopathy.

Recommendation
▶ AHA/ASA 2014

–In patients with ischemic stroke or TIA in sinus rhythm who have left atrial or left ventricular thrombus demonstrated by echocardiography or other imaging modality, anticoagulant therapy with a VKA is recommended for ≥3 mo.

Population
–Valvular heart disease.

Recommendations
▶ AHA/ASA 2014

–For patients with ischemic stroke or TIA who have rheumatic mitral valve disease and AF, long-term VKA therapy with an INR target of 2.5 (range 2.0–3.0) is recommended.
–For patients with ischemic stroke or TIA and native aortic or nonrheumatic mitral valve disease who do not have AF or another indication for anticoagulation, antiplatelet therapy is recommended.

Population
–Prosthetic heart valve.

Recommendations
▶ AHA/ASA 2014

–For patients with a mechanical aortic valve and a history of ischemic stroke or TIA before its insertion, VKA therapy is recommended with an INR target of 2.5 (range, 2.0–3.0).
–For patients with a mechanical mitral valve and a history of ischemic stroke or TIA before its insertion, VKA therapy is recommended with an INR target of 3.0 (range, 2.5–3.5).
–For patients with a mechanical mitral or aortic valve who have a history of ischemic stroke or TIA before its insertion and who are at low risk for bleeding, the addition of aspirin 75 to 100 mg/d to VKA therapy is recommended.
–For patients with a bioprosthetic aortic or mitral valve, a history of ischemic stroke or TIA before its insertion, and no other indication for anticoagulation therapy beyond 3 to 6 mo from the valve placement, long-term therapy with aspirin 75 to 100 mg/d is recommended in preference to long-term anticoagulation.

Population

–Aortic arch atheroma.

Recommendation

▶ AHA/ASA 2014

–For patients with an ischemic stroke or TIA and evidence of aortic arch atheroma, antiplatelet therapy is recommended.

Population

–PFO.

Recommendations

▶ AHA/ASA 2014

–For patients with an ischemic stroke or TIA and a PFO who are not undergoing anticoagulation therapy, antiplatelet therapy is recommended.

–For patients with an ischemic stroke or TIA and both a PFO and a venous source of embolism, anticoagulation is indicated, depending on stroke characteristics. When anticoagulation is contraindicated, an inferior vena cava filter is reasonable.

–For patients with a cryptogenic ischemic stroke or TIA and a PFO without evidence for DVT, available data do not support a benefit for PFO closure.

–In the setting of PFO and DVT, PFO closure by a transcatheter device might be considered, depending on the risk of recurrent DVT.

Population

–Homocysteinemia.

Recommendation

▶ AHA/ASA 2014

–Routine screening for hyperhomocysteinemia among patients with a recent ischemic stroke or TIA is not indicated.

Population

–Hypercoagulation.

Recommendations

▶ AHA/ASA 2014

–The usefulness of screening for thrombophilic states in patients with ischemic stroke or TIA is unknown.

–Antiplatelet therapy is recommended in patients who are found to have abnormal findings on coagulation testing after an initial ischemic stroke or TIA if anticoagulation therapy is not administered.

Population

–Sickle cell disease.

Recommendation

▶ AHA/ASA 2014

- For patients with sickle cell disease ad prior ischemic stroke or TIA, chronic blood transfusions to reduce hemoglobin S to <30% of total hemoglobin are recommended.

Population

–Pregnancy.

Recommendations

▶ AHA/ASA 2014

1. In the presence of a high-risk condition that would require anticoagulation outside of pregnancy, the following options are reasonable:
   a. LMWH twice daily throughout pregnancy, with dose adjusted to achieve the LMWH manufacturer's recommended peak anti-Xa level 4 h after injection, **OR**
   b. Adjusted-dose UFH throughout pregnancy, administered subcutaneously every 12 h in doses adjusted to keep the midinterval aPTT at least twice control or to maintain an anti-Xa heparin level of 0.35 to 0.70 U/mL, **OR**
   c. UFH or LMWH (as above) until the 13th week, followed by substitution of a VKA until close to delivery, when UFH or LMWH is resumed

2. For pregnant women receiving adjusted-dose LMWH therapy for a high-risk condition that would require anticoagulation outside of pregnancy, and when delivery is planned, it is reasonable to discontinue LMWH ≥24 h before induction of labor or cesarean section.

3. In the presence of a low-risk situation in which antiplatelet therapy would be the treatment recommendation outside of pregnancy, UFH or LMWH, or no treatment may be considered during the first trimester of pregnancy depending on the clinical situation.

Population

–Breast-feeding

Recommendations

▶ AHA/ASA 2014

–In the presence of a high-risk condition that would require anticoagulation outside of pregnancy, it is reasonable to use warfarin, UFH, or LMWH.

–In the presence of a low-risk situation in which antiplatelet therapy would be the treatment recommendation outside of pregnancy, low-dose aspirin use may be considered.

Sources

–Guidelines for the Prevention of Stroke in Patients with Stroke and Transient Ischemic Attack: a guideline for healthcare professionals from the American Heart Association/American Stroke Association. *Stroke.* 2014;45.

–http://stroke.ahajournals.org

AHA/ASA ISCHEMIC STROKE GUIDELINES 2013

- Physicians should use *stroke assessment tools* like the Cincinnati Prehospital Stroke Scale or the Los Angles Prehospital Stroke Screen to aid in prompt assessment.
- The role of *9-1-1 emergency systems* should be recommended to ensure prompt transport of patients to the appropriate emergency system.
- Physicians should encourage their local hospitals to become *Primary Care Centers* or *Comprehensive Care Centers.*
- *Neurology imaging* is essential. If not available, teleradiology systems should be encouraged to allow for prompt diagnosis.
- A multidisciplinary *stroke team* should be established including physicians, nurses, and laboratory and radiology personnel.
- An emergency department *stroke protocol* should exist to allow prompt evaluation and initiation of fibrinolytic treatment within 60 min. This should include a stroke severity scale such as NIHSS.
- Noncontrast CT of the head is the first imaging test suggested to exclude intracerebral hemorrhage. A noncontrast CT or MRI is recommended before fibrinolysis is started. These tests should be interpreted within 45 min of patient's arrival.
- Consideration of intravenous recombinant tissue-type plasminogen activator (rtPA) should be considered in all ischemic stroke patients who meet the indications and have no exclusion criteria.
- Imaging with noncontrast CT or MRI is indicated in all patients presenting with transient neurologic symptoms (TIA). The MRI is the test of choice. The test should be performed within 24 h of presentation.
- Sources of hyperthermia should be investigated and treatment should be started.

- Hypertension for hypertension during a stroke should be withheld until BP 220/120 mm Hg. If the BP exceeds that level, it should be lowered by 15% during the first 24 h. BP goals are lower if the patient is to receive rtPA.
- Treat persistent hyperglycemia at ranges of 140–180 mg/dL.
- Intravenous rtPA should be administered to all eligible patients even if intraarterial treatments are being considered. Intraarterial fibrinolysis should be considered with major strokes of <6 h duration involving the middle cerebral artery. This procedure should be performed only in stroke centers.
- Urgent anticoagulation to prevent recurrent stroke or improve symptoms is not recommended.
- Aspirin within 24–48 h after stroke is recommended. ASA administration within 24 h postfibrinolysis is not recommended.
- Stroke Units, which give comprehensive specialized stroke care, are recommended.

Source: Jauch EC, Saver JL, Adams HP, et al. Guidelines for the early management of patients with acute ischemic stroke. Guideline for healthcare professionals from the American Heart Association/American Stroke Association. *Stroke.* 2013;44:870-947.

INTRACRANIAL STROKE AHA/ASA GUIDELINES 2014

- For patients with recent (<30 d) stroke or TIA attributable to severe stenosis (70%–99%) of a major intracranial artery, the addition of clopidogrel 75 mg daily in addition to ASA for 90 d might be reasonable.
- The combination of aspirin and clopidogrel might be considered for initiation within 24 h of a minor ischemic stroke or TIA and for continuation for 90 d.
- For patients with a stroke or TIA attributable to 50%–99% stenosis of a major intracranial artery, maintenance of SBP <140 mm Hg, and high-intensity statin therapy are recommended.
- For patients with a stroke or TIA attributable to moderate stenosis (50%–69%) of a major intracranial artery, angioplasty or stenting is not recommended given the low rate of stroke on medical management and the inherent periprocedural risk of endovascular treatment.
- For patients with stroke or TIA attributable to severe stenosis (70%–99%) of a major intracranial artery, stenting with the Wingspan stent system is not recommended as an initial treatment, even for patients who were taking an antithrombotic agent at the time of the stroke or TIA.
- For patients with stroke or TIA attributable to severe stenosis (70%–99%) of a major intracranial artery, the usefulness of angioplasty alone or placement of stents other than the Wingspan stent is unknown and is considered investigational.
- For patients with severe stenosis (70%–99%) of a major intracranial artery and recurrent TIA or stroke after institution of aspirin and clopidogrel therapy, achievement of systolic BP <140 mm Hg, and high-intensity statin therapy, the usefulness of angioplasty alone or placement of a Wingspan stent or other stents is unknown and is considered investigational.

Source: Bushnell C, McCullough LD, Awad IA, et al. Guidelines for the prevention of stroke in women: a statement for healthcare professionals from the American Heart Association/American Stroke Association. *Stroke.* 2014;45. doi:10.1161/01.str.0000442009.06663.48.

SYNCOPE

Population
–Adults presenting with syncope.

Recommendations
▶ ACC/AHA 2017

ADDITIONAL EVALUATION AND DIAGNOSIS FOR SYNCOPE

Initial Evaluation of Syncope

HISTORICAL CHARACTERISTICS ASSOCIATED WITH INCREASED PROBABILITY OF CARDIAC AND NONCARDIAC CAUSES OF SYNCOPE

More Often Associated with Cardiac Causes of Syncope
• Older age (>60 y)
• Male sex
• Presence of known ischemic heart disease, structural heart disease, previous arrhythmias, or reduced ventricular function
• Brief prodrome, such as palpitations, or sudden loss of consciousness without prodrome
• Syncope during exertion
• Syncope in the supine position

- Low number of syncope episodes (1 or 2)
- Abnormal cardiac examination
- Family history of inheritable conditions or premature SCD (<50 y of age)
- Presence of known congenital heart disease

More Often Associated with Noncardiac Causes of Syncope

- Younger age
- No known cardiac disease
- Syncope only in the standing position
- Positional change from supine or sitting to standing
- Presence of prodrome: nausea, vomiting, feeling warmth
- Situational triggers: cough, laugh, micturition, defecation, deglutition
- Frequent recurrence and prolonged history of syncope with similar characteristics

SCD, sudden cardiac death.

Historical Features of Cardiac vs. Non-cardiac Syncope

EXAMPLE OF SERIOUS MEDICAL CONDITIONS THAT MIGHT WARRANT CONSIDERATION OF FURTHER EVALUATION AND THERAPY IN HOSPITAL SETTING		
Cardiac Arrhythmic Conditions	Cardiac or Vascular Nonarrhythmtc Conditions	Noncardiac Conditions
• Sustained or symptomatic VT • Symptomatic conduction system disease or Mobitz II or third-degree heart block • Symptomatic bradycardia or sinus pauses not related to neurally mediated syncope • Symptomatic SVT • Pacemaker, ICD malfunction • Inheritable cardiovascular conditions predisposing to arrhythmias	• Cardiac ischemia • Severe aortic stenosis • Cardiac tamponade • HCM • Severe prosthetic valve dysfunction • Pulmonary embolism • Aortic dissection • Acute HF • Moderate-to-severe LV dysfunction	• Severe anemia/ gastrointestinal bleeding • Major traumatic injury due to syncope • Persistent vital sign abnormalities

Serious Medical Conditions Associated with Syncope

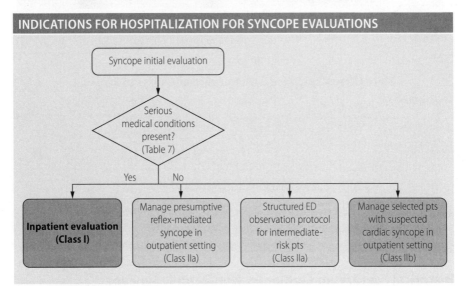

INDICATIONS FOR HOSPITALIZATION FOR SYNCOPE EVALUATIONS

Source: *Circulation*. 2017;136(5):e25-e59.

Recommended Tests for Syncope

–EKG.

–Complete blood count, basic metabolic panel, and other targeted labs based on clinical assessment.

–Echocardiogram if structural heart disease is suspected.

–Stress test if exertional syncope of unclear etiology.

–Continuous telemetry monitoring for patients admitted to hospital.

–Prolonged cardiac monitoring if arrhythmic syncope is suspected.

–Electrophysiologic study if syncope of suspected arrhythmic etiology with negative cardiac monitoring.

Other Interventions for Syncope

–Implantable cardioverter-defibrillator (ICD) implantation is recommended in patients with arrhythmogenic right ventricular cardiomyopathy who present with syncope and have a documented sustained ventricular arrhythmia.

Sources

–2017 AHA/ACC focused update of the 2014 AHA/ACC guideline for the management of patients with valvular heart disease: a report of the American College of Cardiology/American Heart Association Task Force on clinical practice guidelines. *Circulation*. 2017;135:e1159–e1195.

SYPHILIS

Population
–Adults.

Recommendations
▶ IDSA 2011

–Penicillin G 2.4 million units is drug of choice for early syphilis.
–Cerebrospinal fluid (CSF) analysis is indicated if:
  • Early syphilis infection and neurologic symptoms.
  • Late latent syphilis.
–HIV-infected patients with rapid plasma reagent (RPR) titer ≥1:32 or CD4 <350 cells/mm³.
–Patients with early syphilis do not achieve a ≥4-fold decline in RPR titers within 12 mo.
–Doxycycline is second-line therapy for early syphilis in penicillin-allergic patients.
–Ceftriaxone is second-line therapy for neurosyphilis in penicillin-allergic patients.

Source
–http://cid.oxfordjournals.org/content/53/suppl_3/S110.abstract

Comment
–Avoid doxycycline in pregnancy.

THROMBOCYTOPENIA-IMMUNE MEDIATED

Population
–Adults.

Recommendations
▶ American Society of Hematology (ASH)—Evidence-Based Practice Guidelines for ITP 2011

Diagnosis
• Diagnosis of exclusion—no reliable diagnostic test (including antiplatelet antibody studies). Bone marrow examination not necessary irrespective of age in patients with typical immune thrombocytopenia purpura (ITP) (healthy with isolated thrombocytopenia with large normal-appearing platelets on peripheral blood smear). Testing patients for underlying hepatitis C and HIV is recommended. Testing for another underlying illness (rheumatologic disorders, lymphoproliferative disease, *Helicobacter pylori* infection, antiphospholipid syndrome) is based on history and physical exam.

–**Treatment of newly diagnosed ITP:** Treat if platelet count <30,000 with or without bleeding. Longer courses of corticosteroids (prednisone 0.5-2 mg/kg daily with taper) is preferred over shorter courses of high-dose corticosteroids (40 mg of decadron daily x 4) or intravenous immune globulin (IVIG). IVIG should be used with corticosteroids when a more rapid rise in platelet countIf platelets <30,000, second-line therapy (Rituxan is required. Either IVIG or anti-D immune globulin (in patients that are Rh(+) and spleen in place) can be used as first-line therapy if corticosteroids are contraindicated. Dose of IVIG should be 1 g/kg as a one-time dose that may be repeated as necessary. (*Lancet Haematol.* 2016;3:e489) (*Blood.* 2016;127:296)(see Table V).

–**Treatment of patients who are unresponsive or relapse after initial therapy:** Splenectomy, either laparoscopic or open, should be done at least 2 to 4 wk after vaccination with pneumococcal, meningococcal, and *Haemophilus influenzae* b vaccine. Splenectomy is significantly more effective in patients less than 40 y old compared to the elderly. Thrombopoietin receptor agonists (romiplostim or eltrombopag) are used often in second-line therapy after steroids and IVIG failure or after splenectomy relapse to maintain an adequate platelet count. (*Blood.* 2012;120:960. *J Thromb Haemost.* 2015;13:457. *Lancet.* 2008;371:395. *Blood.* 2013;121:537)

• Thrombopoietin receptor agonists can be used in patients at risk for bleeding who have failed one line of therapy but have not had a splenectomy. Response rate is 80%-.90%. Rituximab may be considered in patients at risk of bleeding who have failed one line of therapy, including splenectomy. (*N Engl J Med.* 2011;366:734. *Blood.* 2014;124:3228)

TABLE V

FIRST-LINE THERAPY FOR ITP		
CORTICOSTEROIDS	**RR**	**% WITH SUSTAINED RESPONSE**
Prednisone 0.5–2 mg/kg/d for 2 wk followed by taper	70%–80%	10-y disease-free—13%–15%
Dexamethasone 40 mg daily for 4 d every 2–4 wk for 1–4 cycles	90%	As high as 50% (2–5 y follow-up)
IV anti-D immune globulin 50–75 µg/kg—warning regarding brisk hemolysis and rare DIC	80%	Usually lasts 3–4 wk, but may persist for months in some patients
IVIG 0.4 g/kg/d × 5 d or 1 g/kg/d for 1–2 d	80%	Transient benefit lasting 2–4 wk

–**Treatment of ITP after splenectomy**

- No further treatment is indicated in asymptomatic patients with platelet count >30,000.
- If platelets <30,000, second-line therapy (Rituxan, thrombopoietin receptor agonists, and immunosuppression) should be used (see Table VI).

–**Treatment of ITP in pregnancy**

- In pregnant patients requiring therapy, corticosteroids or IVIG should be used. Romiplostim and eltrombopag are not approved for use in pregnant women.
- For refractory patients, splenectomy can be performed during second trimester. For pregnant women with ITP, method of delivery is based upon obstetrical indications.

–**Treatment of specific forms of secondary ITP** (see Table VII).

- **HCV-associated:** Antiviral therapy should be considered in absence of contraindications. Initial therapy in this setting should be IVIG.
- **HIV-associated:** HIV treatment should be considered first unless patient has significant bleeding complications. If ITP therapy is required use corticosteroids, IVIG, anti-D immune globulin, and romiplostim or eltrombopag. Refractory patients should have a splenectomy.
- **H. pylori-associated:** Eradication therapy of newly diagnosed active *H. pylori* infection (stool antigen, urea breath test, endoscopic biopsy) will result in resolution of ITP in 25%-35% of patients.

Sources
–*Blood.* 2016;128:1547
–*Blood.* 2011;117:4190-4207
–*Blood.* 2010;115:168-186

TABLE VI

SELECTED SECOND-LINE THERAPY OPTIONS IN ADULT ITP	
TPO RECEPTOR AGONIST	**RR**
Eltrombopag 25–75 mg orally daily	70%–80%
Romiplostim 1–10 µg/kg SQ weekly	80%–90%
Immunosuppression	
Azathioprine 1–2 mg/kg	40%
Cyclosporine 5 mg/kg/d for 6 d then 2.5–3 m/kg/d to titrate blood levels of 100 to 200 mg/mL	50%–60%
Cytoxan 1–2 mg/kg orally or IV (0.3–1 g/m²) for 113 doses every 2–4 wk	30%–60%
Rituximab 375 mg/m² weekly × 4	50%–60% respond—sustained >3–5 y in 10%–15%

SELECTED SECOND-LINE THERAPY OPTIONS IN ADULT ITP (*Continued*)	
TPO RECEPTOR AGONIST	**RR**
Uncertain Mechanism	
Danazol 200 mg 2–4× daily (orally)	~50%
Vinca alkaloid 1–2 mg IV weekly to max of 6 mg	~30% variable

TABLE VII

UNDERLYING CAUSES ASSOCIATED WITH ITP

- Drug induced (trimethoprim-sulfa, rifampin, carbamazepine, vancomycin, quinine derivatives, and many more).
- Systemic lupus/Sjögren syndrome, and other rheumatologic diseases.
- Infections—hepatitis C, HIV, cytomegalovirus (CMV), *Helicobacter pylori*, Epstein-Barr virus (EBV), varicella.
- Indolent lymphomas, breast and colon cancer.
- Vaccinations—mostly in children.
- Common variable immunodeficiency—almost exclusively in children.

Comment

–Clinical Information

- Be aware of autosomal dominant hereditary macrothrombocytopenia. Platelets are large, hypogranular, and misshapen with counts between 30 and 60,000. Bleeding is modest but is often confused with ITP. The treatment is with platelet transfusion for significant bleeding. Treatment for ITP is ineffective.
- TTP (thrombotic thrombocytopenic purpura) should always be excluded. These patients will be ill with low-grade fever, muscle aches, chest pain, and altered mental status. They will have thrombocytopenia and a hemolytic anemia with red cell fragmentation, elevated reticulocyte count, and significant elevation of lactate dehydrogenase. This is a medical emergency and should be treated urgently with plasma exchange.
- In the elderly, myelodysplastic syndrome is common, but isolated thrombocytopenia occurs in <10%. ITP is by far the most common cause of isolated thrombocytopenia, even in elderly patients.
- Treating patients for active *H. pylori* infection with new-onset ITP will result in a durable complete remission in up to 50% of patients.
- Be alert to pseudothrombocytopenia caused by platelet clumping in response to ethylenediaminetetraacetic acid (EDTA). Reviewing the peripheral smear or repeating the platelet count in a citrated or heparinized tube is needed to make the diagnosis.
- Platelet transfusion should be considered along with standard therapy when there is life-threatening hemorrhage (usually brain or

GI tract). The platelet count usually will not rise significantly, but bleeding can be slowed. Do not give prophylactic platelets based on platelet counts <5000 or for minor bleeding.

- Anti-D immune globulin therapy (WinRho) is associated with a small percentage of patients developing disseminated intravascular coagulation (DIC) and resultant death. Close monitoring of patients is required. This therapeutic approach is used much less frequently because of complications and more effective new drugs.

Population
–Pediatric.

Recommendations
▶ ASH

–**Diagnosis:** Bone marrow (BM) examination unnecessary in children and adolescents with typical features of ITP (isolated thrombocytopenia, large, morphologically normal platelets, asymptomatic except for bleeding). BM also not necessary in patients failing intravenous IVIG therapy or before splenectomy.

–**Initial management:** Children with no or mild bleeding (bruising, petechiae) can be managed with observation alone *regardless* of platelet count. For patients requiring therapy, a single dose of IVIG (0.8–1 g/kg) or short-course corticosteroid should be used as first-line therapy. Anti-D immune globulin (WinRho) can be used as first-line therapy in Rh-positive, nonsplenectomized children needing treatment.

–**Second-line treatment for pediatric ITP:** Rituximab can be considered if bleeding ongoing despite IVIG, anti-D immune globulin, and steroids. Rituximab can be considered an alternative to splenectomy or in patients not responding to splenectomy. High-dose dexamethasone (0.6/kg/d × 4 d q 4 wk) may be considered for patients with bleeding and persistent thrombocytopenia despite appropriate therapy.

–**Splenectomy:** Consider for children and adolescents with chronic ITP who have significant or persistent bleeding and lack of responsiveness or intolerance to other standard therapies. It is recommended not to do splenectomy for at least 12 mo after start of ITP treatment unless severe disease with significant serious bleeding risks. Splenectomy in patients over 45 y old has a significant risk of recurrence of thrombocytopenia compared to splenectomy in patients younger than 45 y. (*Blood.* 2013;121:4457-4462. *Blood.* 2010;115:168-186. *Pediatr Blood Cancer.* 2009;53:652-654. *Blood.* 2014;124:3295)

Comments
Clinical Considerations
–Measurement of immunoglobulin to exclude common variable immune deficiency (CVID) is common practice as ITP can be the presenting feature of CVID.

–In a study of 332 children with typical ITP with bone marrow—no leukemia—only 1 child was found with BM aplasia.

–Recommendation for treatment focuses on severity of bleeding, not platelet cell count. In a study of 505 children with platelets <20,000 and skin bleeding, only 3 patients developed severe bleeding and none had intracranial hemorrhage.

–The older the child or adolescent, the more likely they are to have chronic ITP (defined as platelet count <150,000 at 6-mo follow-up). Rate for children age 3–12 mo = 23%; children >12 mo and <10 y = 28%; and children >10 y = 47%.

–Anti-D immune globulin therapy more effective at 75 vs. 50 μg/kg, but increased toxicity including small percentage with DIC. Drop in hemoglobin averages 1.6 g/dL.

–Response rate to splenectomy is 70%-80%, but unless a child has severe unresponsive disease, delay the splenectomy for at least 12 mo since 20 to 30% will have spontaneous remission.

–Patients undergoing splenectomy should be immunized at least 2 wk before surgery with pneumococcal, meningococcal, and *H. influenzae* type b vaccine.

–Effectiveness of rituximab varies from 30% to 50% in different trials. Serious side effects include serum sickness, severe hepatitis in hepatitis B carriers, and rare cases of multifocal leukoencephalopathy.

–MMR (measles, mumps, rubella) vaccination-induced ITP occurs in 2.6 per 100,000 vaccine doses. ITP following natural measles or rubella infection ranges from 600 to 1200 per 100,000 cases, justifying the overall clinical benefit of the vaccine.

–Thrombopoietin receptor agonists (romiplostim and eltrombopag) are active agents for ITP in adults but have not been adequately studied in children. Ongoing studies show benefit but not yet approved by FDA.

THROMBOCYTOPENIA, HEPARIN-INDUCED

Population
–Adults.

Recommendation
▶ ACCP 2012, ASH 2016
   –**Diagnosis and Therapy**
      • **Diagnosis:** Maintain high suspicion. If no prior heparin in the last 90 d, monitor platelet count in patients receiving heparin every 2 d from days 4 to 14. If previous exposure to heparin within 90 d, monitor from day 1. If platelets drop 30%–50%, suspect HIT and use 4Ts scoring model (see Table VIII) to assess likelihood of

HIT. If intermediate-to-high probability, treat for HIT and send immunologic (enzyme-linked immunosorbent assay [ELISA]) and functional testing (platelet serotonin release assay).

- **Treatment:** Stop all sources of heparin and give vitamin K if the patient is on warfarin to restore proteins C and S. Begin a direct thrombin inhibitor (argatroban or danaparoid). Fondaparinux is also a safe and effective alternative. (*N Engl J Med.* 2013;368:737-744) Avoid platelet transfusion unless life-threatening bleeding. DO NOT start warfarin until platelet count is >150,000 and overlap with argatroban is for at least 5 d with the INR therapeutic for the last 2 d.
- Patients who have not had clot should be anticoagulated for 6–8 wk.
- In patients with clot, systemic anticoagulation should be continued for a minimum of 3 mo.
- Patients with renal insufficiency should be treated with argatroban, and in patients with liver dysfunction, fondaparinux and danaparoid are preferred. In patients with acute HIT and those who are antibody-positive should be treated with bivalirudin if urgent cardiac surgery is needed, but it is preferable to delay surgery if possible.
- Patients with a past history of HIT with acute thrombosis with negative heparin antibodies should be treated with fondaparinux at full therapeutic dose until transition to warfarin. (*Blood.* 2012;119:2209-2218. *Annu Rev Med.* 2010;61:77-90)
- A direct oral anticoagulant (DOAC) can be substituted for warfarin to complete the course of anticoagulation.

TABLE VIII

DIAGNOSTIC TOOL FOR DIAGNOSIS OF HIT			
4Ts	**2 POINTS**	**1 POINT**	**0 POINT**
Thrombocytopenia	• Fall in platelet count >50% and nadir of ≥20,000 **AND** • No surgery in preceding 3 d	• >50% fall in platelets but with surgery in preceding 3 d • 30%–50% platelet fall with nadir 10–19,000	• <30% fall in platelets • Any platelet fall with nadir <10,000
Timing of platelet fall	• 5–10 d after start of heparin • Platelet fall <5 d with heparin exposure within past 30 d	• Platelet fall after day 10 • Platelet fall <5 d with heparin exposure in past 100 d	• Platelet fall ≤ day 4 without exposure to heparin in last 100 d

DIAGNOSTIC TOOL FOR DIAGNOSIS OF HIT *(Continued)*			
4Ts	**2 POINTS**	**1 POINT**	**0 POINT**
Thrombosis or other sequelae	• Confirmed new venous or arterial thrombosis • Skin necrosis at heparin injection sites • Anaphylactoid reaction to IV heparin	• Progressive or recurrent thrombosis while on heparin • Erythematous skin reaction at heparin injection sites	Thrombosis suspected
Other causes of thrombocytopenia	• No alternative cause of platelet drop evident	• At least one other possible cause of drop in platelet count	Definite or highly likely cause present • Sepsis • Chemotherapy within 20 d • DIC • Drug-induced ITP • Posttransfusion purposes

High probability: 6–8 points; intermediate probability: 4–5 points; low probability: ≤3 points.

Comment

–Clinical Input

- Highest risk for HIT is in postsurgical patients treated with UFH.
- UFH is 8 to 10 fold more likely to cause HIT compared to LMWH. Low molecular weight heparin is equal if not better than UFH. UFH should be used only in patients with significant renal insufficiency.
- Fondaparinux (Arixtra®)—Synthetic pentasaccharide inhibiting factor X activity and is safe to be used in HIT, although direct thrombin inhibitors have previously been the anticoagulants of choice.
- Platelet counts can mildly decrease in the first 4 d after starting heparin but this is not immunologically mediated and is not associated with thrombosis. (*Blood*. 2016; 128:348)
- HIT is an immune-mediated disorder triggered by the formation of antibodies to a heparin/platelet factor 4 antigen complex. The complex binds to platelet FC receptors, causing activation of the platelet microparticle release and increased risk of clotting.
- Both VTE and arterial clotting occur in the HIT syndrome in a ratio of 3:1. Adrenal infarction with shock from arterial thrombosis has been reported.

- HIT occurs very rarely in patients <40 y old. HIT is increased in females 2.4-fold compared to males.
- The median platelet count in HIT is 60,000 and seldom falls below 20,000. HIT-associated thrombosis shows a propensity to occur in areas of vessel injury (sites of central venous catheter, arterial line insertion, or other vascular interventions).
- The development of HIT is not related to the degree of exposure to heparin. A single flush of an IV line or 1 dose of prophylactic heparin can trigger the HIT syndrome. If HIT is not recognized, further administration of heparin will lead to significant increased risk of clot, morbidity, and mortality. (*N Engl J Med*. 2006;355:809-817. *JAMA*. 2004;164:361-369)
- The 4T scoring system is most accurate in the low-risk subset, with a negative predictive value of 0.998. (*Blood*. 2012;120: 4160-4167) (See Table VIII)

THROMBOCYTOPENIA, THROMBOTIC PURPURA (TTP)

Population
–Acquired TTP in adults and children.

Recommendations
▶ British Committee for Standards in Haematology (*Br J Haematol*. 150:323) 2012
–**Approach to Diagnosis and Therapy**
- Diagnosis of TTP should be made on clinical history, laboratory tests, and review of the peripheral blood smear. Diagnosis is suspected if evidence of Coombs-negative microangiopathic hemolytic anemia (MAHA), elevated lactate dehydrogenase (LDH), and thrombocytopenia.
- TTP should be treated as a medical emergency. ADAMTS-13 (von Willebrand factor [vWF] cleaving enzyme) is low in >90% of patients with TTP, but treatment should be started as rapidly as possible and not wait for test results to return.
- Three units of fresh-frozen plasma should be given while a large-bore catheter is placed for plasma exchange, which should begin within 6 h of presentation.
- Serologic testing for HIV, hepatitis B and hepatitis C viruses, and autoantibodies should be done. Young women should have a pregnancy test.
- Plasma exchange (PEX) should be started with 40 mL/kg body weight plasma volume (PV) exchanges. The volume of exchange

can be reduced to 30 mL/kg body weight as clinical conditions and lab studies improve.

- Intensification in frequency of PEX to twice a day should be considered if platelet count is not rising and LDH remains high. (*Transfusion*. 2008;48:349)
- Daily PEX should continue for a minimum of 2 d after platelet count >150,000 and then stopped. Steroids (usually 1 mg/kg of prednisone equivalent) is often given, although benefits are uncertain.
- In patients with neurologic and/or cardiac pathology (associated with increased mortality), rituximab should be used at a dose of 375 mg/m^2 weekly for 4 doses. (*Blood*. 2011;118:1746. *N Engl J Med*. 2014;370:847)
- Cyclosporin or tacrolimus should be considered in patients with acute and chronic relapsing TTP. The benefit of aspirin in TTP is uncertain, but it is safe at a dose of 81 mg/d with a platelet count >50,000. In patients who relapse, 20%–25% repeat the plasma exchange protocol and add rituximab weekly. The majority of relapses occur in first 30 d after remission.
- PEX should be restarted if platelets <50,000 with the addition of rituximab. If ADAMTS-13 level drops to <5% without a drop in platelets, rituximab alone should be considered. (*Blood*. 2010;116:4060)

–**Supportive Therapy**

- Red-cell transfusion as clinically indicated.
- Folate supplementation during active hemolysis.
- Platelet transfusions are CONTRAINDICATED in TTP unless life-threatening hemorrhage (brain or GI tract).
- Thromboprophylaxis with LMWH once platelet count >50,000.
- Caplacizumab is a monoclonal antibody to VWD protein interfering with platelet binding and improves course of TTP. (*N Engl J Med*. 2016;374:511)

Sources

–*Sem Throm Haemot*. 2006;32:81, *Blood*. 2015; 125:3860
–*N Engl J Med*. 354:1927
–*Br J Haematol*. 2008;142:819
–*Transfusion*. 2010;50:868
–*Br J Haematol*. 2011;153:277

Comment

–**Clinical Insight**

- Classic pentad of microangiopathic hemolytic anemia (MAHA), thrombocytopenia, fever, CNS symptoms, hematuria—now most commonly MAHA and thrombocytopenia only at diagnosis. Time is critical to outcome. Expedited treatment associated with better survival.

- Autoimmune disease with IgG antibody to ADAMTS-13 which prevents cleavage of large high-molecular-weight vWF. vWF binds to platelet receptor GPIB and the resulting complex obstructs the microvasculature leading to red cell fragmentation, thrombocytopenia, and organ ischemia.

- Plasma exchange is not a curative therapy, but protects the patient until antibody levels decline either spontaneously or with use of corticosteroids and rituximab.

- Mortality prior to intervention of plasma exchange in the early 1980s was 85%–90%; today the mortality is 10%–15%.

- Prognosis can be predicted using the Wyllie index of adverse features including age >40 y, hemoglobin <9.0, and fever >100.5°F (38°C) at time of diagnosis. Predictions based on 0,1, 2, or 3 of these features resulted in mortality at 6 mo of 12.5%, 14.0%, 31.3%, and 61%, respectively. (*Br J Haematol.* 2005;132:204)

- Precipitating factors associated with the onset of acquired TTP include drugs (quinine, ticlopidine, clopidogrel, simvastatin, trimethoprim, and interferon), HIV infection, and pregnancy (usually in the second trimester). Removal of the fetus has not been shown to affect the course of TTP in pregnancy.

- Congenital TTP is rare, with <200 patients described worldwide. Onset usually is in later infancy or childhood. Patients may present as adults, with pregnancy as a common precipitant. Diagnosis is made by ADAMTS-13 activity <5%, with absence of antibody and confirmation of mutations in ADAMTS-13 gene. Treatment is with fresh-frozen plasma administration prophylactically every 10–20 d.

- Responding patients with acquired TTP will relapse at a rate of 20%–30%, most commonly in the first month following successful therapy. Studies show monitoring ADAMTS-13 levels and instituting rituximab proactively can decrease the rate of disease relapse. (*Br J Haematol* 2007; 136-145. *Blood.* 2011;118:1746)

- Hemolytic uremic syndrome (HUS) clinically resembles TTP, but has a different pathophysiology, and PEX is of minimal benefit. This illness is commonly caused by bacterial toxins (*Shiga*-like toxin from *Escherichia coli*) or drugs (quinine, gemcitabine, mitomycin C). It is also associated with malignancy and autoimmune disease. In HUS, there is disruption of the endothelium and release of high-molecular-weight vWF that overwhelms the cleaving capacity of ADAMTS-13. An antibody to ADAMTS-13 is not involved. Renal failure dominates the clinical picture and 15%–20% succumb to the disease. (*Br J Haematol.* 2010;148:37. *N Engl J Med.* 2014;371:654)

THYROID DISEASE, HYPERTHYROIDISM

Population
–Adults.

Recommendations

▶ American Thyroid Association 2016

–The etiology of thyrotoxicosis should be determined. If the diagnosis is not apparent, consider obtaining a thyroid receptor antibody level (TRAb) +/- determination of the radioactive iodine uptake (RAIU).

–Beta-adrenergic blockade is recommended in all patients with symptomatic thyrotoxicosis.

–Patients with overt Graves' hyperthyroidism should be treated with either radioiodine (RAI) therapy, antithyroid drugs (ATDs), or thyroidectomy.

–A pregnancy test should be obtained within 48 h prior to treatment in any woman with childbearing potential who is to be treated with RAI.

–Recheck a T4, T3, and TSH level in 4–8 wk after RAI therapy.

–Prior to initiating ATD therapy for Graves' disease (GD), we suggest that patients have a baseline complete blood count with differential (CBCD), and a liver profile.

–Obtain a CBCD for patients on ATD therapy with a febrile illness or a sore throat.

–If near-total or total thyroidectomy is chosen as treatment for GD, patients should be rendered euthyroid prior to the procedure with ATD pretreatment, with beta-adrenergic blockade. Potassium iodide should be given in the immediate preoperative period.

–Wean beta-blockers following thyroidectomy.

–Thyroid multinodular goiters or thyroid adenomas with hyperthyroidism should be treated with surgery or RAI.

–Subclinical hyperthyroidism should be treated in all individuals >65 of age, and in patients with cardiac disease, osteoporosis, or symptoms of hyperthyroidism when the TSH is persistently <0.1 mU/L.

Source
–2016 American Thyroid Association guidelines for diagnosis and management of hyperthyroidism and other causes of thyrotoxicosis. *Thyroid.* 2016 Oct;26(10):1343-1421.

▶ AACE 2011

–Radioactive iodine uptake scan should be performed when the etiology of thyrotoxicosis is unclear.

–β-blockade should be prescribed to elderly patients and considered for all patients with symptomatic thyrotoxicosis.

–Graves' disease.
- Options for Graves' disease treatment:
  ◦ ^{131}I therapy.
  ◦ Antithyroid medications.
  ◦ Thyroidectomy.
–Patients with Graves' disease and increased risk of complications should be pretreated with methimazole and beta-blockers prior to ^{131}I therapy.
- Advise smoking cessation.
- Graves' ophthalmopathy should have steroids and ^{131}I therapy.
–^{131}I therapy.
- A pregnancy test should be checked within 48 h of administering ^{131}I therapy.
- Assess patients 1–2 mo after ^{131}I therapy with a free T_4 and total triiodothyronine (T_3) level.
- Consider retreatment with ^{131}I therapy if hyperthyroidism persists 6 mo after ^{131}I treatment.
–Antithyroid drug therapy.
- Methimazole is the preferred antithyroid drug except during the first trimester of pregnancy.
- A CBC with differential should be obtained whenever a patient taking antithyroid drugs develops a febrile illness or pharyngitis.
- Recommend measurement of TSH receptor antibody level prior to stopping antithyroid drug therapy.
–Thyroidectomy.
- Indicated for toxic multinodular goiter or toxic adenoma.
- Wean beta-blockers postoperative.
- Follow serial calcium or intact PTH levels postoperative.
- Start levothyroxine 1.6 µg/kg/d immediately postoperative.
- Check a serum TSH level 6–8 wk postoperative.
–Thyroid storm should be treated with β-blockers, antithyroid drugs, inorganic iodide, corticosteroid therapy, volume resuscitation, and acetaminophen.

Source
–https://www.aace.com/files/hyper-guidelines-2011.pdf

Recommendations

▶ **AACE 2012**

–Replacement dosing of levothyroxine is 1.6 µg/kg/d.

–Recommends checking antithyroid peroxidase antibodies (TPOAb) in patients with subclinical hypothyroidism or recurrent miscarriages.

–Recommends treating hypothyroid patients with levothyroxine if:
  • TSH >10 mIU/L.
  • Symptomatic.
  • Positive TPOAb.

Source

–https://www.aace.com/files/hypothyroidism_guidelines.pdf

▼ THYROID DISEASE, PREGNANCY AND POSTPARTUM

Population

–Women during and immediately after pregnancy.

Recommendations

▶ **ATA 2011, ATA 2017**

–Hypothyroidism in pregnancy is defined as:
  • An elevated TSH (>2.5 mIU/L) and a suppressed free thyroxine (FT_4).
  • TSH ≥10 mIU/L (irrespective of FT_4).
  • Subclinical hypothyroidism is defined as a TSH 2.5–9.9 mIU/L) and a normal FT_4

–Insufficient evidence to support treatment of subclinical hypothyroidism in pregnancy.

–Goal therapy is to normalize TSH levels.

–PTU is the preferred antithyroid drug (ATD) in pregnancy.

–Monitor TSH levels every 4 wk when treating thyroid disease in pregnancy.

–Measure a TSH receptor antibody level at 20–24 wk for any history of Graves' disease.

–All pregnant and lactating women should ingest at least 250-µg iodine daily.

–All pregnant women with thyroid nodules should undergo thyroid ultrasound and TSH testing.

–Patients found to have thyroid cancer during pregnancy would ideally undergo surgery during second trimester.

–Transient hCG-mediated TSH suppression in early pregnancy should not be treated with ATD therapy.

–GD during pregnancy should be treated with the lowest possible dose of ATD needed to keep the mother's thyroid hormone levels at or slightly above the reference range for total T4 and T3 values in pregnancy (1.5 times above nonpregnant reference ranges in the second and third trimesters), and the TSH below the reference range for pregnancy.

–Pregnancy is a relative contraindication to thyroidectomy and should only be used when medical management has been unsuccessful or ATDs cannot be used.

Sources

–2016 American Thyroid Association guidelines for diagnosis and management of hyperthyroidism and other causes of thyrotoxicosis. *Thyroid.* 2016 Oct;26(10):1343-1421

–2017 Guidelines of the American Thyroid Association for the Diagnosis and Management of Thyroid Disease During Pregnancy and the Postpartum. *Thyroid.* 2017;27(3):315-390

–http://thyroidguidelines.net/sites/thyroidguidelines.net/files/file/thy.2011.0087.pdf

Comment

–Surgery for well-differentiated thyroid carcinoma can often be deferred until postpartum period.

THYROID NODULES

MANAGEMENT OF THYROID NODULES

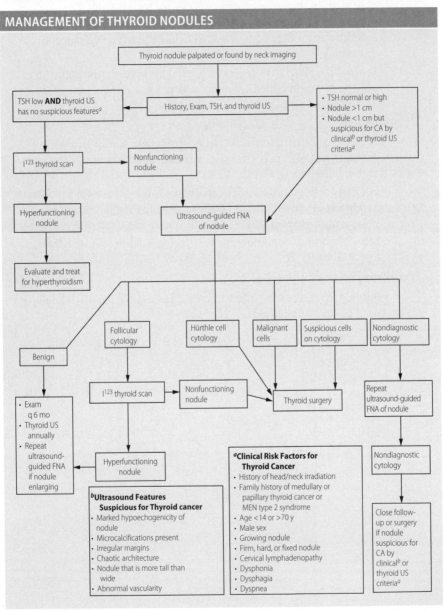

Thyroid nodule palpated or found by neck imaging

History, Exam, TSH, and thyroid US

TSH low **AND** thyroid US has no suspicious features[a]

- TSH normal or high
- Nodule >1 cm
- Nodule <1 cm but suspicious for CA by clinical[b] or thyroid US criteria[a]

I[123] thyroid scan

Nonfunctioning nodule

Hyperfunctioning nodule

Ultrasound-guided FNA of nodule

Evaluate and treat for hyperthyroidism

Follicular cytology

Hürthle cell cytology

Malignant cells

Suspicious cells on cytology

Nondiagnostic cytology

Benign

I[123] thyroid scan

Nonfunctioning nodule

Thyroid surgery

Repeat ultrasound-guided FNA of nodule

- Exam q 6 mo
- Thyroid US annually
- Repeat ultrasound-guided FNA if nodule enlarging

Hyperfunctioning nodule

Nondiagnostic cytology

[b]Ultrasound Features Suspicious for Thyroid cancer
- Marked hypoechogenicity of nodule
- Microcalcifications present
- Irregular margins
- Chaotic architecture
- Nodule that is more tall than wide
- Abnormal vascularity

[a]Clinical Risk Factors for Thyroid Cancer
- History of head/neck irradiation
- Family history of medullary or papillary thyroid cancer or MEN type 2 syndrome
- Age <14 or >70 y
- Male sex
- Growing nodule
- Firm, hard, or fixed nodule
- Cervical lymphadenopathy
- Dysphonia
- Dysphagia
- Dyspnea

Close follow-up or surgery if nodule suspicious for CA by clinical[b] or thyroid US criteria[a]

FNA, fine-needle aspiration; MEN, multiple endocrine neoplasia; TSH, thyroid-stimulating hormone; US, ultrasound.

Sources: AACE, June 2010; ATA, November 2009.

TINNITUS

Population
–Adults and children.

Recommendations
▶ AAO-HNS 2014
–Recommend a thorough history and exam on patients with tinnitus.
–Recommend a comprehensive audiologic examination for unilateral or persistent tinnitus or any associated hearing impairment.
–Recommend imaging studies only for unilateral tinnitus, pulsatile tinnitus, asymmetric hearing loss, or focal neurological abnormalities.
–Recommend a hearing aid for tinnitus with hearing loss.
–Consider cognitive behavioral training or sound therapy for persistent, bothersome tinnitus.
–Recommend against medical or herbal therapy or transcranial magnetic stimulation for tinnitus.

Source
–http://www.guideline.gov/content.aspx?id=48751

TOBACCO ABUSE, SMOKING CESSATION

Population
–Adults, including pregnant women who smoke tobacco.

Recommendations
▶ USPSTF 2015
–Current evidence is insufficient to recommend electronic nicotine delivery systems for tobacco cessation in adults, including pregnant women.
–Current evidence is insufficient to assess the benefits and harms of pharmacotherapy interventions for tobacco cessation in pregnant women.

Source
–https://guidelines.gov/summaries/summary/49684

TOBACCO CESSATION TREATMENT ALGORITHM

Five A's

1. Ask about tobacco use.
2. Advise to quit through clear, personalized messages.
3. Assess willingness to quit.
4. Assist to quit,[a] including referral to Quit Lines (eg, 1-800-NO-BUTTS).
5. Arrange follow-up and support.

[a]Physicians can assist patients to quit by devising a quit plan, providing problem-solving counseling, providing intratreatment social support, helping patients obtain social support from their environment/friends, and recommending pharmacotherapy for appropriate patients. Use caution in recommending pharmacotherapy in patients with medical contraindications, those smoking <10 cigarettes per day, pregnant/breast-feeding women, and adolescent smokers. As of March 2005, Medicare covers costs for smoking cessation counseling for those who (1) have a smoking-related illness; (2) have an illness complicated by smoking; or (3) take a medication that is made less effective by smoking. (http://www.cms.hhs.gov/mcd/viewdecisionmemo.asp?id=130).

Source: Fiore MC, Jaén CR, Baker TB, et al. *Treating Tobacco Use and Dependence. Quick Reference Guide for Clinicians.* Rockville, MD: U.S. Department of Health and Human Services. Public Health Service; 2008 (http://www.ahrq.gov/legacy/clinic/tobacco/tobaqrg.pdf).

MOTIVATING TOBACCO USERS TO QUIT

Five R's

1. Relevance: personal
2. Risks: acute, long term, environmental
3. Rewards: have patient identify (eg, save money, better food taste)
4. Road blocks: help problem-solve
5. Repetition: at every office visit

TOBACCO CESSATION TREATMENT OPTIONS[a]

Pharmacotherapy	Precautions/ Contraindications	Side Effects	Dosage	Duration	Availability
First-Line Pharmacotherapies (approved for use for smoking cessation by the FDA)					
Bupropion SR	History of seizure History of eating disorder	Insomnia Dry mouth	150 mg every morning for 3 d, then 150 mg bid (Begin treatment 1–2 wk prequit)	7–12 wk maintenance up to 6 mo	Zyban (prescription only)
Nicotine gum	—	Mouth soreness Dyspepsia	1–24 cigarettes/d: 2-mg gum (up to 24 pieces/d) 25+ cigarettes/d: 4-mg gum (up to 24 pieces/d)	Up to 12 wk	Nicorette, Nicorette Mint (OTC only)
Nicotine inhaler	—	Local irritation of mouth and throat	6–16 cartridges/d	Up to 6 mo	Nicotrol Inhaler (prescription only)
Nicotine nasal spray	—	Nasal irritation	8–40 doses/d	3–6 mo	Nicotrol NS (prescription only)
Nicotine patch	—	Local skin reaction Insomnia	21 mg/24 h 14 mg/24 h 7 mg/24 h 15 mg/16 h	4 wk Then 2 wk Then 2 wk 8 wk	NicoDerm CQ (OTC only), generic patches (prescription and OTC) Nicotrol (OTC only)

TOBACCO CESSATION TREATMENT OPTIONS[a] *(Continued)*

Pharmacotherapy	Precautions/ Contraindications	Side Effects	Dosage	Duration	Availability
Varenicline	Renal impairment	Nausea Abnormal dreams	0.5 mg qd for 3 d, then 0.5 mg bid for 4 d, then 1.0 mg PO bid	12 wk or 24 wk	Chantix (prescription only)
Second-Line Pharmacotherapies (not approved for use for smoking cessation by the FDA)					
Clonidine	Rebound hypertension	Dry mouth Drowsiness Dizziness Sedation	0.15–0.75 mg/d	3–10 wk	Oral clonidine—generic, Catapres (prescription only), transdermal Catapres (prescription only)
Nortriptyline	Risk of arrhythmias	Sedation Dry mouth	75–100 mg/d	12 wk	Nortriptyline HCL–generic (prescription only)

bid, twice daily; FDA, Food and Drug Administration; OTC, over-the-counter; PO, by mouth; qd, every day.

[a]The information contained within this table is not comprehensive. Please see package inserts for additional information.

Source: U.S. Public Health Service.

TONSILLECTOMY

Population
–Children.

Recommendations
▶ AAO-HNS 2011

–Recommends against routine perioperative antibiotics for tonsillectomy.

–Tonsillectomy indicated for:
- Tonsillar hypertrophy with sleep-disordered breathing.
- Recurrent throat infections for ≥7 episodes of recurrent throat infection in last year; ≥5 episodes of recurrent throat infection per year in last 2 y; or ≥3 episodes of recurrent throat infection per year in last 3 y.

–Recommends posttonsillectomy pain control.

Source

–http://www.entnet.org/HealthInformation/upload/CPG-TonsillectomyInChildren.pdf

TRANSFUSION THERAPY, ALTERNATIVES TO RED BLOOD CELL TRANSFUSION

Population
–Adults and children over 1 y.

Recommendation
▶ NICE 2015

–Alternatives to blood transfusion
- Do not recommend erythropoietin therapy for surgical patients unless patient has anemia and meets the criteria for blood transfusion, but declines it because of religious beliefs.
- Iron therapy is recommended for all patients before and after surgery to patients with iron-deficiency anemia.
  ◦ Oral iron therapy is standard.
  ◦ Intravenous iron can be considered for patients:
    i. Who cannot tolerate oral iron.
    ii. Who cannot absorb oral iron.
    iii. When the time interval before surgery is too short for oral iron to be effective.

- Offer tranexamic acid (TXA) for people undergoing surgery who are expected to have at least moderate blood loss.
- Consider cell salvage with TXA for patients undergoing surgery who are expected to have a very high volume of blood loss.

Source
  –https://guidelines.gov/summaries/summary/49905

Comment
  –Consider cell salvage therapy for cardiac surgery, complex vascular surgery, major obstetrical procedures, and pelvic reconstruction or scoliosis surgery.

TRANSFUSION THERAPY, CRYOPRECIPITATE

Population
  –Adults and children over 1 y.

Recommendations
▶ NICE 2015
  –Recommends cryoprecipitate for patients with significant bleeding and fibrinogen level <150 mg/dL.
  –Consider cryoprecipitate for patients who require an invasive procedure or surgery with high risk of bleeding and fibrinogen level <100 mg/dL.

Source
  –https://guidelines.gov/summaries/summary/49905

TRANSFUSION THERAPY, FRESH FROZEN PLASMA (FFP)

Population
  –Adults and children over 1 y.

Recommendations
▶ NICE 2015
  –Consider FFP transfusion for patients with active bleeding and prothrombin time or activated partial thromboplastin time ratios above 1.5.
  –Do not recommend FFP transfusions for patients with an abnormal coagulation profile who are not actively bleeding.

Source
–https://guidelines.gov/summaries/summary/49905

Comment
–Typical dose of FFP is 15 mL/kg.

TRANSFUSION THERAPY, PLATELET TRANSFUSION

Population
–Adults and children over 1 y.

Recommendations

▶ NICE 2015

–Recommend single-unit platelet transfusion for patients with bleeding and platelet count $<30 \times 10^9$ per liter.
–Consider higher threshold (up to 100×10^9 per liter) for:
  • Major hemorrhage.
  • CNS or ocular bleeding.
–Prophylactic platelet transfusions for:
  • Platelet count $<10 \times 10^9$ per liter.
–Consider platelet transfusion for patients having invasive procedures or surgery and have a platelet count $<50 \times 10^9$ per liter.
  • Threshold for transfusion may be as high as 100×10^9 per liter for CNS or eye surgery.

Source
–https://guidelines.gov/summaries/summary/49905

Comment
–Prophylactic platelet transfusions not necessarily recommended for:
  • Chronic bone marrow failure.
  • Autoimmune thrombocytopenia.
  • Heparin-induced thrombocytopenia.
  • Thrombotic thrombocytopenic purpura.

TRANSFUSION THERAPY, PROTHROMBIN COMPLEX CONCENTRATE

Population
–Adults and children over 1 y.

Recommendation

▶ NICE 2015

–Recommend for emergency reversal of warfarin anticoagulation in patients with:
  • Severe bleeding.
  • Suspected intracranial hemorrhage.

Source
–https://guidelines.gov/summaries/summary/49905

TRANSFUSION THERAPY, RED BLOOD CELL TRANSFUSION

Population
–Adults and children over 1 y.

Recommendations

▶ NICE 2015

–Recommend a restrictive red blood cell transfusion threshold at a hemoglobin 7 g/dL for most patients.
–Consider a red blood cell transfusion threshold at a hemoglobin 8 g/dL for:
  • Acute coronary syndrome.
–Consider single unit transfusions for adults with no active bleeding.

Source
–https://guidelines.gov/summaries/summary/49905

TRAUMATIC BRAIN INJURY

Recommendation

▶ ACEP 2013

–Avoid CT scan of head for minor head trauma in patients who are low risk based on validated decision rules.

Source
–http://www.choosingwisely.org/societies/american-college-of-emergency-physicians/

TREMOR, ESSENTIAL

Population
–Adults.

Recommendations

▶ AAN 2011

–Recommends treatment with propranolol or primidone.
–Alternative treatment options include alprazolam, atenolol, gabapentin, sotalol, or topiramate.
–Recommends against treatment with levetiracetam, pindolol, trazodone, acetazolamide, or 3,4-diaminopyridine.

Source
–http://www.neurology.org/content/77/19/1752.full.pdf+html

Comment
–Unilateral thalamotomy may be effective for severe refractory essential tremors.

TUBERCULOSIS (TB), DIAGNOSIS

Population
–Adults suspected of having active TB.

Recommendations

▶ NICE 2016

–Perform a chest X-ray in all patients.
–Obtain three early-morning sputum samples for AFB smear and culture.

Source
–https://guidelines.gov/summaries/summary/49964

Comment
–Consider sputum for nucleic acid amplification for mycobacterium tuberculosis complex if the person has HIV disease, need for a large contact tracing, or need for rapid diagnosis.

TUBERCULOSIS (TB), EXTRAPULMONARY DIAGNOSIS

Population
–Adults suspected of having extrapulmonary TB.

Recommendations
▶ NICE 2016
–To diagnose TB send fluid for adenosine deaminase and nucleic acid amplification for mycobacterium tuberculosis complex (pleural fluid, cerebrospinal fluid, ascitic fluid, pericardial fluid, synovial fluid).
–Option for TB diagnosis is tissue biopsy.
  • Bone biopsy for osteomyelitis.
  • Pleural biopsy for pleural TB.
  • Peritoneal biopsy for peritoneal TB.
  • Pericardial biopsy for pericardial TB.
  • Synovial biopsy for synovial TB.

Source
–https://guidelines.gov/summaries/summary/49964

TUBERCULOSIS (TB), EXTRA-PULMONARY MANAGEMENT

Population
–Adults suspected of having extra-pulmonary TB.

Recommendations
▶ NICE 2016
–Refer the patient to a clinician with expertise in TB management.
–Report suspect to local public health office for case management and contact screening.
–Start patients on RIPE (rifampin, isoniazid, pyrazinamide, and ethambutol) therapy.
–Consider adjunctive corticosteroids for TB with CNS or pericardial involvement.

Source
–https://guidelines.gov/summaries/summary/49964

Comments
1. TB treatment regimens are modified based on TB sensitivities.
2. Typical duration of treatment for TB with CNS involvement is 12 mo.

TUBERCULOSIS (TB), MANAGEMENT

Population
–Adults suspected of having active TB.

Recommendations
▶ ATS/CDC/IDSA 2016

WHEN TO INITIATE ANTI-TUBERCULOSIS MEDICATION

		Favors Treatment Initiation	Favors Delayed or No Treatment
Patient		Risk for progression/dissemination (eg, HIV, TNF alpha inhibitor)	Elevated concern for adverse treatment events (eg, severe liver disease, pregnancy)
		Age < 2years — TB exposure risk (eg, contact, born in higher TB incidence country)	No TB exposure risk
Laboratory/ Radiographic		Radiographic imaging consistent with TB — Evidence of Mtb infection (ie, positive TST or IGRA)	Radiographic imaging not consistent with TB
		Extended time to microbiologic confirmation (eg, Rapid molecular test not available)	
		Pathologic findings consistent with TB	
		AFB smear positive Rapid molecular test positive	AFB smear positive, Rapid molecular test negative
		AFB smear negative, Rapid molecular test positive	AFB smear negative, Rapid molecular test negative
Clinical status/ Suspicion		Life-threatening disease	Clinically stable
		Symptoms typical for TB	Symptoms not typical for TB
		Alternative diagnosis less likely	Alternative diagnosis
Public Health		Concern for loss to follow-up — High transmission risk (eg, congregate setting, corrections)	Low transmission risk

TREATMENT OF DRUG-SUSCEPTIBLE TUBERCULOSIS

Table 2.　Drug Regimens for Microbiologically Confirmed Pulmonary Tuberculosis Caused by Drug-Susceptible Organisms

	Intensive Phase		Continuation Phase				
Regimen	Drug[a]	Interval and Dose[b] (Minimum Duration)	Drugs	Interval and Dose[b,c] (Minimum Duration)	Range of Total Doses	Comments[c,d]	Regimen Effectiveness
1	INH RIF PZA EMB	7 d/wk for 56 doses (8 wk), or 5 d/wk for 40 doses (8 wk)	INH RIF	7 d/wk for 126 doses (18 wk), or 5 d/wk for 90 doses (18 wk)	182–130	This is the preferred regimen for patients with newly diagnosed pulmonary tuberculosis.	Greater
2	INH RIF PZA EMB	7 d/wk for 56 doses (8 wk), or 5 d/wk for 40 doses (8 wk)	INH RIF	3 times weekly for 54 doses (18 wk)	110–94	Preferred alternative regimen in situations in which more frequent DOT during continuation phase is difficult to achieve.	
3	INH RIF PZA EMB	3 times weekly for 24 doses (8 wk)	INH RIF	3 times weekly for 54 doses (18 wk)	78	Use regimen with caution in patients with HIV and/or cavitary disease. Missed doses can lead to treatment failure, relapse, and acquired drug resistance.	
4	INH RIF PZA EMB	7 d/wk for 14 doses then twice weekly for 12 doses[e]	INH RIF	Twice weekly for 36 doses (18 wk)	62	Do not use twice-weekly regimens in HIV-infected patients or patients with smear-positive and/or cavitary disease. If doses are missed, then therapy is equivalent to once weekly, which is inferior.	Lesser

Abbreviations: DOT, directly observed therapy; EMB, ethambutol; HIV, human immunodeficiency virus; INH, isoniazid; PZA, pyrazinamide; RIF, rifampin.

[a] Other combinations may be appropriate in certain circumstances; additional details are provided in the section "Recommended Treatment Regimens."

[b] When DOT is used, drugs may be given 5 days per week and the necessary number of doses adjusted accordingly. Although there are no studies that compare 5 with 7 daily doses, extensive experience indicates this would be an effective practice. DOT should be used when drugs are administered <7 days per week.

[c] Based on expert opinion, patients with cavitation on initial chest radiograph and positive cultures at completion of 2 months of therapy should receive a 7-month (31-week) continuation phase.

[d] Pyridoxine (vitamin B6), 25–50 mg/day, is given with INH to all persons at risk of neuropathy (eg, pregnant women; breastfeeding infants; persons with HIV; patients with diabetes, alcoholism, malnutrition, or chronic renal failure; or patients with advanced age). For patients with peripheral neuropathy, experts recommend increasing pyridoxine dose to 100 mg/day.

[e] See [426]. Alternatively, some US tuberculosis control programs have administered intensive-phase regimens 5 days per week for 15 doses (3 weeks), then twice weekly for 12 doses.

Source

　–Official American Thoracic Society/Centers for Disease Control and Prevention/Infectious Diseases Society of America Clinical Practice Guidelines: treatment of drug-susceptible tuberculosis. *Clin Infect Dis.* 2016;63(7):853–867.

▶ NICE 2016

　–Refer the patient to a clinician with expertise in TB management.
　–Report suspect to local public health office for case management and contact screening.
　–Isolate patients in negative pressure rooms within the hospital.
　–Start patients on RIPE therapy (rifampin, isoniazid, pyrazinamide, and ethambutol).

Source

　–https://guidelines.gov/summaries/summary/49964

Comments

1. TB treatment regimens are modified based on TB sensitivities.
2. Typical duration of treatment for pulmonary TB is 6 mo.
3. Consider de-escalation of hospital isolation after 2 wk of therapy if:
   - Resolution of cough.
   - Afebrile for a week.
   - Immunocompetent patient.
   - No extensive disease by x-ray.
   - Initial smear grade was 2+ or less.

TUBERCULOSIS (TB), MANAGEMENT OF LATENT TB

Population
–Adults and children who have latent TB.

Recommendations
▶ NICE 2016
–High-risk individuals younger than 35 y with latent TB should be offered:
  • 3 mo of rifampin and isoniazid (with pyridoxine).
  • 6 mo of isoniazid (with pyridoxine).
–Offer adults HIV, HBV, and HCV testing before starting treatment for latent TB.
–Offer high-risk individuals between 35 and 65 y latent TB therapy if hepatotoxicity is not a concern.

Source
–https://guidelines.gov/summaries/summary/49964

Comment
–**High-risk patients with latent TB:**
  • HIV-positive.
  • Younger than 5 y.
  • Excessive alcohol intake.
  • Injection drug users.
  • Solid organ transplant recipients.
  • Hematologic malignancies.
  • Undergoing chemotherapy.
  • Prior jejunoileal bypass.
  • Diabetes.
  • Chronic kidney disease.
  • Prior gastrectomy.
  • Receiving treatment with anti-tumor necrosis factor med or other biologic agents.

TUBERCULOSIS (TB), MULTIDRUG-RESISTANT (MDR-TB)

Population

–Patients with suspected or proven drug-resistant tuberculosis.

Recommendations

▶ WHO 2011

–Rapid drug susceptibility testing of isoniazid and rifampicin is recommended at the time of TB diagnosis.

–Recommends sputum smear microscopy and culture to monitor patients with MDR-TB.

–Recommends addition of a later-generation fluoroquinolone, ethionamide, pyrazinamide, and a parenteral agent ± cycloserine for ≥8 mo.

–Recommends total treatment duration of 20 mo.

Source

–http://whqlibdoc.who.int/publications/2011/9789241501583_eng.pdf

TYMPANOSTOMY TUBES

Population

–Children 6 mo to 12 y.

Recommendations

▶ AAO 2013

–Clinicians should not perform tympanostomy tube insertion for children with:

- A single episode of otitis media with effusion (OME) of <3 mo duration.
- Recurrent acute otitis media without effusion.

–Clinicians should obtain a hearing test if OME persists for at least 3 mo or if tympanostomy tube insertion is being considered.

–Clinicians should offer bilateral tympanostomy tube insertion to children with:

- Bilateral OME for at least 3 mo **AND** documented hearing impairment.
- Recurrent acute otitis media with effusions.
- Tympanostomy tube insertion is an option for chronic symptomatic OME associated with balance problems, poor school performance, behavioral problems, or ear discomfort **thought to be due to OME.**

Source

–http://www.guideline.gov/content.aspx?id=46909

Comment

–No need for prophylactic water precautions (avoidance of swimming or water sports or use of earplugs) for children with tympanostomy tubes.

ULCERS, STRESS

Recommendation

▶ SHM 2013

–Do not prescribe medications for stress ulcer prophylaxis to medical inpatients unless they are at high risk for GI complications.

Source

–http://www.choosingwisely.org/societies/society-of-hospital-medicine-adult/

URINARY INCONTINENCE, OVERACTIVE BLADDER

Population

–Adults.

Recommendations

▶ American Urologic Association 2014

–Rule out a urinary tract infection.

–Recommend checking a post-void residual to rule out overflow incontinence.

–First-line treatments:

  • Bladder training.

  • Bladder control strategies.

  • Pelvic floor muscle training.

–Second-line treatments:

  • Antimuscarinic meds.

–Darifenacin, fesoterodine, oxybutynin, solifenacin, tolterodine, or trospium.

–Contraindicated with narrow-angle glaucoma or gastroparesis.

–Third-line treatments:
- Sacral neuromodulation.
- Peripheral tibial nerve stimulation.
- Intradetrusor botulinum toxin A.

–Recommend against indwelling urinary catheters.

Source

–http://www.guideline.gov/content.aspx?id=48226

URINARY INCONTINENCE, STRESS

Population

–Adult women.

Recommendations

▶ AUA 2017

Source:

–http://www.auanet.org/guidelines/stress-urinary-incontinenVALVULAR ADULT HEART DISEASE 2014 ACC/AHA GUIce-(sui)-new-(aua/sufu-guideline-2017)

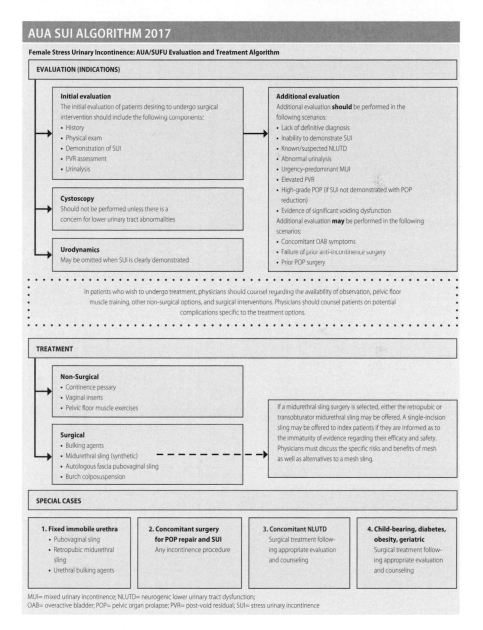

AUA SUI ALGORITHM 2017

Female Stress Urinary Incontinence: AUA/SUFU Evaluation and Treatment Algorithm

EVALUATION (INDICATIONS)

Initial evaluation
The initial evaluation of patients desiring to undergo surgical
intervention should include the following components:
- History
- Physical exam
- Demonstration of SUI
- PVR assessment
- Urinalysis

Cystoscopy
Should not be performed unless there is a
concern for lower urinary tract abnormalities

Urodynamics
May be omitted when SUI is clearly demonstrated

Additional evaluation
Additional evaluation **should** be performed in the
following scenarios:
- Lack of definitive diagnosis
- Inability to demonstrate SUI
- Known/suspected NLUTD
- Abnormal urinalysis
- Urgency-predominant MUI
- Elevated PVR
- High-grade POP (if SUI not demonstrated with POP
  reduction)
- Evidence of significant voiding dysfunction
Additional evaluation **may** be performed in the following
scenarios:
- Concomitant OAB symptoms
- Failure of prior anti-incontinence surgery
- Prior POP surgery

In patients who wish to undergo treatment, physicians should counsel regarding the availability of observation, pelvic floor
muscle training, other non-surgical options, and surgical interventions. Physicians should counsel patients on potential
complications specific to the treatment options.

TREATMENT

Non-Surgical
- Continence pessary
- Vaginal inserts
- Pelvic floor muscle exercises

Surgical
- Bulking agents
- Midurethral sling (synthetic)
- Autologous fascia pubovaginal sling
- Burch colposuspension

If a midurethral sling surgery is selected, either the retropubic or
transobturator midurethral sling may be offered. A single-incision
sling may be offered to index patients if they are informed as to
the immaturity of evidence regarding their efficacy and safety.
Physicians must discuss the specific risks and benefits of mesh
as well as alternatives to a mesh sling.

SPECIAL CASES

1. Fixed immobile urethra	2. Concomitant surgery for POP repair and SUI	3. Concomitant NLUTD	4. Child-bearing, diabetes, obesity, geriatric
• Pubovaginal sling • Retropubic midurethral sling • Urethral bulking agents	Any incontinence procedure	Surgical treatment following appropriate evaluation and counseling	Surgical treatment following appropriate evaluation and counseling

MUI= mixed urinary incontinence; NLUTD= neurogenic lower urinary tract dysfunction;
OAB= overactive bladder; POP= pelvic organ prolapse; PVR= post-void residual; SUI= stress urinary incontinence

▶ ACP 2014
   – Recommends pelvic floor muscle training and bladder training for
     urinary incontinence in women.

Source
   – http://www.guideline.gov/content.aspx?id=48543

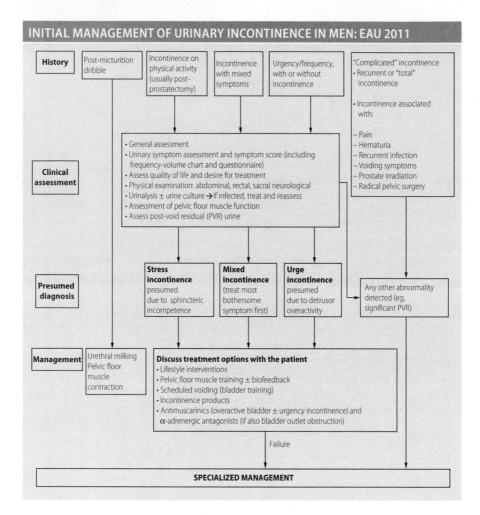

INITIAL MANAGEMENT OF URINARY INCONTINENCE IN MEN: EAU 2011

History
- Post-micturition dribble
- Incontinence on physical activity (usually post-prostatectomy)
- Incontinence with mixed symptoms
- Urgency/frequency, with or without incontinence
- "Complicated" incontinence
  - Recurrent or "total" incontinence
  - Incontinence associated with:
    – Pain
    – Hematuria
    – Recurrent infection
    – Voiding symptoms
    – Prostate irradiation
    – Radical pelvic surgery

Clinical assessment
- General assessment
- Urinary symptom assessment and symptom score (including frequency-volume chart and questionnaire)
- Assess quality of life and desire for treatment
- Physical examination: abdominal, rectal, sacral neurological
- Urinalysis ± urine culture → if infected, treat and reassess
- Assessment of pelvic floor muscle function
- Assess post-void residual (PVR) urine

Presumed diagnosis
- **Stress incontinence** presumed due to sphincteric incompetence
- **Mixed incontinence** (treat most bothersome symptom first)
- **Urge incontinence** presumed due to detrusor overactivity
- Any other abnormality detected (eg, significant PVR)

Management
- Urethral milking Pelvic floor muscle contraction
- **Discuss treatment options with the patient**
  - Lifestyle interventions
  - Pelvic floor muscle training ± biofeedback
  - Scheduled voiding (bladder training)
  - Incontinence products
  - Antimuscarinics (overactive bladder ± urgency incontinence) and α-adrenergic antagonists (if also bladder outlet obstruction)

Failure

SPECIALIZED MANAGEMENT

INITIAL MANAGEMENT OF URINARY INCONTINENCE IN WOMEN: EAU 2011

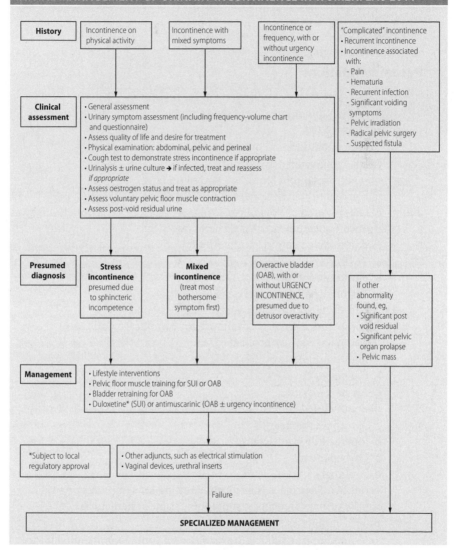

URINARY TRACT INFECTIONS (UTIS)

Population

–Adult women.

Recommendations

▶ ACOG 2008, EAU 2010, IDSA 2011, ACOG 2008, IDSA 2011

1. Screening for and treatment of asymptomatic bacteriuria are not recommended.
2. Recommend duration of antibiotics:
   a. Uncomplicated cystitis: 3 d.
      i. Nitrofurantoin requires 5–7 d of therapy.
   b. Uncomplicated pyelonephritis: 7–10 d.
   c. Complicated pyelonephritis or UTI: 3–5 d after control/elimination of complicating factors and defervescence.
3. Recommended empiric antibiotics for uncomplicated cystitis:[a]
   a. TMP-SMX.
   b. Fluoroquinolones.
   c. Nitrofurantoin macrocrystals.
   d. Beta-lactam antibiotics are alternative agents.[b]
4. Recommended empiric antibiotics for complicated UTI or uncomplicated pyelonephritis:
   a. Fluoroquinolones.
   b. Ceftriaxone.
   c. Aminoglycosides.
5. Recommended empiric antibiotics for complicated pyelonephritis:
   a. Fluoroquinolones.
   b. Piperacillin-tazobactam.
   c. Carbapenem.
   d. Aminoglycosides.
   –Recommend a urinalysis or dipstick testing for symptoms of a UTI: dysuria, urinary frequency, suprapubic pain, or hematuria.
   –Empiric antibiotics for UTI.
     • Trimethoprim-sulfamethoxazole × 3 d (not recommended if local resistance rate >20%).
     • Nitrofurantoin monohydrate × 5 d.
     • Fosfomycin 3 g PO × 1.
   –Consider a fluoroquinolone for symptoms of pyelonephritis or for refractory UTI.

---

[a]TMP-SMX only if regional *Escherichia coli* resistance is <20%; fluoroquinolones include ciprofloxacin, ofloxacin, or levofloxacin.
[b]Amoxicillin-clavulanate, cefdinir, cefaclor, or cefpodoxime-proxetil. Cephalexin may be appropriate in certain settings.

Sources
–http://www.guidelines.gov/content.aspx?id=12628
–http://www.uroweb.org/gls/pdf/Urological%20Infections%202010.pdf
–http://www.guidelines.gov/content.aspx?id=25652
–http://guidelines.gov/content.aspx?id=12628
–http://cid.oxfordjournals.org/content/52/5/e103.full.pdf+html

Comments
1. EAU recommends 7 d of antibiotics for men with uncomplicated cystitis.
2. EAU suggests the following options for antimicrobial prophylaxis of recurrent uncomplicated UTIs in nonpregnant women:
   a. Nitrofurantoin 50 mg PO daily.
   b. TMP-SMX 40/200 mg/d.
3. EAU suggests the following options for antimicrobial prophylaxis of recurrent uncomplicated UTIs in pregnant women:
   a. Cephalexin 125 mg PO daily.
4. Once urine culture and sensitivity results are known, antibiotics can be adjusted to the narrowest spectrum antibiotic.

Population
–Febrile children 2–24 mo.

Recommendations
▶ AAP 2011
–Diagnosis of a UTI if:
   • Pyuria ≥50,000 colonies/mL single uropathogenic organism.
   • Recommend a renal and bladder ultrasound in all infants 2–24 mo with a febrile UTI.
–Treat febrile UTIs with 7–14 d of antibiotics.
–Antibiotic prophylaxis is not indicated for a history of febrile UTI.
–A voiding cystourethrogram (VCUG) is indicated if ultrasound reveals hydronephrosis, renal scarring, or other findings of high-grade vesicoureteral reflux, and for recurrent febrile UTIs.

Source
–http://pediatrics.aappublications.org/content/128/3/595.full.pdf+html?sid=c1de42b3-c89b-4fd2-9592-359087823171

Comments
1. Urine obtained through catheterization has a 95% sensitivity and 99% specificity for UTI.
2. Bag urine cultures have a specificity of approximately 63% with an unacceptably high false-positive rate. **Only useful if the cultures are negative.**

URINARY TRACT SYMPTOMS, LOWER

Population

–Adult men.

Recommendations

▶ NICE 2010, EAU 2011

–All men with LUTS should have a thorough history and exam, including a prostate examination, and a review of current medications.

–Recommends supervised bladder training exercises and consider anticholinergic medications for symptoms suggestive of an overactive bladder.

–Recommends an α-blocker for men with moderate-to-severe LUTS.[a]

–Consider a 5-α-reductase inhibitor for men with LUTS with prostate size larger than 30 g.

–For men with refractory obstructive urinary symptoms despite medical therapy, offer 1 of 3 surgeries: transurethral resection, transurethral vaporization, or laser enucleation of the prostate.

Sources

–http://www.nice.org.uk/nicemedia/live/12984/48557/48557.pdf
–http://www.uroweb.org/gls/pdf/12_Male_LUTS.pdf

[a]Alfuzosin, doxazosin, tamsulosin, or terazosin.

VALVULAR HEART DISEASE

Population
–Adults with valvular heart disease.

Recommendations for Aortic Stenosis
▶ ACC/AHA 2017

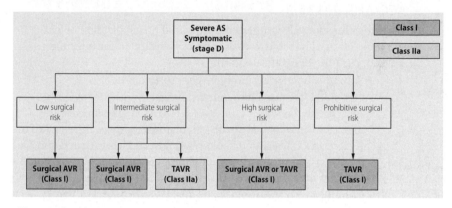

AVR = aortic valve replacement
TAVR = transcatheter aortic valve replacement

AVR, aortic valve replacement; TAVR, transcatheter aortic valve replacement.

Recommendations for Mitral Regurgitation
▶ ACC/AHA 2017

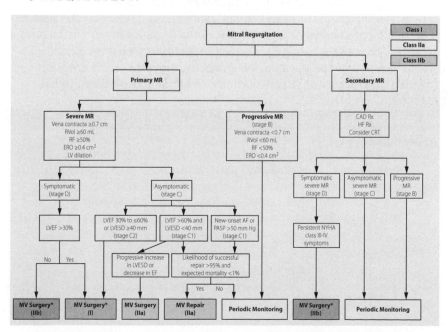

'MV repair is preferred over MV replacement when possible.

AF, atrial fibrillation; CAD, coronary artery disease; CRT, cardiac resynchronization therapy; EF, ejection fraction; ERO, effective regurgitant orifice; HF, heart failure; LV, left ventricular; LVEF, left ventricular ejection fraction; LVESD, left ventricular end-systolic diameter; MR, mitral regurgitation; MV, mitral valve; NYHA, New York Heart Association; PASP, pulmonary artery systolic pressure; RF, regurgitant fraction; RVol, regurgitant volume; Rx, therapy.

Recommendations
▶ ACC/AHA 2017

–Indications for valve surgery during initial hospitalization before completion of full course of antibiotics is indicated for infective endocarditis (IE) associated with:
  • Valve dysfunction resulting in symptoms of HF.
  • Left-sided IE caused by *S. aureus*, fungal, or oth2017 AHA/ACC focused update of the 2014 AHA/ACC guideline for the management of patients with valvular heart disease: a report of the American College of Cardiology/American Heart Association Task Force on Clinical Practice Guidelines. Circulation. 2017;135:e1159–e1195.er highly resistant organisms.
  • Complicated by heart block, annular or aortic abscess, or destructive penetrating lesions.
  • Evidence of persistent infection as manifested by persistent bacteremia or fevers lasting longer than 5 to 7 d after onset of appropriate antimicrobial therapy.
–Surgery is recommended for patients with prosthetic valve endocarditis and relapsing infection (defined as recurrence of bacteremia after a complete course of appropriate antibiotics and subsequently negative blood cultures) without other identifiable source for portal of infection.
–Complete removal of pacemaker or defibrillator systems, including all leads and the generator, is indicated as part of the early management plan in patients with IE with documented infection of the device or leads.

VALVULAR ADULT HEART DISEASE 2014 ACC/AHA GUIDELINES

Aortic Stenosis (AS)
• Transthoracic echocardiogram (TTE) is recommended as initial evaluation with known or suspected aortic stenosis to establish the diagnosis and to determine the severity of the stenosis.
• Exercise treadmill testing is rarely indicated but helpful to evaluate patients who have discordant echo/clinical findings (ie, moderate or severe stenosis in the absence of expected symptoms). Previously undetected symptoms of chest pain, shortness of breath, exertional dizziness, or syncope may be identified to prevent sudden death.
• Hypertension should be treated in the presence of significant AS.
• Statin therapy does not prevent the progression of the AS.

- No medical therapy is available to address symptoms or disease progression.
- Aortic valve replacement (AVR) is indicated in symptomatic patients with a mean gradient >40 mm Hg; aortic valve replacement is indicated in asymptomatic patients with decreased systolic function (EF50%) and mean gradient >40 mm Hg (valve gradient is underestimated with systolic dysfunction).
- Transcatheter aortic valve replacement (TAVR) should be considered in patients with a high surgical risk, marked frailty, associated comorbidities, and minimal associated coronary artery disease who have the same indication for AVR and have a 12-mo life expectancy.
- Percutaneous aortic balloon dilation procedure should be considered a "bridging therapy" to AVR or TAVR therapy.

Aortic Insufficiency (AI)

- Transthoracic echocardiogram is recommended as initial evaluation with known or suspected aortic insufficiency to establish the diagnosis and to determine the severity if there is insufficiency.
- Cardiac magnetic resonance (CMR) is an alternative form of evaluation if the TTE is nondiagnostic or suboptimal.
- Hypertension should be treated to keep SBP <140 mm Hg with nondihydropyridine calcium channel blocker, ACE inhibitor, or ARB agent.
- Aortic valve replacement: symptomatic person with severe AI regardless of the systolic function; asymptomatic patient with severe AI and systolic dysfunction <50% or with end systolic volume (ESD) >50 mm.

Mitral Stenosis (MS)

- Transthoracic echocardiogram is recommended as initial evaluation with known or suspected mitral stenosis to establish the diagnosis and to determine the severity if there is stenosis.
- Transesophageal echocardiogram (TEE) should be considered prior to sending the patient for percutaneous mitral balloon commissurotomy (PMBC) to exclude the presence of left atrial thrombus.
- Warfarin is indicated in patients with mitral stenosis and atrial fibrillation, prior embolic event, or intracardiac thrombus.
- Heart rate control in atrial fibrillation is imperative to allow optimal diastolic filling time across the stenotic valve.
- PMBC is indicated in symptomatic patients with severe mitral stenosis (MVA <1.5 cm^2) with no atrial thrombus and no or minimal mitral insufficiency.
- Mitral valve replacement is indicated if balloon commissurotomy is contraindicated in a patient with severe symptoms and severe mitral stenosis.

Mitral Regurgitation (MR)

- Transthoracic echocardiogram is recommended as initial evaluation with known or suspected mitral regurgitation to establish the diagnosis and to determine the severity if there is insufficiency, left atrial and ventricular size, and right ventricular function.
- Cardiac magnetic resonance (CMR) is an alternative form of evaluation if the TTE is nondiagnostic or suboptimal.

VALVULAR ADULT HEART DISEASE 2014 ACC/AHA GUIDELINES   (*Continued*)

• Mitral valve replacement or repair is indicated in a symptomatic patient with severe regurgitation if the systolic function (EF) is >30%.
• Mitral valve replacement is indicated in an asymptomatic patient with severe mitral regurgitation if the systolic function (EF) is between 30% and 60% or the left ventricular end systolic dimension (LVESD) >40%.

Source: Nishimura RA, Otto CM, Bonow RO. 2014 AHA/ACC guidelines for the management of patients with valvular heart disease: a report of the American College of Cardiology/American Heart Association Task Force on Practice Guidelines. *J Am Coll Cardiol.* 2014 Jun 10;63(22):e57. doi:10.1016/jack.2014.02.536.

Source
–2017 AHA/ACC focused update of the 2014 AHA/ACC guideline for the management of patients with valvular heart disease: a report of the American College of Cardiology/American Heart Association Task Force on Clinical Practice Guidelines. *Circulation.* 2017;135:e1159–e1195.

▼ VENOUS THROMBOEMBOLISM, DEEP VENOUS THROMBOSIS (DVT)

Population
–Patients with DVT (lower and upper extremity).

Recommendations

▶ ACCP 2016, ACP 2012
–**For diagnostic work-up of DVT/PE, see Figures I–III.**
–**Treatment Variables**
• Initial heparin based regimen with unfractionated heparin (UFH) 80 units/kg bolus, then 18 units/kg/h titrated to partial thromboplastin time (PTT), enoxaparin 1 mg/kg SQ q12h or 1.5 mg/kg SQ daily.
• Fondaparinux 5 mg (<50 kg), 7.5 mg (50–100 kg) or 10 mg (>100 kg) SQ daily.
• Start warfarin (≤10 mg) on day 1 and overlap with heparin for at least 5 d with therapeutic INR for last 2 d. Rivaroxaban, dabigatran, apixaban and edoxaban are all now approved by FDA to treat acute DVT and PE history (DOACs—direct oral anticoagulants)—see Table IX. Extended treatment has shown protection from further clot with minimal bleeding risk. Rivaroxaban is now approved in acute coronary syndrome. (*N Engl J Med.* 2010;363:2499-2510. *N Engl J Med.* 2012;366:1287-1297. *Am J Coll Cardiol.* 2013; 62:286) In setting of unprovoked DVT or PE men have a 50% increased risk of recurrent clot compared to women. (*Medicine.* 2014;93:309)

- Outpatient management of VTE with rivaroxaban, apixaban, edoxaban, or dabigitran is acceptable if the patient does not have any of the following: >80 y old, history of cancer, hx of COPD, CHF, pulse >110, BP <100, O_2 sat <90.
- Knee-high GCS (graduated compression stockings) with 30-40 mm Hg pressure at ankles for 2 y will reduce postthrombotic syndrome risk by 50%).

Source
–*Chest*. 2016;149:315-352

Comments

1. Clinical findings alone are poor predictors of DVT.
2. Early ambulation on heparin is safe.
3. With iliofemoral thrombosis and significant swelling, thrombolysis or surgical thrombectomy not recommended unless significant symptoms.
4. Inferior vena cava (IVC) filter indicated if DVT and significant uncontrolled bleeding precluding anticoagulation. (*Chest*. 2016; 150:1182)

FIGURE I

DIAGNOSIS AND TREATMENT OF VENOUS THROMBOEMBOLISM (VTE) WELLS CRITERIA				
DVT			**PE**	
Variable	**Score**		**Variable**	**Score**
Active cancer	1		Clinical evidence of DVT	3.0
Paralysis/immobilization	1		Other dx less likely than PE	3.0
Bedridden for >3 d or major surgery within 4 wk	1		Heart rate >100	1.5
Entire leg swollen	1		Immobile >3 d or major surgery within 4 wk	1.5
Tenderness along deep vein	1		Previous DVT/PE	1.5
Calf swelling >3 cm	1		Hemoptysis	1.0
Pitting edema (unilateral)	1		Malignancy	1.0
Collateral superficial veins	1			
Alternative dx more likely than DVT	−2			
Score and Probability—DVT			**Score and Probability—PE**	
High—3 or greater (75% risk of DVT) Moderate—1 or 2 (20% risk of DVT) Low—0 (3% risk of DVT)			High—6 or greater (>70% risk of PE) Moderate—2–6 (20–30% risk of PE) Low—less than 2 (2–3% risk of PE)	

Note: Pretest probability (PTP) of VTE guides clinical evaluation–Wells criteria for PTP of DVT and PE.

Source: Goldhaber SZ, Bounameaux H. Pulmonary embolism and deep vein thrombosis. *Lancet.* 2012;379:1835.

FIGURE II

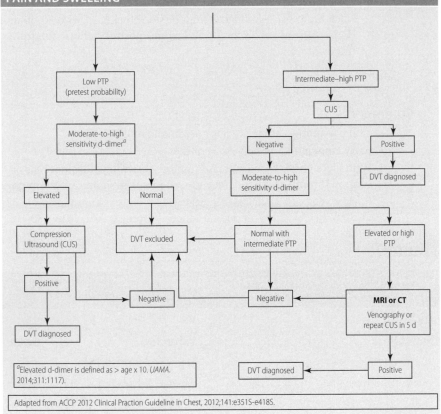

CLINICAL SUSPICION FOR DVT BASED ON PRETEST PROBABILITY (PTP)—LEG PAIN AND SWELLING

[a]Elevated d-dimer is defined as > age x 10. (*JAMA.* 2014;311:1117).

Adapted from ACCP 2012 Clinical Praction Guideline in Chest, 2012;141:e351S-e418S.

5. With provoked clot, anticoagulate for 3 mo if precipitating problem solved.[a]

6. Continue anticoagulation indefinitely if provoking problem continues.

7. In cancer-related clots, continue low-molecular-weight heparin (LMWH), do not transition to warfarin if cancer still active. (*Blood.* 2014;123:3972)

8. In unprovoked clot, anticoagulate for 3 mo then weigh risk of bleeding to benefit of prolonged anticoagulation to prevent clot; consider thrombophilia evaluation, including hereditary factors and

[a]Surgery, cancer, hormones, pregnancy, travel, inflammatory bowel disease, nephritic syndrome, hemolytic anemia, immobilization, trauma, CHF, myeloproliferative disorders, stroke, central venous catheter, rheumatologic disorders.

FIGURE III

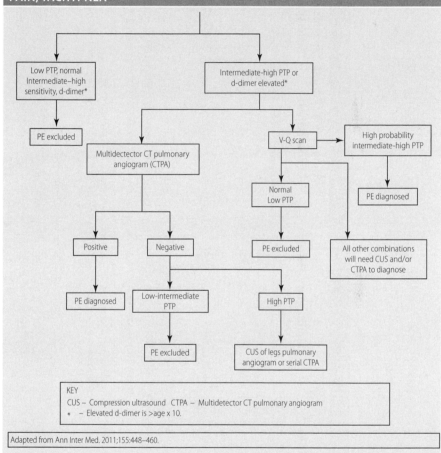

CLINICAL SUSPICION FOR PULMONARY EMBOLUS (PE)—DYSPNEA, CHEST PAIN, TACHYPNEA

KEY
CUS – Compression ultrasound   CTPA – Multidetector CT pulmonary angiogram
* – Elevated d-dimer is >age x 10.

Adapted from Ann Inter Med. 2011;155:448–460.

CUS, compression ultrasound; CTPA, multidetector CT pulmonary angiogram.
* elevated d-dimer is >age x 10.
Source: Ann Intern Med. 2011;155:448.

antiphospholipid antibody syndrome. Men have a 50% increase in recurrent clot compared to women and if first clot is a PE indefinite anticoagulation is advised because of high risk of the next event being a PE (60% vs. 20%) compared to those with VTE only.

9. Rivaroxaban and other DOACs should not be used in pregnancy or in patients with liver disease.

10. Risk factors for warfarin bleeding—age >65 y, history of stroke, history of GI bleed, and recent comorbidity (MI, Hct <30, creatinine

TABLE IX

NEW ORAL ANTICOAGULANTS[a] AND WARFARIN

Agent	Target	Dosing	Monitoring	Half-life	Time to Peak Plasma Concentration	Specific Reversible Agent
Warfarin[b]	Vitamin K epoxide	Once daily	INR–adjusted	40 h	72–96 h	Vitamin K PCC
Dabigatran[a,c]	Thrombin	Fixed—once or twice daily	None	14–17 h	2 h	Idarucizumab
Rivaroxaban[c]	Factor Xa	Fixed—once or twice daily	None	5–9 h (50 y old) 9–13 h (elderly)	2.5–4 h	Developed—needs FDA approved
Apixaban[c]	Factor Xa	Fixed twice daily	None	8–15 h	3 h	None
Edoxaban	Factor Xa	Give once daily	None	10-14 h	1-2 h	None

[a]Do not use new oral anticoagulants in patients with mechanical valves. Warfarin is superior. Warfarin is likely superior to new oral anticoagulants in patients with antiphospholipid antibody syndrome.

[b]If significant bleed on warfarin, give vitamin K, and 4-factor prothrombin complex concentrate (PCC/K - centra) or recombinant FVIIa if not controlled.

[c]If significant bleed, no standard of care. Aggressively treat source of bleed; consider 4-factor PCC or recombinant FVIIa. Agents to reverse anticoagulation with new oral anticoagulants will be available soon.

>1.5, diabetes). If all 4 factors present, 40% risk of significant bleed in 12 mo; 0.4% of patients on warfarin die of bleeding yearly. (*Chest.* 2016;149:315. *Am J Med.* 2011;124:111)

11. Patients with mild symptoms and good support system can be treated as outpatient with rivaroxaban (direct factor Xa inhibitor), other DOACs, or with lovenox and warfarin.

12. Calf and iliofemoral thrombosis have increased incidence of false-negative compression ultrasound—recommend CT or MR venogram or venography for suspected iliofemoral thrombosis, and for calf thrombosis follow-up compression ultrasound (CUS) in 5–7 d is acceptable.

13. Normal d-dimer with abnormal CUS in leg with previous DVT makes new clot unlikely. (*J Thromb Haemost.* 2007;5:1076)

14. Consider high thrombophilic risk in patients with recurrent VTE or patients with first unprovoked VTE who have the following characteristics:
    - Are <50 y old.
    - Family history of VTE.
    - Unusual site of thrombosis.
    - Massive venous thrombosis.

15. In unprovoked VTE 3% of patients are found to have associated malignancy with another 10% diagnosed with cancer over the next 2 y. (*N Engl J Med.* 1998;338:1169. *Ann Intern Med.* 2008;149:323. *N Engl J Med.* 2015; 373:697)

16. In patients with the antiphospholipid antibody syndrome and a new venous thrombosis, transition to warfarin is superior to using the new oral anti-coagulants. (*Am J Hematol.* 2014;89:1017)

VENOUS THROMBOEMBOLISM, PULMONARY EMBOLUS (PE)

Population
–Diagnosed pulmonary embolism.

Recommendations

▶ ACCP 2016, ACP 2011

–Approach to initial anticoagulation is the same as DVT.

–If patient is hypotensive without high bleeding risk and tachycardiac, systemically administered thrombolytic therapy is recommended.

–In a patient with acute PE associated with hypotension with contraindications to or failed thrombolysis or in shock that is likely to lead to rapid death, catheter-assisted thrombus removal is indicated if appropriate expertise and resources are available.

–In patients whose first episode of VTE is an unprovoked PE, extended anticoagulation beyond 3 mo is preferred unless high risk of bleeding.

Source

–*Chest.* 2016;149:315-352

Comments

Clinical Observations

–Patients whose first VTE is a PE will have a 3-fold increased risk of a second clot being a PE compared to patients with DVT only. (*N Engl J Med.* 2010;363:266)

–In patients with unprovoked PE or DVT elevated d-dimer at the time of discontinuation of warfarin or 2–3 wk after stopping anticoagulants predicts for a 3- to 5-fold increase in risk of clot over the next 12 mo. (*Blood.* 2010;115:481)

–The presence of a permanent IVC filter does not mandate continuous anticoagulation unless documented recurrent clot problems

–Unprovoked clot has risk of recurrent clot in first 12 mo of 8%–12% vs. 3% for patients with provoked clot. (*JAMA.* 2011;305:1336)

–Patients with intermediate or high pretest probability (PTP) of PE should be treated with heparin before diagnostic work-up is complete.

–Asymptomatic PE (found incidentally on chest CT) should be treated with same protocol as symptomatic PE. (*Blood.* 2015; 125:1877)

–Emerging data suggest the use of aspirin (100 mg PO daily) may reduce the risk of recurrent clot in patients with unprovoked VTE after 6 to 12 mo of warfarin therapy. (*N Engl J Med.* 2012;366:1959)

–Patients with significant risk of recurrent clot, on long term anticoagulation with reduced dose of a DOAC have continued protection from clot and reduced risk of bleeding (rivaroxiban—10 mg/d, apixaban 2.5 mg bid. (*N Engl J Med.* 2017;376:1279. *N Engl J Med.* 2017;376:1211)

VERTIGO, BENIGN PAROXYSMAL POSITIONAL (BPPV)

Population

–Adults.

Recommendations

▶ AAO-HNS 2008

–Recommends the Dix-Hallpike maneuver to diagnose posterior semicircular canal BPPV.

–Recommends treatment of posterior semicircular canal BPPV with a particle repositioning maneuver.

–If the Dix-Hallpike test result is negative, recommends a supine roll test to diagnose lateral semicircular canal BPPV.

–Recommends offering vestibular rehabilitation exercises for the initial treatment of BPPV.

–Recommends evaluating patients for an underlying peripheral vestibular or central nervous system disorder if they have an initial treatment failure of presumed BPPV.

–Recommends against routine radiologic imaging for patients with BPPV.

–Recommends against routine vestibular testing for patients with BPPV.

–Recommends against routine use of antihistamines or benzodiazepines for patients with BPPV.

Source

–http://www.guideline.gov/content.aspx?id=13403

Comment

–BPPV is the most common vestibular disorder in adults, afflicting 2.4% of adults at some point during their lives.

VITAMIN DEFICIENCIES

Population

–All patients with or suspected of having serum cobalamin and folate deficiency.

Recommendations

▶ BCSH 2014

- Serum cobalamin <200 ng/L suggests cobalamin deficiency.
- Patients with normal cobalamin level but high suspicion of cobalamin deficiency should undergo methylmalonic acid (MMA) testing.
- Patients with cobalamin deficiency or unexplained anemia, neuropathy, or glossitis (regardless of cobalamin level) should have an anti-intrinsic factor antibody test to rule out pernicious anemia.
- Initial therapy for cobalamin deficiency is vitamin B_{12} 1 mg IM TIW for 3 wk and then maintenance therapy.
- Maintenance therapy is either 1 mg IM every 3 mo (if no neurologic symptoms) or every 2 mo (if neurologic symptoms) or vitamin B_{12} 2 mg PO daily.
- Serum folate level <7 nmol/L (<3 µg/L) indicates folate deficiency.

Source

–http://www.guideline.gov/content.aspx?id=48197

Comment

–Recommends against anti-parietal cell antibody to test for pernicious anemia.

Appendices

SENSITIVITY AND SPECIFICITY OF SCREENING TESTS FOR PROBLEM DRINKING

SCREENING INSTRUMENTS: ALCOHOL ABUSE

Instrument Name	Screening Questions/Scoring	Threshold Score	Sensitivity/Specificity (%)	Source
CAGE[a]	See page 501	>1	77/58	*Am J Psychiatry.* 1974;131:1121
		>2	53/81	*J Gen Intern Med.* 1998;13:379
		>3	29/92	
AUDIT	See pages 501-502	>4	87/70	*BMJ.* 1997;314:420
		>5	77/84	*J Gen Intern Med.* 1998;13:379
		>6	66/90	

[a]The CAGE may be less applicable to binge drinkers (eg, college students), the elderly, and minority populations.

SCREENING INSTRUMENTS: ALCOHOL ABUSE

SCREENING PROCEDURES FOR PROBLEM DRINKING

1. CAGE screening test[a]

Have you ever felt the need to	Cut down on drinking?
Have you ever felt	Annoyed by criticism of your drinking?
Have you ever felt	Guilty about your drinking?
Have you ever taken a morning	Eye opener?

INTERPRETATION: Two "yes" answers are considered a positive screen. One "yes" answer should arouse a suspicion of alcohol abuse.

2. The Alcohol Use Disorder Identification Test (AUDIT)[b] (Scores for response categories are given in parentheses. Scores range from 0 to 40, with a cutoff score of ≥ 5 indicating hazardous drinking, harmful drinking, or alcohol dependence.)

1. How often do you have a drink containing alcohol?

   (0) Never   (1) Monthly or less   (2) Two to four times a month   (3) Two or three times a week   (4) Four or more times a week

2. How many drinks containing alcohol do you have on a typical day when you are drinking?

   (0) 1 or 2   (1) 3 or 4   (2) 5 or 6   (3) 7 to 9   (4) 10 or more

3. How often do you have 6 or more drinks on 1 occasion?

   (0) Never   (1) Less than monthly   (2) Monthly   (3) Weekly   (4) Daily or almost daily

4. How often during the last year have you found that you were not able to stop drinking once you had started?

   (0) Never   (1) Less than monthly   (2) Monthly   (3) Weekly   (4) Daily or almost daily

5. How often during the last year have you failed to do what was normally expected of you because of drinking?

   (0) Never   (1) Less than monthly   (2) Monthly   (3) Weekly   (4) Daily or almost daily

6. How often during the last year have you needed a first drink in the morning to get yourself going after a heavy drinking session?

   (0) Never   (1) Less than monthly   (2) Monthly   (3) Weekly   (4) Daily or almost daily

7. How often during the last year have you had a feeling of guilt or remorse after drinking?

   (0) Never   (1) Less than monthly   (2) Monthly   (3) Weekly   (4) Daily or almost daily

SCREENING INSTRUMENTS: ALCOHOL ABUSE

SCREENING PROCEDURES FOR PROBLEM DRINKING　(Continued)

8. How often during the last year have you been unable to remember what happened the night before because you had been drinking?

    (0) Never　　(1) Less than monthly　　(2) Monthly　　(3) Weekly　　(4) Daily or almost daily

9. Have you or has someone else been injured as a result of your drinking?

    (0) No　　　　　　(2) Yes, but not in the last year　　　　　　(4) Yes, during the last year

10. Has a relative or friend or a doctor or other health worker been concerned about your drinking or suggested you cut down?

    (0) No　　　　　　(2) Yes, but not in the last year　　　　　　(4) Yes, during the last year

[a]Modified from Mayfield D, McLeod G, Hall P. The CAGE questionnaire: validation of a new alcoholism screening instrument. *Am J Psychiatry.* 1974;131:1121.
[b]From Piccinelli M, Tessari E, Bortolomasi M, et al. Efficacy of the alcohol use disorders identification test as a screening tool for hazardous alcohol intake and related disorders in primary care: a validity study. *BMJ.* 1997;314:420.

SCREENING INSTRUMENTS: DEPRESSION

SCREENING TESTS FOR DEPRESSION

Instrument Name	Screening Questions/Scoring	Threshold Score	Source
Beck Depression Inventory (short form)	See pages 506-507	0–4: None or minimal depression 5–7: Mild depression 8–15: Moderate depression >15: Severe depression	*Postgrad Med.* 1972;81
Geriatric Depression Scale	See page 508	≥15: Depression	*J Psychiatr Res.* 1983;17:37
PRIME-MD© (mood questions)	1. During the last month, have you often been bothered by feeling down, depressed, or hopeless? 2. During the last month, have you often been bothered by little interest or pleasure in doing things?	"Yes" to either question[a]	*JAMA.* 1994;272:1749 *J Gen Intern Med.* 1997;12:439
Patient Health Questionnaire (PHQ-9)©	http://www.pfizer.com/phq-9/ See pages 504-505	*Major depressive syndrome:* if answers to #1a or b and ≥5 of #1a–i are at least "More than half the days" (count #1i if present at all) *Other depressive syndrome:* if #1a or b and 2–4 of #1a–i are at least "More than half the days" (count #1i if present at all) 5–9: mild depression 10–14: moderate depression 15–19: moderately severe depression 20–27: severe depression	*JAMA.* 1999;282:1737 *J Gen Intern Med.* 2001;16:606

[a]Sensitivity 86%–96%; specificity 57%–75%.

Source: ©Pfizer Inc.

SCREENING INSTRUMENTS: DEPRESSION

PHQ-9 DEPRESSION SCREEN, ENGLISH

Over the past 2 weeks, how often have you been bothered by any of the following problems?

	Not at all	Several days	>Half the days	Nearly every day
a. Little interest or pleasure in doing things	0	1	2	3
b. Feeling down, depressed, or hopeless	0	1	2	3
c. Trouble falling or staying asleep, or sleeping too much	0	1	2	3
d. Feeling tired or having little energy	0	1	2	3
e. Poor appetite or overeating	0	1	2	3
f. Feeling bad about yourself—or that you are a failure or that you have let yourself or your family down	0	1	2	3
g. Trouble concentrating on things, such as reading the newspaper or watching television	0	1	2	3
h. Moving or speaking so slowly that other people could have noticed? Or the opposite—being so fidgety or restless that you have been moving around a lot more than usual?	0	1	2	3
i. Thoughts that you would be better off dead or of hurting yourself in some way	0	1	2	3
For office coding: Total Score	—	= ___	+ ___	+ ___

Major depressive syndrome: If ≥5 items present scored ≥2 and one of the items is depressed mood (b) or anhedonia (a). If item "i" is present, then this counts, even if score = 1.

Depressive screen positive: If at least one item ≥2 (or item "i" is ≥1).

SCREENING INSTRUMENTS: DEPRESSION

PHQ-9 DEPRESSION SCREEN, SPANISH

Durante las últimas 2 semanas, ¿con qué frecuencia le han molestado los siguientes problemas?

	Nunca	Varios días	>La mitad de los días	Casi todos los días
a. Tener poco interés o placer en hacer las cosas	0	1	2	3
b. Sentirse desanimada, deprimida, o sin esperanza	0	1	2	3
c. Con problemas en dormirse o en mantenerse dormida, o en dormir demasiado	0	1	2	3
d. Sentirse cansada o tener poca energía	0	1	2	3
e. Tener poco apetito o comer en exceso	0	1	2	3
f. Sentir falta de amor propio—o qe sea un fracaso o que decepcionara a sí misma o a su familia	0	1	2	3
g. Tener dificultad para concentrarse en cosas tales como leer el periódico o mirar la televisión	0	1	2	3
h. Se mueve o habla tan lentamente que otra gente se podría dar cuenta—o de lo contrario, está tan agitada o inquieta que se mueve mucho más de lo acostumbrado	0	1	2	3
i. Se le han ocurrido pensamientos de que se haría daño de alguna manera	0	1	2	3
For office coding: Total Store	___ =	___ +	___ +	___

Source: From the Primary Care Evaluation of Mental Disorders Patient Health Questionnaire (PRIME-MD PHQ). The PHQ was developed by Drs. Robert L., et al. For research information, contact Dr. Spitzer at rls8@columbia.edu. PRIME-MD® is a trademark of Pfizer Inc. Copyright © 1999 Pfizer Inc. All rights reserved. Reproduced with permission. For office coding: Maj Dep Syn if answer to #2a or b and ≥5 of #2a–i are at least "More than half the days" (count #2i if present at all). Other Dep Syn if #2a or b and 2, 3, or 4 of #2a–i are at least "More than half the days" (count #2i if present at all).

SCREENING INSTRUMENTS: DEPRESSION

BECK DEPRESSION INVENTORY, SHORT FORM

Instructions: This is a questionnaire. On the questionnaire are groups of statements. Please read the entire group of statements in each category. Then pick out the one statement in that group that best describes the way you feel today, that is, right now! Circle the number beside the statement you have chosen. If several statements in the group seem to apply equally well, circle each one. Sum all numbers to calculate a score.

Be sure to read all the statements in each group before making your choice.

A. Sadness

3 I am so sad or unhappy that I can't stand it.
2 I am blue or sad all the time and I can't snap out of it.
1 I feel sad or blue.
0 I do not feel sad.

B. Pessimism

3 I feel that the future is hopeless and that things cannot improve.
2 I feel I have nothing to look forward to.
1 I feel discouraged about the future.
0 I am not particularly pessimistic or discouraged about the future.

C. Sense of failure

3 I feel I am a complete failure as a person (parent, husband, wife).
2 As I look back on my life, all I can see is a lot of failures.
1 I feel I have failed more than the average person.
0 I do not feel like a failure.

D. Dissatisfaction

3 I am dissatisfied with everything.
2 I don't get satisfaction out of anything anymore.
1 I don't enjoy things the way I used to.
0 I am not particularly dissatisfied.

E. Guilt

3 I feel as though I am very bad or worthless.
2 I feel quite guilty.
1 I feel bad or unworthy a good part of the time.
0 I don't feel particularly guilty.

F. Self-dislike

3 I hate myself.
2 I am disgusted with myself.
1 I am disappointed in myself.
0 I don't feel disappointed in myself.

G. Self-harm

3 I would kill myself if I had the chance.
2 I have definite plans about committing suicide.
1 I feel I would be better off dead.
0 I don't have any thoughts of harming myself.

H. Social withdrawal

3 I have lost all of my interest in other people and don't care about them at all.

2 I have lost most of my interest in other people and have little feeling for them.

1 I am less interested in other people than I used to be.

0 I have not lost interest in other people.

I. Indecisiveness

3 I can't make any decisions at all anymore.

2 I have great difficulty in making decisions.

1 I try to put off making decisions.

0 I make decisions about as well as ever.

J. Self-image change

3 I feel that I am ugly or repulsive looking.

2 I feel that there are permanent changes in my appearance and they make me look unattractive.

1 I am worried that I am looking old or unattractive.

0 I don't feel that I look worse than I used to.

K. Work difficulty

3 I can't do any work at all.

2 I have to push myself very hard to do anything.

1 It takes extra effort to get started at doing something.

0 I can work about as well as before.

L. Fatigability

3 I get too tired to do anything.

2 I get tired from doing anything.

1 I get tired more easily than I used to.

0 I don't get any more tired than usual.

M. Anorexia

3 I have no appetite at all anymore.

2 My appetite is much worse now.

1 My appetite is not as good as it used to be.

0 My appetite is no worse than usual.

Source: Reproduced with permission from Beck AT, Beck RW. Screening depressed patients in family practice: a rapid technic. *Postgrad Med.* 1972;52:81-85.

GERIATRIC DEPRESSION SCALE

Choose the best answer for how you felt over the past week

1. Are you basically satisfied with your life?	yes/no
2. Have you dropped many of your activities and interests?	yes/no
3. Do you feel that your life is empty?	yes/no
4. Do you often get bored?	yes/no
5. Are you hopeful about the future?	yes/no
6. Are you bothered by thoughts you can't get out of your head?	yes/no
7. Are you in good spirits most of the time?	yes/no
8. Are you afraid that something bad is going to happen to you?	yes/no
9. Do you feel happy most of the time?	yes/no
10. Do you often feel helpless?	yes/no
11. Do you often get restless and fidgety?	yes/no
12. Do you prefer to stay at home, rather than going out and doing new things?	yes/no
13. Do you frequently worry about the future?	yes/no
14. Do you feel you have more problems with memory than most?	yes/no
15. Do you think it is wonderful to be alive now?	yes/no
16. Do you often feel downhearted and blue?	yes/no
17. Do you feel pretty worthless the way you are now?	yes/no
18. Do you worry a lot about the past?	yes/no
19. Do you find life very exciting?	yes/no
20. Is it hard for you to get started on new projects?	yes/no
21. Do you feel full of energy?	yes/no
22. Do you feel that your situation is hopeless?	yes/no
23. Do you think that most people are better off than you are?	yes/no
24. Do you frequently get upset over little things?	yes/no
25. Do you frequently feel like crying?	yes/no
26. Do you have trouble concentrating?	yes/no
27. Do you enjoy getting up in the morning?	yes/no
28. Do you prefer to avoid social gatherings?	yes/no
29. Is it easy for you to make decisions?	yes/no
30. Is your mind as clear as it used to be?	yes/no

One point for each is response suggestive of depression. (Specifically "no" responses to questions 1, 5, 7, 9, 15, 19, 21, 27, 29, and 30, and "yes" responses to the remaining questions are suggestive of depression.)
A score of ≥15 yields a sensitivity of 80% and a specificity of 100%, as a screening test for geriatric depression. *Clin Gerontol.* 1982;1:37.

Source: Reproduced with permission from Yesavage JA, Brink TL, Rose TL, et al. Development and validation of a geriatric depression screening scale: a preliminary report. *J Psychiatr Res.* 1982–1983;17:37.

MODIFIED CHECKLIST FOR AUTISM IN TODDLERS, REVISED WITH FOLLOW-UP (M-CHAT-R/F)

Instructions: Please answer these questions about your child. Keep in mind how your child usually behaves. If you have seen your child do the behavior a few times, but he or she does not usually do it, then please answer no. Please circle YES or NO for every question. Thank you very much!

1. If you point at something across the room, does your child look at it? YES or NO
   (FOR EXAMPLE, if you point at a toy or an animal, does your child look at the toy or animal?)

2. Have you ever wondered if your child might be deaf? YES or NO

3. Does your child play pretend or make-believe? YES or NO
   (FOR EXAMPLE, pretend to drink from an empty cup, pretend to talk on a phone, or pretend to feed a doll or stuffed animal?)

4. Does your child like climbing on things? YES or NO
   (FOR EXAMPLE, furniture, playground equipment, or stairs)

5. Does your child make unusual finger movements near his or her eyes? YES or NO
   (FOR EXAMPLE, does your child wiggle his or her fingers close to his or her eyes?)

6. Does your child point with one finger to ask for something or to get help? YES or NO
   (FOR EXAMPLE, pointing to a snack or a toy that is out of reach)

7. Does your child point with one finger to show you something interesting? YES or NO
   (FOR EXAMPLE, pointing to an airplane in the sky or a big truck in the road)

8. Is your child interested in other children? YES or NO
   (FOR EXAMPLE, does your child watch other children, smile at them, or go to them?)

9. Does your child show you things by bringing them to you or holding them up for you to see—not to get help, but just to share? YES or NO
   (FOR EXAMPLE, showing you a flower, a stuffed animal, or a toy truck)

10. Does your child respond when you call his or her name? YES or NO
    (FOR EXAMPLE, does he or she look up, talk or babble, or stop what he or she is doing when you call his or her name?)

11. When you smile at your child, does he or she smile back at you? YES or NO

12. Does your child get upset by everyday noises? YES or NO
    (FOR EXAMPLE, does your child scream or cry to noise such as a vacuum cleaner or loud music?)

13. Does your child walk? YES or NO

14. Does your child look you in the eye when you are talking to him or her, playing with him or her, or dressing him or her? YES or NO

MODIFIED CHECKLIST FOR AUTISM IN TODDLERS, REVISED WITH FOLLOW-UP (M-CHAT-R/F)   *(Continued)*

15. Does your child try to copy what you do? (FOR EXAMPLE, wave bye-bye, clap, or make a funny noise when you do)	YES or NO
16. If you turn your head to look at something, does your child look around to see what you are looking at?	YES or NO
17. Does your child try to get you to watch him or her? (FOR EXAMPLE, does your child look at you for praise, or say "look" or "watch me"?)	YES or NO
18. Does your child understand when you tell him or her to do something? (FOR EXAMPLE, if you don't point, can your child understand "put the book on the chair" or "bring me the blanket"?)	YES or NO
19. If something new happens, does your child look at your face to see how you feel about it? (FOR EXAMPLE, if he or she hears a strange or funny noise, or sees a new toy, will he or she look at your face?)	YES or NO
20. Does your child like movement activities? (FOR EXAMPLE, being swung or bounced on your knee)	YES or NO

Scoring: For all items except 2, 5, and 12, 'NO' response indicates autism spectrum disorder risk.
Low-risk: 0–2; no further action required.
Medium-risk: 3–7; administer the follow-up (M-CHAT-R/F); if score remains ≥2, screening is positive.
High-risk: ≥8; refer immediately for diagnostic evaluation and early intervention.
Source: https://www.m-chat.org/_references/mchatDOTorg.pdf.

FUNCTIONAL ASSESSMENT SCREENING IN THE ELDERLY

Target Area	Assessment Procedure	Abnormal Result	Suggested Intervention
Vision	Inquire about vision changes, Snellen chart testing.	Presence of vision changes; inability to read >20/40	Refer to ophthalmologist.
Hearing	Whisper a short, easily answered question such as "What is your name?" in each ear while the examiner's face is out of direct view. Use audioscope set at 40 dB; test using 1000 and 2000 Hz. Brief hearing loss screener.	Inability to answer question Inability to hear 1000 or 2000 Hz in both ears or inability to hear frequencies in either ear Brief hearing loss screen score ≥3	Examine auditory canals for cerumen and clean if necessary. Repeat test; if still abnormal in either ear, refer for audiometry and possible prosthesis.
Balance and gait	Observe the patient after instructing as follows: "Rise from your chair, walk 10 ft, return, and sit down." Check orthostatic blood pressure and heart rate.	Inability to complete task in 15 s	Performance-Oriented Mobility Assessment (POMA). Consider referral for physical therapy.
Continence of urine	Ask, "Do you ever lose your urine and get wet?" If yes, then ask, "Have you lost urine on at least 6 separate days?"	"Yes" to both questions	Ascertain frequency and amount. Search for remediable causes, including local irritations, polyuric states, and medications. Consider urologic referral.
Nutrition	Ask, "Without trying, have you lost 10 lb or more in the last 6 mo?" Weigh the patient. Measure height.	"Yes" or weight is below acceptable range for height	Do appropriate medical evaluation.

FUNCTIONAL ASSESSMENT SCREENING IN THE ELDERLY (Continued)

Mental status	Instruct as follows: "I am going to name three objects (pencil, truck, and book). I will ask you to repeat their names now and then again a few minutes from now."	Inability to recall all three objects after 1 min	Administer Folstein Mini-Mental State Examination. If score is <24, search for causes of cognitive impairment. Ascertain onset, duration, and fluctuation of overt symptoms. Review medications. Assess consciousness and affect. Do appropriate laboratory tests.
Depression	Ask, "Do you often feel sad or depressed?" or "How are your spirits?"	"Yes" or "Not very good, I guess"	Administer Geriatric Depression Scale or PHQ-9. If positive, check for antihypertensive, psychotropic, or other pertinent medications. Consider appropriate pharmacologic or psychiatric treatment.
ADL-IADL[a]	Ask, "Can you get out of bed yourself?" "Can you dress yourself?" "Can you make your own meals?" "Can you do your own shopping?"	"No" to any question	Corroborate responses with patient's appearance; question family members if accuracy is uncertain. Determine reasons for the inability (motivation compared with physical limitation). Institute appropriate medical, social, or environmental interventions.

Home environment	Ask, "Do you have trouble with stairs inside or outside of your home?" Ask about potential hazards inside the home with bathtubs, rugs, or lighting.	"Yes"	Evaluate home safety and institute appropriate countermeasures.
Social support	Ask, "Who would be able to help you in case of illness or emergency?"	—	List identified persons in the medical record. Become familiar with available resources for the elderly in the community.
Pain	Inquire about pain.	Presence of pain	Pain inventory.
Dentition	Oral examination.	Poor dentition	Dentistry referral.
Falls	Inquire about falls in past year and difficulty with walking or balance.	Presence of falls or gait/balance problems	Falls evaluation.

[a]Activities of Daily Living–Instrumental Activities of Daily Living.

Source: Modified from Fleming KC, Evans JM, Weber DC, Chutka DS. Practical functional assessment of elderly persons: a primary-care approach. *Mayo Clin Proc.* 1995;70(9):890-910.

VULNERABLE SENIORS: PREVENTING ADVERSE DRUG EVENTS

For older adults, minimize exposure to potentially inappropriate medications. Below is a summary of the 2015 American Geriatric Society Beers Criteria to prevent adverse drug events in older patients.

SELECTED MEDICATIONS TO AVOID IN OLDER ADULTS

These medications carry risks specific to an older population and should be avoided except in specific situations.

Class of Medications	Reason to Avoid	Exceptions
First Generation Antihistamines (ie, diphenhydramine, hydroxyzine, promethazine, etc.)	Clearance is reduced as age advances; risk of confusion and other anticholinergic effects	Diphenhydramine for acute allergic reaction may be appropriate
Antiparkinsonian agents (ie, benztropine, trihexyphenidyl)	More effective agents exist for Parkinson's disease	
Antispasmodics (ie, atropine, belladonna alkaloids, dicyclomine, etc)	Risk of confusion and other anticholinergic effects	
Nitrofurantoin	Pulmonary, hepato-, and neurotoxicity with long-term use; safer alternatives exist for UTI ppx.	
Alpha-1 blockers, peripheral (ie, doxazosin, prazosin, terazosin)	High risk of orthostatic hypotension	
Alpha blockers, central (ie, clonidine, guanfacine, methyldopa)	Risk of CNS effect, bradycardia, orthostatic hypotension.	Clonidine may be appropriate in some cases as adjunctive agent in refractory HTN.
Digoxin	AFib: more effective alternatives exist and mortality may increase.	May be appropriate in some cases as adjunctive agent for refractory symptomatic atrial fibrillation or heart failure. If used, avoid doses >0.125 mg/d.
	Heart failure: Benefit is arguable; mortality may increase.	

Nifedipine	Risk of hypotension, myocardial ischemia	
Amiodarone	Afib: More toxicity than other agents	May be appropriate for rhythm control if LVH or significant heart failure
Antidepressants with anticholinergic profile *(ie, amitriptyline, nortriptyline, paroxetine)*	Sedating; orthostatic hypotension; anticholinergic effects including confusion	
Antipsychotics, 1st & 2nd generation	Risk of CVA, cognitive decline.	Schizophrenia, bipolar disorder Dementia/delirium: only appropriate if nonpharmacologic options fail and patient threatens significant harm to self or others
Barbiturates *(ie, phenopabital, butalbital)*	Risk of overdose at low dosages, dependence, escalating dose due to tolerance	
Benzodiazepines	Increased sensitivity with age, slower metabolism of longer-acting agents. Risk of cognitive impairment, falls, delirium.	Seizure disorders, alcohol withdrawal, severe generalized anxiety, anesthesia.
Nonbenzodiazepine hypnotics *(ie, zolpidem, zaleplon, eszopiclone)*	Similar to benzodiazepine risk; minimal improvement in sleep	
Androgens *(ie, testosterone, methyltestosterone)*	Cardiac problems; contraindicated in prostate cancer	Lab-verified symptomatic hypogonadism.
Estrogen, +/- progestin	Risk of breast and endometrial cancer; no evidence for cardioprotection or cognitive protection in elderly.	Vaginal estrogens safe/effective for vaginal dryness.
Insulin on a sliding scale	Hypoglycemia risk; no outcome benefit in outpatient or inpatient settings.	
Megestrol	Does not improve weight; higher risk of VTE and death.	

SELECTED MEDICATIONS TO AVOID IN OLDER ADULTS   (Continued)

Sulfonylureas of longer duration *(ie, glyburide, chlorpropamide)*	Severe prolonged hypoglycemia
Metoclopramide	Extrapyramidal effects
Proton pump inhibitors	*Clostridium difficile* infection; osteopenia/osteoporosis	Short-courses (ie, <8 wk). May be appropriate to treat severe conditions such as erosive esophagitis, Barrett's esophagus, or for prevention in high-risk patients (ie, NSAID or corticosteroid use)
NSAIDs *(ie, high-dose aspirin, ibuprofen, naproxen, indomethacin, ketorolac, etc.)*	GI bleed or peptic ulcer disease. Some (ie, indomethacin, ketorolac) carry higher risk of AKI.	Only use if alternative treatments are exhausted and patient can take PPI or misoprostol for gastroprotection (which reduces but does not eliminate risk)
Muscle relaxants *(ie, cyclobenzaprine, methocarbamol, carisoprodol)*	Anticholinergic effects, sedation, fracture risk; minimal efficacy	Urinary retention

*Source:*https://www.ncbi.nlm.nih.gov/pubmed/26446832.

SELECT MEDICATIONS TO AVOID IN OLDER ADULTS WITH CHRONIC CONDITIONS

These medications carry risk of exacerbating or provoking certain chronic diseases.

Condition	Drug(s) to Avoid	Potential Risk
Heart Failure	–NSAIDs, COX-2 inhibitors –Calcium channel blockers, nondihydropyridine –Thiazolidinediones –Cilostazol –Dronedarone	Heart failure exacerbation due to fluid retention
Syncope	–Acetylcholinesterase inhibitors –Alpha-1 blockers, peripheral (ie, terazosin, prazosin, doxazosin) –Tricyclic antidepressants –Olanzapine	Bradycardia, orthostatic hypotension
Epilepsy	–Chlorpromazine –Clozapine –Olanzapine –Tramadol	Lower seizure threshold
Delirium	–Anticholinergics –Antipsychotics –Benzodiazepines –Chlorpromazine –Corticosteroids –H2-receptor antagonists (ie, ranitidine, famotidine, cimetidine) –Meperidine –Sedative hypnotics	Delirium

SELECT MEDICATIONS TO AVOID IN OLDER ADULTS WITH CHRONIC CONDITIONS *(Continued)*		
Dementia/cognitive impairment	–Anticholinergics –Benzodiazepines –H2-receptor antagonists *(ie, ranitidine, famotidine, cimetidine)* –Nonbenzodiazepine hypnotics *(ie, zolpidem, zaleplon, eszopiclone)* –Antipsychotics	Adverse CNS effects
Fractures or falls	–Anticonvulsants –Antipsychotics –Benzoadiazepines –Nonbenzodiazepine hypnotics *(ie, zolpidem, zaleplon, eszopiclone)* –Tricyclic antidepressants –SSRIs –Opioids	More fall risk due to ataxia, impaired psychomotor function, syncope
Insomnia	–Oral decongestants *(ie, pseudoephedrine, phenylephrine)* –Stimulants *(ie, modafinil, methylphenidate, amphetamine)* –Theobromides *(ie, caffeine, theophylline)*	CNS stimulants
Parkinson's disease	–Antipsychotics (exceptions: aripiprazole, quetiapine, clozapine) –Antiemetics *(ie, metoclopramide, promethazine)*	Worsened Parkinson's symptoms due to dopamine-receptor antagonization

Ulcers, gastric or duodenal	–Aspirin (>325 mg/d or higher) –NSAIDs (except COX-2 selective inhibitors)	Exacerbation or new ulcers
CKD	–NSAIDs (all)	Risk of AKI and further decline
Urinary incontinence, women	–Estrogen *(except intravaginal)* –Peripheral alpha-1 antagonists *(ie, doxazosin, prazosin, terazosin)*	Aggravation of incontinence
Lower urinary tract symptoms, BPH	–Anticholinergics *(except: antimuscarinics when used for urinary incontinence)*	

SELECT MEDICATIONS TO USE WITH CAUTION IN OLDER ADULTS

These medications carry increased risk of adverse events in patients of older age.

Medication(s)	Risk
Aspirin (for primary prevention of cardiovascular events)	Evidence does not support that the benefit is greater than risk in patients older than 80 y
Dabigatran	Increased risk of GI bleed vs. warfarin in adults older than 75 y old
Prasugrel	Increased risk of bleeding in adults older than 75 y old
–Antipsychotics –Diuretics –Carbamazepine –Carboplatin –Cyclophosphamide –Cisplatin –Mirtazipine –Oxcarbazepine –SNRIs –SSRIs –TCAs –Vincristine	SIADH or hyponatremia
Vasodilators	Syncope

SCREENING AND PREVENTION GUIDELINES IN PERSPECTIVE: PGPC 2012

The following tables highlight areas where differences exist between various organizations' guideline recommendations and areas where a new direction appears to be developing as a result of new or updated guidelines.

1. Areas of significant difference in guideline recommendations

Guidelines	Organization	Recommendations
Adolescent Alcohol Abuse	USPSTF/AAFP	Evidence insufficient
	Bright Futures/NIAAA	Screen annually
Breast CA Screening, Women Age 40–49 y	UK-NHS	Routine screening not recommended
	ACP	Mammogram and CBE yearly starting at age 40 y—high-risk patients (>20% lifetime risk of breast CA) add annual MRI
	USPSTF/AAFP	Mammography ± breast examination every 2 y beginning at age 50 y and stop at age 75. In women age 40–50 y, counsel regarding risks and benefits; it should no longer be done routinely
Breast CA Screening, Women Age 50–70 y	UK-NHS	Mammography screening every 3 y
	USPSTF/AAFP	Mammography screening every 2 y
	ACS	Annual mammography screening
Cervical CA Screening, Women Age <50 y	UK-NHS	Begin screening every 3 y after age 25 y
	ACS	Screen beginning at age 21 y no matter when sexual activity started; screen annually (or every 2 y if liquid-based Pap smear) until age 30, then every 3 y if consecutive negative Pap smear results. HPV testing can be added after age 30 y. If Pap smears and HPV testing are both negative, the frequency of testing can be every 5 y

SCREENING AND PREVENTION GUIDELINES IN PERSPECTIVE: PGPC 2012 (Continued)		
Prostate CA Screening, Men Age >50 y	USPSTF/AAFP UK-NHS ACS	Do not use PSA-based screening for prostate cancer at any age—evidence suggests harms outweigh benefits Informed decision making Discuss screening PSA and digital rectal examination. Discuss risks and benefits including treatment options and side effects of treatment. Do not do PSA screen unless patient desires
Testicular CA Screening	USPSTF/AAFP ACS	Recommend against screening Perform testicular examination as part of routine CA-related checkup
Depression, Children and Adolescents	USPSTF/AAFP/CTF/NICE Bright Futures	Insufficient evidence to recommend for or against screening Annual screening for behaviors/emotions that indicate depression or risk of suicide
Family Violence and Abuse, Children and Adolescents	USPSTF/AAFP Family Violence Prevention Fund	Insufficient evidence to recommend for or against screening Assess caregivers/parents and adolescent patients at least annually
Hearing Loss, Newborns	USPSTF/AAFP Joint Committee on Infant Hearing	Insufficient evidence to recommend for or against screening during the postpartum hospitalization All infants should be screened for neonatal or congenital hearing loss
Thyroid Screening, Adults	USPSTF/AAFP ATA	Evidence insufficient to recommend for or against screening Screen all women age >35 y at 5-y intervals
Glaucoma, Adults	USPSTF/AAFP AOA	Evidence insufficient to recommend for or against screening Comprehensive eye examination every 2 y age 18–60 y, then every year age >60
Diabetes Mellitus, Gestational	USPSTF/AAFP ADA	Evidence insufficient to recommend for or against screening asymptomatic pregnant women Risk assess all women at first prenatal visit

2. New directions resulting from new or updated guidelines

HIV screening: Opt-out screening for practically everyone, actively recommended against written informed consent.

Endocarditis prophylaxis: Now targets those at increased risk of complications from endocarditis, rather than risk of endocarditis.

Perioperative guidelines: New data have emerged on beta blockade that is not reflected in current guidelines. Two randomized trials of perioperative metoprolol found that perioperative metoprolol does not appear to be effective in reducing postoperative death rates among unselected patients.

Osteoporosis:
• WHO Fracture Risk Algorithm (FRAX) developed to calculate the 1-y probability of fracture to guide treatment decisions.
• Screening recommendations for men.
• Recommendation to measure and supplement serum 25-OH vitamin D levels.

Diabetes type 2 prevention: New recommendation to consider metformin for those at very high risk of developing diabetes.

CA, cancer; CBE, clinical breast examination; HIV, human immunodeficiency syndrome; HPV, human papillomavirus; MRI, magnetic resonance imaging; PSA, prostate-specific antigen.

95TH PERCENTILE OF BLOOD PRESSURE FOR BOYS

Age (y)	Systolic Blood Pressure (mm Hg) by Percentile of Height							Diastolic Blood Pressure (mm Hg) by Percentile of Height						
	5%	10%	25%	50%	75%	90%	95%	5%	10%	25%	50%	75%	90%	95%
3	104	105	107	109	110	112	113	63	63	64	65	66	67	67
4	106	107	109	111	112	114	115	66	67	68	69	70	71	71
5	108	109	110	112	114	115	116	69	70	71	72	73	74	74
6	109	110	112	114	115	117	117	72	72	73	74	75	76	76
7	110	111	113	115	117	118	119	74	74	75	76	77	78	78
8	111	112	114	116	118	119	120	75	76	77	78	79	79	80
9	113	114	116	118	119	121	121	76	77	78	79	80	81	81
10	115	116	117	119	121	122	123	77	78	79	80	81	81	82
11	117	118	119	121	123	124	125	78	78	79	80	81	82	82
12	119	120	122	123	125	127	127	78	79	80	81	82	82	83
13	121	122	124	126	128	129	130	79	79	80	81	82	83	83
14	124	125	127	128	130	132	132	80	80	81	82	83	84	84
15	126	127	129	131	133	134	135	81	81	82	83	84	85	85
16	129	130	132	134	135	137	137	82	83	83	84	85	86	87
17	131	132	134	136	138	139	140	84	85	86	87	87	88	89

95TH PERCENTILE OF BLOOD PRESSURE FOR GIRLS

Age (y)	Systolic Blood Pressure (mm Hg) by Percentile of Height							Diastolic Blood Pressure (mm Hg) by Percentile of Height						
	5%	10%	25%	50%	75%	90%	95%	5%	10%	25%	50%	75%	90%	95%
3	104	104	105	107	108	109	110	65	66	66	67	68	68	69
4	105	106	107	108	110	111	112	68	68	69	70	71	71	72
5	107	107	108	110	111	112	113	70	71	71	72	73	73	74
6	108	109	110	111	113	114	115	72	72	73	74	74	75	76
7	110	111	112	113	115	116	116	73	74	74	75	76	76	77
8	112	112	114	115	116	118	118	75	75	75	76	77	78	78
9	114	114	115	117	118	119	120	76	76	76	77	78	79	79
10	116	116	117	119	120	121	122	77	77	77	78	79	80	80
11	118	118	119	121	122	123	124	78	78	78	79	80	81	81
12	119	120	121	123	124	125	126	79	79	79	80	81	82	82
13	121	121	123	124	126	127	128	80	80	80	81	82	83	83
14	123	123	125	126	127	129	129	81	81	82	82	83	84	84
15	124	125	126	127	129	130	131	82	82	82	83	84	85	85
16	125	126	127	128	130	131	132	82	82	83	84	85	85	86
17	125	126	127	129	130	131	132	82	83	83	84	85	85	86

Source: Blood Pressure Tables for Children and Adolescents from the Fourth Report on the Diagnosis, Evaluation, and Treatment of High Blood Pressure in Children and Adolescents. http://www.nhlbi.nih.gov/guidelines/hypertension/child_tbl.htm. Accessed June 3, 2008.

BODY MASS INDEX (BMI) CONVERSION TABLE

Height in Inches (cm)	BMI 25 kg/m^2	BMI 27 kg/m^2	BMI 30 kg/m^2
	Body weight in pounds (kg)		
58 (147.32)	119 (53.98)	129 (58.51)	143 (64.86)
59 (149.86)	124 (56.25)	133 (60.33)	148 (67.13)
60 (152.40)	128 (58.06)	138 (62.60)	153 (69.40)
61 (154.94)	132 (59.87)	143 (64.86)	158 (71.67)
62 (157.48)	136 (61.69)	147 (66.68)	164 (74.39)
63 (160.02)	141 (63.96)	152 (68.95)	169 (76.66)
64 (162.56)	145 (65.77)	157 (71.22)	174 (78.93)
65 (165.10)	150 (68.04)	162 (73.48)	180 (81.65)
66 (167.64)	155 (70.31)	167 (75.75)	186 (84.37)
67 (170.18)	159 (72.12)	172 (78.02)	191 (86.64)
68 (172.72)	164 (74.39)	177 (80.29)	197 (89.36)
69 (175.26)	169 (76.66)	182 (82.56)	203 (92.08)
70 (177.80)	174 (78.93)	188 (85.28)	207 (93.90)
71 (180.34)	179 (81.19)	193 (87.54)	215 (97.52)
72 (182.88)	184 (83.46)	199 (90.27)	221 (100.25)
73 (185.42)	189 (85.73)	204 (92.53)	227 (102.97)
74 (187.96)	194 (88.00)	210 (95.26)	233 (105.69)
75 (190.50)	200 (90.72)	216 (97.98)	240 (108.86)
76 (193.04)	205 (92.99)	221 (100.25)	246 (111.59)

Metric conversion formula = weight (kg)/ height (m^2)

Example of BMI calculation:
A person who weighs 78.93 kg and is 177 cm tall has a BMI of 25:
weight (78.93 kg)/height (1.77 m^2) = **25**

BMI categories:
Underweight = <18.5
Normal weight = 18.5–24.9
Overweight = 25–29.9
Obesity = ≥30

Nonmetric conversion formula = [weight (lb)/height (in^2)] × 704.5

Example of BMI calculation:
A person who weighs 164 lb and is 68 in. (or 5′8″) tall has a BMI of 25:
[weight (164 lb)/height (68 in.^{2})] × 704.5 = 25

Sources: Adapted from NHLBI Obesity Guidelines in Adults. http://www.nhlbi.nih.gov/guidelines/obesity/bmi_tbl.htm. Accessed October 13, 2011.
BMI online calculator. http://www.nhlbisupport.com/bmi/bmicalc.htm. Accessed October 13, 2011.

ESTIMATE OF 10-Y CARDIAC RISK FOR MEN[a]

Age (y)	Points
20–34	−9
35–39	−4
40–44	0
45–49	3
50–54	6
55–59	8
60–64	10
65–69	11
70–74	12
75–79	13

Total Cholesterol	Points				
	Age 20–39	Age 40–49	Age 50–59	Age 60–69	Age 70–79
<160	0	0	0	0	0
160–199	4	3	2	1	0
200–239	7	5	3	1	0
240–279	9	6	4	2	1
≥280	11	8	5	3	1

	Points				
	Age 20–39	Age 40–49	Age 50–59	Age 60–69	Age 70–79
Nonsmoker	0	0	0	0	0
Smoker	8	5	3	1	1

ESTIMATE OF 10-Y CARDIAC RISK FOR MEN[a] (Continued)

High-Density Lipoprotein (mg/dL)	Points
≥60	−1
50–59	0
40–49	1
<40	2

Systolic Blood Pressure (mm Hg)	If Untreated	If Treated
<120	0	0
120–129	0	1
130–139	1	2
140–159	1	2
≥160	2	3

Point Total	10-y Risk %	Point Total	10-y Risk %
<0	<1	9	5
0	1	10	6
1	1	11	8
2	1	12	10
3	1	13	12
4	1	14	16
5	2	15	20
6	2	16	25
7	3	≥17	≥30
8	4		

10-y Risk _____ %

[a]Framingham point scores.

Source: U.S. Department of Health and Human Services, Public Health Service, National Institutes of Health, National Heart, Lung, and Blood Institute. NIH Publication No. 01–3305, May 2001. https://www.nhlbi.nih.gov/files/docs/guidelines/atglance.pdf.

ESTIMATE OF 10-Y CARDIAC RISK FOR WOMEN[a]

Age (y)	Points
20–34	−7
35–39	−3
40–44	0
45–49	3
50–54	6
55–59	8
60–64	10
65–69	12
70–74	14
75–79	16

Total Cholesterol	Points				
	Age 20–39	Age 40–49	Age 50–59	Age 60–69	Age 70–79
<160	0	0	0	0	0
160–199	4	3	2	1	1
200–239	8	6	4	2	1
240–279	11	8	5	3	2
≥280	13	10	7	4	2

	Points				
	Age 20–39	Age 40–49	Age 50–59	Age 60–69	Age 70–79
Nonsmoker	0	0	0	0	0
Smoker	9	7	4	2	1

ESTIMATE OF 10-Y CARDIAC RISK FOR WOMEN[a] (Continued)

High-Density Lipoprotein (mg/dL)	Points
≥60	-1
50–59	0
40–49	1
<40	2

Systolic Blood Pressure (mm Hg)	If Untreated	If Treated
<120	0	0
120–129	1	3
130–139	2	4
140–159	3	5
≥160	4	6

Point Total	10-y Risk %	Point Total	10-y Risk %
<9	<1	17	5
9	1	18	6
10	1	19	8
11	1	20	11
12	1	21	14
13	2	22	17
14	2	23	22
15	3	24	27
16	4	≥25	≥30

10-y Risk _____ %

[a]Framingham point scores.

Source: U.S. Department of Health and Human Services, Public Health Service, National Institutes of Health, National Heart, Lung, and Blood Institute. NIH Publication No. 01-3305, May 2001. https://www.nhlbi.nih.gov/files/docs/guidelines/atglance.pdf.

ESTIMATE OF 10-Y STROKE RISK FOR MEN

Age (y)	Points
54–56	0
57–59	1
60–62	2
63–65	3
66–68	4
69–72	5
73–75	6
76–78	7
79–81	8
82–84	9
85	10

Untreated Systolic Blood Pressure (mm Hg)	Points
97–105	0
106–115	1
116–125	2
126–135	3
136–145	4
146–155	5
156–165	6
166–175	7
176–185	8
186–195	9
196–205	10

Treated Systolic Blood Pressure (mm Hg)	Points
97–105	0
106–112	1
113–117	2
118–123	3
124–129	4
130–135	5
136–142	6
143–150	7
151–161	8
162–176	9
177–205	10

History of Diabetes	Points
No	0
Yes	2

ESTIMATE OF 10-Y STROKE RISK FOR MEN (Continued)

Cigarette Smoking	Points
No	0
Yes	3

Cardiovascular Disease	Points
No	0
Yes	4

Atrial Fibrillation	Points
No	0
Yes	4

Left Ventricular Hypertrophy on Electrocardiogram	Points
No	0
Yes	5

Point Total	10-y Risk %	Point Total	10-y Risk %
1	3	16	22
2	3	17	26
3	4	18	29
4	4	19	33
5	5	20	37
6	5	21	42
7	6	22	47
8	7	23	52
9	8	24	57
10	10	25	63
11	11	26	68
12	13	27	74
13	15	28	79
14	17	29	84
15	20	30	88

10-y Risk _____ %

Source: Modified Framingham Stroke Risk Profile. Circulation. 2006;113:e873–e923.

ESTIMATE OF 10-Y STROKE RISK FOR WOMEN

Age (y)	Points	Untreated Systolic Blood Pressure (mm Hg)	Points
54–56	0	95–106	1
57–59	1	107–118	2
60–62	2	119–130	3
63–64	3	131–143	4
65–67	4	144–155	5
68–70	5	156–167	6
71–73	6	168–180	7
74–76	7	181–192	8
77–78	8	193–204	9
79–81	9	205–216	10
82–84	10		

Treated Systolic Blood Pressure (mm Hg)	Points	History of Diabetes	Points
95–106	1	No	0
107–113	2	Yes	3
114–119	3		
120–125	4		
126–131	5		
132–139	6		
140–148	7		
149–160	8		
161–204	9		
205–216	10		

ESTIMATE OF 10-Y STROKE RISK FOR WOMEN (Continued)

Cigarette Smoking	Points
No	0
Yes	3

Cardiovascular Disease	Points
No	0
Yes	2

Atrial Fibrillation	Points
No	0
Yes	6

Left Ventricular Hypertrophy on Electrocardiogram	Points
No	0
Yes	4

Point Total	10-y Risk %	Point Total	10-y Risk %
1	1	16	19
2	1	17	23
3	2	18	27
4	2	19	32
5	2	20	37
6	3	21	43
7	4	22	50
8	4	23	57
9	5	24	64
10	6	25	71
11	8	26	78
12	9	27	84
13	11		
14	13		
15	16		

10-y Risk _____ %

Source: Modified Framingham Stroke Risk Profile. *Circulation*. 2006;113:e873-e923.

IMMUNIZATION SCHEDULE

Figure 1. Recommended immunization schedule for children and adolescents aged 18 y or younger – United States, 2017. (FOR THOSE WHO FALL BEHIND OR START LATE, SEE THE CATCH-UP SCHEDULE [FIGURE 2]).

These recommendations must be read with the footnotes that follow. For those who fall behind or start late, provide catch-up vaccination at the earliest opportunity as indicated by the green bars in Figure 1. To determine minimum intervals between doses, see the catch-up schedule (Figure 2). School entry and adolescent vaccine age groups are shaded in gray.

Vaccine	Birth	1 mo	2 mos	4 mos	6 mos	9 mos	12 mos	15 mos	18 mos	19-23 mos	2-3 yrs	4-6 yrs	7-10 yrs	11-12 yrs	13-15 yrs	16 yrs	17-18 yrs
Hepatitis B[1] (HepB)	1st dose	←2nd dose→			←————————— 3rd dose —————————→												
Rotavirus[2] (RV) RV1 (2-dose series); RV5 (3-dose series)			1st dose	2nd dose	See footnote 2												
Diphtheria, tetanus, & acellular pertussis[3] (DTaP: <7 yrs)			1st dose	2nd dose	3rd dose		←———— 4th dose ————→					5th dose					
Haemophilus influenzae type b[4] (Hib)			1st dose	2nd dose	See footnote 4		3rd or 4th dose, See footnote 4										
Pneumococcal conjugate[5] (PCV13)			1st dose	2nd dose	3rd dose		←—— 4th dose ——→										
Inactivated poliovirus[6] (IPV: <18 yrs)			1st dose	2nd dose	←————————— 3rd dose —————————→							4th dose					
Influenza[7] (IIV)							Annual vaccination (IIV) 1 or 2 doses							Annual vaccination (IIV) 1 dose only			
Measles, mumps, rubella[8] (MMR)					See footnote 8		←——— 1st dose ———→					2nd dose					
Varicella[9] (VAR)							←——— 1st dose ———→					2nd dose					
Hepatitis A[10] (HepA)							←———— 2-dose series, See footnote 10 ————→										
Meningococcal[11] (Hib-MenCY ≥6 weeks; MenACWY-D ≥9 mos; MenACWY-CRM ≥2 mos)							See footnote 11							1st dose		2nd dose	
Tetanus, diphtheria, & acellular pertussis[12] (Tdap: ≥7 yrs)														Tdap			
Human papillomavirus[13] (HPV)														See footnote 13			
Meningococcal B[14]														See footnote 14			
Pneumococcal polysaccharide[15] (PPSV23)													See footnote 5				

Range of recommended ages for all children

Range of recommended ages for catch-up immunization

Range of recommended ages for certain high-risk groups

Range of recommended ages for non-high-risk groups that may receive vaccine, subject to individual clinical decision making

No recommendation

NOTE: The above recommendations must be read along with the footnotes of this schedule.

Figure 2. Catch-up immunization schedule for persons age 4 mo through 18 y who start late or who are more than 1 mo behind—United States, 2017.

The figure below provides catch-up schedules and minimum intervals between doses for children whose vaccinations have been delayed. A vaccine series does not need to be restarted, regardless of the time that has elapsed between doses. Use the section appropriate for the child's age. Always use this table in conjunction with Figure 1 and the footnotes that follow.

Vaccine	Minimum Age for Dose 1	Minimum Interval Between Doses			
		Dose 1 to Dose 2	Dose 2 to Dose 3	Dose 3 to Dose 4	Dose 4 to Dose 5
Children age 4 months through 6 years					
Hepatitis B[2]	Birth	4 weeks	8 weeks *and at least 16 weeks after first dose.* Minimum age for the final dose is 24 weeks.		
Rotavirus[3]	6 weeks	4 weeks	4 weeks[3]		6 months[3]
Diphtheria, tetanus, and acellular pertussis[4]	6 weeks	4 weeks	4 weeks	6 months	6 months[4]
Haemophilus influenzae type b[5]	6 weeks	4 weeks if first dose was administered before the 1st birthday. 8 weeks (as final dose) if first dose was administered at age 12 through 14 months. No further doses needed if first dose was administered at age 15 months or older.	4 weeks[5] if current age is younger than 12 months and first dose was administered at younger than age 7 months, and at least 1 previous dose was PRP-T (ActHIB, Pentacel, Hiberix) or unknown. 8 weeks (as final dose)[5] • if current age is younger than 12 months and first dose was administered at age 7 through 11 months; OR • if current age is 12 through 59 months and first dose was administered before the 1st birthday, and second dose administered before the 1st birthday; OR • if both doses were PRP-OMP (PedvaxHIB, Comvax) and were administered before the 1st birthday. No further doses needed if previous dose was administered at age 15 months or older.	8 weeks (as final dose) This dose only necessary for children age 12 through 59 months who received 3 doses before the 1st birthday.	
Pneumococcal[6]	6 weeks	4 weeks if first dose administered before the 1st birthday. 8 weeks (as final dose for healthy children) if first dose was administered at the 1st birthday or after. No further doses needed for healthy children if first dose was administered at age 24 months or older.	4 weeks if current age is younger than 12 months and previous dose given at <7 months old. 8 weeks (as final dose for healthy children) if previous dose given between 7–11 months (wait until at least 12 months old); OR if current age is 12 months or older and at least 1 dose was given before age 12 months. No further doses needed for healthy children if previous dose administered at age 24 months or older.	8 weeks (as final dose) This dose only necessary for children aged 12 through 59 months who received 3 doses before age 12 months or for children at high risk who received 3 doses at any age.	
Inactivated poliovirus[8]	6 weeks	4 weeks[8]	4 weeks if current age is younger than 4 years. 6 months (as final dose) if current age is 4 years or older.	6 months[8] (minimum age 4 years for final dose).	
Measles, mumps, rubella[9]	12 months	4 weeks			
Varicella[10]	12 months	3 months			
Hepatitis A[11]	12 months	6 months			
Meningococcal[13] (Hib-MenCY ≥6 weeks; MenACWY-D ≥9 mos; MenACWY-CRM ≥2 mos)	6 weeks	8 weeks[13]	See footnote 11	See footnote 11	
Children and adolescents age 7 through 18 years					
Meningococcal[13] (MenACWY-D ≥9 mos; MenACWY-CRM ≥2 mos)	Not Applicable (N/A)	8 weeks[13]			
Tetanus, diphtheria; tetanus, diphtheria, and acellular pertussis[7]	7 years[7]	4 weeks	4 weeks if first dose of DTaP/DT was administered before the 1st birthday. 6 months (as final dose) if first dose of DTaP/DT or Tdap/Td was administered at or after the 1st birthday.	6 months if first dose of DTaP/DT was administered before the 1st birthday.	
Human papillomavirus[12]	9 years	Routine dosing intervals are recommended.[12]			
Hepatitis A[10]	N/A	6 months			
Hepatitis B[10]	N/A	4 weeks	8 weeks and at least 16 weeks after first dose.		
Inactivated poliovirus[8]	N/A	4 weeks	4 weeks[8]	6 months[8]	
Measles, mumps, rubella[9]	N/A	4 weeks			
Varicella[9]	N/A	3 months if younger than age 13 years. 4 weeks if age 13 years or older.			

NOTE: The above recommendations must be read along with the footnotes of this schedule.

VACCINE ▼ INDICATION ▶	Pregnancy	Immunocompromised status (excluding HIV infection)	HIV infection CD4+ count (cells/μL) <15% of total CD4 cell count	HIV infection CD4+ count (cells/μL) ≥15% of total CD4 cell count	Kidney failure, end-stage renal disease, on hemodialysis	Heart disease, chronic lung disease	CSF leaks/ cochlear implants	Asplenia and persistent complement component deficiencies	Chronic liver disease	Diabetes
Hepatitis B[1]										
Rotavirus[2]		SCID*								
Diphtheria, tetanus, & acellular pertussis[3] (DTaP)										
Haemophilus influenzae type b[4]										
Pneumococcal conjugate[5]										
Inactivated poliovirus[6]										
Influenza[7]										
Measles, mumps, rubella[8]										
Varicella[9]										
Hepatitis A[10]										
Meningococcal ACWY[11]										
Tetanus, diphtheria, & acellular pertussis[12] (Tdap)										
Human papillomavirus[13]										
Meningococcal B[11]										
Pneumococcal polysaccharide[6]										

Legend:
- Vaccination according to the routine schedule recommended
- Recommended for persons with an additional risk factor for which the vaccine would be indicated
- Vaccination is recommended, and additional doses may be necessary based on medical condition. See footnotes.
- No recommendation
- Contraindicated
- Precaution for vaccination

*Severe Combined Immunodeficiency

NOTE: The above recommendations must be read along with the footnotes of this schedule.

Footnotes — Recommended Immunization Schedule for Children and Adolescents Aged 18 Years or Younger, UNITED STATES, 2017

For further guidance on the use of the vaccines mentioned below, see: www.cdc.gov/vaccines/hcp/acip-recs/index.html.
For vaccine recommendations for persons 19 years of age and older, see the Adult Immunization Schedule.

Additional information

- For information on contraindications and precautions for the use of a vaccine and for additional information regarding that vaccine, vaccination providers should consult the ACIP General Recommendations on Immunization and the relevant ACIP statement, available online at www.cdc.gov/vaccines/hcp/acip-recs/index.html.
- For purposes of calculating intervals between doses, 4 weeks = 28 days. Intervals of 4 months or greater are determined by calendar months.
- Vaccine doses administered ≤4 days before the minimum interval are considered valid. Doses of any vaccine administered ≥5 days earlier than the minimum interval or minimum age should not be counted as valid doses and should be repeated as age-appropriate. The repeat dose should be spaced after the invalid dose by the recommended minimum interval. For further details, see Table 1, *Recommended and minimum ages and intervals between vaccine doses*, in *MMWR, General Recommendations on Immunization and Reports / Vol. 60 / No. 2*, available online at www.cdc.gov/mmwr/pdf/rr/rr6002.pdf.
- Information on travel vaccine requirements and recommendations is available at wwwnc.cdc.gov/travel/.
- For vaccination of persons with primary and secondary immunodeficiencies, see Table 13, *Vaccination of persons with primary and secondary immunodeficiencies*, in *General Recommendations on Immunization* (ACIP), available at www.cdc.gov/mmwr/pdf/rr/rr6002.pdf.; and Immunization in Special Clinical Circumstances, (American Academy of Pediatrics). In: Kimberlin DW, Brady MT, Jackson MA, Long SS, eds. *Red Book: 2015 report of the Committee on Infectious Diseases. 30th ed.* Elk Grove Village, IL: American Academy of Pediatrics, 2015:68-107.
- The National Vaccine Injury Compensation Program (VICP) is a no-fault alternative to the traditional legal system for resolving vaccine injury petitions. Created by the National Childhood Vaccine Injury Act of 1986, it provides compensation to people found to be injured by certain vaccines. All vaccines within the recommended childhood immunization schedule are covered by VICP except for pneumococcal polysaccharide vaccine (PPSV23). For more information, see www.hrsa.gov/vaccinecompensation/index.html.

1. **Hepatitis B (HepB) vaccine. (Minimum age: birth)**

   Routine vaccination:

   At birth:

   - Administer monovalent HepB vaccine to all newborns within 24 hours of birth.
   - For infants born to hepatitis B surface antigen (HBsAg)-positive mothers, administer HepB vaccine and 0.5 mL of hepatitis B immune globulin (HBIG) within 12 hours of birth. These infants should be tested for HBsAg and antibody to HBsAg (anti-HBs) at age 9 through 12 months (preferably at the next well-child visit) or 1 to 2 months after completion of the HepB series if the series was delayed.
   - If mother's HBsAg status is unknown, within 12 hours of birth, administer HepB vaccine regardless of birth weight. For infants weighing less than 2,000 grams, administer HBIG in addition to HepB vaccine within 12 hours of birth. Determine mother's HBsAg status as soon as possible and, if mother is HBsAg-positive, also administer HBIG to infants weighing 2,000 grams or more as soon as possible, but no later than age 7 days.

   Doses following the birth dose:

   - The second dose should be administered at age 1 or 2 months. Monovalent HepB vaccine should be used for doses administered before age 6 weeks.
   - Infants who did not receive a birth dose should receive 3 doses of a HepB-containing vaccine on a schedule of 0, 1 to 2 months, and 6 months, starting as soon as feasible (see Figure 2).
   - Administer the second dose 1 to 2 months after the first dose (minimum interval of 4 weeks); administer the third dose at least 8 weeks after the second dose AND at least 16 weeks after the **first** dose. The final (third or fourth) dose in the HepB series should be administered **no earlier than age 24 weeks.**

   - Administration of a total of 4 doses of HepB vaccine is permitted when a combination vaccine containing HepB is administered after the birth dose.

   Catch-up vaccination:

   - Unvaccinated persons should complete a 3-dose series.
   - A 2-dose series (doses separated by at least 4 months) of adult formulation Recombivax HB is licensed for use in children aged 11 through 15 years.
   - For other catch-up guidance, see Figure 2.

2. **Rotavirus (RV) vaccines. (Minimum age: 6 weeks for both RV1 [Rotarix] and RV5 [RotaTeq])**

   Routine vaccination:

   Administer a series of RV vaccine to all infants as follows:

   1. If Rotarix is used, administer a 2-dose series at ages 2 and 4 months.
   2. If RotaTeq is used, administer a 3-dose series at ages 2, 4, and 6 months.
   3. If any dose in the series was RotaTeq or vaccine product is unknown for any dose in the series, a total of 3 doses of RV vaccine should be administered.

   Catch-up vaccination:

   - The maximum age for the first dose in the series is 14 weeks, 6 days; vaccination should not be initiated for infants aged 15 weeks, 0 days, or older.
   - The maximum age for the final dose in the series is 8 months, 0 days.
   - For other catch-up guidance, see Figure 2.

3. **Diphtheria and tetanus toxoids and acellular pertussis (DTaP) vaccine. (Minimum age: 6 weeks. Exception: DTaP-IPV [Kinrix, Quadracel]: 4 years)**

   Routine vaccination:

   - Administer a 5-dose series of DTaP vaccine at ages 2, 4, 6, 15 through 18 months, and 4 through 6 years. The fourth dose may be administered as early as age 12 months,

   provided at least 6 months have elapsed since the third dose.
   - Inadvertent administration of fourth DTaP dose early: If the fourth dose of DTaP was administered at least 4 months after the third dose of DTaP and the child was 12 months of age or older, it does not need to be repeated.

   Catch-up vaccination:

   - The fifth dose of DTaP vaccine is not necessary if the fourth dose was administered at age 4 years or older.
   - For other catch-up guidance, see Figure 2.

4. ***Haemophilus influenzae* type b (Hib) conjugate vaccine. (Minimum age: 6 weeks for PRP-T [ActHIB, DTaP-IPV/Hib (Pentacel), Hiberix, and Hib-MenCY (MenHibrix)], PRP-OMP [PedvaxHIB])**

   Routine vaccination:

   - Administer a 2- or 3-dose Hib vaccine primary series and a booster dose (dose 3 or 4, depending on vaccine used in primary series) at age 12 through 15 months to complete a full Hib vaccine series.
   - The primary series with ActHIB, MenHibrix, Hiberix, or Pentacel consists of 3 doses and should be administered at ages 2, 4, and 6 months. The primary series with PedvaxHIB consists of 2 doses and should be administered at ages 2 and 4 months; a dose at age 6 months is not indicated.
   - One booster dose (dose 3 or 4, depending on vaccine used in primary series) of any Hib vaccine should be administered at age 12 through 15 months.
   - For recommendations on the use of MenHibrix in patients at increased risk for meningococcal disease, refer to the meningococcal vaccine footnotes and also to *MMWR* February 28, 2014 / 63(RR01):1-13, available at www.cdc.gov/mmwr/PDF/rr/rr6301.pdf.

For further guidance on the use of the vaccines mentioned below, see: www.cdc.gov/vaccines/hcp/acip-recs/index.html.

Catch-up vaccination:
- If dose 1 was administered at ages 12 through 14 months, administer a second (final) dose at least 8 weeks after dose 1, regardless of Hib vaccine used in the primary series.
- If both doses were PRP-OMP (PedvaxHIB or COMVAX) and were administered before the first birthday, the third (and final) dose should be administered at age 12 through 59 months and at least 8 weeks after the second dose.
- If the first dose was administered at age 7 through 11 months, administer the second dose at least 4 weeks later and a third (and final) dose at age 12 through 15 months or 8 weeks after second dose, whichever is later.
- If first dose is administered before the first birthday and second dose administered at younger than 15 months, a third (and final) dose should be administered 8 weeks later.
- For unvaccinated children aged 15–59 months, administer only 1 dose.
- For other catch-up guidance, see Figure 2. For catch-up guidance related to MenHibrix, see the meningococcal vaccine footnotes and also *MMWR* February 28, 2014 / 63(RR01):1–13, available at www.cdc.gov/mmwr/PDF/rr/rr6301.pdf.

Vaccination of persons with high-risk conditions:
Children aged 12 through 59 months who are increased risk for Hib disease, including chemotherapy recipients and those with anatomic or functional asplenia (including sickle cell disease), human immunodeficiency virus (HIV) infection, immunoglobulin deficiency, or early component complement deficiency, who have received either no doses or only 1 dose of Hib vaccine before age 12 months, should receive 2 additional doses of Hib vaccine, 8 weeks apart; children who received 2 or more doses of Hib vaccine before age 12 months should receive 1 additional dose.
- For patients younger than age 5 years undergoing chemotherapy or radiation treatment who received a Hib vaccine dose(s) within 14 days of starting therapy or during therapy, repeat the dose(s) at least 3 months following therapy completion.
- Recipients of hematopoietic stem cell transplant (HSCT) should be revaccinated with a 3-dose regimen of Hib vaccine starting 6 to 12 months after successful transplant, regardless of vaccination history; doses should be administered at least 4 weeks apart.
- A single dose of any Hib-containing vaccine should be administered to unimmunized* children and adolescents 15 months of age and older undergoing an elective splenectomy; if possible, vaccine should be administered at least 14 days before procedure.
- Hib vaccine is not routinely recommended for patients 5 years or older. However, 1 dose of Hib vaccine should be administered to unimmunized* persons aged 5 years or older who have anatomic or functional asplenia (including sickle cell disease) and unimmunized* persons 5 through 18 years of age with HIV infection.

* Patients who have not received a primary series and booster dose or at least 1 dose of Hib vaccine after 14 months of age are considered unimmunized.

5. **Pneumococcal vaccines. (Minimum age: 6 weeks for PCV13, 2 years for PPSV23)**
Routine vaccination with PCV13:
- Administer a 4-dose series of PCV13 at ages 2, 4, and 6 months and at age 12 through 15 months.
Catch-up vaccination with PCV13:
- Administer 1 dose of PCV13 to all healthy children aged 24 through 59 months who are not completely vaccinated for their age.
- For other catch-up guidance, see Figure 2.
Vaccination of persons with high-risk conditions with PCV13 and PPSV23:
- All recommended PCV13 doses should be administered prior to PPSV23 vaccination if possible.
- For children aged 2 through 5 years with any of the following conditions: chronic heart disease (particularly cyanotic congenital heart disease and cardiac failure); chronic lung disease (including asthma if treated with high-dose oral corticosteroid therapy); diabetes mellitus; cerebrospinal fluid leak; cochlear implant; sickle cell disease and other hemoglobinopathies; anatomic or functional asplenia; HIV infection; chronic renal failure; nephrotic syndrome; diseases associated with treatment with immunosuppressive drugs or radiation therapy, including malignant neoplasms, leukemias, lymphomas, and Hodgkin disease; solid organ transplantation; or congenital immunodeficiency:
  1. Administer 1 dose of PCV13 if any incomplete schedule of 3 doses of PCV13 was received previously.
  2. Administer 2 doses of PCV13 at least 8 weeks apart if unvaccinated or any incomplete schedule of fewer than 3 doses of PCV13 was received previously.
  3. The minimum interval between doses of PCV13 is 8 weeks.
  4. For children with no history of PPSV23 vaccination, administer PPSV23 at least 8 weeks after the most recent dose of PCV13.
- For children aged 6 through 18 years who have cerebrospinal fluid leak; cochlear implant; sickle cell disease and other hemoglobinopathies; anatomic or functional asplenia; congenital or acquired immunodeficiencies; HIV infection; chronic renal failure; nephrotic syndrome; diseases associated with treatment with immunosuppressive drugs or radiation therapy, including malignant neoplasms, leukemias, lymphomas, and Hodgkin disease; generalized malignancy; solid organ transplantation; or multiple myeloma:
  1. If neither PCV13 nor PPSV23 has been received previously, administer 1 dose of PCV13 now and 1 dose of PPSV23 at least 8 weeks later.
  2. If PCV13 has been received previously but PPSV23 has not, administer 1 dose of PPSV23 at least 8 weeks after the most recent dose of PCV13.
  3. If PPSV23 has been received but PCV13 has not, administer 1 dose of PCV13 at least 8 weeks after the most recent dose of PPSV23.
- For children aged 6 through 18 years with chronic heart disease (particularly cyanotic congenital heart disease and cardiac failure), chronic lung disease (including asthma if treated with high-dose oral corticosteroid therapy), diabetes mellitus, alcoholism, or chronic liver disease, who have not received PPSV23, administer 1 dose of PPSV23. If PCV13 has been received previously, then PPSV23 should be administered at least 8 weeks after any prior PCV13 dose.
- A single revaccination with PPSV23 should be administered 5 years after the first dose to children with sickle cell disease or other hemoglobinopathies; anatomic or functional asplenia; congenital or acquired immunodeficiencies; HIV infection; chronic renal failure; nephrotic syndrome; diseases associated with treatment with immunosuppressive drugs or radiation therapy, including malignant neoplasms, leukemias, lymphomas, and Hodgkin disease; generalized malignancy; solid organ transplantation; or multiple myeloma.

6. **Inactivated poliovirus vaccine (IPV). (Minimum age: 6 weeks)**
Routine vaccination:
- Administer a 4-dose series of IPV at ages 2, 4, 6 through 18 months, and 4 through 6 years. The final dose in the series should be administered on or after the fourth birthday and at least 6 months after the previous dose.
Catch-up vaccination:
- In the first 6 months of life, minimum age and minimum intervals are only recommended if the person is at risk of imminent exposure to circulating poliovirus (i.e., travel to a polio-endemic region or during an outbreak).
- If 4 or more doses are administered before age 4 years, an additional dose should be administered at age 4 through 6 years and at least 6 months after the previous dose.
- A fourth dose is not necessary if the third dose was administered at age 4 years or older and at least 6 months after the previous dose.
- If both oral polio vaccine (OPV) and IPV were administered as part of a series, a total of 4 doses should be administered, regardless of the child's current age.
- If only OPV was administered, and all doses were given prior to age 4 years, 1 dose of IPV should be given at 4 years or older, at least 4 weeks after the last OPV dose.
- IPV is not routinely recommended for U.S. residents aged 18 years or older.
- For other catch-up guidance, see Figure 2.

For further guidance on the use of the vaccines mentioned below, see: www.cdc.gov/vaccines/hcp/acip-recs/index.html.

7. **Influenza vaccines. (Minimum age: 6 months for inactivated influenza vaccine [IIV], 18 years for recombinant influenza vaccine [RIV])**

Routine vaccination:

- Administer influenza vaccine annually to all children beginning at age 6 months. For the 2016–17 season, use of live attenuated influenza vaccine (LAIV) is not recommended.

For children aged 6 months through 8 years:

- For the 2016–17 season, administer 2 doses (separated by at least 4 weeks) to children who are receiving influenza vaccine for the first time or who have not previously received ≥2 doses of trivalent or quadrivalent influenza vaccine before July 1, 2016. For additional guidance, follow dosing guidelines in the 2016–17 ACIP influenza vaccine recommendations (see *MMWR* August 26, 2016;65(5):1–54, available at www.cdc.gov/mmwr/volumes/65/rr/pdfs/rr6505.pdf).
- For the 2017–18 season, follow dosing guidelines in the 2017–18 ACIP influenza vaccine recommendations.

For persons aged 9 years and older:

- Administer 1 dose.

8. **Measles, mumps, and rubella (MMR) vaccine. (Minimum age: 12 months for routine vaccination)**

Routine vaccination:

- Administer a 2-dose series of MMR vaccine at ages 12 through 15 months and 4 through 6 years. The second dose may be administered before age 4 years, provided at least 4 weeks have elapsed since the first dose.
- Administer 1 dose of MMR vaccine to infants aged 6 through 11 months before departure from the United States for international travel. These children should be revaccinated with 2 doses of MMR vaccine, the first at age 12 through 15 months (12 months if the child remains in an area where disease risk is high), and the second dose at least 4 weeks later.

Catch-up vaccination:

- Administer 2 doses of MMR vaccine to children aged 12 months and older before departure from the United States for international travel. The first dose should be administered on or after age 12 months and the second dose at least 4 weeks later.

9. **Varicella (VAR) vaccine. (Minimum age: 12 months)**

Routine vaccination:

- Administer a 2-dose series of VAR vaccine at ages 12 through 15 months and 4 through 6 years. The second dose may be administered before age 4 years, provided at least 3 months have elapsed since the first dose. If the second dose was administered at least 4 weeks after the first dose, it can be accepted as valid.

Catch-up vaccination:

- Ensure that all school-aged children and adolescents have had 2 doses of VAR vaccine; the minimum interval between the 2 doses is 4 weeks.

Catch-up vaccination:

- Ensure that all persons aged 7 through 18 years without evidence of immunity (see *MMWR* 2007;56[No. RR-4], available at www.cdc.gov/mmwr/pdf/rr/rr5604.pdf) have 2 doses of varicella vaccine. For children aged 7 through 12 years, the recommended minimum interval between doses is 3 months (if the second dose was administered at least 4 weeks after the first dose, it can be accepted as valid); for persons aged 13 years and older, the minimum interval between doses is 4 weeks.

10. **Hepatitis A (HepA) vaccine. (Minimum age: 12 months)**

Routine vaccination:

- Initiate the 2-dose HepA vaccine series at ages 12 through 23 months; separate the 2 doses by 6 to 18 months.
- Children who have received 1 dose of HepA vaccine before age 24 months should receive a second dose 6 to 18 months after the first dose.
- For any person aged 2 years and older who has not already received the HepA vaccine series, 2 doses of HepA vaccine separated by 6 to 18 months may be administered if immunity against hepatitis A virus infection is desired.

Catch-up vaccination:

- The minimum interval between the 2 doses is 6 months.

Special populations:

- Administer 2 doses of HepA vaccine at least 6 months apart to previously unvaccinated persons who live in areas where vaccination programs target older children, or who are at increased risk for infection. This includes persons traveling to or working in countries that have high or intermediate endemicity of infection; men having sex with men; users of injection and non-injection illicit drugs; persons who work with HAV-infected primates or with HAV in a research laboratory; persons with clotting-factor disorders; persons with chronic liver disease; and persons who anticipate close, personal contact (e.g., household or regular babysitting) with an international adoptee during the first 60 days after arrival in the United States from a country with high or intermediate endemicity. The first dose should be administered as soon as the adoption is planned, ideally, 2 or more weeks before the arrival of the adoptee.

11. **Meningococcal vaccines. (Minimum age: 6 weeks for Hib-MenCY [MenHibrix], 2 months for MenACWY-CRM [Menveo], 9 months for MenACWY-D [Menactra], 10 years for serogroup B meningococcal [MenB] vaccines: MenB-4C [Bexsero] and MenB-FHbp [Trumenba])**

Routine vaccination:

- Administer a single dose of Menactra or Menveo vaccine at age 11 through 12 years, with a booster dose at age 16 years.
- For children aged 2 months through 18 years with high-risk conditions, see "Meningococcal conjugate ACWY vaccination of persons at increased risk" and other persons at increased risk" and "Meningococcal B

vaccination of persons with high-risk conditions and other persons at increased risk of disease below.

Catch-up vaccination:

- Administer Menactra or Menveo vaccine at age 13 through 18 years if not previously vaccinated.
- If the first dose is administered at age 13 through 15 years, a booster dose should be administered at age 16 through 18 years, with a minimum interval of at least 8 weeks between doses.
- If the first dose is administered at age 16 years or older, a booster dose is not needed.
- For other catch-up guidance, see Figure 2.

Clinical discretion:

- Young adults aged 16 through 23 years (preferred age range is 16 through 18 years) who are not at increased risk for meningococcal disease may be vaccinated with a 2-dose series of either Bexsero (0, ≥1 month) or Trumenba (0, 6 months) vaccine to provide short-term protection against most strains of serogroup B meningococcal disease. The two MenB vaccines are not interchangeable; the same vaccine product must be used for all doses.
- If the second dose of Trumenba is given at an interval of <6 months, a third dose should be given at least 6 months after the first dose; the minimum interval between the second and third doses is 4 weeks.

Meningococcal conjugate ACWY vaccination of persons with high-risk conditions and other persons at increased risk:

Children with anatomic or functional asplenia (including sickle cell disease), children with HIV infection, or children with persistent complement component deficiency (includes persons with inherited or chronic deficiencies in C3, C5–9, properdin, factor D, factor H, or taking eculizumab [Soliris]):

- Menveo
  - *Children who initiate vaccination at 8 weeks.* Administer doses at ages 2, 4, 6, and 12 months.
  - *Unvaccinated children who initiate vaccination at 7 through 23 months.* Administer 2 primary doses, with the second dose at least 12 weeks after the first dose AND after the first birthday.
  - *Children 24 months and older who have not received a complete series.* Administer 2 primary doses at least 8 weeks apart.
- MenHibrix
  - *Children who initiate vaccination at 6 weeks.* Administer doses at ages 2, 4, 6, and 12 through 15 months.
  - If the first dose of MenHibrix is given at or after age 12 months, a total of 2 doses should be given at least 8 weeks apart to ensure protection against serogroups C and Y meningococcal disease.

Figure 3. Vaccines that might be indicated for children and adolescents age 18 yr or younger based on medical indications.

For further guidance on the use of the vaccines mentioned below, see: www.cdc.gov/vaccines/hcp/acip-recs/index.html.

Menactra

o **Children with anatomic or functional asplenia or HIV infection**

- *Children 24 months and older who have not received a complete series.* Administer 2 primary doses at least 8 weeks apart. If Menactra is administered to a child with asplenia (including sickle cell disease) or HIV infection, do not administer Menactra until age 2 years and at least 4 weeks after the completion of all PCV13 doses.

o **Children with persistent complement component deficiency**

- *Children 9 through 23 months.* Administer 2 primary doses at least 12 weeks apart.
- *Children 24 months and older who have not received a complete series.* Administer 2 primary doses at least 8 weeks apart.

o **All high-risk children**

- If Menactra is to be administered to a child at high risk for meningococcal disease, it is recommended that Menactra be given either before or at the same time as DTaP.

Meningococcal B vaccination of persons with high-risk conditions and other persons at increased risk of disease:

Children with anatomic or functional asplenia (including sickle cell disease) or children with persistent complement component deficiency (includes persons with inherited or chronic deficiencies in C3, C5-9, properdin, factor D, factor H, or taking eculizumab [Soliris]):

- **Bexsero or Trumenba**

o *Persons 10 years or older who have not received a complete series.* Administer a 2-dose series of Bexsero, with doses at least 1 month apart, or a 3-dose series of Trumenba, with the second dose at least 1–2 months after the first and the third dose at least 6 months after the first. The two MenB vaccines are not interchangeable; the same vaccine product must be used for all doses.

For children who travel to or reside in countries in which meningococcal disease is hyperendemic or epidemic, including countries in the African meningitis belt or the Hajj:

- Administer an age-appropriate formulation and series of Menactra or Menveo for protection against serogroups A and W meningococcal disease. Prior receipt of MenHibrix is not sufficient for children traveling to the meningitis belt or the Hajj because it does not contain serogroups A or W.

For children at risk during an outbreak attributable to a vaccine serogroup:

- For serogroup A, C, W, or Y: Administer or complete an age- and formulation-appropriate series of MenHibrix, Menactra, or Menveo.

- For serogroup B: Administer a 2-dose series of Bexsero, with doses at least 1 month apart, or a 3-dose series of Trumenba, with the second dose at least 1–2 months after the first and the third dose at least 6 months after the first. The two MenB vaccines are not interchangeable; the same vaccine product must be used for all doses.

For MenACWY booster doses among persons with high-risk conditions, refer to *MMWR* 2013;62(RR02):1-22, at www.cdc.gov/mmwr/preview/mmwrhtml/rr6202a1.htm, *MMWR* June 20, 2014 / 63(24);527-530, at www.cdc.gov/mmwr/pdf/wk/mm6324.pdf, and *MMWR* November 4, 2016 / 65(43):1189-1194, at www.cdc.gov/mmwr/volumes/65/wr/pdfs/mm6543a3.pdf.

For other catch-up recommendations for these persons and complete information on use of meningococcal vaccines, including guidance related to vaccination of persons at increased risk of infection, see meningococcal *MMWR* publications, available at: www.cdc.gov/vaccines/hcp/acip-recs/vacc-specific/mening.html.

12. **Tetanus and diphtheria toxoids and acellular pertussis (Tdap) vaccine. (Minimum age: 10 years for both Boostrix and Adacel)**

Routine vaccination:

- Administer 1 dose of Tdap vaccine to all adolescents aged 11 through 12 years.
- Tdap may be administered regardless of the interval since the last tetanus and diphtheria toxoid-containing vaccine.
- Administer 1 dose of Tdap vaccine to pregnant adolescents during each pregnancy (preferably during the early part of gestational weeks 27 through 36), regardless of time since prior Td or Tdap vaccination.

Catch-up vaccination:

- Persons aged 7 years and older who are not fully immunized with DTaP vaccine should receive Tdap vaccine as 1 dose (preferably the first) in the catch-up series; if additional doses are needed, use Td vaccine. For children 7 through 10 years who receive a dose of Tdap as part of the catch-up series, an adolescent Tdap vaccine dose at age 11 through 12 years may be administered.
- Persons aged 11 through 18 years who have not received Tdap vaccine should receive a dose, followed by tetanus and diphtheria toxoids (Td) booster doses every 10 years thereafter.

- Inadvertent doses of DTaP vaccine:

- If administered inadvertently to a child aged 7 through 10 years, the dose may count as part of the catch-up series. This dose may count as the adolescent Tdap dose, or the child may receive a Tdap booster dose at age 11 through 12 years.
- If administered inadvertently to an adolescent aged 11 through 18 years, the dose should be counted as the adolescent Tdap booster.

- For other catch-up guidance, see Figure 2.

13. **Human papillomavirus (HPV) vaccines. (Minimum age: 9 years for 4vHPV [Gardasil] and 9vHPV [Gardasil 9])**

Routine and catch-up vaccination:

- Administer a 2-dose series of HPV vaccine on a schedule of 0, 6-12 months to all adolescents aged 11 or 12 years. The vaccination series can start at age 9 years.
- Administer HPV vaccine to all adolescents through age 18 years who were not previously adequately vaccinated. The number of recommended doses is based on age at administration of the first dose.
- For persons initiating vaccination before age 15, the recommended immunization schedule is 2 doses of HPV vaccine at 0, 6-12 months.
- For persons initiating vaccination at age 15 years or older, the recommended immunization schedule is 3 doses of HPV vaccine at 0, 1–2, 6 months.
- A vaccine dose administered at a shorter interval should be readministered at the recommended interval.

- In a 2-dose schedule of HPV vaccine, the minimum interval is 5 months between the first and second dose. If the second dose is administered at a shorter interval, a third dose should be administered a minimum of 12 weeks after the second dose and a minimum of 5 months after the first dose.

- In a 3-dose schedule of HPV vaccine, the minimum intervals are 4 weeks between the first and second dose, 12 weeks between the second and third dose, and 5 months between the first and third dose. If a vaccine dose is administered at a shorter interval, it should be readministered after another minimum interval has been met since the most recent dose.

Special populations:

- For children with history of sexual abuse or assault, administer HPV vaccine beginning at age 9 years.
- Immunocompromised persons*, including those with human immunodeficiency virus (HIV) infection, should receive a 3-dose series at 0, 1–2, and 6 months, regardless of age at vaccine initiation.
- Note: HPV vaccination is not recommended during pregnancy, although there is no evidence that the vaccine poses harm. If a woman is found to be pregnant after initiating the vaccination series, no intervention is needed; the remaining vaccine doses should be delayed until after the pregnancy. Pregnancy testing is not needed before HPV vaccination.

*See *MMWR* December 16, 2016;65(49):1405-1408, available at www.cdc.gov/mmwr/volumes/65/wr/pdfs/mm6549a5.pdf.

CS270497-C

Figure 1. Recommended immunization schedule for adults aged 19 years or older by age group, United States, 2017.

Vaccine	19–21 years	22–26 years	27–59 years	60–64 years	≥65 years
Influenza[1]	1 dose annually				
Td/Tdap[2]	Substitute Tdap for Td once, then Td booster every 10 yrs				
MMR[3]	1 or 2 doses depending on indication				
VAR[4]	2 doses				
HZV[5]				1 dose	
HPV–Female[6]	3 doses	3 doses			
HPV–Male[6]	3 doses	3 doses			
PCV13[7]				1 dose	
PPSV23[7]	1 or 2 doses depending on indication				1 dose
HepA[8]	2 or 3 doses depending on vaccine				
HepB[9]	3 doses				
MenACWY or MPSV4[10]	1 or more doses depending on indication				
MenB[10]	2 or 3 doses depending on vaccine				
Hib[11]	1 or 3 doses depending on indication				

Recommended for adults who meet the age requirement, lack documentation of vaccination, or lack evidence of past infection

Recommended for adults with additional medical conditions or other indications

No recommendation

Vaccine	Pregnancy[1,6,9]	Immuno-compromised (excluding HIV infection)[3-7,11]	HIV infection CD4+ count (cells/µL)[3-7,9-11] <200	HIV infection CD4+ count (cells/µL)[3-7,9-11] ≥200	Asplenia, persistent complement deficiencies[7,10,11]	Kidney failure, end-stage renal disease, on hemodialysis[7,9]	Heart or lung disease, chronic alcoholism[7]	Chronic liver disease[7,9]	Diabetes[7,9]	Health care personnel[3,4,9]	Men who have sex with men[6,8,9]
Influenza[1]	1 dose annually										
Td/Tdap[2]	1 dose Tdap each pregnancy	Substitute Tdap for Td once, then Td booster every 10 yrs									
MMR[3]		contraindicated	contraindicated	1 or 2 doses depending on indication							
VAR[4]		contraindicated	contraindicated	2 doses							
HZV[5]		contraindicated	contraindicated		1 dose						
HPV–Female[6]		3 doses through age 26 yrs									
HPV–Male[6]		3 doses through age 26 yrs				3 doses through age 21 yrs					3 doses through age 26 yrs
PCV13[7]							1 dose				
PPSV23[7]							1, 2, or 3 doses depending on indication				
HepA[8]							2 or 3 doses depending on vaccine				
HepB[9]							3 doses				
MenACWY or MPSV4[10]					1 or more doses depending on indication						
MenB[10]					2 or 3 doses depending on vaccine						
Hib[11]		3 doses post-HSCT recipients only			1 dose						

Recommended for adults who meet the age requirement, lack documentation of vaccination, or lack evidence of past infection

Recommended for adults with additional medical conditions or other indications

Contraindicated

No recommendation

Footnotes. Recommended immunization schedule for adults aged 19 years or older, United States, 2017

1. Influenza vaccination

General information

- All persons aged 6 months or older who do not have a contraindication should receive annual influenza vaccination with an age-appropriate formulation of inactivated influenza vaccine (IIV) or recombinant influenza vaccine (RIV).
- In addition to standard-dose IIV, available options for adults in specific age groups include: high-dose or adjuvanted IIV for adults aged 65 years or older, intradermal IIV for adults aged 18 through 64 years, and RIV for adults aged 18 years or older.
- Notes: Live attenuated influenza vaccine (LAIV) should not be used during the 2016–2017 influenza season. A list of currently available influenza vaccines is available at www.cdc.gov/flu/protect/vaccine/vaccines.htm.

Special populations

- Adults with a history of egg allergy who have only hives after exposure to egg should receive age-appropriate IIV or RIV.
- Adults with a history of egg allergy other than hives, e.g., angioedema, respiratory distress, lightheadedness, or recurrent emesis; or who required epinephrine or another emergency medical intervention, may receive age-appropriate IIV or RIV. The selected vaccine should be administered in an inpatient or outpatient medical setting and under the supervision of a healthcare provider who is able to recognize and manage severe allergic conditions.
- Pregnant women and women who might become pregnant in the upcoming influenza season should receive IIV.

2. Tetanus, diphtheria, and acellular pertussis vaccination

General information

- Adults who have not received tetanus and diphtheria toxoids and acellular pertussis vaccine (Tdap) or for whom pertussis vaccination status is unknown should receive 1 dose of Tdap followed by a tetanus and diphtheria toxoids (Td) booster every 10 years. Tdap should be administered regardless of when a tetanus or diphtheria toxoid-containing vaccine was last received.
- Adults with an unknown or incomplete history of a 3-dose primary series with tetanus and diphtheria toxoid-containing vaccines should complete the primary series that includes 1 dose of Tdap. Unvaccinated adults should receive the first 2 doses at least 4 weeks apart and the third dose 6–12 months after the second dose.
- Notes: Information on the use of Td or Tdap as tetanus prophylaxis in wound management is available at www.cdc.gov/mmwr/preview/mmwrhtml/rr5517a1.htm.

Special populations

- Pregnant women should receive 1 dose of Tdap during each pregnancy, preferably during the early part of gestational weeks 27–36, regardless of prior history of receiving Tdap.

3. Measles, mumps, and rubella vaccination

General information

- Adults born in 1957 or later without acceptable evidence of immunity to measles, mumps, or rubella (defined below) should receive 1 dose of measles, mumps, and rubella vaccine (MMR) unless they have a medical contraindication to the vaccine, e.g., pregnancy or severe immunodeficiency.
- Notes: Acceptable evidence of immunity to measles, mumps, or rubella in adults is: born before 1957, documentation of receipt of MMR, or laboratory evidence of immunity or disease. Documentation of healthcare provider-diagnosed disease without laboratory confirmation is not acceptable evidence of immunity.

Special populations

- Pregnant women who do not have evidence of immunity to rubella should receive 1 dose of MMR upon completion or termination of pregnancy and before discharge from the healthcare facility; non-pregnant women of childbearing age without evidence of rubella immunity should receive 1 dose of MMR.
- Adults with primary or acquired immunodeficiency including malignant conditions affecting the bone marrow or lymphatic system, systemic immunosuppressive therapy, or cellular immunodeficiency should not receive MMR.
- Adults with human immunodeficiency virus (HIV) infection and CD4+ T-lymphocyte count ≥200 cells/µL for at least 6 months who do not have evidence of measles, mumps, or rubella immunity should receive 2 doses of MMR at least 28 days apart. Adults with HIV infection and CD4+ T-lymphocyte count <200 cells/µL should not receive MMR.
- Adults who work in healthcare facilities should receive 2 doses of MMR at least 28 days apart; healthcare personnel born before 1957 who are unvaccinated or lack laboratory evidence of measles, mumps, or rubella immunity, or laboratory confirmation of disease should be considered for vaccination with 2 doses of MMR at least 28 days apart for measles or mumps, or 1 dose of MMR for rubella.
- Adults who are students in postsecondary educational institutions or plan to travel internationally should receive 2 doses of MMR at least 28 days apart.
- Adults who received inactivated (killed) measles vaccine or measles vaccine of unknown type during years 1963–1967 should be revaccinated with 1 or 2 doses of MMR.
- Adults who were vaccinated before 1979 with either inactivated mumps vaccine or mumps vaccine of unknown type who are at high risk for mumps infection, e.g., work in a healthcare facility, should be considered for revaccination with 2 doses of MMR at least 28 days apart.

4. Varicella vaccination

General information

- Adults without evidence of immunity to varicella (defined below) should receive 2 doses of single-antigen varicella vaccine (VAR) 4–8 weeks apart, or a second dose if they have received only 1 dose.
- Persons without evidence of immunity for whom VAR should be emphasized are: adults who have close contact with persons at high risk for serious complications, e.g., healthcare personnel and household contacts of immunocompromised persons; adults who live or work in an environment in which transmission of varicella zoster virus is likely, e.g., teachers, childcare workers, and residents and staff in institutional settings; adults who live or work in environments in which varicella transmission has been reported, e.g., college students, residents and staff members of correctional institutions, and military personnel; non-pregnant women of childbearing age; adolescents and adults living in households with children; and international travelers.
- Notes: Evidence of immunity to varicella in adults is: U.S.-born before 1980 (for pregnant women and healthcare personnel, U.S.-born before 1980 is not considered evidence of immunity); documentation of 2 doses of VAR at least 4 weeks apart; history of varicella or herpes zoster diagnosis or verification of varicella or herpes zoster disease by a healthcare provider; or laboratory evidence of immunity or disease.

Special populations

- Pregnant women should be assessed for evidence of varicella immunity. Pregnant women who do not have evidence of immunity should receive the first dose of VAR upon completion or termination of pregnancy and before discharge from the healthcare facility, and the second dose 4–8 weeks after the first dose.
- Healthcare institutions should assess and ensure that all healthcare personnel have evidence of immunity to varicella.
- Adults with malignant conditions, including those that affect the bone marrow or lymphatic system or who receive systemic immunosuppressive therapy, should not receive VAR.

5. Herpes zoster vaccination

General information

- Adults aged 60 years or older should receive 1 dose of herpes zoster vaccine (HZV), regardless of whether they had a prior episode of herpes zoster.

Special populations

- Adults aged 60 years or older with chronic medical conditions may receive HZV unless they have a medical contraindication, e.g., pregnancy or severe immunodeficiency.
- Adults with malignant conditions, including those that affect the bone marrow or lymphatic system or who receive systemic immunosuppressive therapy, should not receive HZV.
- Adults with human immunodeficiency virus (HIV) infection and CD4+ T-lymphocyte count <200 cells/µL should not receive HZV.

6. Human papillomavirus vaccination

General information

- Adult females through age 26 years and adult males through age 21 years who have not received any human papillomavirus (HPV) vaccine should receive a 3-dose series of HPV vaccine at 0, 1–2, and 6 months.
- Males aged 22 through 26 years may be vaccinated with a 3-dose series of HPV vaccine at 0, 1–2, and 6 months.
- Adult males through age 26 years, and adult males through age 21 years (and males aged 22 through 26 years who may receive HPV vaccination) who initiated the HPV vaccination series before age 15 years and received 2 doses at least 5 months apart are considered adequately vaccinated and do not need an additional dose of HPV vaccine.
- Adult females through age 26 years and adult males through age 21 years (and males aged 22 through 26 years who may receive HPV vaccination) who initiated the HPV vaccination series before age 15 years and received only 1 dose, or 2 doses less than 5 months apart, are not considered adequately vaccinated and should receive 1 additional dose of HPV vaccine.
- Notes: HPV vaccination is routinely recommended for children at age 11 or 12 years. For adults who had initiated but did not complete the HPV vaccination series, consider their age at first HPV vaccination (described above) and other factors (described below) to determine if they have been adequately vaccinated.

Special populations

- Men who have sex with men through age 26 years who have not received any HPV vaccine should receive a 3-dose series of HPV vaccine at 0, 1–2, and 6 months.
- Adult females and males through age 26 years with immunocompromising conditions (described below), including those with human immunodeficiency virus (HIV) infection, should receive a 3-dose series of HPV vaccine at 0, 1–2, and 6 months.
- Pregnant women are not recommended to receive HPV vaccine, although there is no evidence that the vaccine poses harm. If a woman is found to be pregnant after initiating the HPV vaccination series, delay the remaining doses until after the pregnancy. No other intervention is needed. Pregnancy testing is not needed before administering HPV vaccine.
- Notes: Immunocompromising conditions for which a 3-dose series of HPV vaccine is indicated are primary or secondary immunocompromising conditions that might reduce cell-mediated or humoral immunity, e.g., B-lymphocyte antibody deficiencies, complete or partial T-lymphocyte defects, HIV infection, malignant neoplasm, transplantation, autoimmune disease, and immunosuppressive therapy.

7. Pneumococcal vaccination

General information

- Adults who are immunocompetent and aged 65 years or older should receive 13-valent pneumococcal conjugate vaccine (PCV13) followed by 23-valent pneumococcal polysaccharide vaccine (PPSV23) at least 1 year after PCV13.
- Notes: Adults are recommended to receive 1 dose of PCV13 and 1, 2, or 3 doses of PPSV23 depending on indication. When both PCV13 and PPSV23 are indicated, PCV13 should be administered at least 1 year (after PPSV23. When two or more doses of PPSV23 are indicated, the interval between PPSV23 doses should be at least 5 years. Supplemental information on pneumococcal vaccine timing for adults aged 65 years or older and adults aged 19 years or older at high risk for pneumococcal disease (described below) is available at www.cdc.gov/vaccines/vpd-vac/pneumo/downloads/adult-vax-clinician-aid.pdf. No additional doses of PPSV23 are indicated for adults who received PPSV23 at age 65 years or older. When indicated, PCV13 and PPSV23 should be administered to adults whose pneumococcal vaccination history is incomplete or unknown.

Special populations

- Adults aged 19 through 64 years with chronic heart disease including congestive heart failure and cardiomyopathies (excluding hypertension); chronic lung disease including chronic obstructive lung disease, emphysema, and asthma; chronic liver disease including cirrhosis; alcoholism; or diabetes mellitus; or who smoke cigarettes should receive PPSV23. At age 65 years or older, they should receive 1 dose of PCV13 and another dose of PPSV23 at least 1 year after PCV13 and at least 5 years after the most recent dose of PPSV23.
- Adults aged 19 years or older with immunocompromising conditions or anatomical or functional asplenia (described below) should receive PCV13 and a dose of PPSV23 at least 8 weeks after PCV13, followed by a second dose of PPSV23 at least 5 years after the first dose of PPSV23. If the most recent dose of PPSV23 was administered before age 65 years, at age 65 years or older, administer another dose of PPSV23 at least 8 weeks after PCV13 and at least 5 years after the most recent dose of PPSV23.
- Adults aged 19 years or older with cerebrospinal fluid leak or cochlear implant should receive PCV13 followed by PPSV23 at least 8 weeks after PCV13. If the most recent dose of PPSV23 was administered before age 65 years, at age 65 years or older, administer another dose of PPSV23 at least 8 weeks after PCV13 and at least 5 years after the most recent dose of PPSV23.
- Notes: Immunocompromising conditions that are indications for pneumococcal vaccination are congenital or acquired immunodeficiency including B- or T-lymphocyte deficiency, complement deficiencies, and phagocytic disorders excluding chronic granulomatous disease; human immunodeficiency virus (HIV) infection; chronic renal failure and nephrotic syndrome; leukemia, lymphoma, Hodgkin disease, generalized malignancy, and multiple myeloma; solid organ transplant; and iatrogenic immunosuppression including long-term systemic corticosteroid and radiation therapy. Anatomical or functional asplenia that are indications for pneumococcal vaccination are sickle cell disease and other hemoglobinopathies, congenital or acquired asplenia, splenic dysfunction, and splenectomy. Pneumococcal vaccines should be given at least 2 weeks before immunosuppressive therapy or an elective splenectomy, and as soon as possible to adults who are diagnosed with HIV infection.

8. Hepatitis A vaccination

General information

- Adults who seek protection from hepatitis A virus infection may receive a 2-dose series of single-antigen hepatitis A vaccine (HepA) at either 0 and 6–12 months (Havrix) or 0 and 6–18 months (Vaqta). Adults may also receive a combined hepatitis A and hepatitis B vaccine (HepA-HepB) (Twinrix) as a 3-dose series at 0, 1, and 6 months. Acknowledgment of a specific risk factor by those who seek protection is not needed.

Special populations

- Adults with any of the following indications should receive a HepA series: have chronic liver disease, receive clotting factor concentrates, men who have sex with men, use injection or non-injection drugs, or work with hepatitis A virus-infected primates or in a hepatitis A research laboratory setting.
- Adults who travel in countries with high or intermediate levels of endemic hepatitis A infection or anticipate close personal contact with an international adoptee, e.g., reside in the same household or regularly babysit, from a country with high or intermediate level of endemic hepatitis A infection within their first 60 days of arrival in the United States should receive a HepA series.

9. Hepatitis B vaccination

General information

- Adults who seek protection from hepatitis B virus infection may receive a 3-dose series of single-antigen hepatitis B vaccine (HepB) (Engerix-B, Recombivax HB) at 0, 1, and 6 months. Adults may also receive a combined hepatitis A and hepatitis B vaccine (HepA-HepB) (Twinrix) at 0, 1, and 6 months. Acknowledgment of a specific risk factor by those who seek protection is not needed.

Special populations

- Adults at risk for hepatitis B virus infection by sexual exposure should receive a HepB series, including sex partners of hepatitis B surface antigen (HBsAg)-positive persons, sexually active persons who are not in a mutually monogamous relationship, persons seeking evaluation or treatment for a sexually transmitted infection, and men who have sex with men (MSM).
- Adults at risk for hepatitis B virus infection by percutaneous or mucosal exposure to blood should receive a HepB series, including adults who are recent or current users of injection drugs, household contacts of HBsAg-positive persons, residents and staff of facilities for developmentally disabled persons, incarcerated, healthcare and public safety workers at risk for exposure to blood or blood-contaminated body fluids, younger than age 60 years with diabetes mellitus, and age 60 years or older with diabetes mellitus at the discretion of the treating clinician.
- Adults with chronic liver disease including, but not limited to, hepatitis C virus infection, cirrhosis, fatty liver disease, alcoholic liver disease, autoimmune hepatitis, and an alanine aminotransferase (ALT) or aspartate aminotransferase (AST) level greater than twice the upper limit of normal should receive a HepB series.
- Adults with end-stage renal disease including those on pre-dialysis care, hemodialysis, peritoneal dialysis, and home dialysis should receive a HepB series. Adults on hemodialysis should receive a 3-dose series of 40 µg Recombivax HB at 0, 1, and 6 months or a 4-dose series of 40 µg Engerix-B at 0, 1, 2, and 6 months.
- Adults with human immunodeficiency virus (HIV) infection should receive a HepB series.
- Pregnant women who are at risk for hepatitis B virus infection during pregnancy, e.g., having more than one sex partner during the previous six months, been evaluated or treated for a sexually transmitted infection, recent or current injection drug use, or had an HBsAg-positive sex partner, should receive a HepB series.
- International travelers to regions with high or intermediate levels of endemic hepatitis B virus infection should receive a HepB series.
- Adults in the following settings are assumed to be at risk for hepatitis B virus infection and should receive a HepB series: sexually transmitted disease treatment facilities, HIV testing and treatment facilities, facilities providing drug-abuse treatment and prevention services, healthcare settings targeting services to persons who inject drugs, correctional facilities, healthcare settings targeting services to MSM, hemodialysis facilities and end-stage renal disease programs, and institutions and nonresidential day care facilities for developmentally disabled persons.

10. Meningococcal vaccination

Special populations

- Adults with anatomical or functional asplenia or persistent complement component deficiencies should receive a 2-dose primary series of serogroups A, C, W, and Y meningococcal conjugate vaccine (MenACWY) at least 2 months apart and revaccinate every 5 years. They should also receive a series of serogroup B meningococcal vaccine (MenB) with either a 2-dose series of MenB-4C (Bexsero) at least 1 month apart or a 3-dose series of MenB-FHbp (Trumenba) at 0, 1–2, and 6 months.
- Adults with human immunodeficiency virus (HIV) infection who have not been previously vaccinated should receive a 2-dose primary series of MenACWY at least 2 months apart and revaccinate every 5 years. Those who previously received 1 dose of MenACWY should receive a second dose at least 2 months after the first dose. Adults with HIV infection are not routinely recommended to receive MenB because meningococcal disease in this population is caused primarily by serogroups C, W, and Y.
- Microbiologists who are routinely exposed to isolates of Neisseria meningitidis should receive 1 dose of MenACWY and revaccinate every 5 years if the risk for infection remains, and either a 2-dose series of MenB-4C at least 1 month apart or a 3-dose series of MenB-FHbp at 0, 1–2, and 6 months.
- Adults at risk because of a meningococcal disease outbreak should receive 1 dose of MenACWY if the outbreak is attributable to serogroup A, C, W, or Y, or either a 2-dose series of MenB-4C at least 1 month apart or a 3-dose series of MenB-FHbp at 0, 1–2, and 6 months if the outbreak is attributable to serogroup B.
- Adults who travel to or live in countries with hyperendemic or epidemic meningococcal disease should receive 1 dose of MenACWY and revaccinate every 5 years if the risk for infection remains. MenB is not routinely indicated because meningococcal disease in these countries is generally not caused by serogroup B.
- Military recruits should receive 1 dose of MenACWY and revaccinate every 5 years if the increased risk for infection remains.
- First-year college students aged 21 years or younger who live in residence halls should receive 1 dose of MenACWY if they have not received MenACWY at age 16 years or older.
- Young adults aged 16 through 23 years (preferred age range is 16 through 18 years) who are healthy and not at increased risk for serogroup B meningococcal disease (described above) may receive either a 2-dose series of MenB-4C at least 1 month apart or a 2-dose series of MenB-FHbp at 0 and 6 months for short-term protection against most strains of serogroup B meningococcal disease.
- For adults aged 56 years or older who have not previously received serogroups A, C, W, and Y meningococcal vaccine and need only 1 dose, meningococcal polysaccharide serogroups A, C, W, and Y vaccine (MPSV4) is preferred. For adults who previously received MenACWY or anticipate receiving multiple doses of serogroups A, C, W, and Y meningococcal vaccine, MenACWY is preferred.
- Notes: MenB-4C and MenB-FHbp are not interchangeable, i.e., the same vaccine should be used for all doses to complete the series. There is no recommendation for MenB revaccination at this time. MenB may be administered at the same time as MenACWY but at a different anatomic site, if feasible.

11. Haemophilus influenzae type b vaccination

Special populations

- Adults who have anatomical or functional asplenia or sickle cell disease, or are undergoing elective splenectomy should receive 1 dose of Haemophilus influenzae type b conjugate vaccine (Hib) if they have not previously received Hib. Hib should be administered at least 14 days before splenectomy.
- Adults with a hematopoietic stem cell transplant (HSCT) should receive 3 doses of Hib in at least 4 week intervals 6–12 months after transplant regardless of their Hib history.
- Notes: Hib is not routinely recommended for adults with human immunodeficiency virus infection because their risk for Haemophilus influenzae type b infection is low.

Figure 2. Recommended immunization schedule for adults aged 19 years or older by medical condition and other indications, United States, 2017.

Table. Contraindications and precautions for vaccines recommended for adults aged 19 years or older*

The Advisory Committee on Immunization Practices (ACIP) recommendations and package inserts for vaccines provide information on contraindications and precautions related to vaccines. Contraindications are conditions that increase chances of a serious adverse reaction in vaccine recipients and the vaccine should not be administered when a contraindication is present. Precautions should be reviewed for potential risks and benefits for vaccine recipient. For a person with a severe allergy to latex, e.g., anaphylaxis, vaccines supplied in vials or syringes that contain natural rubber latex should not be administered unless the benefit of vaccination clearly outweighs the risk for a potential allergic reaction. For latex allergies other than anaphylaxis, vaccines supplied in vials or syringes that contain dry, natural rubber or natural rubber latex may be administered.

Contraindications and precautions for vaccines routinely recommended for adults

Vaccine	Contraindications	Precautions
All vaccines routinely recommended for adults	• Severe reaction, e.g., anaphylaxis, after a previous dose or to a vaccine component	• Moderate or severe acute illness with or without fever

Additional contraindications and precautions for vaccines routinely recommended for adults

Vaccine	Additional Contraindications	Additional Precautions
IIV†		• History of Guillain-Barré Syndrome within 6 weeks after previous influenza vaccination • Egg allergy other than hives, e.g., angioedema, respiratory distress, lightheadedness, or recurrent emesis; or required epinephrine or another emergency medical intervention (IIV may be administered in an inpatient or outpatient medical setting and under the supervision of a healthcare provider who is able to recognize and manage severe allergic conditions)
RIV†		• LAIV should not be used during 2016–2017 influenza season
LAIV†	• LAIV should not be used during 2016–2017 influenza season	• History of Guillain-Barré Syndrome within 6 weeks after previous influenza vaccination
Tdap/Td	• For pertussis-containing vaccines: encephalopathy, e.g., coma, decreased level of consciousness, or prolonged seizures, not attributable to another identifiable cause within 7 days of administration of a previous dose of a vaccine containing tetanus or diphtheria toxoid or acellular pertussis	• Guillain-Barré Syndrome within 6 weeks after a previous dose of tetanus toxoid-containing vaccine • History of Arthus-type hypersensitivity reactions after a previous dose of tetanus or diphtheria toxoid-containing vaccine. Defer vaccination until at least 10 years have elapsed since the last tetanus toxoid-containing vaccine • For pertussis-containing vaccine, progressive or unstable neurologic disorder, uncontrolled seizures, or progressive encephalopathy (until a treatment regimen has been established and the condition has stabilized)
MMR§	• Severe immunodeficiency, e.g., hematologic and solid tumors, chemotherapy, congenital immunodeficiency or long-term immunosuppressive therapy*, human immunodeficiency virus (HIV) infection with severe immunocompromise • Pregnancy	• Recent (within 11 months) receipt of antibody-containing blood product (specific interval depends on product)* • History of thrombocytopenia or thrombocytopenic purpura • Need for tuberculin skin testing†
VAR†	• Severe immunodeficiency, e.g., hematologic and solid tumors, chemotherapy, congenital immunodeficiency or long-term immunosuppressive therapy*, HIV infection with severe immunocompromise • Pregnancy	• Recent (within 11 months) receipt of antibody-containing blood product (specific interval depends on product)* • Receipt of specific antiviral drugs (acyclovir, famciclovir, or valacyclovir) 24 hours before vaccination (avoid use of these antiviral drugs for 14 days after vaccination)
HZV†	• Severe immunodeficiency, e.g., hematologic and solid tumors, chemotherapy, congenital immunodeficiency or long-term immunosuppressive therapy*, HIV infection with severe immunocompromise • Pregnancy	• Receipt of specific antiviral drugs (acyclovir, famciclovir, or valacyclovir) 24 hours before vaccination (avoid use of these antiviral drugs for 14 days after vaccination)
HPV vaccine		• Pregnancy
PCV13	• Severe allergic reaction to any vaccine containing diphtheria toxoid	

1. For additional information on use of influenza vaccines among persons with egg allergy, see: CDC. Prevention and control of seasonal influenza with vaccines: recommendations of the Advisory Committee on Immunization Practices—United States, 2016–17 influenza season. MMWR 2016;65(RR-5):1–54. Available at www.cdc.gov/mmwr/volumes/65/rr/rr6505a1.htm.
2. MMR may be administered together with VAR or HZV on the same day; if not administered on the same day, separate live vaccines by at least 28 days.
3. Immunosuppressive steroid dose is considered to be daily receipt of 20 mg or more prednisone or equivalent for two or more weeks. Vaccination should be deferred for at least 1 month after discontinuation of immunosuppressive steroid therapy. Providers should consult ACIP recommendations for complete information on the use of specific live vaccines among persons on immune-suppressing medications or with immune suppression because of other reasons.
4. Vaccine should be deferred for the appropriate interval if replacement immune globulin products are being administered. See: CDC. General recommendations on immunization: recommendations of the Advisory Committee on Immunization Practices (ACIP). MMWR 2011;60(No. RR-2). Available at www.cdc.gov/mmwr/preview/mmwrhtml/rr6002a1.htm.
5. Measles vaccination may temporarily suppress tuberculin reactivity. Measles-containing vaccine may be administered on the same day as tuberculin skin testing, or should be postponed for at least 4 weeks after vaccination.

* Adapted from: CDC, Table 6, Contraindications and precautions to commonly used vaccines. General recommendations on immunization: recommendations of the Advisory Committee on Immunization Practices. MMWR 2011;60(No. RR-2):40–41 and from: Hamborsky J, Kroger A, Wolfe S, eds. Appendix A. Epidemiology and prevention of vaccine preventable diseases. 13th ed. Washington, DC: Public Health Foundation, 2015. Available at www.cdc.gov/vaccines/pubs/pinkbook/index.html.

Acronyms of vaccines recommended for adults

HepA	hepatitis A vaccine	LAIV	live attenuated influenza vaccine
HepA-HepB	hepatitis A and hepatitis B vaccines	MenACWY	serogroups A, C, W, and Y meningococcal conjugate vaccine
HepB	hepatitis B vaccine		
Hib	*Haemophilus influenzae* type b conjugate vaccine	MenB	serogroup B meningococcal vaccine
HPV vaccine	human papillomavirus vaccine	MMR	measles, mumps, and rubella vaccine
HZV	herpes zoster vaccine	MPSV4	serogroups A, C, W, and Y meningococcal polysaccharide vaccine
IIV	inactivated influenza vaccine		

PCV13	13-valent pneumococcal conjugate vaccine
PPSV23	23-valent pneumococcal polysaccharide vaccine
RIV	recombinant influenza vaccine
Td	tetanus and diphtheria toxoids
Tdap	tetanus toxoid, reduced diphtheria toxoid, and acellular pertussis vaccine
VAR	varicella vaccine

CS270457-A

PROFESSIONAL SOCIETIES AND GOVERNMENTAL AGENCIES

Abbreviation	Full Name	Internet Address
AACE	American Association of Clinical Endocrinologists	http://www.aace.com
AAD	American Academy of Dermatology	http://www.aad.org
AAFP	American Academy of Family Physicians	http://www.aafp.org
AAHPM	American Academy of Hospice and Palliative Medicine	http://www.aahpm.org
AAN	American Academy of Neurology	http://www.aan.com
AAO	American Academy of Ophthalmology	http://www.aao.org
AAO-HNS	American Academy of Otolaryngology—Head and Neck Surgery	http://www.entnet.org
AAOS	American Academy of Orthopaedic Surgeons and American Association of Orthopaedic Surgeons	http://www.aaos.org
AAP	American Academy of Pediatrics	http://www.aap.org
ACC	American College of Cardiology	http://www.acc.org
ACCP	American College of Chest Physicians	http://www.chestnet.org
ACIP	Advisory Committee on Immunization Practices	http://www.cdc.gov/vaccines/acip/index.html
ACOG	American Congress of Obstetricians and Gynecologists	http://www.acog.com
ACP	American College of Physicians	http://www.acponline.org
ACR	American College of Radiology	http://www.acr.org
ACR	American College of Rheumatology	http://www.rheumatology.org
ACS	American Cancer Society	http://www.cancer.org
ACSM	American College of Sports Medicine	http://www.acsm.org
ADA	American Diabetes Association	http://www.diabetes.org
AGA	American Gastroenterological Association	http://www.gastro.org
AGS	American Geriatrics Society	http://www.americangeriatrics.org
AHA	American Heart Association	http://www.americanheart.org
ANA	American Nurses Association	http://www.nursingworld.org
AOA	American Optometric Association	http://www.aoa.org

PROFESSIONAL SOCIETIES AND GOVERNMENTAL AGENCIES (Continued)

Abbreviation	Full Name	Internet Address
ASA	American Stroke Association	http://www.strokeassociation.org
ASAM	American Society of Addiction Medicine	http://www.asam.org
ASCCP	American Society for Colposcopy and Cervical Pathology	http://www.asccp.org
ASCO	American Society of Clinical Oncology	http://www.asco.org
ASCRS	American Society of Colon and Rectal Surgeons	http://www.fascrs.org
ASGE	American Society for Gastrointestinal Endoscopy	http://asge.org
ASHA	American Speech-Language-Hearing Association	http://www.asha.org
ASN	American Society of Neuroimaging	http://www.asnweb.org
ATA	American Thyroid Association	http://www.thyroid.org
ATS	American Thoracic Society	http://www.thoracic.org
AUA	American Urological Association	http://auanet.org
BASHH	British Association for Sexual Health and HIV	http://www.bashh.org
	Bright Futures	http://brightfutures.org
BGS	British Geriatrics Society	http://www.bgs.org.uk/
BSAC	British Society for Antimicrobial Chemotherapy	http://www.bsac.org.uk
CDC	Centers for Disease Control and Prevention	http://www.cdc.gov
COG	Children's Oncology Group	http://www.childrensoncologygroup.org
CSVS	Canadian Society for Vascular Surgery	http://canadianvascular.ca
CTF	Canadian Task Force on Preventive Health Care	http://canadiantaskforce.ca
EASD	European Association for the Study of Diabetes	http://www.easd.org
EAU	European Association of Urology	http://www.uroweb.org
ERS	European Respiratory Society	http://ersnet.org
ESC	European Society of Cardiology	http://www.escardio.org
ESH	European Society of Hypertension	http://www.eshonline.org

ARC	International Agency for Research on Cancer	http://screening.iarc.fr
ICSI	Institute for Clinical Systems Improvement	http://www.icsi.org
IDF	International Diabetes Federation	http://www.idf.org
NAPNAP	National Association of Pediatric Nurse Practitioners	http://www.napnap.org
NCCN	National Comprehensive Cancer Network	http://www.nccn.org/cancer-guidelines.html
NCI	National Cancer Institute	http://www.cancer.gov/cancerinformation
NEI	National Eye Institute	http://www.nei.nih.gov
NGC	National Guideline Clearinghouse	http://www.guidelines.gov
NHLBI	National Heart, Lung, and Blood Institute	http://www.nhlbi.nih.gov
NIAAA	National Institute on Alcohol Abuse and Alcoholism	http://www.niaaa.nih.gov
NICE	National Institute for Health and Clinical Excellence	http://www.nice.org.uk
NIDCR	National Institute of Dental and Craniofacial Research	http://www.nidr.nih.gov
NIHCDC	National Institutes of Health Consensus Development Program	http://www.consensus.nih.gov
NIP	National Immunization Program	http://www.cdc.gov/vaccines
NKF	National Kidney Foundation	http://www.kidney.org
NOF	National Osteoporosis Foundation	http://www.nof.org
NTSB	National Transportation Safety Board	http://www.ntsb.gov
SCF	Skin Cancer Foundation	http://www.skincancer.org
SGIM	Society of General Internal Medicine	http://www.sgim.org
SKI	Sloan-Kettering Institute	http://www.mskcc.org/mskcc/html/5804.cfm
SVU	Society for Vascular Ultrasound	http://www.svunet.org
UK-NHS	United Kingdom National Health Service	http://www.nhs.uk
USPSTF	United States Preventive Services Task Force	http://www.ahrq.gov/clinic/uspstfix.htm
WHO	World Health Organization	http://www.who.int/en

Index